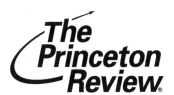

Cracking the
USMLE®
STEP 1

Dustin Y. Yoon, MD, MS and Jubina Bhaijee, MD

PrincetonReview.com

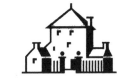

Random House, Inc. New York

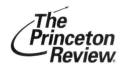

The Princeton Review, Inc.
111 Speen Street, Suite 550
Framingham, MA 01701
E-mail: editorialsupport@review.com
1-800-2-Review

ISBN: 978-0-307-94506-8

The Princeton Review is not affiliated with Princeton University.

Editor: Liz Rutzel
Production Coordinators: Craig Patches, Keith Kinsella, Keren Peysakh, and
Debbie Silvestrini
Production Editors: Kiley Pulliam, Jim Melloan, and Dustin Helmer

Printed in the United States of America on partially recycled paper.

10   9   8   7   6   5   4   3   2   1

Editorial

Rob Franek, VP Test Prep Books, Publisher
Selena Coppock, Senior Editor
Calvin Cato, Editor
Meave Shelton, Editor
Kristen O'Toole, Editor

Random House Publishing Team

Tom Russell, Publisher
Nicole Benhabib, Publishing Manager
Ellen L. Reed, Production Manager
Alison Stoltzfus, Associate Managing Editor

Acknowledgments

Authors

Ankur Bakshi, BS Biochemistry

Jubina Bhaijee, MD Reproductive, Editor

Anthony Choi, BS Endocrinology; Renal; Reproductive

Sharmistha Dev, MD Hematology

Denise Fabian Microbiology

Joel Fantanarosa Genetics

Abhishek Ganta, BA Musculoskeletal

Andrew Gonzalez, MD Hematology

Mustafa Gulam Neurology & Neuroanatomy

Stephen Hart, MD Cardiology

Christopher Holbrook, MD Pharmacology; Psychiatry

Esther Kim, MS Microbiology

Anny Hsu, MD, MS Musculoskeletal

Cindy Meerim Kim, MD Neurology & Neuroanatomy

Neel Mansukhani, MD Genetics

Nancy Pham, MD Gastrointestinal

Akshata Pandit Microbiology

Marissa Schwartz, BS Skin & Connective Tissue

Joseph F. Styron, MD, PhD Biostatistics; Epidemiology

Patrick Sylvester Immunology; Pulmonary & Respiratory

Joyce H. Wang Cell Biology

Dustin Y. Yoon, MD MS Editor

Paul Yi Musculoskeletal

Content Reviewers

Nida F. Degesys

Cindy Meerim Kim, MD

Esther Kim, MS

Michael Lee, MD

Euna Lhee, MS

James Lieu, MS

Alfred Liu

Patrick Hughes

Alejandro Marquez-Lara, MD

Eduardo Moili, MD, PhD

Acknowledgments

To my wife, Jung, for asking for hugs, even though, at times, I needed it more than you did. To my parents and Heidi... thank you for supporting my dreams. To Darcy for her unconditional love and licks. Shekeeeeeeee... "How are you?!"

To the Vascular Surgery staff at Northwestern Memorial Hospital, Drs. Yao, Pearce, Eskandari, Rodriguez, Kibbe, Hoel, and war team Mancona, Leslie, Rita, Jan, and of course Sara, and fellows CJ Hyung, Marlon, Suman, Mila, Courtney, and Neel—thank you for giving me a chance to become a surgeon.

To my mentors at the Cleveland Clinic, Dr. Blackstone, a genius in the guise of a gentleman, and Dean Franco, always the den mother. And most importantly, thanks be to God.

DYY

To my friend, my confidant, and the leader of my cheering section, my loving husband Adam—Thank you for believing in me, and for helping me to believe in myself. To my dear parents, my brother Rajeev, and my closest loved ones who have encouraged and supported me through and through. You are all crucial to my happiness, and therefore to any success that comes with it.

To my mentor Richard H. Smith, M.D., F.A.C.C.—Thank you for turning a pivotal moment in my life into the life changing experience that inspired me to follow my dreams. To M.H. Zarrabi M.D. M.A.C.P., for taking me under your wing and for sharing your wealth of wisdom. To my colleague, Zuhair Ali, M.D., who has been an invaluable friend throughout my journey in medicine.

Above all, to the one who gives me courage every day—I give thanks to God.

JB

Contents

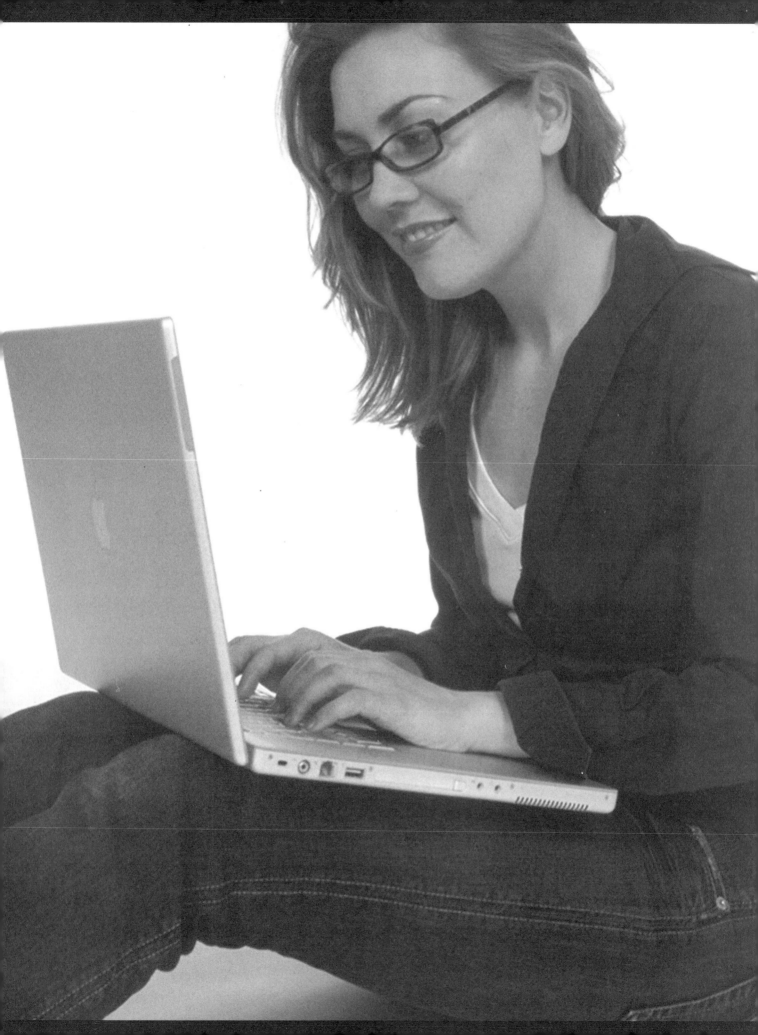

...So Much More Online!

More Practice...

- 2 full-length practice USMLEs

  - Score reports

    - Interactive, click-through learning

Register Your Book Now!

- Go to PrincetonReview.com/cracking

- You'll see a Welcome page where you should register your book by ISBN (the ISBN for this book is 9780307945068).

- Next you will see a Sign Up/Sign In page where you will type in your e-mail address (username) and choose a password.

- Now you're good to go!

CHAPTER 1

INTRODUCTION

Take a deep breath and relax.

If you're reading this book, it probably means that you are about to embark on one of the most stressful times in your life, studying for the USMLE Step 1. We recently attended a medical education conference that said in a national survey of fourth year medical students, the second year of medical school was considered most stressful. In reply to that, we say "relax and take heart!" If you've made it this far, you can make it all the way! Remember, you've gotten into medical school and you're living the dream now. It has been said that balance is the key to success in life. While you're preparing for this exam, remember that you need to balance your life with exercise, time with friends and family, and extracurricular activities outside of medicine—otherwise, you'll likely to feel burnt-out and succumb to the stress. Trust us, we've been there.

So why buy this book? We know that there are many review books out there already, so you might be wondering why we wrote yet another one. In our preparation for the United States Medical Licensing Examination (USMLE), we never found a review book that had everything we wanted, and all of us ended up buying way too many books. The so-called "Bibles" of USMLE prep were often books of facts that didn't make sense during our first couple of years and didn't teach us the concepts behind the facts until we learned them further on in medical school. We wanted to write a book that might approach the "perfect" boards review book.

What makes a review book good? A comprehensive review book should cover all the topics you are required to know for the exam, but be concise enough so that you can actually read the entire thing. This book serves as a primary source of information, your home base. Obviously, we can't cover everything you've learned (and might have forgotten) in your preclinical courses, so use your course notes, syllabi, and textbooks for reference. The entire outline provided by the USMLE for Step 1 is covered in this book.

In keeping with the current style of the exam standards, our book primarily uses an organ system approach to presenting and synthesizing the material. We have chapters on general principles (e.g., biochemistry, pharmacology, microbiology), but pathology, physiology, histology, anatomy, microbiology, and pharmacology are discussed in the context of each organ system. The USMLE has now moved toward using clinical vignettes and case presentations to test your knowledge of the material. This is probably a good thing because that's how you will take care of your patients in the real world.

Where possible, we've also tried to present the material in an intuitive fashion because we feel that such an approach makes the material much easier to remember than list after list of facts to memorize. We've used bullets to describe signs and symptoms, diagnosis, and treatment of disease entities, and key points are highlighted or emphasized in the margins.

Just a few words of advice. Realize that your medical school's curriculum may have seemed exhaustive, but chances are that the USMLE will pose some questions that your courses didn't cover. This may become apparent as you're studying and doing practice questions. There are many strategies for studying: reading books, study guides, old notes and syllabi, doing lots of practice questions, and many more. We believe that nothing will prepare you more than adequately understanding the concepts and doing practice questions. Don't wait too long to start doing practice questions. Invest in a question bank and practice early. We recommend making a strategic plan to cover all of the material with associated questions about six months before your exam.

DESCRIPTION OF THE USMLE STEP 1

The USMLE Step 1 is the first part of a three-step process to gain medical licensure in the United States. It is offered as a one-day computerized-based test (CBT) administered by authorized Thompson Prometric Centers and can be taken throughout the year, with the exception of major holidays and the first two weeks of January.

The subjects tested on the USMLE Step 1 include anatomy (gross anatomy, embryology, neuroanatomy, and histology), biochemistry, behavioral sciences (including biostatistics and epidemiology), microbiology, immunology, pathology, pharmacology, and physiology. Over the years, the exam has become more inter-disciplinary in nature, with many questions being posed in the format of clinical vignettes that span different fields of knowledge. In addition, integrative topics such as nutrition, genetics, and aging will be covered.

To register for the exam, students can obtain registration materials at the NBME website. Students and graduates of United States and Canadian medical schools accredited by the Liaison Committee on Medical Education (LCME) or the American Osteopathic Association (AOA) may refer to the following for further information:

> National Board of Medical Examiners (NBME)
> Department of Licensing Examination Services
> 3750 Market Street
> Philadelphia, PA 19104
> Telephone: (215) 590-9700
> Internet: www.nbme.org

> USMLE Secretariat
> 3750 Market Street
> Philadelphia, PA 19104
> Telephone: (215) 590-9700
> Internet: www.usmle.org

Students and graduates of foreign medical schools should also consult:

> Education Commission for Foreign Medical Graduates (ECFMG)
> 3624 Market Street
> Philadelphia, PA 19104-2685
> Telephone: (215) 386-5900
> Internet: www.ecfmg.org

Additional information on the examination can be obtained from the registration packet or the web site www.usmle.org. Test site information can be obtained from the web site www.prometric. com. Be sure to read the latest copy of the USMLE Bulletin of Information for further details.

The USMLE Step 1 scores are reported three to six weeks within the date of the exam, at which time they are sent to the examinee. The score report includes the pass/fail status, two overall scores, and a graphic depiction of performance in each subject area. The first test score is a three-digit number with a mean of about 225 and standard deviation of about 20. The second test score is a two-digit number with 75 as the minimum passing score (equivalent to a score of 188 on the first scale). A passing USMLE Step 1 score corresponds to answering 60–70% of questions correctly.

U.S. Seniors

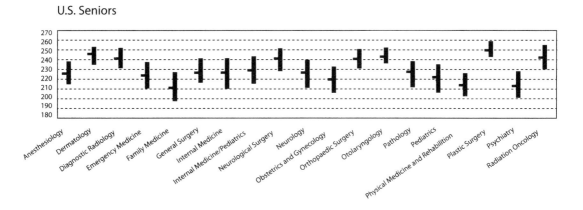

Figure 1 Mean USMLE Step 1 score for matched U.S. seniors (www.nrmp.org)

TEST FORMAT

The USMLE Step 1 Computer Based Test (CBT) exam consists of seven question blocks of 46 questions each for a total of 322 questions, with 1 hour allotted for each block. The test begins with a short tutorial of the CBT features and tools that is 15 minutes long. Should you already be familiar with these tools (which we recommend you be prior to the exam), then you can skip this section and add this time to your allotted break time. Be warned that once you finish a specific block, you cannot go back and change your answers. You can, however, change answers within a block as long as it is within the 1 hour allotted time. All questions are multiple choice, with a "one best answer" format. There is no penalty for wrong answers so don't leave any questions unanswered! Approximately 75% of the time, a brief clinical vignette is followed by a variable number of options. At times, a photograph, diagram, histology slide, radiograph, or an audio clip accompanies the question. If necessary, a "Lab" icon is available that shows you the normal ranges of clinically relevant laboratory values of blood, cerebrospinal fluid, urine, and sweat.

ABSOLUTES AND PEARLS OF WISDOM

Different students have different goals, so the amounts of time students spend studying for the examination differs greatly. Informal surveys of medical students nationwide show study times ranging from two weeks to a year! Obviously, the right amount of time to study depends on your experience, your strengths, and your goals (not to mention the amount of time available). Regardless of your goals, we know from surveys of Program Directors across the country that USMLE Step 1 scores are critical (Figure 2), and in fact, may be the most important factor in the interview selection process.

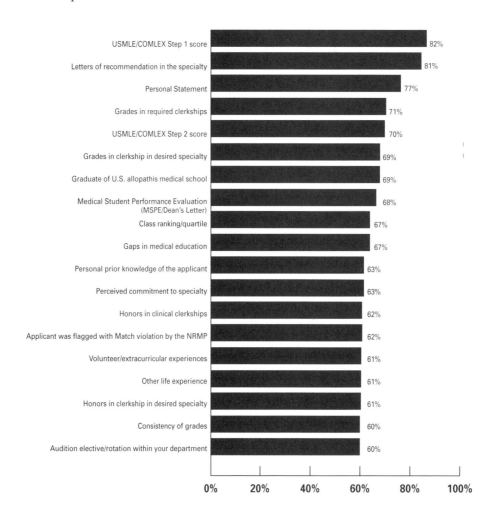

Figure 2 NRMP Program Director Survey of Applicant Factors Evaluated for Interview Selection (www.nrmp.org), shown as percentages

Here are some recommendations that we have for you:

- Make a schedule for yourself! Once you've determined your goals, map out a schedule of your study plan. Most students spend approximately four to six weeks of full time study to prepare for the exam. Stick to your deadline and avoid pushing back the exam date. We know from the exam statistics that taking the test later does not translate into a better score.

- Use the USMLE practice exams, such as those that come with this book. The NBME also provides practice tests on their website. Practice tests contain several hundred Step 1 questions that are excellent study tools. Many medical schools keep an old copy of these questions for students to use during Step 1 study, and "big sibs" often pass old copies from one class to the next. Locating one of these question sets is definitely worth the effort!

- The sample items are similar to those that appear on the Step 1 and may even have been pulled from previous administrations of the test. Some students take the sample examination before they begin studying to reveal their areas of weakness, whereas others prefer to use it toward the end to simulate the examination and practice their pacing. Either way, you'll get a feel for the content, style, and pace of the test.

- Get comfortable with the computerized table of lab values; if you have the time, you might even want to memorize a few key values. The computerized format requires you to scroll through the table to find the value you want. If you don't know where to look, precious seconds may be lost during your search.

- Sleep regular hours. In weeks prior to the exam, you should be waking up at the same time that you will need to for the exam. Get in a pattern of training yourself to be alert during these hours. Keep a balanced study schedule with time for exercise and healthy eating habits. Try to avoid excessive caffeine and energy drinks. This is an eight-hour test, which is a marathon, not a sprint. If you feel frustrated, take a small break. If you get discouraged, remember why you are doing this and get inspired! You're living the dream!

Good luck, keep your head up, and keep the faith!

"My advice to you is this… shut up and work hard."

—James S.T. Yao, MD, PhD
Northwestern University Professor Emeritus
Division of Vascular Surgery

With much admiration,

Dustin & Jubina

CHAPTER 2

BIOCHEMISTRY

DNA

The central dogma of molecular biology (Figure 1) postulates that the general flow of information starts from DNA, which is transcribed to RNA, which itself is translated to proteins. DNA must be replicated to pass on the information it stores.

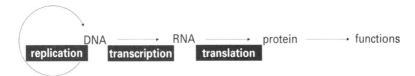

Figure 1 Central dogma of molecular biology

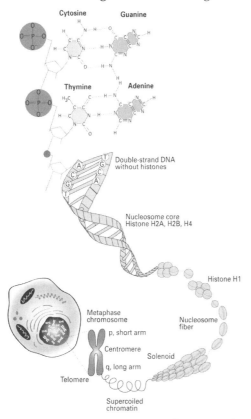

DNA is double helix molecule that has a deoxyribose sugar backbone with phosphate-linked bases. The bases are characterized by their ring structure. The purines—adenine and guanine—have two rings. The pyrimidines—cytosine, thymine, and uracil—have one ring. Thymine is only found in DNA, while uracil is only found in RNA. In DNA, adenine pairs with thymine and guanine pairs with cytosine (Figure 2). You might notice in Figure 2 that adenine forms two hydrogen bonds with thymine and guanine forms 3 hydrogen bonds with cytosine. As a result of the number of hydrogen bonds, DNA with more G-C pairings requires a higher temperature to denature than DNA with more A-T pairings.

Figure 2 Base pairing of DNA and organization and condensation of DNA (Adapted from *Harrison's Principles of Internal Medicine*)

Pyramids CUT PURe AG:
Pyrimidines—Cytosine, Uracil, Thymine

Purines—Adenosine, Guanine

Amino Acid Precursors for Purines: GAG (glycine, aspartate, glutamine), Amino Acid precursors for Pyrimidines: Aspartate

DNA melting point: More G-C = more hydrogen bonds = higher denaturing temperature

Nucleosides are composed of a base and either a deoxyribose (for DNA) or ribose (for RNA) sugar. A nucleotide is a nucleoside with one to three phosphates linked to the 5′ position of the sugar (Figure 3). Strands are formed when the phosphate forms a bond with a 3′ hydroxyl group on another sugar.

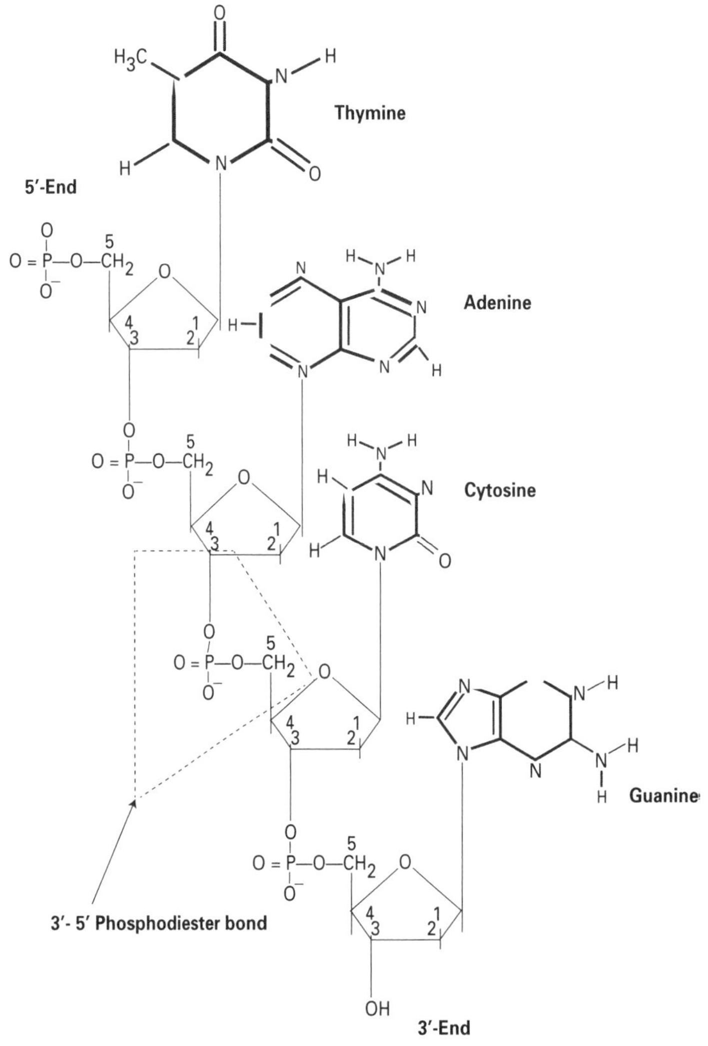

Figure 3 Nucleotides linked together by 3′ to 5′ phosphodiester bond

In eukaryotes, DNA is compacted to fit into the nucleus. This process is depicted in Figure 2. This is accomplished by histones, positively charged proteins which bind to the negatively charged sugar-phosphate backbone. Histones mostly consist of the positively charged amino acids lysine and arginine. Two each of H2A, H2B, H3, and H4 histones form a nucleosome core. DNA wraps around each nucleosome twice. H1 histones bind between the nucleosomes to further pack DNA. Heterochromatin is DNA that has been highly condensed and transcriptionally inactive. Histone methylation promotes heterochromatin formation. Euchromatin is transcriptionally active DNA. Acetylation of lysine in heterochromatin promotes formation of euchromatin and promotes transcription.

Nucleotide Biosynthesis

The de novo purine and pyrimidine nucleotide synthesis pathway can be seen in Figure 4. This pathway initially synthesizes ribonucleotides and requires ribonucleotide reductase to convert the ribonucleotide to a deoxyribonucleotide for DNA. This pathway is a target for various drugs, particularly antineoplastic drugs, as rapidly dividing cells require a large supply of pyrimidines and purines to synthesize new DNA.

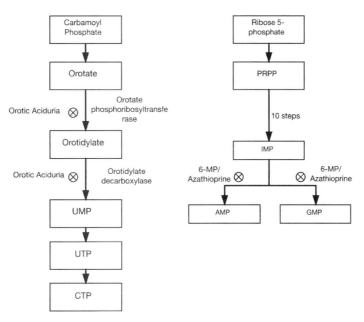

Figure 4 Purine and pyrimidine synthesis. This forms ribonucleotides for RNA. Individual steps are not as important as the clinical correlates. UMP is uridylate, UTP is uridine 5'-triphosphage, CTP is Cyridine 5'-phosphate, PRPP is 5-phosphoriboxyl 1-pyrophosphate, IMP is inosinate, AMP is Adenylate, GMP is guanylate.

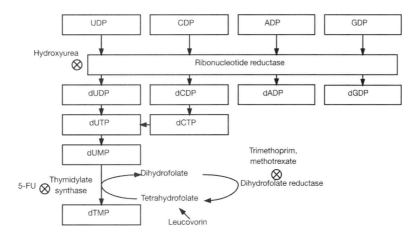

Figure 5 Synthesis of deoxyribonucleotides for synthesis of DNA. The d in front of some of the names represents deoxy.

Hydroxyurea is a drug used for treatment of myeloproliferative diseases, such as chronic myelogenous leukemia (CML), by inhibiting ribonucleotide reductase. It also works by an unknown mechanism to increase Hemoglobin F production and is used as a treatment for patients with sickle cell disease. 5-fluorouracil (5-FU) is a uracil analog that binds to and irreversibly inhibits thymidylate synthase. 6-mercaptopurine (6-MP) is a purine analog that inhibits purine synthesis. It has been used to treat conditions like acute lymphoblastic leukemia (ALL) and inflammatory bowel diseases. Azathioprine is a prodrug that is metabolized to 6-MP. Methotrexate inhibits dihydrofolate reductase in humans. Trimethoprim is an antibiotic that inhibits bacterial dihydrofolate reductase. Leucovorin is a folate analog that is converted to tetrahydrofolate by enzymes other than dihydrofolate reductase. As a result, it can be used to reverse the effects of methotrexate by providing tetrahydrofolate for the body to use. This is known as a leucovorin rescue.

Rapidly dividing cells require new nucleotides to continue synthesizing DNA for replication. These drugs inhibit their ability to create new nucleotides, leading to cell death. White blood cells are rapidly proliferating cells, so these drugs (with the exception of trimethoprim) are immunosuppressive.

Orotic aciduria is a disease where orotic acid cannot be converted to UMP due to a defect in orotic acid phosphoribosyltransferase or orotidine 5'-phosphate decarboxylase. It is an autosomal recessive disease. It results in an accumulation of orotic acid and hypochromic megaloblastic anemia due to pyrimidine deficiency. The megaloblastic anemia is refractory to vitamin B_{12} and folic acid supplementation since the defect occurs before the steps of pyrimidine synthesis involving folic acid and Vitamin B_{12}. It can also result in failure to thrive and neurologic abnormalities if untreated. Unlike ornithine transcarbamylase deficiency, it does not result in hyperammonemia.

The purine salvage pathway (Figure 6) is a way for cells to recycle purines. Hypoxanthine-guanine PRPP transferase (HGPRT) replenishes mononucleotides from ribonucleosides. This pathway alone is not enough to replenish purines. A deficiency in HGPRT results in Lesch Nyhan Disease. Patients with this disease have behavioral deficits and develop mental retardation. Purines are metabolized rather than salvaged, leading to hyperuricemia, which causes gout. Self mutilation is characteristic for this disease. The disease is X-linked.

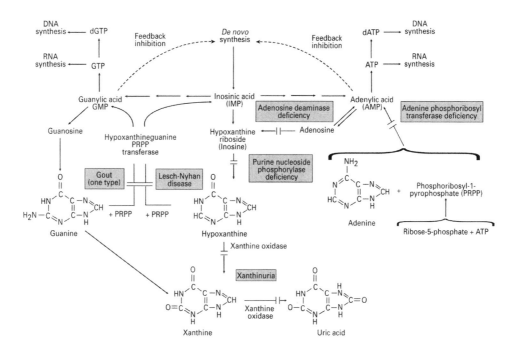

Figure 6 Purine salvage and metabolism. Individual steps are not as important as pathologies that are discussed (Adapted from Nelson's Textbook of Pediatrics).

Disease	Enzyme deficient	Metabolic Effects	Results in	Notes
Gout	Many causes, affecting uric acid metabolism (uric acid is the product of purine degradation)	High uric acid levels in serum (hyperuricemia)	Uric acid crystals in joint, causing arthritis	Treatment: allopurinol, which inhibits xanthine oxidase to lower uric acid production
Lesch Nyhan syndrome	Hypoxanthineguanine phosphoribosyl-transferase (purine salvage)	Accumulation of hypoxanthine and guanine Excess uric acid production because salvage inhibition increases purine metabolism	Self-mutilation and aggression Mental and physical retardation Spastic cerebral palsy	Rare X-linked recessive disease, seen only in males Sometimes gouty arthritis develops
Adenosine deaminase (ADA) deficiency	ADA (purine degradation)	Accumulation of dATP, which inhibits ribonucleotide reductase (and DNA synthesis)	Severe combined immunodeficiency	Presents in neonatal period Children die from infection before age 2 Autosomal recessive

Table 1 High yield summary of purine salvage/metabolism related diseases

DNA Replication

DNA replication is a semiconservative process, meaning that after DNA replication, the product contains one original strand and one new strand. The process begins at an origin of replication. Prokaryote DNA only has one origin while eukaryote DNA has multiple origins. DNA replication is initiated when proteins bind to these origins and cause the DNA at the origin to unwind. DNA helicase is a protein that assists with unwinding of DNA by breaking its hydrogen bonds. The replication fork is the area where DNA helicase unwinds DNA and leading and lagging strands of DNA are synthesized. Single strand binding proteins prevent separated strands of DNA from reannealing.

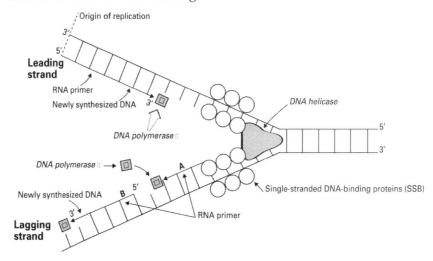

Figure 7 Schematic of DNA replication

Fluoroquinolones
Target DNA gyrase, the -floxacins

During DNA synthesis, the DNA can become supercoiled. DNA topoisomerases are used to create nicks in the phosphate backbone to prevent supercoiling. The topoisomerases can also reanneal nicks that they create in DNA. In prokaryotes, this enzyme is known as DNA gyrase. It is a target for the flouroquinolone antibiotic class. Antibiotics in this class include ciprofloxacin and levofloxacin."

The following steps of DNA synthesis apply to prokaryotic cells, but eukaryotic cells have similar proteins and steps. DNA synthesis starts with the creation of an RNA primer by the primase. This RNA primer serves as the starting point for DNA polymerase III to add nucleotides to the 3' position. It synthesizes DNA from 5' to 3'. There are no polymerases that synthesize DNA from 3' to 5'. On the leading strand, this replication is a continuous process. On the lagging strand, DNA is synthesized until DNA polymerase encounters the RNA primer of a previously synthesized segment. Lagging strand synthesis is created in a step-wise fashion. The segments of DNA in the lagging strand are called Okazaki fragments. DNA polymerase I uses 5' to 3' exonuclease activity to remove RNA primers and then uses 5' to 3' synthesis to replace the RNA primers with

DNA. Ligase enzymes seal DNA strands. Telomeres, the end caps of DNA, cannot be synthesized by DNA polymerase and must be synthesized by telomerase.

DNA Proofreading and Repair

Throughout the course of a cell's life cycle, its DNA is exposed to a large variety of stresses. UV exposure can result in cross linking of DNA by formation of thymidine dimers. *Xeroderma pigmentosum* is a rare, autosomal recessive disease that results in people who lack the ability to repair these thymidine dimers due to mutations in the nucleotide excision repair system. Patients with the disease have dry, parchment-like skin and are at increased risk of all the skin cancers (melanoma, basal cell, and squamous cell). Deamination of cytosine to uracil and depurination of nucleotides are also common spontaneous DNA alterations.

During DNA replication, DNA polymerase I, II, and III all have proofreading and DNA repair activity. DNA polymerase III has 3' to 5' proofreading and proofreads while it synthesizes DNA. Outside of replication, DNA repair enzymes exist for nucleotide excision repair, base excision repair and mismatch repair. For nucleotide excision repair, endonucleases identify and remove damaged nucleotides and nucleotides around them. DNA polymerase and ligase then fill the created gap and seal it. For base excision repair, glycosylases remove damaged bases, allowing AP endonucleases to remove the empty sugar. As with nucleotide excision repair, DNA polymerase and ligase fill and seal the gap. In prokaryotes, mismatched DNA is unmethylated. This unmethylated DNA is recognized and excised. Patients with *hereditary nonpolyposis colorectal cancer* (also known as HNPCC or Lynch syndrome) have a defect in mismatch repair enzymes, increasing their likelihood of having various cancers, including colorectal and endometrial cancer.

RNA

There are four types of RNA: rRNA, mRNA, tRNA, and small RNA. Ribosomal RNA (rRNA) is used to create ribosomes, which participate in protein translation. Messenger RNA (mRNA) is the product of DNA transcription and is used by ribosomes to synthesize proteins. Transfer RNA (tRNA) carries amino acids for use in protein synthesis. Small RNAs modulate mRNA to effect gene expression.

Transcription

Transcription is the process of converting DNA to RNA. In prokaryotes, there is a single RNA polymerase which converts DNA to various types of RNA. In eukaryotes, RNA polymerase I transcribes rRNA, RNA polymerase II transcribes mRNA, and RNA polymerase III transcribes tRNA. RNA polymerase II and III can transcribe small RNAs as well. RNA synthesis and DNA synthesis are similar. RNA synthesis does not require the primase to start the process. As is the case with DNA polymerases, RNA polymerases can only add nucleotides in a 5' to 3' direction.

Xeroderma Pigmentosum: Inability to repair thymidine dimers leading to skin cancers

HNPCC/Lynch Syndrome: Mismatch repair enzyme, commonly MSH2, defect resulting in increased incidence of colorectal and endometrial cancer

DNA Repair: NBME— Nucleotide, Base, and Mismatch Excisors

Therefore the template strand (from the DNA) or antisense strand is in the 3' to 5' direction. The RNA synthesized is similar to the 5' to 3' DNA strand or coding strand or sense strand, with the exception of containing ribonucleotides instead of deoxyribonucleotides and uracil instead of thymine.

Transcription is regulated by the organization of genes themselves. Transcription must begin at a promoter. Near the promoter is the TATA box. Enhancers increase the rate of RNA synthesis while repressors or silencers decrease the rate of RNA synthesis. Enhancers and silencers do not necessarily need to be near the promoter. Due to the twisting and winding of DNA, they may be in close contact with the promoters without being next to them.

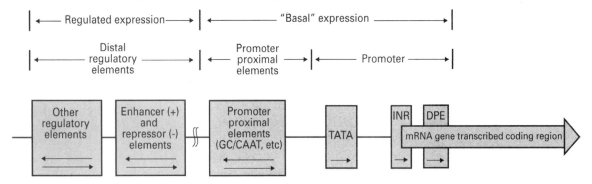

Figure 8 Schematic of gene organization
(Adapted from *Harper's's Illustrated Biochemistry*)

Post-transcriptional Modification of mRNA

Synthesized mRNA of eukaryotes must undergo modification before it is usable. In eukaryotes, coding sequences in the DNA are called exons while noncoding sequences are called introns. Both are transcribed to RNA, but introns must be removed in a process called splicing. A spliceosome is a complex of proteins and RNAs that forms to splice out introns. Splicing can also remove exons in a process called alternative splicing, yielding variations of proteins from one gene. Splicing is implicated in the pathology of one form of β-thalassemia. A nucleotide change in the β-globin gene, a component of hemoglobin, leads to an inability to remove an intron. A 7-methylguanosine cap is added to the 5' terminal end of mRNA and a poly-A tail to the 3' end. The 5' cap protects the mRNA from enzymatic degradation.

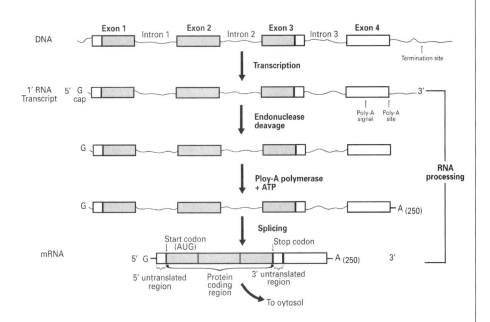

Figure 9 Summary of post-transcriptional modification of mRNA

PROTEIN

Translation

Translation is the process of converting mRNAs to proteins. Proteins are composed of amino acids. Codons are sequences of three nucleic acids, which code for a single amino acid. There are 64 possible codons and only 20 amino acids used in proteins. The codon code is degenerate, as multiple codons can specify the same amino acid. Important codons include the start and stop codons. There is only one start codon, AUG, which codes for methionine in eukaryotes and formyl-methionine in prokaryotes. UGA, UAA, and UAG are stop codons. As their name implies, start codons signal the beginning of translation while stop codons signal the end of translation. Note: Only try to memorize the stop and start codons. It is not important to memorize other codons.

Mutations in DNA can alter codon meaning, resulting in various degrees of impairment. Silent mutations result in a change of a codon but code for the same amino acid. Missense mutations result in a different amino acid. Nonsense mutations result in the introduction of a stop codon, truncating the protein. Since codons consist of three nucleic acids, addition or loss of nucleic acids that are not in multiples of three will result in frameshift mutations. These mutations create all new groups of codons.

For translation to occur, tRNA must carry the proper amino acids. Transfer RNAs are cloverleaf shaped RNAs which carry the amino acid on their 3' end. The anticodon is responsible for detecting the codon on the mRNA. It is located on the opposite side of the amino acid. Aminoacyl-

Methionine inAUGurates protein synthesis
UGA: **U G**o **A**way,
UAA: **U A**re **A**way,
UAG: **U A**re **G**one
(alternatively, start with UAA and swap a G for either A).

Stop the nonsense (stop codon introduced in nonsense mutation)

tRNA synthetase is the protein responsible for pairing amino acids with their appropriate tRNAs. This process is known as charging and is ATP dependent. Due to degeneracy of codons, the codon and anti-codon only need to match the first two nucleic acids. This is a phenomenon known as wobble.

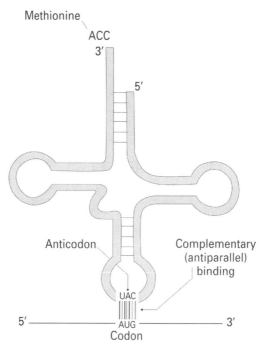

Figure 10 Structure of tRNA

Prokaryotes are odd (30, 50, 70)

Ribosomes catalyze protein synthesis. In eukaryotes, 40S and 60S ribosomes combine to form 80S ribosomes. In prokaryotes, 30S and 50S ribosomes combine to form 70S ribosomes. For protein synthesis to begin, the smaller subunit, initiation factors, and the initiator tRNA (containing methionine) scan mRNA until the start codon is found. Once this occurs, the larger ribosome combines with the complex, and the initiator tRNA in the P (peptidyl tRNA) site. New tRNAs bind to the A site and the new amino acid is added to the peptide in a reaction catalyzed by the ribosome. The ribosome progresses to the next codon and moves the peptide to the P position. The process of tRNA recruitment (gripping) and protein translocation is GTP mediated. The process continues until release factors detect a stop codon. At this point, the protein is released.

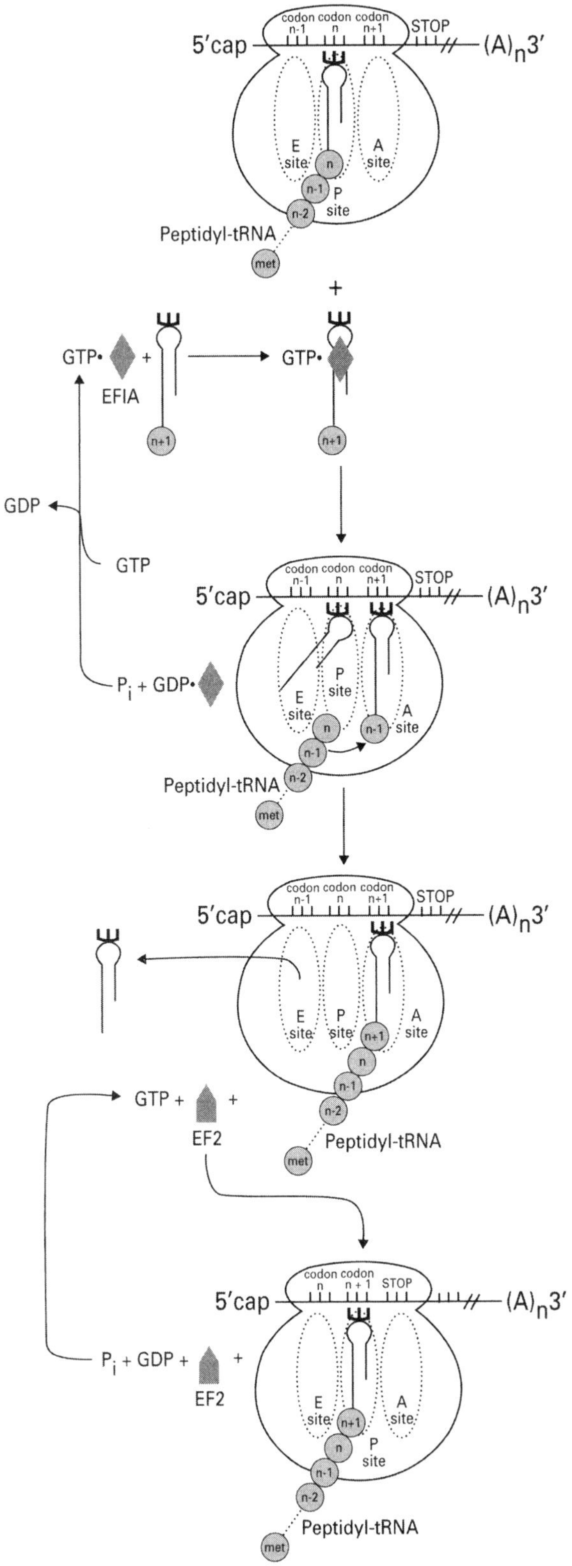

Figure 11 Depiction of protein synthesis
(Adapted from *Harper's's Illustrated Biochemistry*)

Tetracyline:
Thirty S, **t**RNA
attachment

Chloramphenicol:
Pifty (50) S
peptidyltransferase

The **MC** blocks Fiddy
(50S) from
translocating
(MC = Macrolide,
Clindamycin)

Aminoglycosides
Abort Initiation Complex

Minoglycosides
Misread **m**RNA

The process of translation is a target for antibiotics. Antibiotics can be specific for a bacteria given the difference in eukaryote and prokaryote ribosomes. Tetracylines block tRNAs from binding to 30S. Chloramphenicol inhibits 50S peptidyltransferase. Macrolides and clindamycin prevent 50S from translocating. Aminoglycosides have multiple mechanisms, including inhibiting the formation of the initiation complex and causing the ribozyme to misread mRNA.

Proteins are subject to various post-translational modifications including trimming by zymogens into mature proteins, phosphorylation, glycosylation, hydroxylation, and degradation by ubiquination.

The endoplasmic reticulum is one site of protein synthesis. Rough endoplasmic reticulum (RER) consists of ribosomes attached to endoplasmic reticulum. Proteins synthesized here are destined for lysosomes, peroxisomes, cell surface, or for excretion. As a result, cells that secrete proteins, such as goblet cells and plasma cells, contain a large quantity of RER. The rough endoplasmic reticulum is the site of N-linked glycosylation which leads to the formation of glycoproteins. Paroxysmal nocturnal hemoglobinuria (PNH) is a disease where patients have a defect in glycosylphosphatidylinositol (GPI, a glycoprotein) anchor. As a result of this defect, decay accelerating factor (DAF) and CD59 (inhibitor of reactive lysis) are not expressed on the surface of red blood cells. These proteins inhibit complement-mediated hemolysis. Patients with this rare disease will present with "cola-colored" urine that they notice when they wake up.

PNH = no DAF,CD59

Nissl bodies are RER found in neurons. They are responsible for synthesizing enzymes and peptide neurotransmitters. Smooth endoplasmic reticulum is the site of steroid synthesis and drug detoxification. As a result, hepatocytes and adrenal-cortex cells contain a large quantity of smooth endoplasmic reticulum.

The golgi body is involved in protein transport and modification. It is involved in the addition of mannose-6-phosphate to proteins destined for lysosomes. Mannose-6-phosphate is detected by receptors in the golgi apparatus, resulting in transport of the protein to a lysosome. When mannose-6-phosphate addition is defective, patients suffer from I-Cell disease (inclusion cell disease). The proteins are excreted into the plasma, rather than transported to lysosomes. As a result of the defect, the lysosomes are unable to properly function, leading to accumulation of lysosomes full of material that was destined to be degraded. These accumulated lysosomes form inclusion bodies. Patients with this rare disease present with coarse facial features, restricted joint movement, and cardiac involvement. They may also present with corneal clouding.

I-**CCC**Cell disease:
Coarse Facies,
Can't move fully,
Cardiac Involvement,
Clouded Cornea

Protein Structure and Function

The structure of proteins can be described at four levels. The primary structure describes the amino acids that the protein contains. The secondary structure describes the local conformation of the amino acids; it is dictated by hydrogen bonding. The tertiary structure is the overall structure of the protein. The quaternary structure describes the interaction of the protein with other proteins. Chaperone proteins found in the endoplasmic reticulum ensure the proper folding of proteins. These chaperone proteins also tag misfolded proteins and prevent them from being exported.

Collagen synthesis is an example of the effect of protein posttranslational modification and structure on its function. In the endoplasmic reticulum, the pro-α-chains undergo hydroxylation of proline and lysine. This step requires ascorbic acid or Vitamin C. This increases the hydrogen bonding capacity of the proteins. The proteins also undergo glycosylation at some of the hydroxylated lysines. As a result of these modifications, three pro-α-chains spontaneously organize into a triple helix pattern to form procollagen. This triple helix is a tertiary structure. The procollagen is secreted. In the extracellular matrix it undergoes cleavage of the amino and carboxy ends to form tropocollagen, the monomer of collagen fibers. Lysyl oxidase then links chains of tropocollagen together to form collagen fibrils. The triple helix structure gives collagen the strength it needs to serve as connective tissue.

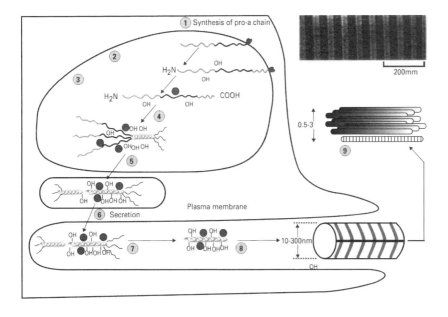

Figure 12 Diagram depicting steps of collagen synthesis
(Adapted from *Sabiston Textbook of Surgery*)

Collagen synthesis steps and defects are high yield!

Defects in collagen synthesis result in disease. *Vitamin C deficiency*, also known as scurvy, leads to an inability to hydroxylate proline and lysine. As a result, collagen of the blood vessels is affected. These patients have hemorrhages and bleeding from their gums. *Osteogenesis imperfecta* (OI) is a defect in the synthesis of type I collagen. Type I collagen is a major component of bone, gives the dermis its strength and is found in most organs. In OI type I, the most common form of OI, patients suffer from multiple fractures, characteristic "blue sclerae," and hearing loss. They may also have irregularities with their teeth. *Ehlers Danlos syndrome* is a set of diseases that are characterized by hyperextendable skin, abnormal

Ehlers Danlos:
Hyperextendibility,
hyperflexibility,
hyperfragility

Alport Syndrome:
"can't pee, can't see,
can't hear"

Alpor: Broken Floor
(basement membrane)

fragility of tissue, and increased joint mobility. Lysyl hydroxylase deficiency and defects in the cleavage of propeptides are two common causes of Ehlers Danlos syndrome. *Alport syndrome* is a group of diseases caused by defects in type IV collagen. This collagen is found in basement membranes. As a result, patients with this disease have nephritis due to defects in the kidney basement membrane. This presents as microscopic or gross hematuria. Bilateral sensorineural hearing loss also occurs. Ocular abnormalities may also be associated with Alport Syndrome. The most common mutation is X-linked. A summary of collagen synthesis defects can be found in Table 2.

Disease	Defect	Symptoms
Scurvy	Vitamin C deficiency, Can not hydroxylate proline and lysine	Hemorrhage, bleeding from gums
Osteogenesis Imperfecta	Type I collagen synthesis defect	Easy fractures, blue sclera, hearing loss, abnormal teeth
Alport syndrome	Type IV collagen synthesis defect	Hematuria, sensorineural deafness, ocular abnormalities
Ehler-Danlos syndrome	Various	Hyperextendibility, hypermobility, hyperfragility

Table 2 High yield summary of collagen synthesis defects

Sickle cell is high yield!

Acute Chest Syndrome: "White out" on chest X-ray

Possible presentation of patients with sickle cell: Pain crisis, sequestration crisis, acute chest syndrome, bone infarcts, sepsis from encapsulated bacteria

Various hemoglobinopathies are caused by mutations and misfolding of the globin proteins. *Sickle cell anemia* is a disease caused by the substitution of valine for glutamine in the beta-hemoglobin chain. In a deoxygenated state, Hb S, the hemoglobin type made in patients with sickle cell, polymerizes. Initially, oxygenation may help reverse the sickling; however, this sickling eventually becomes unreversible. Since deoxygenation is important in causing the sickling, factors that affect hemoglobin oxygenation, such as pH, temperature and 2,3-bisphosphoglycerate, will affect the rate and severity of the sickling. Increased Hb S is also another important factor in sickling. The disease is characterized by increased adhesion to endothelium by sickled cells as well as an inflammatory process. Patients with sickle cell anemia can have sickle crisis or vasoocclusive crisis, where sickling leads to intense pain and anemia. These patients can also have sequestration crisis, where the spleen sequesters sickled cells, leading to autoinfarction of the spleen. Patients with sickle cell often undergo splenectomy or are termed "functionally asplenic." Asplenic patients require vaccinations against encapsulated bacteria. Acute chest syndrome is fever, cough, and dyspnea with infiltrates found on chest X-ray. Patients can be treated with hydroxyurea to increase production of Hb F.

Chaperone proteins are implicated in the pathophysiology of cystic fibrosis. *Cystic fibrosis* is an autosomal recessive genetic defect in the cystic fibrosis transmembrane conductance regulator (CFTR) gene which codes for a chloride channel. The most common mutation is a deletion of the codon for phenylalanine at the 508 position. The mutation leads to misfolding of the protein. Chaperone proteins prevent the CFTR protein from being expressed on the cell surface. The defect leads to an inability to secrete chloride in the lungs and GI tract and an inability to reabsorb chloride in the skin. As a result of a defect, mucus is thickened and its clearance is decreased. The inability to clear mucus results in chronic bronchitis, bronchiectasis, and recurrent *Pseudomonas* and *Staphylococcus* aureus infections. The defect in the gene leads to an inability to secrete bicarbonate in the pancreas, leading to retention of pancreatic enzymes. Patients have pancreatic insufficiency leading to malabsorption of fat soluble vitamins and steatorrhea. Infants with the disease can present with a meconium ileus. Male patients with the disease are infertile, as the vas deferens does not form. Diagnosis of the disease can be done by measuring the concentration of chloride (> 60 mEq/L) in sweat performed on two separate days. Treatment for the disease is symptomatic relief. It includes supplementation of pancreatic enzymes, vitamin and nutrient supplementation, n-acetyl-cysteine for loosening of respiratory plugs, and treatment of respiratory infections.

ENERGY METABOLISM

Energy metabolism utilizes catabolic pathways to breakdown complex molecules to simple molecules. This breakdown process releases energy which is stored in various forms, most importantly ATP. Catabolic pathways utilize oxidation with molecules such as NAD+ and FADH as electron acceptors to form NADH and $FADH_2$ which are electron carriers.

Glycolysis

Glycolysis is the most important pathway for glucose metabolism. The pathway begins with glucose and ends with energy in the form of two ATP, two pyruvate, and two NADH. In anaerobic glycolysis, glycolysis that is not in the presence of oxygen, pyruvate is converted to lactate at the expense of two NADH. The first step of the process requires phosphorylation of glucose to glucose-6-phosphate. This step is done by glucokinase (an isozyme of hexokinase) in the liver and beta cells of the pancreas. It sequesters glucose, as glucose-6-posphate can not leave the cell. The enzyme is also induced by glucose. Hexokinase phosphorylates glucose in other tissues; it is product inhibited. Phosphofructokinase-1 is the rate limiting step in glycolysis. It is also the most important regulatory step. It is inhibited by citrate and 5'-AMP which both signal an abundance of energy. Fructose-2,6-bisphosphate plays an important role in the regulation of glycolysis. It is an allosteric activator of phosphofructokinase-1. High levels of fructose-6-phosphate indicate a high level of carbohydrates and upregulate fructose-2,6-bisphosphate synthesis by allosterically activating phosphofructokinase-2 and inhibiting the phosphatase activity on the same protein.

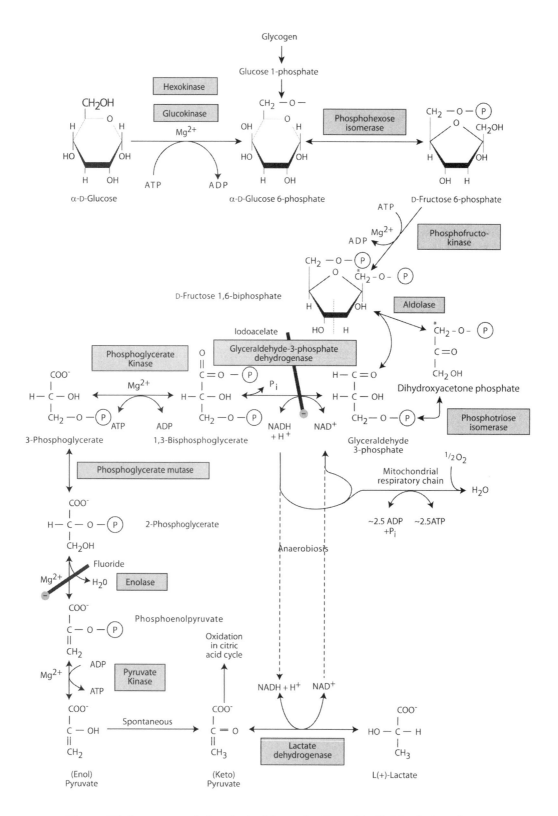

Figure 13 Summary of glycolysis. Memorization of individual steps is not as important as learning the regulation of the system.
(Adapted from *Harper's Illustrated Biochemistry*)

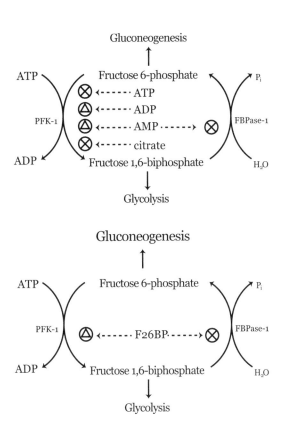

Figure 14 Regulation of Phosphofructokinase-1
(Adapted from *Lehninger Principles of Biochemistry*)

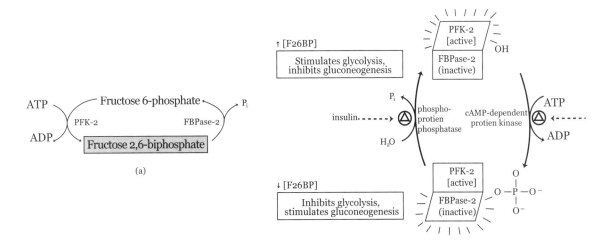

Figure 15 Role of Fructose 2,6-bisphosphate on glycolysis regulation
(Adapted from *Lehininger Principles of Biochemistry*)

Deficiency of pyruvate kinase, the step that catalyzes the conversion of phosphoenolpyruvate to pyruvate, can lead to a common form of hemolytic anemia.

Once pyruvate is created as a product of glycolysis, it has multiple fates. It can be converted to lactate by lactate dehydrogenase for ATP synthesis in anaerobic glycolysis. This path is used by red blood cells, white blood cells, the kidney medulla, the lens, the testes, and the cornea. Pyruvate dehydrogenase, within the cystoplasm of the mitochondria, converts pyruvate to acetyl-CoA which has many uses including the citric acid cycle and lipogenesis. The enzyme requires Vitamin B1, B2, B3, B5 (CoA), and lipoic acid as cofactors. Acetyl-CoA and NADH inhibit pyruvate dehydrogenase. In the liver, pyruvate can be metabolized to alanine and transported to muscle. Pyruvate is also converted to oxaloacetate for various pathways including the Tricarboxylic Acid (TCA) cycle and gluconeogenesis.

Arsenic poisoning: garlic breath, lactic acidosis, liver angiosarcoma

Pyruvate dehydrogenase can be inhibited by arsenic and mercury. As a result, excess pyruvate accumulates and is shunted to the lactate pathway. These patients will have lactic acidosis. Patients with *arsenic poisoning* will also have "garlic breath," vomiting, diarrhea, and Mees lines on nails. Liver angiosarcoma and lung cancer are also sequellae of arsenic poisoning. Congenital deficiencies will also lead to lactic acidosis. Neurologic problems occur because the brain relies on glucose metabolism for energy. A ketogenic diet high in fat, lysine, and leucine can lower the lactic acidosis; however, prognosis of these patients is poor. Thiamine deficiency, seen in alcoholics, is an acquired form of pyruvate dehydrogenase deficiency that leads to lactic acidosis.

The TCA cycle converts acetyl-CoA into H_2O, CO_2, 3 NADH, 1 FADH, and 1 GTP. The GTP is used directly as energy. The NADH and FADH are used in oxidative phosphorylation to create more ATP. Alpha-ketoglutarate dehydrogenase is structurally similar to pyruvate dehydrogenase and uses the same cofactors. As a result, it also is inhibited during arsenic poisoning. Intermediates in the TCA cycle have various uses, including amino acid synthesis.

NADH and $FADH_2$ generated by the TCA cycle generate ATP through the electron transport chain and oxidative phosphorylation. The molecules are used as electron donors to the electron transport chain and help to establish a proton gradient. ATP synthase (complex V) utilizes the proton gradient to convert ADP to ATP. Uncoupling of the electron transport chain can lead to production of heat rather than ATP. This is the mechanism that thermogenin uses in brown adipose tissue to help maintain temperature.

Sodium thiosulfate: cyanide antidote

Carbon monoxide, cyanide, and azide poisoning affect complex IV of the electron transport chain. *Cyanide poisoning* can rapidly result in coma and death. It is treated with sodium nitrite and sodium thiosulfate. Sodium nitrite oxidizes the heme in hemoglobin to form methemoglobin. Cyanide has a greater binding affinity for methemoglobin than it does for complex IV. Sodium thiosulfate is a sulfur donor which helps the body to detoxify cyanide to thiocyanate.

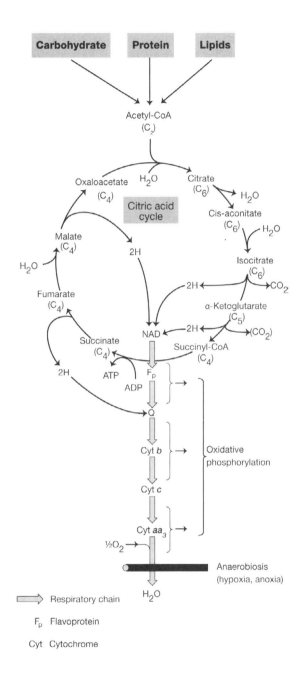

Can I Keep Selling Stuff
For Money Officer?—
TCA Cycle
(citrate, isocitrate,
α-ketoglutarate, succinyl
coa, succinate, fumarate,
malate, oxaloacetate)

Figure 16 Summary of TCA cycle and electron transport chain.
Memorizing the steps of the TCA cycle is high yield.
(Adapted from *Harper's Illustrated Biochemistry*)

The pentose-phosphate pathway (also known as the exose monophosphate shunt) is a pathway synthesizes ribose sugars for nucleotide synthesis and NADPH. NADPH is a source of energy used in anabolic pathways. It is important in the synthesis of glutathione, an antioxidant used in detoxifying free radicals. NADPH is also used in the creation of reactive radicals in neutrophils. The pentose-phosphate pathway has irreversible oxidative reactions and reversible nonoxidative reactions. It is the irreversible oxidative reactions that form NADPH. The reversible reactions allow for the regeneration of glucose-6-phosphate by creating three carbon intermediates. Glucose-6-phosphate dehydrogenase is an important enzyme in this pathway. *Glucose-6-phosphate deficiency* leads to a hemolytic anemia in the presence of increased oxidative stress, since the RBCs can not produce NADPH and therefore glutathione. A typical question stem will describe an African American patient with a hemolytic anemia after ingestion of certain foods or medications. Triggers for hemolysis include fava beans, infection, primaquine, sulfonamides, or TB drugs. A blood smear will show Heinz bodies which are collections of precipitated hemoglobin in red blood cells and bite cells which are red blood cells that look like they have had a portion "bitten" off. This process occurs due to macrophages in the spleen. Asplenic patients will have Heinz bodies but will not have bite cells. The deficiency is thought to confer a survival advantage in malaria-endemic regions, as infection with malaria leads to hemolysis and death of the plasmodium parasite.

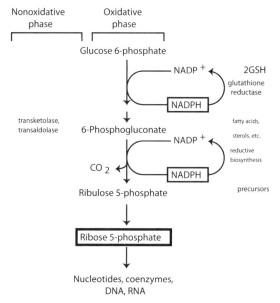

Figure 17 Overview of the pentose phosphate shunt.
It is not high yield to memorize the steps
(Adapted from *Lehninger Principles of Biochemistry*).

NADPH oxidase is an important enzyme in neutrophils, as it creates free radicals for respiratory burst, a release of reactive oxygen intermediates by neutrophils. Patients who have a NADPH oxidase deficiency have a disease called *Chronic Granulomatous Disease*. Neutrophils are still able to fight off disease by releasing hydrogen peroxide. However, the body is susceptible to catalase-positive bacteria like *Staphylococcus aureus*, since catalase can breakdown hydrogen peroxide. These patients tend to form granulomas in the liver, lungs, and lymph nodes. They are treated prophylactically with trimethoprim/sulfamethoxazole and antifungal agents such as itraconazole.

Fructose Metabolism

Fructose is a hexose sugar that is an epimer of glucose. It enters the glycolysis pathway via two enzymes: fructokinase and aldolase B. Fructokinase phosphorylates fructose to fructose 1-phosphate. Unlike glucokinase, fructokinase is not regulated by insulin. Fructose 1-phosphate is then cleaved by aldolase B to dihydroxyacetone-phosphate and glyceraldehyde, entering the glycolysis pathway. Fructose metabolism is not regulated by insulin and is also not regulated by phosphofructokinase, the key regulatory step in glycolysis, as dihydroxyacetone-phosphate and glyceraldehyde enter glycolysis after this step. Excess products of glycolysis created by fructose metabolism typically are used in gluconeogenesis, creating excess glucose. Fructose is an important energy source for sperm.

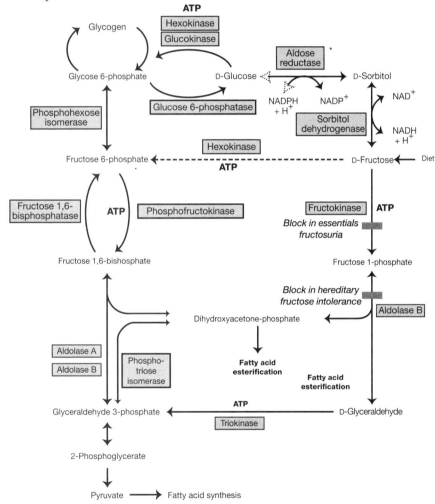

Figure 18 Diagram demonstrating how fructose enters glycolysis. Note the two enzyme blocks that lead to disease. (Adapted from *Harper's Illustrated Biochemistry*)

Deficiency in fructokinase leads to essential or *benign fructosuria*. It is a disease that is found incidentally. A typical scenario will involve the addition of cupric sulfate, a reagent that detects reducable sugars. The blue cupric sulfate will be reduced to red cuprous sulfate. Chromatography will then reveal fructose in the urine. The disease is benign, autosomal recessive, and is characterized by excess fructose in the blood and urine.

Deficiency of aldolase B leads to *Hereditary Fructose Intolerance*. Deficiency in aldolase B results in accumulation of fructose-1-phosphate, the substrate of the enzyme. Patients with this deficiency can exhibit vomiting, abdominal pain, diarrhea, jaundice, hepatomegaly, and signs of hypoglycemia. Symptoms first manifest with the initial intake of fructose from fruits or other fructose-containing foods. Treatment is avoidance of foods with fructose sugars (including foods with sucrose, a disaccharide of glucose, and fructose).

Galactose Metabolism

Galactose is a hexose epimer of glucose. Galactokinase phosphorylates galactose to galactose-1-phosphate. Galactose 1-phosphate uridyl transferase converts galactose-1-phosphate to UDP-galactose. The reaction also results in the creation of glucose-1-phosphate. UDP-galactose is converted to UDP glucose by UDP-Gal 4-epimerase which can be used in glycogen synthesis. Galactose can also be converted to galactitol, a sugar alcohol, by aldose reductase. Galactose is a component of lactose, a disaccharide found in milk.

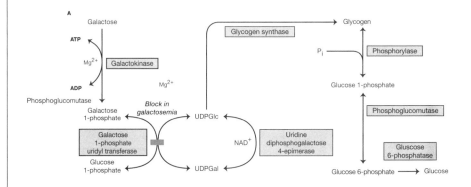

Figure 19 Galactose conversion to glucose. Note the enzyme block leading to galactosemia.
(Adapted from *Harper's Illustrated Biochemistry*)

Galactokinase deficiency leads to conversion of excess galactose to galactitol which can accumulate in the lens of the eye and lead to infantile cataracts. *Classic galactosemia* is a disease caused by the absence of galactose-1-phosphate urdyltransferase. It results in an accumulation of the enzyme's substrate, galactose-1-phosphate, and results in kidney, liver, and brain damage including jaundice, hepatomegaly, and mental retardation. Accumulation of galactitol also leads to infantile cataracts. Vomiting and

Infantile cataracts: think galactokinase deficiency

Infantile cataracts + hypoglycemia + *E coli* sepsis = think classic galactosemia hypoglycemia are also manifestations of the disease. Patients are also susceptible *E. coli* sepsis. The disease can be diagnosed by newborn screening with a reducing agent like cupric sulfate (see explanation under fructosuria). Enzyme activity in patient's red blood cells provides definitive diagnosis. Treatment is avoidance of galactose containing foods and lactose. Hypergonadotrophic hypogonadism is a long term sequelae seen in female patients with the disease.

Sorbitol

Conversion of glucose to sorbitol is an alternative pathway to trapping glucose in the cell. This pathway is mediated by aldose reductase. Sorbitol dehydrogenase converts sorbitol back to glucose. Schwann cells, lens, retina, and kidneys only have aldose reductase. In patients with diabetes, sorbitol can accumulate in these cells and cause damage via osmosis. This may explain why diabetics have blurry vision when acutely hyperglycemic and one of the potential mechanisms behind neuropathy, retinopathy, and cataracts.

ENERGY STORAGE

Gluconeogenesis

Gluconeogenesis is the synthesis of glucose from precursors that are not 6 carbon sugars. Gluconeogenesis occurs in both the liver and kidneys. Gluconeogenesis begins with oxaloacetate. The gluconeogenic amino acids alanine, glutamine, pyruvate, lactate, and propionyl-CoA can be converted to oxaloacetate. Propionyl-CoA is a derivative of odd chain fatty acid metabolism. There are several important and unique steps in gluconeogenesis. Pyruvate is converted to oxaloacetate via pyruvate carboxylase. Oxaloacetate is converted to phosphoenolpyruvate (PEP) via PEP carboxykinase. PEP is eventually converted to fructose-1,6-bisphosphate which is converted to fructose-6 phospate by fructose 1,6-bisphosphatase. Finally, in order to be exported, glucose-6-phosphate must be converted to glucose via glucose-6-phosphatase. These steps are irreversible. Gluconeogenesis is an energetically unfavored process, requiring 4 ATP and 2 GTP to produce a glucose molecule.

Glycogen Synthesis and Metabolism

Glycogen is the storage macromolecule of carbohydrates in humans. It is a highly branched molecule. Recall that carbohydrates tend to grow in a linear fashion with 1 to 4 bonds. Branched bonds are 1 to 6 bonds. Glycogen is mostly synthesized and stored in the liver and muscle. In muscle, the stores are used for rapid release of energy during muscle use, while in the liver the stores are used to maintain blood sugar levels. Glycogen synthesis starts when glucose-6-phosphate is made into glucose-1-phosphate and then UDP-glucose. Glycogenin creates 7 glucose long glycogen primers with 1 to 4 bonds. Glycogen synthase then takes UDP-glucose and lengthens a glycogen chain in the 1 to 4 direction. A branching enzyme creates 1 to 6 bonds by taking at least 6 glucose molecules at the end of a chain and transferring them to a branch point. Glycogen synthase is the key regulated protein in glycogen synthesis. Phosphorylation of glycogen synthase decreases its activity. Glucagon and epinephrine (think as signs for more needed energy) regulate a decrease in the dephosphorylation of the enzyme. Glucose, glucose-6-phosphate, and insulin (think signs of excess energy in the body to be stored) increase the desphosphorylation of the enzyme. Insulin also decreases the amount of phosphorylation of the enzyme.

Glycogen metabolism is mediated by glycogen phosphorylase. It catalyzes the phosphorolysis of glycogen, removing a glucose molecule from the end of glycogen, breaking 1 to 4 bonds to form glucose-1-phosphate. It removes glucose from glycogen until it reaches a point near a branch point. The resulting molecule is called a limit dextran. Then a debranching enzyme transfers all but one glucose molecule from the branch to the glycogen chain. A 1 to 6 glucosidase removes the remaining glucose branched molecule.

Free glucose-1-phosphate is converted to glucose-6-phosphate. In the liver, glucose-6-phosphatase removes the phosphate, allowing for glucose to be exported to the blood. Lysosomes contain both 1,4-glucosidase and 1,6-glucosidase, allowing for them to metabolize glycogen as well. Glycogen phosphorylase is upregulated by phosphorylation. Glucagon, epinephrine, Ca^{2+}, and AMP upregulate phosphorylation of the enzyme. Calcium and AMP in the muscle are signs of muscle activity and that the muscle needs more energy.

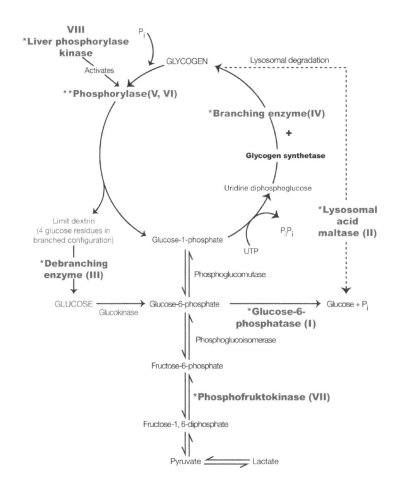

Figure 20 Glycogen metabolism. Steps with asterisk are enzymes affected in different glycogen storage diseases.
(Adapted from *Robbins and Cotran Pathologic Basis of Disease*)

Glycogen storage diseases are caused by defects in the enzymes that mediate the metabolism of glycogen. *Von Gierke's* (type I) disease is caused by a defect in glucose-6-phosphatase. Since this enzyme is found in the liver and is required for the liver to release glucose into the blood, these patients have hypoglycemia. The body must resort to anaerobic metabolism, leading to lactic academia and ketosis. Glycogen accumulates in the liver, leading to hepatomegaly. The enzyme is also found in the kidney. Accumulation of glycogen in the kidneys leads to kidney failure. In *Pompe's* (type II) disease, lysosomal glucosidase is defective. This results in accumulation of glycogen in lysosomes. In the juvenile form, the heart is damaged, leading to heart failure. Patients also have myopathies. In *Cori's* (type III) disease, the debranching enzyme is defective. Hypoglycemia is less severe than Von Gierke's disease, as the liver can still conduct gluconeogenesis. Accumulation of dextrin in the liver and muscle leads to hepatomegaly and myopathies. *McArdle's* (type V) disease is caused by a defect in muscle phosphorylase. Accumulation of glycogen in the muscle leads to muscle cramps while exercising. Muscle destruction leads to myoglobinuria. Myoglobinuria may be described as "tea" colored urine and requires hydration to prevent acute kidney injury.

Disease	Enzyme deficient	Metabolic effects	Results in	
Type I: Von Gierke	Glucose-6-phosphatase	Increased amount of glycogen (normal structure) stored in liver, kidneys	Liver enlargement Sever Hypoglycemia Failure Thrive	Most important example of hepatic glycogenoses Autosomal recessive
Type II: Pompe	Lysosomal α-glucosidase (acid maltase)	Excessive deposition of glycogen (normal structure) in liver, heart, muscle	Massive cardiomegaly Pronounced hypotonia	Autosomal recessive
Type III: Cori	Amylo (1:6) glucosidase (debranching enzyme)	Increased glycogen (short outer branches) in muscle and liver	Cardiorespiratory failure often results in death by age 2	Autosomal recessive
Type V: McArdle	Skeletal muscle glycogen phosphorylase	Increased amounts of glycogen (normal structure) in muscle; cannot be broken down	Painful cramps on strenuous exercise Myoglobinuria	Autosomal recessive

Table 3 Table of high yield facts for glycogen storage diseases

Amino Acid Synthesis and Metabolism

Essential amino acids are amino acids that can not be synthesized and must be consumed from the diet. Essential amino acids include valine, leucine, isoleucine, lysine, methionine, threonine, phenylalanine, and tryptophan. Amino acids are degraded by oxidative deamination, removing the amino group and leaving a carbon skeleton. The amino group is excreted through the urea cycle (see next section). These carbon skeletons can then be used for precursors of other reactions. For example, glutamate is converted to a-ketoglutarate of the TCA cycle. Glucogenic amino acids are used to form intermediates for glycolysis or the TCA cycle. Ketogenic amino acids are converted to ketone bodies which can be further converted to Acyl-CoA or used as an energy source during periods of glucose starvation.

Mousy odor in newborn will be PKU

Phenylalanine is metabolized to tyrosine. This pathway can be seen in Figure 21. *Phenylketonuria* (PKU) is a defect in the phenylalanine hydroxylase enzyme, the first step in this pathway. As a result of a defect in this pathway, excess phenylalanine is shunted to other pathways which result in the synthesis of phenylketones such as phenylactic acid, phenylpyruvatic acid, phenylacetic acid, and hydroxyphenylacetic acid. These ketones are detectable in the urine. They are also neurotoxic, leading to mental retardation and seizures. These patients also characteristically have urine with a "mousy" odor. They will also have fair skin and eczema. Symptoms manifest several days after birth, once phenylalanine has accumulated. Treatment consists of dietary restriction of phenylalanine, found in foods such as artificial sweeteners, and addition of tyrosine rich foods. In pregnant women with PKU, the diet must be followed during pregnancy. Otherwise, the metabolites cross the placenta and cause microcephaly, mental retardation, and possibly congenital heart disease.

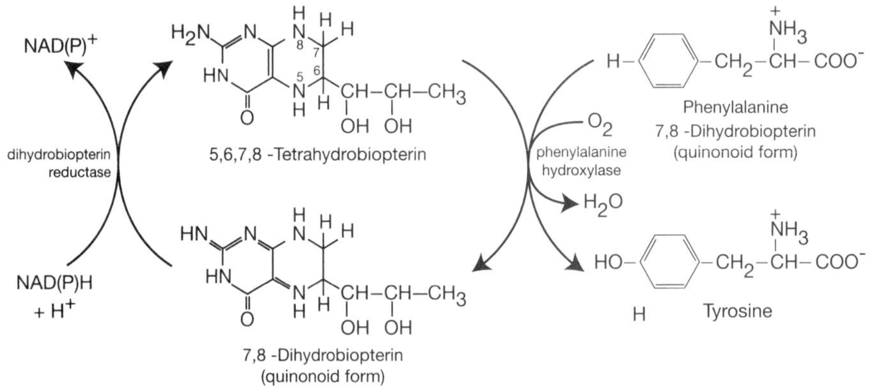

Figure 21 Degradation of phenylalanine to tyrosine mediated by tetrahydrobiopterin (Adapted from *Lehninger Principles of Biochemistry*)

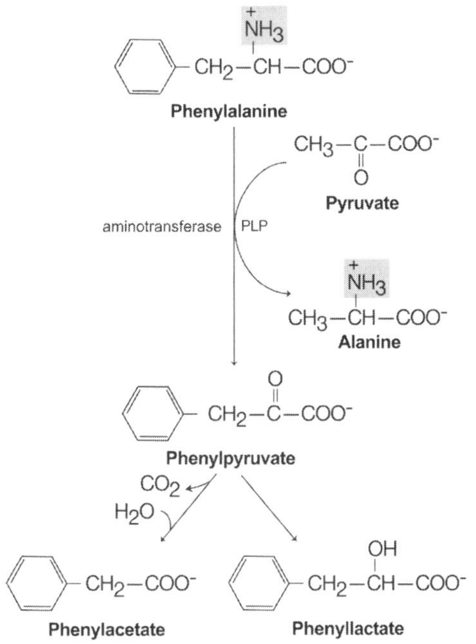

Figure 22 Alternative degradation of phenylalanine
leading to phenylketonuria
(Adapted from *Lehninger Principles of Biochemistry*)

A deficiency in tetrahydrobiopterin (BH_4) can also lead to PKU, as it is a cofactor for phenylalanine hydroxylase. BH_4 is also a cofactor for tyrosine hydroxylase. A decrease in BH_4 will lead to a decrease in Dopa and dopamine. This also results in an increase in prolactin (release of prolactin is suppressed by dopamine). Treatment consists of L-dopa/carbidopa which increases dopamine in the CNS. BH_4 supplementation can also be effective.

Alkaptonuria (also known as ochronosis) is a deficiency in homogentisic oxidase, an enzyme in the tyrosine degradation pathway. It results in the accumulation of homogentisic acid. These patients may present with urine that turns black after a prolonged period of sitting. This is due to the oxidation of excreted homogentisic acid. Homogentisic acid accumulates in connective tissues, tendons, and cartilage, causing black pigmentation. Accumulation in articular cartilage results in arthritis. There is no treatment.

Cystinuria results from a defect of the amino acid transporter in the kidney for cystine, lysine, ornithine, and arginine. As a result, these dibasic amino acids are not reabsorbed in the proximal renal tubule. Cystinuria causes formation of cystine kidney stones. Use hydration to prevent crystallization of cystine, and acetazolamide to alkalinize the urine and make cystine more soluble are treatment for cystinuria.

Homocystinuria is a disease caused by an inability to metabolize homocysteine. As seen in Figure 23, homocystine is metabolized

Remember black urine

Cystinuria:
COLA—Cystine,
Ornithine, Lysine,
Arginine

Homocytinuria:
Marfanoid +
prothrombotic

by two paths. A defect in cystathionine synthase results in "classic homocystinuria." This form leads to shunting of homocysteine to methionine. As a result, these patients will have excess homocysteine and excess methionine. A defect in homocysteine methyltransferase enzyme leads to low levels of methionine and high levels of homocysteine. Methylcobalamin is a cofactor for homocysteine methyltransferase. Defects in the synthesis of methylcobalamin result in high levels of homosytine and low levels of methionine. homocysteine results in endothelial inflammation and dysfunction resulting in thrombosis. It also affects the structure of fibrillin, resulting in a marfanoid appearance (tall stature, lens subluxation, etc.). Mental retardation is common in patients with classical homocystinuria and can occur with homocysteine methyltransferase defects. Treatment for classical homocystinuria includes decreased methionine intake, increased cystine intake, and increased vitamin B6 (pyridoxine). About half of the patients with classical homocystinuria respond to Vitamin B_6 supplementation. Defectsin methylcobalamin synthesis require vitamin B_{12} treatment.

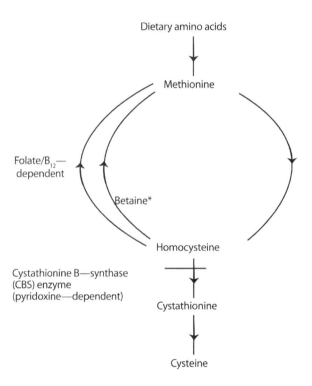

Figure 23 Metabolism of homocysteine
(Adapted from *Clinical Pediatric Neurology*)

Maple Syrup Urine Disease is caused by a defect in α-keto dehydrogenase resulting in an inability to degrade branched amino acids (leucine, isoleucine, valine). As a result, these amino acids are converted to α-keto acids. This results in the characteristic "maple syrup" or "burnt sugar" odor in the urine. Accumulation of the a-ketoacids results in abnormal brain development, mental retardation, and early death. Treatment is diet restriction of leucine, isoleucine, and valine.

Can **LIV** without Maple Syrup (Leucine, Isoleucine, Valine)

Hartnup disorder results from a defect in the neutral amino acid transporter. Most importantly, tryptophan is not absorbed in the gut and is not reabsorbed in the kidney. Tryptophan is needed in the biosynthesis of niacin. Patients are typically asymptomatic. Sun exposure and sun-burn can result in pellagra—a disease caused by niacin deficiency. Patients will have diarrhea, dermatitis, and dementia. Treatment includes niacin supplementation.

Albinism is caused by an inability to synthesize melanin from tyrosine (due to tyrosinase deficiency), defects in the melanosomes that synthesize melanin or a disorder in the migration of melanocytyes that produce melanin. Patients with albinism will have lack of pigmentation to their skin and hair. Lack of pigmentation in the eyes may lead to decreased visual acuity and other visual defects. These patients are susceptible to UV damage and are at an increased risk of skin cancer.

Disease	Enzyme Deficiency	Metabolic Effects	Results in	Notes
Phenyloketonuria	Phenylalanine hydroxylase	Cannot convert phenylalanine to tyrosine	Mental retardation, "mousy odor," eczema	Treatment: Low phenylalanine and high tyrosine
Maple Syrup Urine Disease	Branched-chain α-ketoacid dehydrogenase	Cannot degrade branched chain amino acids	Maple syrup urine, mental retardation	Treatment: Avoid branched amino acids
Alkaptonuria	Homogentisate oxidase	Accumulation of homogentisate	Dark urine, dark connective tissue, arthritis	Urine that turns dark upon standing
Albinism	Tyrosinase	Cannot synthesize melanin from tyrosine	Pigmentation deficiency, visual problems, increased skin cancer risk	—
Homocystinuria	Various	Ammulate homocysteine	Mental retardation, Marfans + Thrombosis	Treatment: Varies based on mutation
Cystinuria	Amino acid transporter	Excretion of COLA amino acids	Cystine kidney stones	Treatment: Alkanize urine
Hartnup Disease	Neutral amino acid transporter	Tryptophan deficiency	Sun-induced pellagra	Mimics niacin deficiency

Table 4 High yield facts about amino acid disorders

Urea Cycle and Nitrogenous Waste Metabolism

The urea cycle is a means for the body to breakdown nitrogenous waste for excretion. It occurs in the mitochondria of hepatocytes of the liver. Ammonia, from amino acids, enters the cycle and is processed into urea. An alanine-glutamate shuttle helps to transport nitrogen from peripheral tissues to the liver. α-ketoglutarate is an intermediate in this shuttle. Excess ammonia can deplete α-ketoglutarate, leading to inhibition of the TCA cycle. Ammonia toxicity will lead to neurologic signs, as the brain depends on glucose for energy. Such signs include asterixis, slurring of speech, somnolence, vomiting, cerebral edema, and blurring of vision. Patients with liver failure have an acquired form of hyperammonemia. Hyperammonemia in these patients can be avoided by limiting the amount of protein consumed. Lactulose can also help decrease the amount of ammonia in the body.

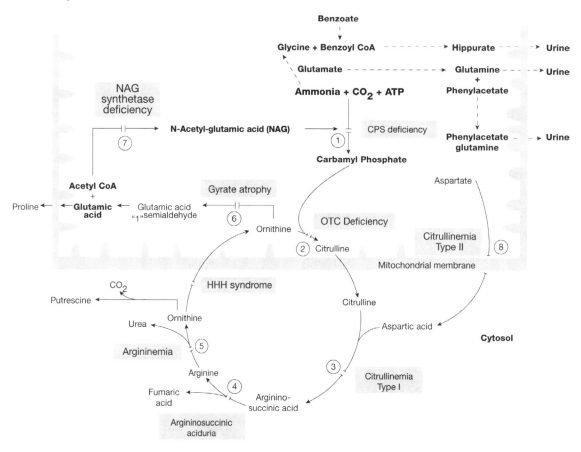

Figure 24 Summary of urea cycle. Ornithine transcarbamylase (OTC) deficiency is the most high yield of the urea cycle disorders.
(Adapted from *Nelson Textbook of Pediatrics*)

OTC deficiency is the most common disorder of the urea cycle. It is an X-linked disease. As a result of OTC deficiency, ammonia will accumulate. It often presents in newborns with symptoms of hyperammonemia. In addition to high levels of ammonia in the blood, patients will also have high levels of orotic acid in the urine.

LIPIDS

In humans, α-linolenic acid and linoleic acid are essential fatty acids and must be ingested through diet. Most lipids, which include triacylglycerols, phospholipids, cholesterol, cholesteryl esters, and free fatty acids, are absorbed through the diet. Ingested lipids form micelles with bile salts and are absorbed by intestinal epithelium. Ezitimibe is a cholesterol lowering drug which inhibits the absorption of these micelles by intestinal epithelium. The intestinal epithelia form the lipids into chylomicrons. Chylomicrons are very large lipid particles which contain all of the lipids and transport the lipids throughout the body through the lymphatic system. They contain apolipoproteins. As the chylomicrons circulate, lipoprotein lipase (LPL) found in endothelium of adipose tissue hydrolyzes triacylglycerol in chylomicrons into free fatty acids which are stored in the adipose tissue. Remnant chylomicrons, rich in cholesterol and triacylglycerols, are absorbed by the liver. Triacylglycerols and cholesterol are then either metabolized by the liver or repackaged into very low density lipoproteins (VLDL) and released into the blood stream to deliver triacylglyerols to peripheral tissues. Extraction of triacylglycerols from VLDL by LPL forms intermediate density lipoproteins (IDL) which is converted to low density lipoproteins (LDL). LDL functions to deliver cholesterol from the liver to peripheral tissues. LDL is also reabsorbed by the liver. High density lipoproteins (HDL), synthesized in the liver and intestines, is responsible for transporting lipoproteins and cholesterol from the peripheral tissues to the liver. Sequestration of cholesterol by HDL is mediated by lecithin cholesterol acyltransferase (LCAT). HDL also transfers cholesterol to LDL and VLDL via cholesterol ester transfer protein (CETP).

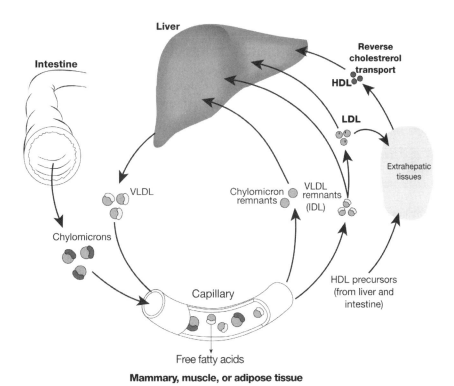

Figure 25 Lipid particle uptake in the body
(Adapted from *Lehninger Principles of Biochemistry*)

Apolipoproteins are important in differentiating lipoproteins and in mediating their actions. Apoprotein A-1, found in HDL, is important in LCAT activation. Apoprotein B-100 is found in LDL and VLDL. It mediates binding to the LDL receptor and is a structural protein in both LDL and VLDL. Apo B-48 is a structural protein for chylomicrons. Apo C-II, found in chylomicrons and VLDL, is a cofactor for LPL. ApoE found in chylomicrons, VLCL, IDL, and HDL mediates uptake by the liver.

Lipase is an important enzyme in lipid metabolism. It is found in the salivary, gastric, and pancreatic secretions and aids in the digestion of lipids. It is found in peripheral tissues as LPL where it aids in metabolism of lipoproteins. Hormone sensitive lipase is found in adipose tissue and aids in the metabolism of stored lipids. Insulin inhibits hormone sensitive lipase but epinephrine, among other hormones, activates it.

Lipoprotein dysfunction leads to various diseases. *Familial hypercholesterolemia* is an autosomal dominant disease of the LDL receptors that results in the elevation of blood LDL concentrations. As a result deposits of cholesterol can be found in various tissues. Xanthomas are deposits on tendons, particularly the Achilles tendon. They may be described as irregular, bumpy tendons. Xanthelasmas are deposits on the surface of the skin, often found on the eyelid. Many of these patients have heart attacks at a very young age and, because it is an autosomal dominant disease, they will have a very strong family history of early heart disease. Homozygotes can have cholesterols in the 600 mg/dL to 1000 mg/dL range (normal < 200 mg/DL). *Familial hypertriglyceridemia* is caused by an overproduction of VLDL by the liver. There is an increase in VLDL and triglycerides with low HDL and LDL. High triglycerides can cause pancreatitis. *Familial hyperchylomicronemia* can be associated with LPL or apo-BII defects. As a result, these patients have high chylomicron levels as well as high triglyceride levels. This results in pancreatitis and xanthomas. *Familial dysbetalipoproteinemia* is caused by a defect in apo-E. As a result, remnant lipoproteins cannot be taken up by the liver. These patients will have elevated chylomicrons and VLDL—these particles become cholesterol rich. This results in xanthomas and elevated risk for heart disease. The xanthomas are characteristically in the palms. *Abetalipoproteinemia* is caused by a defect in the ability to integreate apo-B proteins into lipoproteins. These patients are unable to absorb fat-soluble vitamins (A, D, E, K). At an early age, they present with steatorrhea, mental, and developmental retardation.

Disease	Defect	Elevated lipoprotein	Results in	Notes
Familial hypercholesterolemia	LDL Receptor	LDL: up to 1000 in homozygotes, usually half that in heterozygotes	Xanthomas, xanthelesmas, early MI	—
Familial hypertriglyceridemia	Overproduction of VLCL	VLDL, triglycerides	Pancreatitis	Low HDL and LDL
Familial hyperchylomicronemia	LPL or apoBII	Chylomicron, triglyceride	Pancreatitis, xanthomas	—
Familial dysbetalipoproteinemia	Apo-E	Remnant chylomicron, VLCL	Xanthomas of palms	—
Abetalipoproteinemia	Apo-B	—	Steatorrhea, fat-soluble vitamin deficiency, mental retardation	Can not process lipids

Table 5 Summary of high yield lipid disorders

Cholesterol is also synthesized in the liver. The rate limiting step of cholesterol synthesis is HMG-CoA reductase. Statins are a class of drugs that lower cholesterol levels by inhibiting HMG-CoA reductase.

Fatty Acid Metabolism

Fatty acids are a concentrated source of energy for the body. Most fatty acid metabolism occurs in the mitochondria. In order to transport long chain fatty acids across the mitochondria's double membrane, a carnitine shuttle is used. Once in the mitochondria, β-oxidation cleaves the end of fatty acid chains, resulting in the formation of acyl-CoA, which can be used in the TCA cycle to create ATP. The liver, in certain circumstances, will convert acyl-coa to ketone bodies. It produces acetoacetate (which spontaneously decarboxylates to acetone) and 3-hydroxybutyrate. Ketone bodies are used by muscle and the brain as energy sources. The presence of acetoacetate in the breath yields a "fruity breath" which is characteristic of a ketogenic state. Decreased insulin and increased glucagon promote ketogenesis. In a state of starvation, whether actual starvation or starvation in diabetics due to insufficient insulin, a ketogenic state predominates. Decreased oxaloacetate in starvation states also promotes shunting of acetyl-coa from the TCA cycle towards ketone body production. Increased ketogenesis can result in ketoacidosis.

Carnitine deficiency is caused by a defect in the carnitine transporter, resulting in an inability to shuttle long chain fatty acids. It typically involves the transporters in muscle, heart, and kidneys. These patients develop cardiomyopathy and weakness at a young age. If the liver transporter is also affected, then they will develop fasting hypoketotic hypoglycemia because the liver can not synthesize ketone bodies.

Acyl-CoA dehydrogenase deficiencies are defects that also hinder the body's ability to metabolize fatty acids. The most common is *Medium-chain Acyl-CoA Dehydrogenase deficiency*. These patients, like those with carnitine deficiency, have hypoketotic hypoglycemia during fasting. This results in vomiting, lethargy, seizures, and potentially coma. Treatment consists of dextrose for acute episodes and avoiding fasting for long term control.

LYSOSOMAL STORAGE DISEASES

Lysosomal storage diseases cover a number of diseases focused on defects in enzymes typically found in lysosomes, preventing lysosomes from properly metabolizing certain substrates. As a result, these substrates accumulate within the cells, damaging cells and causing pathology. The organ systems affected depend on the distribution of the substrate throughout the body.

Lysosomal storage diseases are high yield!

Gangliosidosis

Gangliosidoses is a collection of lysosomal storage diseases resulting from the accumulation of gangliosides. *Tay-Sachs disease* is caused by accumulation of ganglioside GM2. The most common manifestation of Tay-Sachs is caused by a defect in the B-hexosaminidase A enzyme. The defect has a high carrier rate amongst Ashkenazy Jews. Ganglioside GM2 accumulates in the central nervous system, autonomic nervous system, and retina. As a result, manifestations of the disease include neurocognitive degeneration starting at 6 months of age and cherry-red spots found in the macula.

Mucopolysaccharidoses

In mucopolysaccharidoses, lysosomal enzymes to degrade glycosaminoglycans (GAGs) are deficient. As a result GAGs like heparin sulfate, dermatan sulfate, and hyaluron accumulate. *Hurler's disease* is a severe mucopolysaccharidoses resulting from a defect in a-L-iduronidase. These patients present with gargoylism, corneal clouding, hepatosplenomegaly, and a large tongue. The large tongue contributes to obstructive airway disease. These patients will have developmental delay. *Hunter's Syndrome* is an X-linked mucopolysacchridoses. It is caused by a defect in iduronate sulfatase. These patients present like patients with Hunter's disease except that they do not have corneal clouding.

Sphingolipidoses

Gaucher disease is caused by a defect in B-glucocerebrosidase. Glucocerebroside accumulates in cells of the reticuloendoethelial system (RES). As a result, pathology reveals a characteristic Gaucher cell which is a macrophage with a "wrinkled paper" appearance. Cells of the RES are also found in the liver, spleen, and bone marrow. As a result, patients will have hepatosplenomegaly, bone pains, and pathologic fractures. Aseptic necrosis of the femur and "Erlenmeyer flask deformities" are seen.

Fabry disease is an X-linked disorder caused by a defect in the a-Galactosidase A enzyme. Ceramide trihexose accumulates in vascular endothelium and smooth muscle. It is classically characterized by angiokeratomas. Angiokeratomas are non-blanching, large red skin lesions. Patients also have debilitating pain of the extremities. Accumulation in vascular endothelium leads to vascular disease and affects the heart and kidneys.

Niemann-pick disease is caused by a sphingomyelinase defect. Sphingomyelin accumulates in the RES and CNS. As a result, patients will have hepatosplenomegaly and "Erlenmeyer flask deformities" as well as neurodegeneration and cherry-red spot on the macula. The lungs are also affected. On pathology, macrophages with lipid-laden vacuoles or "foam cells" can be seen.

Leukodystrophies

The leukodystrophies involve the improper myelination of white matter. *Krabbe Disease* is a deficiency of galactocerebroside B-galactosidase. As a result of this deficiency, galactocerebroside accumulates. There is loss of myelin within the brain and peripheral nervous systems. Patients with this disease have developmental delays, spasticity and hypertonia, and seizures. They later develop optic atrophy. Patients with this disease often do not survive. Pathology demonstrates globoid cells.

Metachromatic leukodystrophy is a leukodsytrophy caused by a deficiency of arylsulfatase A, resulting in accumulation of cerebroside sulfate. These patients present at an older age than patients with Krabbe. They present similarly to patients with Krabbe but may also have nystagmus, ataxia, and peripheral neuropathy. The course of disease is often more indolent.

VITAMIN DEFICIENCIES/EXCESS

Vitamin	Function	Deficiency/ Excess	Signs/ Symptoms	Associated Conditions
A	Involved in synthesis of rhodopsin, bone growth, epithelial cell function	Deficiency	Night blindness, poor bone growth, poor tooth health, hyperkeratosis	Fat soluble vitamin deficiencies
		Excess	Hepatosplenomegaly, alopecia, yellow skin coloration, elevated intracranial pressure (bulging fontanelle, nausea and vomiting)	
B_1: thiamine	Cofactor in various reactions, synthesis of acetylcholine and GABA	Deficiency	Dry beriberi: peripheral neuropathies, ptosis, muscle atrophy Wet beriberi: congestive heart failure, edema Wernicke's Encephalopathy: mental status changes, ophthalmoplegia, ataxia	Polished rice diet, alcoholics

Galactus was krabby after his globe atrophied (Galactocerebrosidase, Krabbe's, Globoid cells, Optic Atrophy).

Fat soluble vitamin deficiency associated with: Inflammatory bowel disease, short guy syndrome, cystic fibrosis, celiac sprue, biliary disease

Fat soluble Vitamins: ADEK

Consider thiamine deficiency in alcoholics

Chvostek sign: tapping on angle of jaw leads to contraction of muscle

Trousseau sign: inflation of blood pressure cuff around arm resulting in involuntary wrist flexion

B₂: riboflavin	Synthesis of FAD	Deficiency	Cheilosis (scaling and fissure on lips), glossitis (sore, red tongue)	
B₃: niacin	Part of NAD and NADP	Deficiency	Pellagra: 4Ds: dermatitis, diarrhea, dementia, death, "raw beef" swollen tongue	Anorexia, corn-based diet
B₆: Pyridoxine	Amino acid metabolism, glycogen metabolism	Deficiency	Peripheral neuritis, cheilosis, glossitis, seborrheic dermatitis	Isoniazid use
B₉: Folic Acid	Carbon transporter in various reactions including purine biosynthesis; needed in times of rapid growth	Deficiency	Megaloblastic anemia, neural tube defects (if low in mom),	Increased utilization (ie hemolytic anemias), decreased absorption (ie celiacs, alcoholics), decreased ability to use (ie convulsants, ethotrexate)
B₁₂: Cobalamin	Methylmalonyl-COA to succinyl-coa, homocysteine to methionine, purine synthesis	Deficiency	Megaloblastic anemia with elevated methylmalonyl-COA, peripheral neuropathy	Vegan diet, Pernicious anemia, Crohn's disease, ileal resection
Biotin	Carboxylase reactions	Deficiency	Alopecia, dermatitis	Raw egg white consumption
C	Hydroxylation of proline and lysine in collagen synthesis	Deficiency	Scurvy: poor wound healing, bleeding gums, petechiae, iron, folate, and B₁₂ deficiency	Lack of fruit in diet

D	When converted to 1,25—hydroxy-vitamin D: Intestinal absorption of calcium, bone resorption (increases serum calcium)	Deficiency	Rickets (children): bowing of legs Osteomalacia (adults): gait instability, bone pain, muscle weakness Paresthesia: muscle cramping, hypocalcemia (can lead to seizures), tetany (Chvostek, Troussea sign)	Lack of sunlight, Fat soluble vitamin deficiencies
		Excess	Hypercalcemia: "Stones (kidney stones), bones (bone pain), groans (constipation, nausea, vomiting), psychiatric overtones (confusion, coma)"	
E	Antioxidant	Deficiency	Hemolysis from increased oxidative stress on red blood cells, truncal ataxia, myopathy	Fat soluble vitamin deficiencies
K	Cofactor in synthesis of clotting factors II, VII, IX, X and anticoagulants protein C and S	Deficiency	Hemorrhage, all newborns are given Vitamin K shot to prevent hemorrhage	Long term broad spectrum antibiotic use

Table 6 Vitamin deficiencies/excess

TECHNIQUES IN BIOCHEMISTRY AND MOLECULAR BIOLOGY

Various techniques have been developed to analyze DNA, RNA, and proteins. Gel electrophoresis is a method using gels to separate mixtures of DNA, RNA, or protein. A gel is made from materials like agarose and a current is run through it. The gel contains pores that slow down bigger molecules. Southern blotting is a technique used to analyze DNA fragments in this fashion. Since DNA is negatively charged, DNA fragments will move towards the positive electrode. Smaller fragments will pass through the gel pores easier and migrate to the positive electrode faster. After the gel has been run, the DNA is transferred to a membrane where it can be radiolabeled with complementary DNA probes. A similar technique is used for RNA and is known as Northern blotting. The technique used for proteins is called Western blotting. Antibodies to the protein of interest are necessary for Western blotting.

Polymerase chain reaction (PCR) is a method used to create copies of DNA sequences. Primers are used to delineate the sequence of interest from a strand of DNA. The first step of PCR is the denaturation of the DNA sequence. This occurs between 92 C and 94 C. Then the temperature is lowered so that the primers can anneal to the strands of DNA. Next, a bacterial polymerase elongates the strand of DNA. Since the process requires very high temperatures, specific heat resistant bacterial polymerases are used. PCR can be used for the diagnosis of diseases such as chlamydia and gonorrhea.

Enzyme-Linked Immunosorbent Assays (ELISA) is a test that can be used to detect the presence of proteins. Clinically, it is used for detection of antigens or antibodies. Antibodies or antigens are linked with a peroxidase enzyme. Serum is added to a plate and then washed away. If the antibody or antigen is found in the serum, it will adhere to the antibody/antigen on the plate. Next, peroxide is added and catalyzed by the peroxidase enzyme. The color created by this enzymatic reaction is then detected. ELISA assays have various diagnostic uses, including for HIV and pregnancy tests.

Microarrays are a method for analyzing large amounts of data quickly. The arrays can contain complementary RNA fragments or RNA probes. If an mRNA is expressed in the cell, then it will link to the probe in the microarray. A scanner can detect how many of the probes are bound and give an estimate of the expression of the RNA. DNA microarrays can detect DNA fragments and give an idea if the cells contain the gene in question.

CHAPTER 3

EPIDEMIOLOGY & BIOSTATISTICS

BIOSTATISTICS TERMINOLOGY

Descriptive statistics summarizes the numerical data contained within a given set. There are various terminologies used in descriptive statistics that are frequently tested in USMLE. Initially, these terminologies can be confusing, as many start with the letter 'M.' It is crucial to familiarize yourself with these terms. As with any new language acquired in medicine, recognition of descriptive statistics and correct use of biostatistics terminologies will guide you through the USMLE exams and your future career.

The USMLE will typically include 1–3 questions in each block of 46 questions dealing with Epidemiology or Biostatistics. While not a huge part of the exam, they are easy points that should not be squandered.

Let us use the following data set to demonstrate key biostatistics terminologies: [1,1,2,3,5,8,13,21,34]

Mean

The mean is the most commonly used biostatistics term. It is commonly referred to as the "average", or the sum of all of the values in a given set, divided by the total number of items in the set.

Mean = Average = Sum total/# of items

For example, applying our set from above:

Mean = (1+1+2+3+5+8+13+21+34)/(9 items) = 88/9 = 9.8

Median

When all of the values in a given set are arranged in numerical order from lowest to highest the median is the value that lies in the middle. The key to finding the median is the placement of numbers in order of increasing value.

Median is like the median of a road—it is what is in the middle.

For example, using our sample data set that has already been arranged in numerical order:

Median = (lowest—1,1,2,3,5,8,13,21,34—highest) = 5 is in the middle

Mode

The mode is the number that appears most frequently in a given set. In our data set the mode would be 1, as it appears twice, while other numbers only appears once.

MODE is the number that there are MORE of in the dataset.

Mode: [1,1,2,3,5,8,13,21,34] = 1 is most frequent

PROBABILITY DISTRIBUTIONS

The USMLE likes to test your familiarity with distribution curves, and you must be comfortable evaluating the information conveyed in graphs. In probability distributions, the x-axis represents the standard deviations from the mean, while the y-axis represents the frequency of values within the data set. Most naturally occurring values tend to be bell-shaped, with the highest frequency in the middle. It is not surprising that probability distributions are often called the bell curve, so named due to the similarity of the outline shape to that of a bell shape. The bell curve is the most frequently tested probability distribution in USMLE, and we are thankful because we can use its symmetric shape to easily predict statistical values.

Mean ±
1SD = 68%

Mean ± 2SD = 95%

Mean ± 3SD = 99.9%

In a bell curve:
mean = median = mode

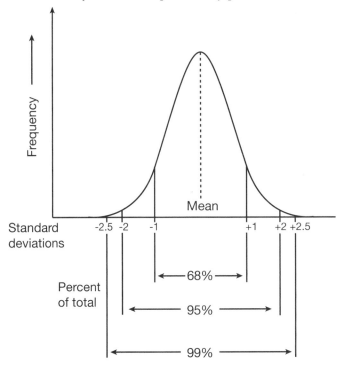

Figure 1 The bell curve. In a normal bell curve, the mean is directly in the middle so it also equals the median, and it appears most frequently, so it is also the mode.
(Adapted from *Prescription for the Boards*)

Variability

Variability is more of a qualitative term than an actual quantitative value. It is used to describe the differences in a given data set. For example, there is far less variability among ages of third grade classmates compared to ages of patients seen in a family physician's clinic. When describing variability, range can be used to measure exactly how different the numbers are in a given data set. The range is calculated by taking the highest value and subtracting the lowest value.

For examples, let us assume the following are the ages of patients seen in a family practice clinic.

Patient's age: 1,1,2,3,5,8,13,21,34,60,65,65,65,70,72,80,85.

Range = (highest value – lowest value)= (85 – 1) = 84

Variance

Variance should not be confused with variability. Variability is a qualitative term used to describe differences in values in a given data set. Variance is a quantitative value that can be calculated. Variance describes the degree to which the values in the dataset are related to each other across a range. Determining variance is also a necessary step in calculating the standard deviation of a data set. The variance is often represented by s^2 since taking the square root of the variance will provide the standard deviation.

$$\text{Variance} = 8^2 = \frac{\Sigma(\text{Average value} - \text{individual value})^2}{\text{Total number of data points} = 1}$$

For example, let's calculate the variance of patients' age in the above family physician's clinic.

The mean age of patients is:

$[(1+1+2+3+5+8+13+21+34+60+65+65+65+70+72+80+85)/17] = 38.23$

In order to calculate the variance, you would subtract each individual's age from the mean and then square the value: $(38.23 – 1)^2 + (38.23 – 1)^2 + (38.23 – 2)^2 + … + (38.23 – 85)^2 = 17,001.06$. This sum of values would then be divided by the total number of patients subtracted by 1: $(17 – 1) = 16$.

The variance in the ages of patients seen in the family medicine clinic would be:

Variance= 17,001.06/16 = 1,062.57

Standard Deviation

The standard deviation is the most commonly used statistic to describe the degree of variation in a distribution of values in a given data set. The standard deviation is often represented represented by the abbreviations SD or Sn. The standard deviation is calculated by taking the square root of the variance. For example, the variance in the ages of patients seen in the family medicine clinic above is 1,062.57. Therefore, the standard deviation would be:

SD = (1,062.57) = 32.60.

Due to the predictable nature of the bell curve, standard deviation provides an easy way of capturing the total percentage of values within each standard deviation. Using figure 1 from above, you can see that within the mean ± 1 standard deviation, 68% of the data can be found.

Let's illustrate the use of standard deviations in naturally occurring values that generally follow a bell curve distribution. In the United States, the mean height of men is 5 feet 10 inches, while the mean height of women is 5 feet 4 inches. The standard deviation in height for both men and women in the United States is approximately 3 inches. Using the bell curve distribution, we know that within the mean ± 1 standard deviation, 68% of the data can be found. Therefore:

Men: mean ± 1 standard deviation= 5'10" ± 3" =

68% of American men's heights are between 5'7" and 6'1"

Women: mean ± 1 standard deviation= 5'4" ± 3" =

68% of American women's heights are between 5'1" and 5'7".

Let's expand on the concept of standard deviation a bit further. As standard deviations increase, total percentage of values also increases. For example, 95% of American men are within two standard deviations from the mean.

Men: 5'10" ± 6" = 98% of American men's heights are between 5'4" and 6'4"

Referring to Figure 1, if 95% of American men are between +2 standard deviation from the mean, then only 5% of men have heights that are less than 5'4" and greater than 6'4". Furthermore, you can predict that 2.5% of American men are shorter than 5'4" while 2.5% of men are taller than 6'4".

Hence, if you are taller than 6'4", you are taller than 95% + 2.5% = 97.5% of American men or in the 97.5th percentile.

Skew/Kurtosis

As with all things in medicine, not all bell curves are identical in shape and size. Statisticians use skewness to describe variations in the bell curve when the bell curve is not symmetric. If a bell curve is not symmetric, it is either positively or negatively skewed. Hence, the middle of the bell curve is no longer the mean, median or mode. If the mode is greater than the mean, then the curve is positively skewed. Remember, the mode is the number that appears most frequently in a given set. Because the y-axis represents the frequency of values within the data set, as the mode becomes greater than the mean the peak of the curve is now to the left of the mean, as the graph becomes positively skewed towards the right side. However, if the mode is less than the mean, the curve is now said to be negatively skewed. This concept is illustrated in Figure 2.

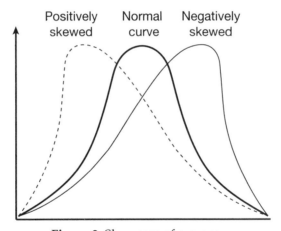

Figure 2 Skewness of a curve

The extreme ends on the left and right sides of the bell curve are commonly known as tails. The thickness of the tails, can also vary. The term used to describe the thickness of the tails is the curve's kurtosis. This concept is rarely tested on the USMLE. Keep in mind that having greater kurtosis, or thicker tails or thicker tails, indicates that the peak of the curve is flattened and that the variability of the data is greater. Moreover, a wider curve with greater kurtosis indicates that the standard deviation is greater when compared to a narrower curve with lesser kurtosis.

Epidemiology

Epidemiology is the study of distributions and patterns of disease and their underlying causes in populations. Epidemiologists revolutionized modern medicine by investigating the outbreak of disease, screening and monitoring of disease progress, as well as treatment effects in populations. Epidemiology remains an integral part of public health and plays a role in identifying risk factors for disease and development of preventative medicine, as well as public policy.

DISEASE MONITORING

Prevalence

Prevalence is a measure of how many individuals have the diagnosis of a specific disease within a given population.

$$Prevalence = \frac{Number\,of\,existing\,cases\,of\,a\,disease}{Total\,population}$$

Prevalence = Popularity = Persistence

Incidence

Incidence measures the rate of diagnosis of a disease within a given population. It is expressed in terms of the number of new cases diagnosed during a specific period of time in a given population. It is important to remember that the period of time needs to be specified in order to calculate incidence. Distinction between prevalence and incidence is a commonly tested question on USMLE, as many confuse the two.

$$Incidence = \frac{Number\,of\,new\,cases\,of\,a\,disease\,over\,a\,given\,period}{Total\,population}$$

Incidence = Initial diagnosis

Remember that incidence measures newly diagnosed cases of a disease in a given time in a population, while prevalence is a snapshot of all cases of a disease within the population.

Let us use an example to illustrate the distinction between prevalence and incidence. Since incidence measures new cases of a disease in a given time, a condition that affects a large portion of the population, but has a short duration would have a high incidence. For example, the incidence of seasonal influenza in winter months is very high in the United States, as there are many new cases of flu in a short time frame. On the other hand, chronic medical disease, such as diabetes mellitus type II, will have high prevalence. The prevalence of diabetes has been increasing over the past few decades in the United States along with the increase in the prevalence of obesity. Remember that prevalence is a snapshot of disease in a given population; as the number of people living with the disease increases, the prevalence of the disease will also increase. For example, with the invention of insulin and oral hypoglycemic agents, people with diabetes are living longer, thereby increasing the prevalence of diabetes in a population.

In short, conditions which affect a large portion of the population, but only for a brief period of time will have a high incidence rate with low prevalence. Chronic conditions that persist for a long period of time will often have low incidence rate with high prevalence.

Causes of Mortality in US

When evaluating causes of death in USMLE, it is important to recognize the different causes of mortality in different age groups. For example, infants are typically born with their cause of death. Middle-aged adults tend to succumb to cancer, while the elderly are more likely to die of cardiac problems. Hence preventive cancer screening, such as mammograms and colonoscopies are recommended for middle-aged adults and not recommended in elderly populations, as risks begin to outweigh the benefits of screening.

You do not need to memorize this chart but look at the trends among the age categories.

	All Ages	**Infant**	**25–44**	**65+**
1	Heart disease	Congenital malformations	Accidents	Heart Disease
2	Cancer	Short gestation or low birth weight issues	Cancer	Cancer
3	Chronic lung disease	Sudden infant death syndrome	Heart disease	Chronic lung disease
4	Cerebrovascular disease	Maternal complications of pregnancy	Suicide	Cerebrovasc. Disease
5	Accidents	Accidents	Assault	Alzheimer's disease
6	Alzheimer's disease	Complications of placenta or umbilical cord	Chronic liver disease & cirrhosis	Diabetes mellitus
7	Diabetes mellitus	Bacterial sepsis	HIV	Influenza & pneumonia
8	Kidney disease	Circulatory system disease	Cerebrovascular Disease	Kidney disease
9	Influenza & pneumonia	Respiratory distress	Diabetes mellitus	Accidents
10	Suicide	Necrotizing enterocolitis	Influenza & pneumonia	Septicemia

Top 10 Causes of Death in the US by age in 2010

Table 1 Top 10 causes of death by age in 2010

TYPES OF STUDIES

There are two fundamental types of research studies: observational and experimental studies. In an observational study, a population is simply observed in its natural setting without any intervention. In an experimental study, the researcher will actively intervene and change an aspect of a population in an attempt to examine its effects.

TYPES OF OBSERVATIONAL STUDIES

Cohort Studies

Cohort studies are the backbone of epidemiology research. Cohort studies follow a population and monitor disease outbreak, progression, and outcome in a specified period of time. It is important to note that cohort studies could be either prospective or retrospective. A prospective study looks into the future, while a retrospective study examines the past of a population with shared disease exposure. For example, a prospective study could enroll the medical school class of 2012 and follow them for 20 years to see how many people develop renal failure. Researchers can then assess common characteristics of renal failure group in order to establish risk factors. A retrospective study could examine all of the medical school graduates of the class of 1992 with current renal failure and reversibly establish risk factors for renal failure. The distinguishing characteristic of cohort studies is that they select patients based on exposure status. In our example, the exposure status was attending medical school.

The term 'cohort' comes from the Roman army as this was a tactical unit that worked together. Remember that in a cohort study, the participants share the same initial event then travel together in the study to its conclusion.

Case-control Studies

Case-control studies enroll patients based on disease status. For example, a case-control study can enroll 100 subjects who have renal failure as compared to 100 control subjects without renal failure who are matched with the renal failure group based on common characteristics such as living in the same neighborhood, having the same education level, age, and/or race. These two groups are then compared to identify characteristics more common in one group than the other. For example, the renal failure group may be more likely to have diabetes mellitus as compared to the matched control group. Since these groups are not examined prior to disease progression, you cannot identify causation from a case-control study, only association. Due to its design, a case-control study also has a real advantage in the research of rare disorders. For example, if you want to identify a cause of a rare brain tumor with an incidence of 1 in 1,000,000, you would have the daunting and very expensive task of enrolling 10 million individuals in a cohort study to have a likelihood of 10 individuals with the disease.

Remember that participants in a case-control study are selected based on whether or not they have the disease/condition of interest, not an exposure as in the cohort group. Therefore, you cannot calculate incidence rates from a case-control study.

Cross-sectional

Cross-sectional studies do not follow patients over time but are a snapshot of a disease in a population. Cross-sectional studies are helpful preliminary studies to identify potential associations between variables, which can then be further studied in cohort or cross-sectional studies.

A researcher analyzing health care costs and mortality in different states may want to compare the total amount of healthcare expenditure and life expectancy in Ohio and Virginia. If more money is spent on healthcare in Virginia and residents of Virginia live longer than residents of Ohio, it may be tempting for the researcher to say increased healthcare spending leads to greater life expectancy. However, it is impossible to identify causation with a case-control study. For example, one can argue that as people live longer, they spend more money on health care. Thus, increased life expectancy causes the increased health care spending.

Case Study

Case studies are simply descriptive studies in which researchers examine either a single individual or a small number of subjects with a specific condition. Case studies are frequently utilized in rare disorders or new and novel therapies. Case studies are like cross-sectional studies, however, on a much smaller scale. Case studies are also helpful for identifying potential factors to examine in depth with a future cohort or case-control study.

TYPES OF EXPERIMENTAL STUDIES

Randomized Clinical Trials

Randomized Clinical Trials as sometimes referred to as Randomized Control Trials, or RCT for short. They are considered the gold standard of research and provide the strongest evidence of a relationship between variables.

These are the "Gold Standard" and preferred type of experimental research study in medicine. In experimental studies, the researcher attempts to alter the natural course of a condition by exposing one set of research participants to an intervention while denying the other group of research participants the same exposure. By randomizing the participants into experimental and control groups, one can potentially eliminate any potential biases and confounders associated with the study. For example, you cannot establish a causal relationship between the type of car a person drives and life expectancy without taking into consideration the potential confounders, such as socioeconomic status. By randomizing the participants between the exposure and control groups, the researcher attempts to eliminate the naturally occurring extraneous variables between two groups.

In a randomized control study, a comparison of the subjects in both groups illustrates how comparable the two groups are after randomization. In order to isolate the effect of the intervention being studied, it is imperative to control for confounders by having both groups match in terms of demographics and risk factors, such as age, geography, and diet. If two randomized treatment and control groups are equal in all respects other than the intervention, causation can be accurately established.

Randomized clinical trials are typically described as being either blind or double-blind. A blind study indicates that the participants do not know if they are randomized to the control or the treatment group. A double-blind study indicates that both the participants and researchers do not know which group subjects are randomized into. Double-blind study removes the temptation of researchers to allocate subjects differently due to the researcher's often unconscious bias towards the treatment being studied.

Cross-over Studies

Cross-over studies initially begin as randomized studies involving a treatment and a control group. However, after a period of time, the groups are switched so that the group initially given the intervention is subsequently denied the intervention, while the control group is then given the intervention. These cross-over studies frequently have a "wash-out" period prior to the switch to eliminate possible lingering effects of the intervention. For example, depending on the half-life of a drug, intervention group participants given a drug as intervention will have to wait for the drug to clear their system prior to being placed in control group. The advantage of a cross-over study is the ability of each subject to act as his/her own control. It is often used when researchers want to perform a randomized control trial but do not have the resources to enroll many participants. Cross-over studies allow the researcher to examine participants without having to enroll similarly matched control subjects.

Intention-to-Treat

Intention-to-treat is a type of analysis rather than a type of study. When research participants are randomized into specific treatment arms, it can be expected that participants will follow the research protocol to varying degrees and may stop taking the treatment prescribed or start taking the treatment on their own, despite being randomized into the control group. Despite potential errors in data, intention-to-treat analysis maintains participants in the groups to which they were initially randomized, regardless of their compliance. Advocates of intention-to-treat emphasize that in the real world patients do not always fill their prescriptions and may take medications they are not prescribed. Therefore, the intention-to-treat method of analysis is a more realistic assessment of the general population. In addition, intention-to-treat is often less biased since it removes the ability of the researcher to decide which patients to include in the final analysis. The opposite approach to intention-to-treat, would be "as-treated," where patients are only included in the treatment group analysis if they finished the pre-determined amount of the treatments prescribed.

RISK FACTORS

Risk factors are characteristics or activities that increase an individual's likelihood of developing a certain condition. For example, smoking is a significant risk factor for development of lung cancer. The USMLE likes to distinguish between *modifiable* risk factors such as smoking and *non-modifiable* risk factors such as genetics and gender.

Risk factors are often based on a correlation between the characteristics or behaviors of a person and their association for the development of a particular disease. Nonetheless, remember that association alone does not lead to causation. For example, statistics indicate that there is a higher crime rate as well as increased ice cream consumption during summer months. Although increased ice cream consumption is associated with higher crime levels in the summer, no one is trying to decrease ice cream sales in an effort to decrease crime rates.

PREVENTION

Primary

Primary prevention involves the preemptive prevention of disease. An example would be high school education program advocating avoidance of drinking alcohol and driving.

Secondary

Secondary prevention focuses on early detection of disease. An example would be utilization of Pap smears to detect abnormal, pre-cancerous cervical cells prior to progression into cervical cancer.

Tertiary

Tertiary prevention is an attempt to prevent further progression of the disease. For example, giving tPA immediately after an ischemic stroke can help to reduce the morbidity and mortality of stroke patients.

TESTING

Screening

Screening detects disease prior to symptoms of the disease. For example, having all patients over 50 years old undergo a colonoscopy is an effective way to screen for early colon cancer before a patient may have symptoms, such as changes in bowel movement or weight loss.

Diagnostic

Diagnostic testing occurs after the patient has already experienced symptoms of a disease. For example, if an elderly man presented to his physician's office complaining of weight loss and blood in the stool, a colonoscopy would now become a diagnostic test to confirm a suspicion of colon cancer.

HYPOTHESIS TESTING

Null hypothesis—A null hypothesis (H_o) states that there is no difference between two groups, while the alternate hypothesis (H_1) states that there is a difference. Researchers design their studies to examine whether or not the null hypothesis is true.

	True difference	No difference
Test positive (Reject H_o)	True positive	False negative Type 1 error (α)
Test negative (Retain H_o)	False positive Type 2 error (β)	True negative

Prevention Levels:
Primary = Prior to onset
Secondary = Soon after onset
Tertiary = Decrease long-term effects

Types of Error

There are 2 types of errors that are frequently tested on the USMLE.

Type 1 error refers to inaccurately stating that the null hypothesis is false when it is actually true. This is also referred to as the alpha (α) error and indicative of a false positive result. Most researchers arbitrarily accept a 5% risk of Type I error.

Type 2 error refers to inaccurately failing to reject the null hypothesis. This is also referred to as the beta (β) error and indicative of a false negative result.

Power

Power refers to the ability of the test to detect a difference if one actually exists. The most common way to boost the power of a study is to increase the number of research participants. Power is calculated as 1 minus the risk of failing to detect a true difference (the β error).

$$\text{Power} = 1 - \beta \text{ error}$$

P-values and Confidence Intervals

The p-value cited in statistical analysis represents the alpha error rate. The most common threshold for accepting a test as being statistically significant is p-value of < 0.05, indicating that the α risk is less than 5%. The confidence intervals are typically 95% confidence intervals, which imply that an individual can be 95% assured that the true value is within the given interval.

RISK 2X2 TABLES

	Disease present	Disease absent
Test positive	A	B
Test negative	C	D

Sensitivity

The sensitivity of a test refers to how likely the test is able to detect if the disease is present:

$$\text{SeNsitivity} = A/(A + C)$$

A significant test is one where the p-value (risk of α error) is < 0.05

The best way to increase the power of a study is to increase the number of participants. With more participants though, there is the chance to inaccurately find a difference that does not truly exist. Thus the type 1 and type 2 errors are always in balance.

You are almost guaranteed to get a question about a 2 x 2 table on the USMLE Step 1.

SeNsitivity—increasing it means you are more likely to capture anyone with the condition → the Negative Predictive Value will increase.

Specificity

The specificity refers to the test's ability to detect when the disease is absent.

$$Specificity = D/(B+D)$$

Positive Predictive Value

(PPV) refers to the likelihood of the patient actually having the disease if the test has a positive result.

$$PPV = A/(A + B)$$

Negative Predictive Value

(NPV) refers to the likelihood of the patient not having the disease if the test has a negative result.

$$NPV = D/(C + D)$$

	Disease present	Disease absent
Exposed group	A	B
Unexposed group	C	D

Relative Risk

Relative risk is the increased likelihood that an exposed population has of contracting a particular disease when compared to an unexposed population. For example, a relative risk of 10 indicates that the population exposed to the risk factor has 10 times the risk of developing the disease than the unexposed population.

Relative risk can be calculated as the risk of developing the disease in the exposed group divided by the risk of developing the disease in the unexposed group:

$$Relative\ Risk\ (RR) = \frac{A/(A + B)}{C/(C + D)}$$

Absolute Risk

Absolute risk is the risk of developing the disease in the exposed group after excluding the baseline risk of developing the disease in the unexposed group. For example, if the risk of developing lung cancer among smokers is 14 per 100 years and 1 in 100 years among non-smokers, then the absolute risk of smoking for developing lung cancer is 13 per 100 years.

SPecificity—increasing it means you are less likely to inaccurately label a person as having the disease/condition who doesn't → the Positive Predictive Value will increase.

Sensitivity and Specificity are actually properties of the test. Changing the thresholds will change the properties of the test. The positive and negative predictive values can change if the population on which the test is used changes and the new population has a different incidence of the condition.

How USMLE tests the idea of sensitivity: You are presented with a bell curve of the distribution of lab results or scores. It is stated that the test-makers lower the value that indicates a positive test. You are asked how this would affect the sensitivity (increase), specificity (decrease), PPV (decrease), and NPV (increase).

Number Needed to Treat

Number needed to treat (NNT) is the number of people who must be treated in order to prevent morbidity or mortality from a disease. It is calculated as the inverse of the absolute risk.

$$NNT = 1/Absolute\ risk$$

Using our earlier example of lung cancer, NNT can be calculated by taking an inverse of absolute risk of 13 per 100 years.

$$NNT = 1/0.13 = 7.7$$

In other words, if you convince approximately 8 people to quit smoking, you would prevent lung cancer in at least 1 patient.

Odds Ratio

The odds ratio is calculated in case-control studies. Remember that case-control studies select subjects based on whether or not they already have the disease being studied. Therefore, you cannot calculate the relative risk of the disease/condition. In case-control studies, the odds ratio is used to estimate the relative risk in a nearly identical manner. The odds of developing the disease in the entire exposed group is divided by the odds of developing the disease in the entire unexposed group. The primary difference between the odds ratio and relative risk is the type of study used to obtain the data (relative risks can only be calculated from cohort studies since they have actual incidence rates; odds ratios are used in case-control studies).

	Disease	No disease
Exposed group	A	B
Unexposed group	C	D

$$Odds\ Ratio\ (OR) = \frac{A/B}{C/D} = \frac{A*D}{C*B}$$

VALIDITY

Precision Versus Accuracy

Precision refers to the consistency of the results. Accuracy refers to how close the result is to the truth. A typical analogy used to distinguish between the two concepts is archery. A tight group of arrows in close proximity demonstrates precision because the archer consistently hits the same spot every time. On the other hand, an arrow directly in the middle of the bulls-eye demonstrates accuracy. Remember that one can be precisely inaccurate if there is a tight cluster of arrows away from the bulls-eye.

The USMLE likes to ask how many people would need to be treated to prevent 1 death so NNT is a helpful short formula to remember.

The odds ratio approximates the relative risk if the rare-disease principle is true (which is usually why you would do a case-control instead of a cohort study).

The odds ratio is sometimes called the cross-product due to how it is calculated.

Thinking of a bulls-eye target is the easiest way to visualize the distinction between accuracy and precision—and the USMLE likes to test this concept.

Face Validity

Face validity is the most superficial type of validity. It is often referred to as a "sniff test" in layman terms. On the initial "sniff test," does the result smell like garbage or does it seem justifiable? Face validity answers this question by applying a simple, common sense approach to test results.

Construct Validity

Construct validity refers to whether or not a test actually measures what it claims to measure. For example, depression screening questionnaires may test for symptoms that overlap with other psychiatric disorders, such as anxiety. A depression test with good construct validity will ask questions that are specific for depression and eliminate other potential psychiatric diagnoses.

External Validity

External validity refers to the generalizability or how applicable the study results are in the real world. This is largely demonstrated by how closely the study population resembles the general population.

Reliability

Reliability refers to the likelihood that a test outcome can be replicated in future studies. There can be different types of reliability, such as **inter-observer** reliability, which represents the likelihood that another researcher can come to the same conclusion. Another type of reliability is **test-retest reliability**, which assesses how likely the same researcher is to obtain the same results.

Bias

The USMLE will typically ask one or two questions about types of biases. The two most commonly tested are selection bias and recall bias. Selection bias is usually described in the way participants are enrolled, while recall bias is described in retrospective studies where participants are asked to complete questionnaires about their conditions.

Biases occur in a variety of ways, from a poorly designed study to a researcher's personal gain, and may be conscious or unconscious in nature. Biases are phenomena that cause inaccurate conclusions due to failure to fully recognize the extraneous variable that exists between the intervention and outcome.

Systematic versus random

Biases do not always result in a false conclusion but may fail to fully identify the differences between the treatment groups. The best analogy to understand systematic versus random biases is a ruler. In a systematic bias, all of the results measured are inaccurate by the same degree. For example, if a meter stick ruler is actually only 90 centimeters, it will create a systemic biased. It will over-estimate all of the ruler's measurements by a uniform amount. Therefore, the relative difference will remain consistent; however, the actual measurements obtained will be inaccurate. In contrast, a random bias is inconsistent and irregular in nature. For example, if two rulers of slightly different lengths were used for a study, you would have unreliable results depending on which ruler was used for measurements.

With systematic biases, the researcher may still find significant differences between the groups, but the effect size may be inaccurate. With random biases, the researcher is often unable to identify a significant difference between the groups because the measurements obtained are inconsistent.

Confounding

Confounding occurs when an unrecognized and unmeasured variable is associated with either the exposure or the outcome. Our example earlier of ice cream sales being associated with crime rates in summer months is a good example. The confounding variable in this example is warm temperature in summer months, as ice cream sales increase in summer and criminal activities increase in warmer weather as well. A naïve researcher might associate ice cream with criminal activity.

Selection

A selection bias occurs when participants enrolled in a study do not represent the population at large. This is a greater risk in a study that is not randomized. For example, a drug trial may claim to enroll cancer patients; however, they may only enroll cancer patients in remission. This drug trial has selection bias as they selected subjects that do not represent the cancer population at large. In another example, healthier patients can preferentially be placed in the treatment group compared to the control group, leading to inaccurate representation of the treatment effect.

Lead-time Bias

Certain diseases have a long prodromal period or early phases without any symptoms. Therefore, if subjects are enrolled in the study at different times in their disease course, the effect of the study may vary solely based on the differences in the natural progression of the disease, rather than on the effects of the treatments being studied. An example of lead-time bias is that of a new screening tool that detects a disease earlier in its natural course, giving the false impression that patients survive longer.

Newer, more accurate screening tests being used more frequently cause the increase in incidence of several cancers—a lead-time bias when historical controls are used.

Length Bias

If patients are not followed long enough to reveal meaningful outcomes, the study may inaccurately report erroneous patient outcomes due to its incomplete nature. On the other hand, length bias can also occur if the patients are identified too late for enrollment. For example, if patients who had more aggressive forms of the disease have already died prior to study enrollment, the study only included patients with more benign forms of the disease.

Volunteer Bias

Many studies request volunteer participants who may not share average characteristics of the general population. For example, many psychology studies rely on freshmen psychology students as subjects in their study. Freshmen college students do not reflect general population as only 56.9% of United States populations have some college education.

Withdrawal

Participants can withdraw from a study for different reasons. If a treatment has undesirable side effects, the treatment group may have more people withdraw from the study than the control group. As a result, drawing any conclusions from the study can be difficult since the characteristics of the subjects that complete the study may no longer be representative of the general population. Often times, the very sick or the very healthy remain, skewing the results.

Compliance

Patients follow study protocols to varying degrees. If patients are required to take a study medication four times a day, it can be very cumbersome. Furthermore, if the drug has undesirable side effects, it is even more likely that patients will not comply with the regimen.

Recall

Retrospective studies that rely on patients' memory is often wrought with recall problems. For example, women who give birth to a child with congenital disorders are far more likely to thoroughly reflect on their pregnancy and identify potential causes of their infant's condition than mothers who gave birth to healthy infants.

Attention

Studies will sometimes involve therapies that require frequent monitoring of the subjects. If some participants are observed more frequently than other participants, those participants receiving more attention are more likely to be identified with disease or complications compared to others. Therefore, it is important for researchers to ensure that participants are monitored to the same extent.

PRINCIPLES OF ETHICAL RESEARCH

Belmont Report

In the mid-20th century, revelations came to light that many physicians were abusing their positions in society as trustworthy caregivers. Physicians were enrolling patients in studies without their knowledge and intentionally misinforming patients about the nature of these study. Such revelations lead to increased pressure to have standardized and ethical oversight of medical research. In order to ensure that research participants are not being manipulated and misinformed for the benefit of research, a commission at Belmont University in Nashville, Tennessee developed the Belmont report stating the essential components of ethical medical research. These principles have largely been adopted and enforced across the country by medical researchers.

Respect for Persons

Researchers must recognize the rights and dignity of all human participants. All research participants deserve to make an INFORMED CONSENT to participate in research. Informed consent includes the complete purpose and nature of the study with its inherent risks and possible benefits. There are rare circumstances in which informed consent is not required. For example, although comatose patients or children cannot consent, a health care proxy or parents can consent on their behalf. The doctrine of implied consent can be applied with the belief that patient would consent if capable.

Beneficence

The Hippocratic Oath states: *"First do no harm."* Medical researchers are expected to follow this philosophy by maximizing the benefits and minimizing the risks to research participants.

Justice

Justice refers to the equitable distribution of risk within research. A group of research participants should not be forced to bear all of the risks of potential harm from the research so that others might benefit. For example, abuse of justice in research can occur when prisoners are forced to participate in a potentially harmful research study to benefit the population at large.

INSTITUTIONAL REVIEW BOARD

The Institutional Review Board (IRB) is a fixture of organizations involved in research ethics. It is comprised of both researchers and people from the community. The IRB reviews research proposals in order to ensure that the principles of the Belmont Report are followed. The IRB has the power to approve or demand changes in the research protocol. The IRB follows the study to completion to ensure that the researcher does not stray from his or her approved research plan.

Confidentiality

Patients are entitled to receive medical care without fear that their medical records will be made public or seen by people who are not directly involved in their care. Confidentiality is essential in the doctor-patient relationship so that patients feel comfortable expressing all of their physical and emotional concerns to their physician. For the USMLE, confidentiality can be waived in two circumstances: 1) Patient waives the right to confidentiality—for example, patients allow the physician to tell their family members about their diagnoses; and 2) If there is a possibility of serious potential harm to the patient or others. For example, if the patient expresses suicidal or homicidal ideation, the physician is required to report the threat to proper authorities to prevent harm which could have occurred by withholding the information. Elderly and child abuse also warrant breach of confidentiality.

Minors are unable to provide an informed consent, it must be provided by their parent or guardian. The minor must give their ASSENT though, indicating they are comfortable with being a part of the research study.

TYPES OF MEDICAL PLANS

Health Maintenance Organizations (HMOs)

HMOs closely monitor health care providers by regulating excessive referrals to specialists and limiting the number of unnecessary tests ordered on patients.

Capitation

For capitation, think of a "CAP"—you wear your cap on your head. With capitation plans, if a physician has a patient with a lot of complications, they can lose their head because they do not get reimbursed for all of the additional treatments required. It is a fixed price paid.

Capitation is a health plan that gives providers a set amount of reimbursement, regardless of the expenses a patient may incur. It is designed to encourage providers to be more cost-effective.

Medicare & Medicaid

Medicare—you CARE for the elderly.

Medicaid—you AID the poor.

Medicare is the federal government insurance plan that covers Americans over 65 years old. Medicaid is federal and state government insurance program for the low-income individuals with limited resources.

CHAPTER 4

CARDIOVASCULAR SYSTEM

ANATOMY

Pericardium

Consists of two layers separated by a small volume of pericardial fluid. Fibrous (*parietal*) pericardium is on the outside. It is anchored to the sternum, diaphragm, and mediastinal pleura. *Visceral* pericardium is on the inside and is adherent to the heart.

Carotid Sheath

There are 3 important structures: the internal jugular vein (vein), the common carotid artery (artery), and the vagus nerve (nerve).

Coronary Arteries

There are 5 major arteries: RCA, PD, LCA, LAD, LCX (Figure 1).

Right coronary artery (RCA)

The RCA supplies the **RA**, **RV**, **SA nod***e*, and **AV node**. In 85% of the population, the RCA supplies the **posterior descending artery** (PD). posterior Interventricular septum; descending artery supplies the *diaphragmatic surface of the heart*. These patients have a "right-dominant circulation". In 10% of patients, the circumflex artery from the left reaches posteriorly and supplies the posterior IV septum; this is known as "left-dominant" circulation. The remaining 5% have "codominant" circulation.

Left coronary artery (LCA)

This splits into the **left anterior descending artery** (**LAD**) and the **left circumflex artery** (**LCX**). The LAD supplies the *apex and anterior 2/3 of the interventricular septum*. A coronary artery occlusion occurs most commonly in the LAD. The LAD sends off several branches: **diagonals** ("D" for LA**D** and diagonal) and septal perforators. The LCX supplies the *posterior* Left venticle (LV). Coronary veins drain into the **coronary sinus**, which drains right ventricle (RV.

VAN: Vein, Artery, Nerve

(medial → lateral)

D: LA**D** sends off **d**iagonals

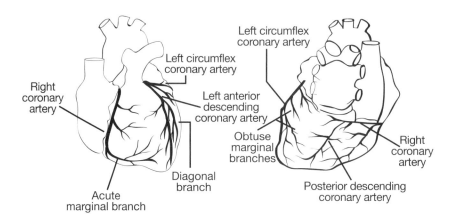

Figure 1 Coronary arteries

Valves

Tricuspid Valve: 3-leaflet valve that separates the right atrium (RA) and the right ventricle (RV). When the ventricles contract, the tricuspid valve closes (**Figure 2**).

Pulmonic Valve: 3-leaflet valve that separates the RV and the pulmonary artery (PA). When the ventricles contract, the pulmonic valve opens.

Mitral Valve: 2-leaflet valve that separates the left atriium (LA) and the left ventricle (LV). When the ventricles contract, the mitral valve closes.

Aoric Valve: 3-leaflet valve that separates the LV and aorta. When the ventricles contract, the aortic valve opens.

When ventricles contract: tricuspid/mitral valves close and pulmonic/aortic valves open

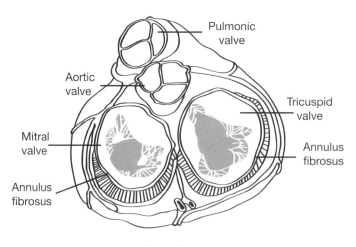

Figure 2 Cardiac calves

Conduction System

All myocardial cells are electrically active and can automatically fire periodically on their own (**automaticity**). Normally, electrical impulses arise from the **sinoatrial (SA) node**, located along the junction between the superior vena cava (SVC) and the RA (Figure 3). Depolarizations initiated at the SA node move outward to stimulate contraction of the LA and RA. The depolarization passes from the atria to the ventricles through the **atrioventricular (AV) node**. After passing through the **AV node**, the wave of depolarization enters and rapidly passes through the ventricular conduction system. This includes, in order of depolarization sequence, **the bundle of His**, the **left** and **right bundle branches**, and, finally, the actual myocytes of the ventricles. The rapid conduction system (bundle of His, left and right bundle branches) is known as the **Purkinje system**. Contraction initiates on depolarization but continues well after depolarization is complete—it takes longer to mechanically contract than it does to conduct an electrical impulse.

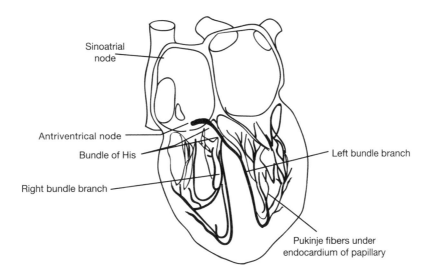

Figure 3 Conduction system

Circulation

Deoxygenated blood (blue blood) returns from the body from the **superior vena cava (SVC)" and "inferior vena cava (IVC)** and empties into the RA. Deoxygenated blood that perfused the heart drains into the coronary sinus which also drains into the RA. Blood travels to the RV and is pumped to the lungs via the pulmonary artery (Figure 4).

Oxygenated blood (red blood) returns from the lungs via 4 pulmonary veins. Blood travels to the LV and is pumped to the body via the aorta.

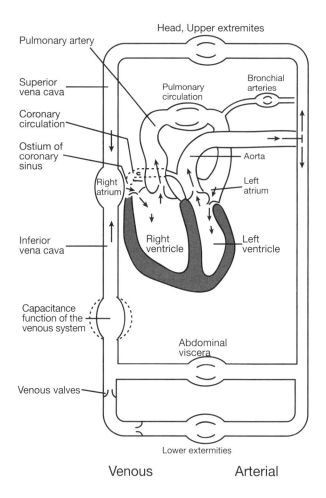

Figure 4 Circulation

Fetal Circulation

In utero, fetal blood is oxygenated by the placenta. The physiological shunts of fetal circulation (Figure 5) are:

1. *Ductus Venosus*—Allows oxygenated blood from umbilical vein to enter the IVC, bypassing the hepatic vasculature.

2. *Foramen Ovale*—Allows blood to pass from the RA directly to the LA bypassing the lungs.

3. *Ductus Arteriosus*—Allows blood to pass from the PA to the aorta also bypassing the lungs.

You can close a patent ductus arteriosus (PDA) in a newborn with **indomethacin** (to prevent pulmonary hypertension). You can keep a PDA open by giving prostaglandins such as **PGE1** (in the case of cyanotic congenital heart disease).

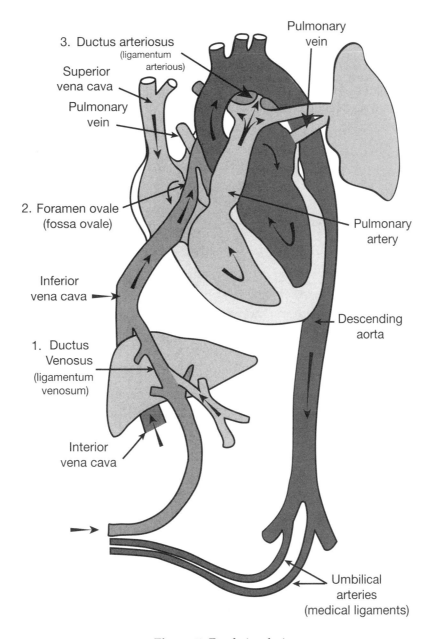

3. Ductus arteriosus
(ligamentum arterious)

Superior vena cava

Pulmonary vein

Pulmonary vein

2. Foramen ovale
(fossa ovale)

Inferior vena cava

1. Ductus Venosus
(ligamentum venosum)

Interior vena cava

Pulmonary vein

Pulmonary artery

Descending aorta

Umbilical arteries
(medical ligaments)

Figure 5 Fetal circulation

HISTOLOGY

Veins

Veins store most of the blood in the body. They are composed of **three layers**: tunica intima, tunica media, and tunica adventitia (Figure 6).

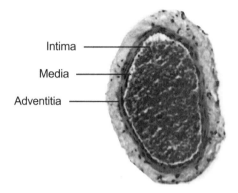

Figure 6 Vein histology

Arteries

Arteries deliver blood to the body. They are also composed of **three layers**: *tunica intima, tunica media,* and *tunica adventitia.* Arteries require their own blood supply called the *vasa recta,* which are located in the adventitia.

Three types of arteries:

1. **Elastic arteries:** Strong and compliant thanks to elastic fibers (aorta and major branches are examples).

2. **Muscular arteries:** Most abundant in the body. Similar to elastic arteries, but elastic tissue are confined to internal and external elastic lamina (Figure 7).

3. **Aterioles**: Small muscular arteries that control peripheral vascular tone.

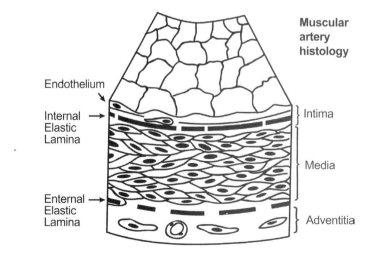

Figure 7 Artery histology

Capillaries

Capillaries are usually a single endothelial cell layer thick and rest on a basement membrane (Figure 8).

Continuous capillaries

This is the most common type of capillary. They have an uninterrupted barrier that allows only small molecules to pass. These are found in nervous tissue, muscle, connective tissue, exocrine glands, blood-brain-barrier, and blood-testes barrier.

Fenestrated capillaries

They have large pores and exchange fluids rapidly across the basement membrane. These are found in the GI tract, endocrine glands, and exocrine glands.

Discontinuous capillaries

Similar to fenestrated capillaries, but have gaps with no endothelium at all. **They are only found in liver sinusoids**.

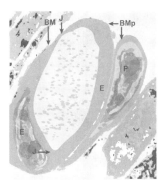

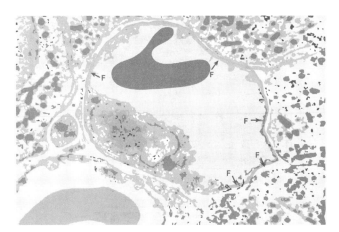

Figure 8 Capillaries
Top: Continuous capillary and Bottom: Fenestrated capillary
BM: basement membrane, E: endothelial cells, J: tight junctions, F: fenestrations, P: pericytes

Heart

Also composed of three layers:

1. **Endocardium:** lines the cardiac chambers and is connected to the endothelium of incoming and outgoing vessel endothelium.

2. **Myocardium:** is the actual heart muscle composed of cardiac myocytes.

3. **Epicardium (visceral pericardium):** is a single layer of epithelial cells that line the outside of the myocardium and is continuous with the parietal pericardium.

Cardiac Myocytes

Cardiac myocytes are specialized muscle cells that depolarize and contract with impeccable timing and coordination, ejecting blood into the lungs and aorta. Cardiac myocytes have sarcomeres like regular muscle cells, but they are also branched and tightly connected to each other at regions called **intercalated discs** (Figure 9). The intercalated discs are composed of cell-cell junctions called **fascia adherens** and **desmosomes**. Other regions have gap junctions, which allow the action potential to spread quickly between cells.

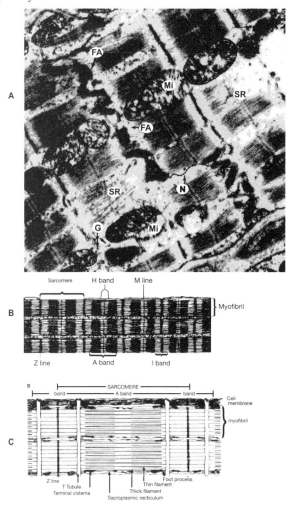

Figure 9 A. Cardiac muscle. (Mi = mitochondria; FA fascua adherens; N = gap junctions; SR = sarcoplasmic reticulum; G = glycogen granule.) **B.** The myofibril.
C. A close-up view of single sacromere

Purkinje cells are modified cardiac myocytes that conduct electrical stimuli from the AV node to the myocardium and coordinate the repeated cycles of contraction and relaxation. T-tubules are found at Z-lines ("TAZ"). They are invaginations of the cell membrane that facilitate the conversion of electrical impulses (depolarization) to physical muscle contractions. The sarcoplasmic reticulum (SR) stores calcium in the cell and is located near the T-tubules. The SR is instrumental in facilitating contraction of cardiac myocytes. Cardiac myocytes require an extraordinary amount of energy in the form of adenosine triphosphate (ATP), which is provided by numerous mitochondria.

EMBRYOLOGY

Myocardium

Myocardium originates from mesenchymal cells in the splanchnic mesoderm.

The heart tube forms from tissue near the prechordal plate (Figure 10).

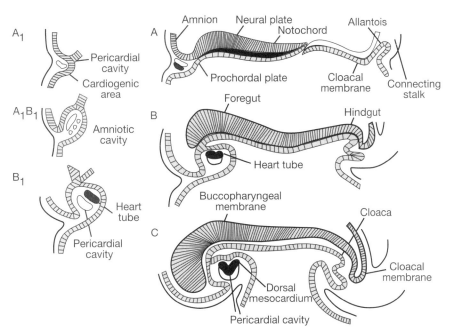

Figure 10 Early cardiac development.
The cardiogenic area starts ventral to the pericardial cavity (A1) then rotates to a dorsal position.
A. 18 days; **B.** 21 days; **C.** 22 days.

The heart begins as a long tube, then folds in half with a twist to create a 4-chamber heart (Figure 11). The atrial and ventricular septa form between days 27 and 37.

Endocardial cushions

Endocardial cushions grow toward each other and eventually meet. They form portions of the tricuspid/mitral valves and the atrial/ventricular septa. Endocardial cushion malformations cause atrial septal defects (ASDs)", "ventricular septal defects (VSDs)" and "atrio-ventricular septal defects (AVSDs)" should all be bold faced, which are common in **Down Syndrome**.

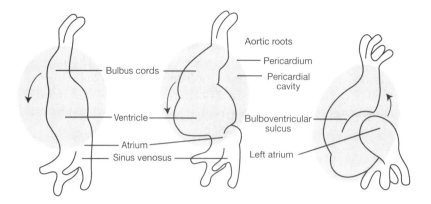

Figure 11 Continued cardiac development at **A.** 22 days; **B.** 23 days; **C.** 24 days.

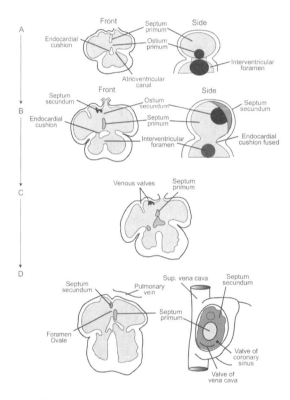

Figure 12 Septal development at **A.** 30 days **B.** 33 days **C.** 37 days **D.** and newborn.

Atrial septum

The **atrial septum** is formed by the overlapping **septum primum and septum secundum** (Figure 12). Failure of the two septa to fuse after birth results in **patent foramen ovale (PFO),** which is present in ~25% of the population. Generally asymptomatic, but can lead to **cryptogenic stroke** whereby venous clots pass from the RA to LA and into the systemic circulation.

Aorticopulmonary septum

The **aorticopulmonary septum** is formed by **neural crest** derived mesenchymal cells. The developing structure undergoes a 180 rotation. Abnormal *rotation* leads to **transposition of the great arteries (TGA)**. Abnormal *septation* leads to **truncus arteriosus**.

Aortic arches (Figure 13)

1—Maxillary arteries

2—Hyoid and stapedial arties

3—Common carotid, external carotid, internal carotid (1ˢᵗ portion) arteries

4—Aortic arch (L) and subclavian artery (R)

5—*Transient (no final structure)*

6—Ductus arteriosus (L) and right pulmonary artery (R)

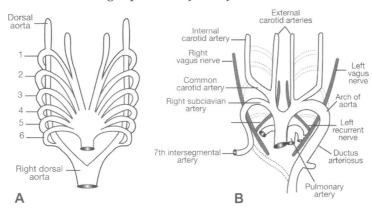

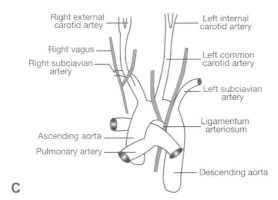

Figure 13 Aortic arches.

A. Original aortic arches.
B. Transformation of arches during development.
C. Adult structures.

PHYSIOLOGY

Cardiac Action Potentials

At rest, the concentrations of **sodium and calcium** are **higher outside** the cell than inside, and the concentration of **potassium** is **higher inside**. Ion channels in the cell membrane allow a small, constant leak of ions down their concentration gradient (Na^+ and Ca^{2+} flow in, K^+ flows out). Counteracting these leaks are ATP-driven Na^+-K^+ exchange pumps that move Na^+ out of the cell and K^+ into the cell to maintain the resting concentration gradient (Figure 14). Ca^{2+} is moved out of the cell by a Na^+/Ca^{2+} exchanger and, to a lesser degree, by an ATP-driven Ca^{2+} pump.

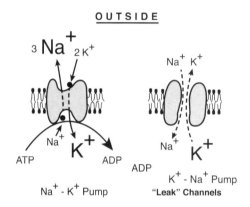

Figure 14 Na-K exchange

The potential of a cell at rest and during activation depends on three factors: 1) the concentration of ions inside the cell, 2) the concentration of ions outside the cell, and 3) the relative permeability of the cell to the different ions. The **Nernst equation** is used to calculate the equilibrium concentration of ion x.

$$V_x = -\left(\frac{RT}{zF}\right)\log\frac{x_{in}}{x_{out}}$$

Where the quotient (RT/zF) is a constant equal to 62, and x is the concentration of the ion inside and outside the cell, respectively. **You don't need to memorize this equation**, just understand the physiology behind it.

Let's use K^+ as an example. The concentration of K^+ inside the cell is much greater than the concentration outside the cell. Based on the concentrations alone, K^+ would tend to flow out until the concentration inside equals the concentration outside. However, K has a positive charge, so as the positive charges leave the cell, a net negative charge develops inside the cell which will tend to pull positively charged K back into the cell. The "VK^+" is the equilibrium membrane potential at which the outward forces drawing K^+ down its concentration gradient are exactly matched by the electrostatic forces drawing the positively charged K^+ into the negatively-charged cell. VK^+ is about -90mV. At rest, Na^+ channels are leaking much more slowly than are the K^+ channels. This explains why the resting membrane potential is only slightly more positive than –90 mV. The opening of voltage-gated Na+ channels during an action potential, which makes the cell transiently more permeable to Na^+ than K^+, explains why the membrane potential shoots up to near the Na^+ equilibrium potential.

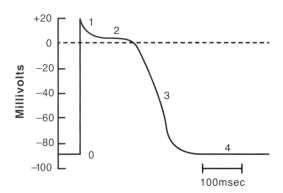

Figure 15 Action potential of myocardial cell

Figure 15 shows the action potential of a myocardial cell. The phases of the action potential are as follows:

- **Phase 0** is called the *rapid upstroke*. Voltage-gated Na^+ channels open, Na^+ flows in, and the cell depolarizes, bringing the cell potential closer to the Na^+ equilibrium potential.

- **Phase 1** is initial repolarization caused by the opening of slow voltage-gated K^+ channels followed by K^+ efflux. At the same time, phase 0 Na^+ channels become inactivated.

- **Phase 2** is called the plateau phase. Voltage-gated Ca^{2+} channels open, causing Ca^{2+} influx. The Ca^{2+} influx balances K^+ efflux, so there is no change in the membrane potential. Ca^{2+} influx is also important because it drives the contraction of the myocytes via actin and myosin interactions.

- **Phase 3** is rapid repolarization. The Ca^{2+} channels close, and the K^+ channels are now open without opposition, causing a relatively massive K^+ efflux. This brings the cell membrane potential back to the resting potential. Repolarization allows the Na^+ channels to recover from inactivation so that they're ready for the next action potential.

- **Phase 4** is the resting state (resting membrane potential). The resting K^+ channels are open, allowing K^+ efflux and bringing the cell close to the K^+ equilibrium membrane potential (–90 mV).

Pacemaker Action Potentials

The cells of the SA node, AV node, and His-Purkinje system all have pacemaker activity. The SA node normally controls the heart rate because it has the fastest pacemaker cycle, but if it fails, the AV node takes over (the next fastest), followed by the His-Purkinje system (the least fastest). Figure 16 shows the action potential of a pacemaker cell. The phases of the action potential are as follows:

- **Phase 0** is the slow upstroke. Slow Ca^{2+} channels open, causing Ca^{2+} influx. Resting K^+ channels close due to this depolarization. There is no phase 1 because voltage-gated Na^+ channels are not involved in phase 0. In pacemaker cells, the resting membrane potential is more positive than normal; therefore the Na^+ channels never recover from their inactive state.

- **Phase 3** is repolarization caused by Ca^{2+} channels closing and K^+ channels opening, which allows unopposed K^+ efflux (no phase 2).

- **Phase 4** is considered diastolic depolarization (or automaticity). This is caused by the slow closure of K^+ channels and by Na^+ channels letting Na^+ leak into the cell. (These Na^+ channels are different from the fast sodium channels responsible for phase 0 cardiac cell depolarization.) The membrane potential gradually becomes more positive until it reaches a threshold and results in an action potential (and heartbeat).

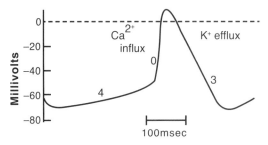

Figure 16 Action potential of pacemaker cell

The phase 4 slope determines the heart rate and is controlled by the sympathetic and vagal tones (Figure 17). Catecholamines or b1-agonists increase the slope by increasing Na^+ influx, so the threshold is reached faster and the heart rate increases. Conduction through the AV node is also faster because of increased Ca^{2+} influx during phase 0 and a steeper phase 0 slope. This is reflected on the ECG by a shorter PR interval. Acetylcholine or muscarinic agonists increase K^+ efflux, lowering the phase 4 slope, prolonging the time to reach threshold and ultimately lowering the heart rate. Conduction velocity through the AV node is slowed, and the PR interval is prolonged.

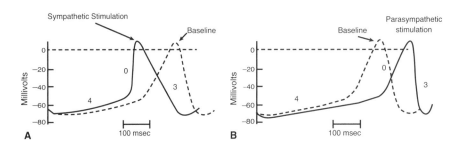

Figure 17 Change in phase 4 slope. **A:** sympathetic stimulation and **B:** parasympathetic stimulation

Refractory periods are part of normal pacemaker activity. The **absolute refractory period** or **effective refractory period** occurs when the cell absolutely refuses to depolarize no matter how much stimulus you give it starting from phase 1 and extending into phase 3 (Figure 18). This inability to depolarize is caused by the temporary mechanical inactivation of voltage-gated channels. The **relative refractory period** occurs close to the end of phase 3, when the cell can depolarize early if given enough stimulus. This occurs because Na^+ channels are able to open again if the membrane potential is raised high enough.

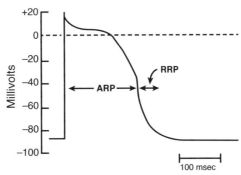

Figure 18 Refractory periods:
ARP: absolute refractory period
RRP: relative refractory period

Excitation-Contraction Coupling

After membrane depolarization, Ca^{2+} influx occurs during phase 2. Ca^{2+} binds to *ryanodine* receptors on the **Sarcoplasmic Reticulum (SR)**, which causes them to open, releasing even more Ca^{2+} in the cell (Figure 19). The available intracellular Ca^{2+} leads to sarcomere contraction.

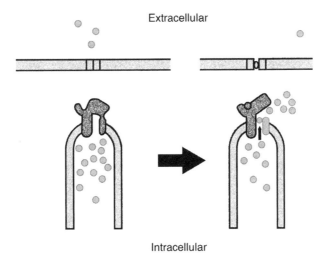

Figure 19 Cardiac muscle contraction

For the myocyte to relax, Ca^{2+} must be removed from the cell. This is done in two ways. The SR has an ATP-dependent Ca^{2+} pump, which brings Ca^{2+} into the SR. If the amount of Ca^{2+} stored in the SR is increased, then the subsequent contractions are even more vigorous. This force of contraction is called **contractility**.

The other calcium removal mechanism is a Na^+-Ca^{2+} exchanger. It depends primarily on the Na^+ gradient across the membrane, so that if there is very little Na^+ inside, three Na^+ can move into the cell quickly in exchange for one Ca^{2+} pushed out. This is important for understanding the effects of digitalis. Because *digitalis* poisons the Na^+/K^+ ATPase, Na^+ accumulates in the myocyte and decreases the Na^+ gradient (Na+ isn't as interested in rushing into the cell because there's already enough Na^+ inside). Ultimately, the Na^+- Ca^{2+} exchanger doesn't work as well as the calcium pump, Ca^{2+} accumulates in the cell and is stored in the SR, and the muscle contracts more vigorously on subsequent beats (Figure 20). Therefore, digitalis increases contractility and is called a **positive inotrope**.

Digitalis

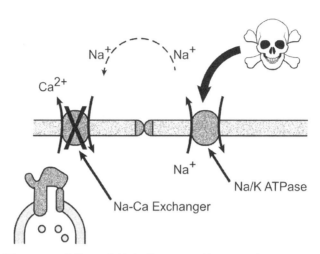

Figure 20 Effect of digitalis on cardiac muscle contraction

Physics of Circulation

The physics governing blood flow through vessels may appear complicated but are intuitive. There are two important concepts to grasp and two important relationships to understand.

Concept 1

The only way blood flows is when a difference in pressure is achieved. Blood always flows from areas of high pressure to areas of low pressure (Think of the how blood flows from the high pressure arterial system to the low pressure venous system).

Concept 2

Pressure will fall across a resistance to flow. Thought of another way, it requires a large pressure differential to overcome a resistance to flow (Think of the pressure the LV must develop to maintain systemic blood pressure in the face of aortic stenosis).

The first relationship that is important to understand simply relates the two concepts above. It states that a pressure differential (P) is proportional to cardiac output (CO) and resistance, in this case systemic vascular resistance (SVR).

$$\Delta P = CO \bullet SVR$$

Cardiac output can also be calculated as heart rate (HR) multiplied by the LV stroke volume (SV).

$$CO = HR \bullet SV$$

The second relationship that is important to understand is that the resistance of a single vessel (R) is inversely proportional to the radius of the vessel (r) and proportional to the viscosity of the fluid (n) and the length of the vessel (l).

$$R = \frac{8nl}{\pi r^4}$$

You don't need to memorize this equation. The only thing you need to remember is that when the **radius of a blood vessel drops in half, the resistance of that vessel will increase by a factor of 16**. Similarly, when the vessel size increases by 2, the resistance will drop by a factor of 16.

Another equation governs fluid flow *across* the blood vessel into the interstitium, known as the **Starling Equation**. The flow across the blood vessel (*F*) is related to the hydrostatic pressure gradient and oncotic pressure gradient between the blood vessel and the interstitium by a permeability constant (*k*).

$$F = k\left[(P_{cap} - P_{Int}) - (\pi_{cap} - \pi_{Int})\right]$$

Where P_{Cap} is the hydrostatic pressure in the blood vessel (capillary) and P_{Int} is the hydrostatic pressure in the interstitium. Similarly, π_{Cap} is the oncotic pressure in the capillary while π_{Int} is the oncotic pressure in the insterstitium.

The Cardiac Cycle

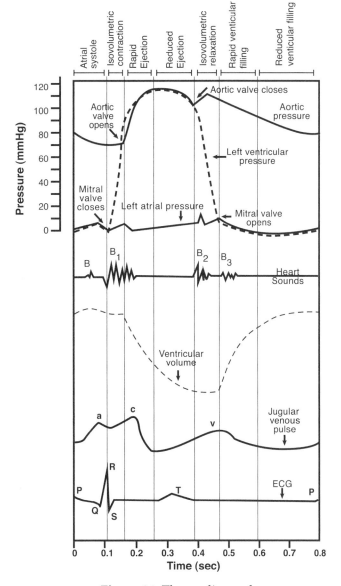

Figure 21 The cardiac cycle

Figure 21 illustrates the cardiac cycle.

Atrial systole comes right after the P wave (depolarization of the atria). It is seen in the venous pulse as the **a-wave**, and in patients with LV hypertrophy, an S4 is heard.

Isovolumetric contraction comes right after the QRS complex (depolarization of the ventricles) and causes the mitral valve to close (S1) when LV pressure exceeds LA pressure. The aortic valve is still closed at this point because LV pressure has not reached aortic pressure.

Rapid ejection occurs when the LV pressure is greater than the aortic pressure. This is when most of the stroke volume is ejected. The **c-wave** corresponds to RV contraction and the tricuspid valve bulging into the RA.

Reduced ejection occurs as blood continues to be ejected slowly from the ventricle. Ventricular pressure begins to decrease (from ventricular repolarization), and aortic pressure starts to fall as blood quickly flows into the smaller arteries.

Isovolumetric relaxation comes right after the T wave. When LV pressure drops below aortic pressure, the back-flow of blood causes the aortic valve to close (pulmonic valve on the right side), which is heard as S2. The atria continue to fill against a closed tricuspid (and mitral) valve, causing the pressure to increase in the RA (and LA). This is seen as the **v-wave** of the jugular venous pressure (JVP). When the aortic valve closes, the transient increase in aortic pressure is called the **dicrotic notch.**

Rapid ventricular filling occurs when LV pressure drops below LA pressure and the mitral valve opens. An S3 may be heard in normal children but is also heard in patients with dilated CHF.

Reduced ventricular filling (diastasis) is marked by a slower increase in ventricular volume. Diastasis ends with the onset of atrial contraction.

Cardiac Output

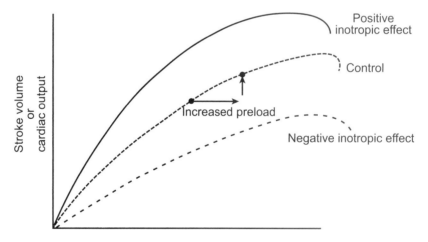

Figure 22 Frank-Starling cardiac function curve

Cardiac output (CO) depends on four parameters: **preload, afterload, heart rate** (HR), and **contractility** (or **inotropy**). It is essential to understand these interactions.

Preload is the amount of "stretch" in sarcomeres prior to contraction. As "pre-stretch" (or preload) increases, the number of actin-myosin crossbridges increases resulting in a more vigorous contraction of the myocyte. This is reflected on the **Frank-Starling curve** (Figure 22). Preload is commonly measured as the end-diastolic volume (EDV) because the larger the EDV, the more "stretch" is placed on myocytes. Preload increases with exercise, transfusion, and sympathetic stimulation (venous constriction). It decreases with hypovolemia (dehydration) or venous dilation (nitroglycerin). When preload increases, the ventricle fills with more blood, and the sarcomeres in the myocyte are stretched. As preload increases, the SV increases, which means that CO increases.

Contractility was described earlier and is basically a reflection of the amount of Ca^{2+} stored in the SR. Contractility can be increased (positive inotropic effect) by sympathetic stimulation, digitalis, catecholamines, O_2, increased muscle mass, increased myofibril number, decreased extracellular Na^+, or an increase in HR. As HR increases, the myocyte is stimulated more times per minute, so more Ca^{2+} is released from the SR each minute, leading to increased contractility. As the curve shows, an increase in contractility leads to an increase in CO at any EDV. Contractility is decreased (negative inotropic effect) by myocardial damage (e.g., infarction, heart failure), decreased extracellular Ca^{2+}, beta-adrenergic receptor blockade, hypoxia, acidosis, or decreased HR.

Afterload is pressure the heart has to pump against (essentially aortic pressure), but is a reflection of the SVR (regulated at the level of the arterioles). As afterload increases, the ventricle must eject blood in the face of a higher aortic pressure, resulting in a decreased SV and CO. Afterload increases with sympathetic stimulation, alpha-1-agonists (phenylephrine), coarctation of the aorta, and aortic valve stenosis. Afterload decreases with vasodilation (angiotensin-converting enzyme [ACE] inhibitors; Calcium channel blockers such as nifedipine).

Pressure-Volume Loops

PV loops are simply another representation of the cardiac cycle, but they also reflect preload, afterload, HR, and contractility (Figure 23). When any of these parameters are changed, PV loops diagram the effect on CO.

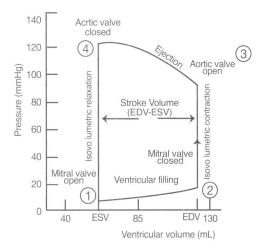

Figure 23 Pressure-volume loop

1 → 2: Ventricular filling begins once LV pressure drops below LA pressure and the mitral valve opens. The ventricular volume increases, and pressure increases slightly as the ventricular wall is passively stretched by blood (preload).

2 → 3: Isovolumetric contraction occurs after the QRS complex, on closure of the mitral valve. LV pressure increases, but ventricular volume doesn't change because both the aortic and mitral valves are closed.

3 → 4: Ventricular ejection occurs once the LV pressure is greater than aortic pressure, forcing the aortic valve to open. As blood is ejected into the aorta, ventricular volume decreases. The stroke volume is thus the difference between the EDV and the end-systolic volume (ESV). Ejection fraction is SV/EDV and should be 50–75%. The point at which the aortic valve opens is a reflection of afterload.

4 → 1: Isovolumetric relaxation occurs after LV pressure drops below aortic pressure, and the aortic valve closes. Because both the aortic and mitral valves are again closed, ventricular volume does not change as the pressure falls.

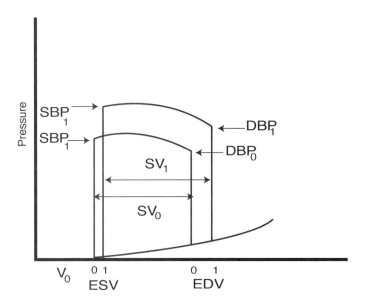

Figure 24 Effect of increased preload moving from 0 to 1.
DBP: diastolic blood pressure
SBP: systolic blood pressure
ESV: end systolic volume
EDV end diastolic volume
SV: stroke volume

If preload increases, the EDV increases on the loop (Figure 24). We already know that the SV increases with increased preload, according to the Frank-Starling relationship (from increased formation of actin and myosin cross-bridges), but now we can see it on the PV loop. If everything else stays constant the resulting loop demonstrates an increased SV. Remember that if SV increases, CO and BP increase (also demonstrated on the loop by an increased **diastolic blood pressure [DBP]** and **systolic blood pressure** [SBP]).

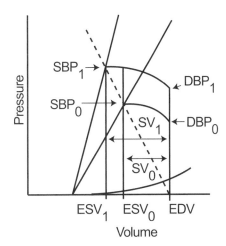

Figure 25 Effect of increased contractility moving from 0 to 1.
DBP: diastolic blood pressure
SBP: systolic blood pressure
ESV: end systolic volume
EDV: end diastolic volume
SV: stroke volume

If contractility increases, the ventricle can develop more pressure and increase SV by ejecting more blood. The new PV loop again demonstrates an increased SV, DBP, and SBP. Intuitively, remember that if the ventricle squeezes harder (increased contractility), SV and CO increase.

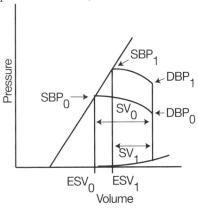

Figure 26 Effect of increased afterload moving from 0 to 1.
DBP: diastolic blood pressure
SBP: systolic blood pressure
ESV: end systolic volume
EDV end diastolic volume

EDV end diastolic volume If afterload increases the SV decreases (because the LV is now trying to eject blood against a greater aortic pressure), but DBP and SBP increase.

Venous Return

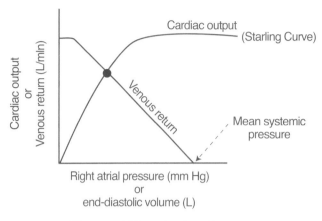

Figure 27 Vascular function curves

The relationship between venous return (VR) to the heart and preload can also be displayed on a Frank-Starling curve. VR is greatest when right atrial pressure (RAP) approaches zero. As RAP increases, VR decreases. VR has to equal CO because the circulation is a closed system (what goes into the heart must come out). The intercept of the two curves is the value at which CO = VR and the "operating point" of the system.

With hemorrhage, the VR curve shifts down and to the left because less blood is returning to the heart. The maximum RAP is lower, and CO is lower. If this patient were transfused, VR and CO would increase (Figure 27).

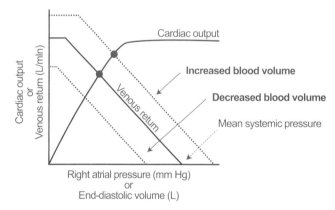

Figure 28 Change in cardiac output and venous return with hemorrhage (decreased blood volume) and with transfusion (increased blood volume)

This translates as a decrease in contractility and a shift to a lower Starling curve (point 0 to 1, Figure 29). The body tries to compensate by saving salt and water and increasing preload, which moves the patient up and along the same Starling curve (point 1 to 2). You then try to increase the patient's contractility and CO with digoxin. An increase in contractility shifts the patient to a higher Starling curve (point 2 to 3). Now that the heart is ejecting blood better, there is less congestion in the heart and a lower RAP (point 3 to 4). Although shifting down this Starling curve may lower CO a tiny bit, this measure is ultimately beneficial because it prevents congestion and further dilation of the heart.

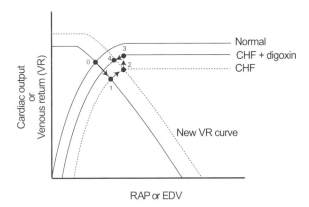

Figure 29 Vascular function curves in heart failure (CHF)

Regulation of Mean Arterial Pressure

The body is extremely smart and is capable of compensating for a BP that is either too high or too low. The fast response is mediated by the nervous system, and the slower one is mediated by the kidneys. Consider the example of a patient who has an acute hemorrhage and consequent drop in BP (Figure 30). The decrease in MAP is sensed by baroreceptors in the aortic arch and the carotid sinus. This message is relayed to the medulla via the vagus and glossopharyngeal nerves. The ultimate effect is to decrease stimulation of the vagal center (and decrease parasympathetic outflow) and increase stimulation of sympathetic outflow. Both mechanisms serve to increase the MAP by increasing HR, contractility, VR, and SVR (vasoconstriction).

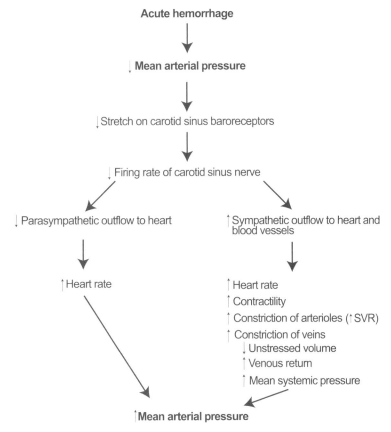

Figure 30 Baroreceptor response to acute hemorrhage

A second, slower method of increasing MAP is via the renin-angiotensin-aldosterone system (Figure 31). The decrease in MAP is sensed by the juxtaglomerular (JG) cells, which then release renin into the blood. Renin converts angiotensinogen to angiotensin I, then angiotensin-converting enzyme (ACE) modifies angiotensin I to angiotensin II in the lungs. Angiotensin II is a potent vasoconstrictor and causes an increase in TPR; it also leads to aldosterone release from the zona glomerulosa of the adrenal cortex. Aldosterone works at the level of the nephron—more specifically, at the distal collecting tubules—to increase retention of Na^+ and water. This increases plasma volume, preload, SV, CO, and ultimately BP.

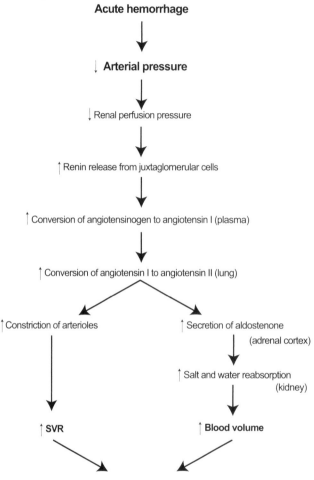

Figure 31 Renin-angiotensin-aldosterone response to acute hemorrhage

Other regulators of the MAP include chemoreceptors peripherally (aortic and carotid bodies) and centrally (the brain). When MAP decreases, less O_2 is delivered to these receptors and blood P_{CO_2} decreases. The aortic and carotid bodies respond mostly to an increase in P_{CO_2} (and the resulting decrease in blood pH) but can also respond to a decrease in P_{O_2}. The central receptors do not respond directly to P_{O_2}. The cumulative effect is to help increase sympathetic tone and decrease vagal tone. A decrease in MAP also stimulates the posterior pituitary to release antidiuretic hormone, which increases water absorption at the collecting tubules.

On the other hand, if MAP increases, everything works in reverse to lower it. In addition, the elevated MAP stretches the atria, which release atrial natriuretic peptide. This peptide inhibits vasoconstriction (TPR decreases), increases Na^+ and water excretion by the kidney, and inhibits the JG cells from releasing renin. The resultant decrease in TPR and blood volume causes a decrease in MAP.

Circulation to Specific Organs

Blood flow to different organ systems is largely regulated on a local level by active metabolites. (Table 1).

- The heart is able to extract a huge amount of O_2 from the blood (large arteriovenous [AV] O_2 difference). If more O_2 is needed (e.g., if HR increases), the only way the muscle can get it is if coronary blood flow increases; **it cannot increase O_2 extraction**.

- The control of blood flow to skeletal muscle depends on its activity level. At rest, sympathetic fibers stimulate alpha-1-receptors, leading to vasoconstriction and increased SVR. If the muscle is actively exercising, however, local metabolites override sympathetic control and cause vasodilation of local blood vessels, which increases blood flow (and O_2) to the hard-working muscle.

- Skin is one of the few team players. If there is sympathetic stimulation, blood vessels to the skin constrict so that blood can be supplied to more critical organs (i.e., brain and muscle) during a "fight-or flight" response.

- **Kidneys receive the largest amount of blood flow per gram of tissue.**

- The lungs must accept the entire CO with each beat.

- The liver accepts the largest percentage of the systemic CO.

- The GI tract also acts as a martyr during a sympathetic response and diverts blood away by constricting splanchnic vessels.

Circulation	% of Resting cardiac output	Control	Vasoactive metabolites
Coronary	5%	Local metabolic	Hypoxia, adenosine
Cerebral	15%	Local metabolic	CO_2H^+
Muscle	20%	Metabolic and sympathetic	Lactate, adenosine, K^+
Pulmonary	100%	Local metabolic	Hypoxia, vasoconstriction
Renal	25%	Local metabolic	—
Skin	5%	Sympathetic	—
Liver	29%	Local metabolic	—

Table 1 Cardiac output to various organ systems

Response to Standing

The behavior of blood during postural change is the perfect example that gravity works on fluid, even when the fluid is in blood vessels. Because veins are not muscular structures, blood pools in leg veins when a person moves from a lying to standing position. If more blood remains in the legs, there is less blood to return to the heart, so VR decreases, as does CO and BP. If the body doesn't respond to this drop by increasing CO, the patient may feel light-headed or faint. This is called **orthostatic hypotension**. In a normal individual, the body responds promptly to maintain BP (and CO) by increasing sympathetic tone, which raises HR and SVR.

Response to Aerobic Exercise

Exercise is extremely complicated physiologically, but a few generalizations can be made. Sympathetic tone increases, which increases HR and contractility. VR increases from muscle contraction (which "milks" venous blood back to the heart) and from venoconstriction (decreases blood pooled in the veins). CO increases mostly from increased HR but also from increased SV and contractility. SVR increases in non-exercising tissues but decreases in active muscles (from local metabolite-induced vasodilation) to give a net decrease in SVR. The AV O_2 difference increases because muscles are consuming more O_2. All these factors serve to increase BP slightly.

ELECTOCARDIOGRAM (ECG OR EKG) AND ARRHYTHMIAS

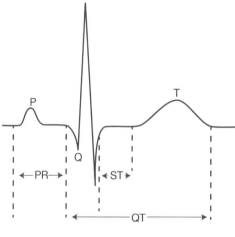

Figure 32

P Wave

P wave—atrial depolarization (RA and LA contract together). Atrial repolarization not seen on EKG as it is "buried" in the QRS complex (Figure 32)

Sinus rhythm: Depolarization starts at the SA node and travels through the AV node.

Atrial fibrillation: Disorganized depolarization of atria. Only a few depolarizations make it through AV node. So called **"irregularly-irregular"** rhythm.

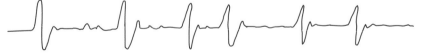

Figure 33 Atrial fibrillation

Atrial flutter: Rapid (but coordinated) atrial rhythm. Characteristic "sawtooth" pattern.

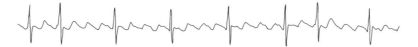

Figure 34 Atrial flutter

PR Interval

PR interval: represents delay in conduction through the AV node. This is required to allow the ventricles to have an appropriate amount of time to fill with blood. AV block occurs when the PR interval is greater than 200 ms (5 small boxes on EKG).

1st degree block: PR interval prolonged

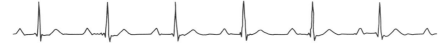

Figure 35 1st degree block

2nd degree block: *Mobitz type I (Wenckebach)* occurs when PR interval gets progressively longer until a QRS is "dropped". Asymptomatic condition.

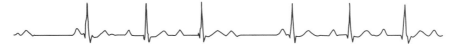

Figure 36 2nd degree block type 1

Mobitz type II occurs when there are dropped beats without lengthening PR intervals. Intervention is always required for Mobitz type II as it can progress to 3rd degree block (BAD!).

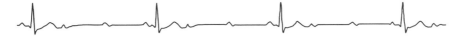

Figure 37 2nd degree block type 2

3rd degree block: "Complete" block occurs when p-waves and QRS complexes are totally unrelated.

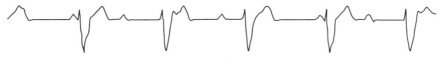

Figure 38 3rd degree block

Wolf-Parkinson-White: A condition associated with an extra conduction pathway between the RA and the ventricular conduction system that "pre-excites" the ventricles. This can be seen on an EKG with a "delta wave".

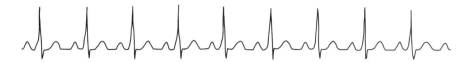

Figure 39 Wolf-Parkinson-White

QRS Complex

QRS complex—represents ventricular depolarization. Normally 120 ms or less (3 small boxes on EKG).

Ventricular tachycardia: Represents ectopic ventricular contractions . "Sustained" ventricular tachycardia is a dire sign and may decompensate into ventricular fibrillation.

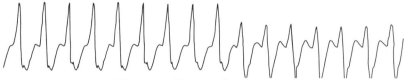

Figure 40 Ventricular tachycardia

Ventricular fibrillation: Completely disorganized rhythm. Leads to death if not converted back to normal rhythm (electrical or pharmacological).

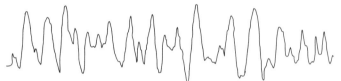

Figure 41 Ventricular fibrillation

Asystole: Cardiac arrest, "flat line".

ST Segment

ST segment—interval of ventricular depolarization. ST segment depression = reversible myocardial ischemia; ST segment elevation = myocardial infarction (MI).

T Wave

T wave—represents ventricular repolarization. "Peaked T waves" commonly represent hyperkalemia.

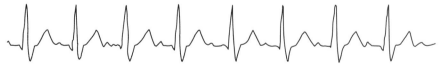

Figure 42 Ventricular repolarization

QT Interval

QT interval—**represents the entire period of systole**. Prolongation may suggest drug toxicity (e.g., quinidine), electrolyte disturbances (e.g., hypocalcemia), or congenital long QT syndrome. Prolonged QT may lead to **Torsades de Pointes** which can deteriorate into ventricular fibrillation.

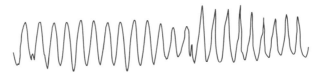

Figure 43 QT

HYPERTENSION

Essential hypertension (95% of all hypertensive patients) occurs when no cause is found. Secondary hypertension has a known cause including:

- **Estrogen** in birth control pills causes hypertension in about 5% of women taking OCPs.

- **Renovascular hypertension**, or renal artery stenosis, is caused by a thickening of the renal artery wall. The juxtaglomerular apparatus senses a decrease in renal blood flow, which prompts the renin-angiotensin-aldosterone system to increase blood pressure.

- **Hyperaldosteronism** and **Cushing's** syndrome often lead to hypertension and are usually due to adrenal adenomas.

- **Pheochromocytoma** is a rare adrenal tumor that secretes epinephrine and norepinephrine.

- **Coarctation** of the aorta causes hypertension and presents in newborns and infants.

Signs and Symptoms

Most patients are asymptomatic. Patients with significant hypertension might show signs of the end-organ damage caused by the disease: blindness, aneurysm, CNS injury (stroke), or coronary artery disease (CAD).

Diagnosis

At least three separate BP readings above 140/90 (or > 95th% based on age and height for children) are required to diagnosis hypertension. Adequate cuff size must be used.

Treatment

Commonly used drug classes include diuretics, β-blockers, angiotensin converting enzyme (ACE) inhibitors, angiotensin receptor blockers (ARB), calcium channel blockers and direct vasodilators (Table 4).

ISCHEMIC HEART DISEASE

Coronary Artery Disease is caused by **atherosclerosis**, or **plaque** formation in the arteries. The steps in plaque formation are as follows:

1. Fatty streak (at the intima)

2. Simple plaque formation

3. Fibrin deposition and calcification

4. Complicated plaque

5. Rupture and thrombosis, which can lead to occlusion

Angina

Angina is transient chest pain, often described by patients as crushing, suffocating, or "like an elephant sitting on my chest." It is substernal, often with radiation to the left arm, neck, or jaw. It can usually be brought on by exercise (hence the use of stress tests for diagnosing cardiac disease). It is relieved by nitrates (e.g., sublingual nitroglycerin) and rest. The pathology of angina is temporary occlusion of the coronary vasculature, either by thrombosis, vasospasm, or embolism.

Several classifications of angina exist. **Stable angina** occurs with a well-specified amount of exertion, regularly, and in an unchanging pattern. **Unstable angina** is angina that is new; that is increasing in frequency, duration, or intensity; or that occurs at rest. **Variant (Prinzmetal's) angina** is caused by coronary vasospasm. It occurs at rest (and at night), is relieved by calcium channel blockers, and is thought to be triggered by cold and factors other than exercise.

Myocardial infarction (MI)

Myocardial infarction is occlusion of a coronary artery lasting long enough to result in ischemia to the myocardium. This can then lead to infarction and necrosis of the involved myocardium. The evolution of an MI is important to know and high yield:

- Day 1: coagulative necrosis begins

- Days 2–4: inflammation, hyperemia, neutrophilic infiltration progresses

- Days 5–10: granulation tissue forms, macrophages, neutrophils

- Day 10–6 weeks: scar formation completed

Several complications may occur after an MI, including:

- Arrhythmias

- CHF, pulmonary edema

- Cardiogenic shock

Granulation phase =
Ventricular rupture

Scar phase =
Ventricular aneurysm

Diffuse ST segment
elevation post-MI =
Dressler's Syndrome

- Ventricular wall rupture, ventricular aneurysm, papillary muscle rupture

- Pericarditis (known as **Dressler's syndrome**)

- Sudden cardiac death, usually due to arrhythmia

Signs and Symptoms

Angina, dyspnea, fatigue, diaphoresis, nausea, and vomiting (from vagal stimulation)

Diagnosis

ECG. It's always best to have an old ECG for comparison. Specifically, look for:

- Signs of ischemia—T wave peaking or inversion

- Signs of injury—ST elevations or depressions in consecutive leads

- Signs of infarction—wide and deep Q waves in consecutive leads

Laboratory tests in MI include the following:

- **Creatine kinase (CK):** Look for a peak in CK levels. CK isoenzymes should be determined. The MB isoenzyme has a cardiac source. Other isoenzymes include MM (skeletal muscle) and BB (CNS source).

- **Lactate dehydrogenase (LDH)**

- **Aspartate aminotransferase (AST)**

- **Troponin I:** serially measured

- **Homocysteine:** High serum levels have recently been found to have an extremely high correlation with the risk for CAD.

Chest X-ray (CXR) may show signs of CHF, such as pulmonary edema.

Treatment

β**-Blockers**—Reduce myocardial oxygen demand by decreasing **inotropy** and HR and cause minimal peripheral vasodilation, leading to some decrease in afterload.

Aspirin—Acts as an antiplatelet factor.

Nitrates—Acts directly on endothelial cells to cause vasodilation, resulting in decreased preload and somewhat decreased afterload. Coronary vasodilation leads to relief of pain.

Oxygen—Maximizes oxygen delivery.

Pain control—Opiates improve comfort but also decrease myocardial demand by relaxing the patient.

ACE inhibitors—After a significant MI, ACE inhibitors improve cardiac remodeling.

MONA: **M**orphine, **O**xygen, **N**itrates, **A**spirin

CONGESTIVE HEART FAILURE

Chronic injury to the myocardium through ischemia or other causes leads to decreased contractility, remodeling of myocardium, and inability of the heart to adequately pump blood. Causes include ischemic injury (MI) and cardiomyopathy (ethanol, viral, toxic, idiopathic).

Systolic failure: The heart can't adequately perfuse the rest of the body, leading to cyanosis, fatigue, and end-organ damage (e.g., renal failure, altered mental status, angina, elevated liver enzymes).

Diastolic failure: A stiff, noncompliant heart can't relax fully and therefore can't fill completely with blood. Blood backs up leading to pulmonary edema, dyspnea on exertion, paroxysmal nocturnal dyspnea, orthopnea, distended neck veins, hepatosplenomegaly, and pedal edema. Compensatory mechanisms include increased sympathetic activity: HR increases, contractility increases slightly, and fluid is retained (the body tries to maximize Starling forces by increasing preload).

LV failure: causes pulmonary edema and elevated left atrial pressures.

The #1 cause of RV failure is LV failure

RV failure: causes increased jugular venous pressure (JVP), pedal edema, and hepatosplenomegaly.

Cor pulmonale: refers to RV failure as a result of pulmonary disease (pulmonary hypertension). The most common underlying pulmonary disorder is reduction of the lung vascular bed. COPD is the most common cause of cor pulmonale.

Signs and Symptoms

Shortness of breath, dyspnea on exertion, orthopnea, paroxysmal nocturnal dyspnea, distended neck veins, hepatosplenomegaly, pedal edema, S3 and S4 gallop.

Diagnosis

ECG may show atrial or ventricular hypertrophy, or both, and possibly conduction abnormalities. Echocardiogram shows depressed myocardial function and may show mural thrombus (from stasis of flow). **Ejection fraction** (EF) can be estimated from Doppler flow studies on echocardiography. An EF less than 20% reveals severe dysfunction (an EF above 50% is considered normal). Coronary catheterization is performed to rule out ischemic causes of cardiomyopathy .

Treatment

Treatment is based on whether the pathology is primarily systolic or diastolic dysfunction. In systolic dysfunction, the goal is to improve CO, limit symptoms, and anticoagulate to prevent embolism from mural thrombus. Diastolic dysfunction causes impaired relaxation, which makes the patient's CO highly dependent on preload. Too much preload and blood backs up into the lungs. Too little preload and the ventricle inadequately fills.

CARDIOMYOPATHIES

Dilated cardiomyopathy occurs when the ventricles become large and inadequately squeeze. Causes include ischemic heart disease, viral infection, and drugs (especially chemotherapy). S3 and S4 may be heard ("gallop"). Treatment is similar to systolic heart failure.

Hypertrophic cardiomyopathy occurs when the ventricle walls become too **thick**. Thickening is often seen in the ventricular septum. At least 50% of cases are familial. **Hypertrophic obstructive cardiomyopathy (HOCM)** occurs when the septum become so thick that it blocks blood leaving the left ventricle. HOCM is a common cause of sudden death in young athletes. Treatment is similar to diastolic heart failure.

Restrictive cardiomyopathy occurs when the pericardium prevents the ventricles from expanding normally. Causes include radiation, amyloidosis, sarcoidosis, and Fabry's disease. Treatment is symptomatic and limited to cardiac transplantation.

Amyloidosis is caused by deposition of extracellular protein called amyloid. The amyloid can accumulate in any tissue of the body but is most commonly found in the joints, subcutaneous tissue, the solid organs (heart, liver, kidney), lungs, brain, nervous tissue, and bowel. In **primary amyloidosis**, the amyloid protein is an immunoglobulin light chain (AL). The disease is associated with multiple myeloma. In **secondary amyloidosis**, serum amyloid (SAA) is the responsible protein, which deposits mainly in the kidneys, liver, spleen, and adrenals.

Hemochromatosis is an autosomal recessive disorder characterized by deposition of iron throughout the body. The classic triad seen is **hepatic cirrhosis**, **diabetes mellitus** (from pancreatic deposition), and **bronze pigmentation** of the skin. Cardiac involvement leads to restrictive cardiomyopathy. Liver biopsy is the diagnostic test of choice. Serum iron studies (total iron-binding capacity, transferrin, ferritin) all indicate iron overload. Intense phlebotomy therapy to unload the body of iron works pretty well. End-stage liver disease requires liver transplantation.

VALVULAR HEART DISEASE

Stenosis is caused by narrowing of the valve orifice or decreased mobility of valve leaflets and causes **decreased flow**.

Regurgitation (insufficiency) is essentially a **leaky valve** allowing blood to move backwards in the heart.

Valve disease may be either congenital or acquired. Common causes of acquired valve disease include cardiomyopathy, CHF, ischemic heart disease, infections (endocarditis), inflammatory or autoimmune disease (rheumatic heart disease), or neoplasms.

Mitral or tricuspid stenosis leads to blood "backing up" in the atria, resulting in atrial enlargement. Mitral or tricuspid regurgitation places an extra volume load on the ventricles. The ventricles pump their stroke volume both forward in the correct direction and backward to the atria through the incompetent valve. On the next stroke, this extra blood gets dumped from the atria back into the ventricles. The result of both volume and pressure overload leads to cardiomyopathy, increased oxygen demand, and impaired hemodynamics.

Mitral stenosis and **mitral regurgitation** are usually due to rheumatic fever. **Mitral valve prolapse** is the result of a floppy valve. Mitral valve prolapse is a common finding that may have no hemodynamic consequences.

Aortic stenosis is most commonly caused by a congenital bicuspid valve that gradually thickens throughout life, becoming symptomatic in the later years. Aortic regurgitation may be caused by aortic root dilation (Marfan's) or rheumatic fever.

Tricuspid and pulmonic valve disease is much less common than the aortic and mitral valve problems.

Tricuspid disease is most often caused by rheumatic fever.

Pulmonic disease is most often due to congenital anomalies.

When the aortic or pulmonic valve is stenotic, the increased resistance leads to increased afterload on the ventricles, which usually leads to a **concentric hypertrophy.** Aortic or pulmonic insufficiency, on the other hand, leads to increased volume load on the heart, as a fraction of the ejected blood leaks back. This leads to **dilation** of the affected ventricle.

Lesion	Symptoms	Signs
Mitral stenosis	Dyspnea, orthopnea, PND	—
Mitral regurgitaiton (MR)	Pulmonary edema, fatigue	Holosystolic blowing murmur at the apex
Mitral prolapse	—	Midsystolic click, late systolic murmur
Aortic stenosis	Chest pain, syncope	—
Aortic regurgitation	—	High pitched diastolic murmur at the right upper sternal border
Tricuspid stenosis	RV failure, lower extremity edema, hepatic congestion	Tricuspid opening snap at the left lower sternal border
Tricuspid regurgitaiton	RV failure, lower extremity edema, hepatic congestion	Large v wave on JVP, blowing systolic murmur at the left lower sternal border

Table 2 Valvular lesions

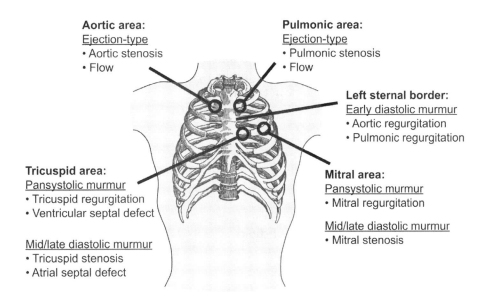

Aortic area:
Ejection-type
• Aortic stenosis
• Flow

Pulmonic area:
Ejection-type
• Pulmonic stenosis
• Flow

Left sternal border:
Early diastolic murmur
• Aortic regurgitation
• Pulmonic regurgitation

Tricuspid area:
Pansystolic murmur
• Tricuspid regurgitation
• Ventricular septal defect

Mid/late diastolic murmur
• Tricuspid stenosis
• Atrial septal defect

Mitral area:
Pansystolic murmur
• Mitral regurgitation

Mid/late diastolic murmur
• Mitral stenosis

Figure 44 Murmur locations

Signs and Symptoms

Please see Table 3.

Diagnosis

Diagnosis is based on echocardiography, with Doppler visualization of the regurgitation or stenosis. In stenosis, valve area can be estimated from the measured velocity of blood flow through that valve.

Treatment

General management involves (1) treating underlying pathology (e.g., endocarditis, rheumatic fever); (2) management of general symptoms and hemodynamic compromise (e.g., CHF); and (3) correction of the valvulopathy (valvuloplasty or valve replacement).

Prosthetic valves are either mechanical or bioprosthetic (bovine or porcine). Bioprostheses have the advantage of not requiring chronic anticoagulation but have a short lifespan of ~10 years. Mechanical valves require chronic anticoagulation but are far more durable than bioprosthetics.

RHEUMATIC FEVER

Following a group A streptococcal infection an autoimmune process may occur called rheumatic fever. Damage of heart valves (especially mitral) is a common consequence. In the underdeveloped world, mitral stenosis from rheumatic fever leads to significant morbidity and mortality.

Signs and Symptoms

The initial prodrome is pharyngitis: sore throat, fever, chills, and cough. Strep throat most often affects young school-aged children. Two to 3 weeks after the prodrome, if untreated, the patient develops one or more of the following: chorea, arthralgias, rash, fever, and malaise. **Aschoff bodies** are the classic lesion seen on the pathologic heart specimen.

Diagnosis

The diagnosis is based on clinical features. Tests include: blood culture, rapid strep antigen test, or antistreptolysin O titer (ASO-Titer).

Treatment

Antibioitcs (penicillin) are the treatment of choice.

BACTERIAL ENDOCARDITIS

Bacterial endocarditis is a bacterial infection of the endocardium and valves, usually by gram-positive cocci. Intravenous drug users are more likely to be infected with staphylococci. Previous valve damage (e.g., rheumatic fever), prosthetic valves, or other niduses for infection predispose to endocarditis.

- **Acute endocarditis** is usually due to *Staphylococcus* spp.

- **Subacute bacterial endocarditis** is usually due to *Streptococcus viridans*.

- **Nonbacterial (marantic) endocarditis** has fibrin deposits. **Libman-Sacks** lesions are nonbacterial endocardial vegetations seen in lupus patients.

Signs and Symptoms

The classic description of clinical findings in endocarditis likely result from microembolism of infectious vegetations to distal end organs. Fever, a new unexplained murmur, cutaneous stigmata (Osler nodes, Janeway lesions, petechiae, splinter hemorrhages), Roth spots (eyes), and end-organ damage (e.g., nephritis, embolic stroke) are all possible.

Diagnosis

Valvular vegetations can be seen on echocardiography, the diagnostic tool of choice. Positive blood cultures are also required.

Treatment

Appropriate antibiotics.

SYSTEMIC SHOCK

Shock can be simply defined as the inadequate delivery of blood flow to the peripheral tissues, resulting in end-organ dysfunction, systemic hypoxia, and eventually death. Shock is classified as follows:

- **Cardiogenic shock**: Pump failure leads to inadequate tissue perfusion. It can result from infarction, valve disease, cardiac tamponade, massive pulmonary embolism, and arrhythmias.

- **Hypovolemic shock**: Exsanguination, diarrhea, vomiting, diabetes with polyuria, burns, pancreatitis, or severe dehydration lead to intravascular volume depletion.

- **Distributive shock**: Lowered systemic vascular resistance leads to decreased perfusion. Distributive shock can arise from (1) sepsis or systemic inflammatory response syndrome, (2) anaphylaxis, or (3) autonomic dysfunction.

The end point of shock is inadequate end-organ perfusion, leading to altered mental status, myocardial ischemia, acute renal failure, bowel ischemia, and ischemia of the extremities. The body has several built-in compensatory mechanisms that kick in with progressive shock:

- **Increased sympathetic tone:** increases CO (increased rate and contractility) and systemic vascular resistance (arteriolar vasoconstriction), but it can lead to increased myocardial demand in the face of decreased coronary perfusion.

- **Hyper-renin state:** leads to retention of intravascular volume but contributes to renal insufficiency

- **Increased peripheral O_2 extraction**

Signs and Symptoms

Blood pressure is normal early in shock. Heart rate increases to match demand (compensated shock) until HR alone is not able to sustain blood pressure and hypotension ensues (uncompensated shock). Flat neck veins, dry mucous membranes, altered mental status, oliguria or anuria, presyncope or syncope, and tachypnea are present. The specific etiology determines other symptoms. Crackles of pulmonary edema suggest cardiogenic shock. Distributive shock typically presents as a "warm" shock with warm feeling skin. Signs of trauma may indicate hypovolemic shock, history of medication or atypical food intake suggests anaphylaxis, and fever may suggest sepsis.

Diagnosis

The etiology of shock must be determined to ensure proper management. Invasive hemodynamic monitoring is indicated if there is any uncertainty about the etiology of shock or about the patient's volume status. This is especially true when initial resuscitation fails to produce significant improvement

Treatment

General principles: ABCs (airway, breathing, circulation), then noninvasive and invasive monitoring:

- Initiate intensive care unit (ICU) or critical care unit monitoring.

- Ensure adequate oxygenation and ventilation (give supplemental O_2).

- Monitor hemodynamic status.

- Ensure vascular access with large-bore peripheral intravenous lines or central venous access or both.

Treatment of cardiogenic shock includes diuresis, inotropic agents, vasodilators if indicated, and intra-aortic balloon pump. Septic shock requires finding the source of infection, covering with appropriate antibiotics, and maintaining fluid status. Hypovolemia requires fluids and blood products. Anaphylactic shock is treated with epinephrine, steroids, and antihistamines. Specific inotropics, vasopressors, and vasodilators are often used; these are discussed under Pharmacology.

ANEURYSMS

Aneurysms are abnormal dilations of the vasculature. Aneurysms can be true aneurysms, when all three vessel wall layers are dilated, or pseudoaneurysms, where the intima dilates into the media and adventitia. In a dissection, a split in the intima lets blood and clot track into the vessel wall between the medial and adventitial layers, forming a **false lumen**.

Aortic aneurysm is an abnormal, localized dilation of the aorta. Most aortic aneurysms occur in the abdomen, with the remainder in the thorax. Abdominal aortic aneurysms (AAAs) are usually caused by atherosclerosis, which gradually weakens the vascular wall. Hypertension, smoking, a family history of abdominal aneurysms, trauma, and vasculitis may contribute. Two other causes of abdominal aortic aneurysm are **Marfan's syndrome** and **syphilis,** which are primary causes of thoracic (ascending) aortic aneurysms.

Signs and Symptoms

Sharp or tearing back pain radiating to the shoulders is the classic presentation for a dissecting aneurysm. Dissection is a true emergency.

Diagnosis

BP of all four limbs is crucial because an aneurysm that involves the artery or left subclavian causes the involved limb BP to be lower than the BP of other limbs. The patient may present in frank hypotensive shock. Ultrasound is a good means of imaging abdominal aortic aneurysms because the liver provides good acoustic access to the abdominal aorta. Thoracic aneurysms can be diagnosed best with angiography or CT. MRI is also a good diagnostic tool.

Treatment

Surgical candidates need to be taken immediately to the OR. BP must be controlled because excessive hypertension can worsen a possible dissection. Mortality is very high.

DISEASES INVOLVING THE PERICARDIUM

Cardiac Tamponade

Cardiac tamponade is caused by fluid accumulation in the pericardial space. The fluid collection prevents the ventricles from filling properly, leading to a **restrictive filling pattern**, which can cause hemodynamic collapse. The causes are trauma, ventricular wall rupture, malignant effusion, infectious effusion, and rheumatologic effusion.

Signs and Symptoms

Decreased intensity of heart sounds, decreased pulse pressure, neck vein distention, pulsus paradoxus.

Diagnosis

CXR may show increased cardiac silhouette size, and ECG may show decreased voltage or electrical alternans. Echocardiography is the diagnostic tool of choice. PA catheterization shows equalization of diastolic pressures because the tamponade compresses the heart chambers and equalizes filling pressures.

Treatment

Tamponade is a medical emergency requiring drainage of the fluid either percutaneously or surgically.

Pericarditis

Pericarditis is inflammation of the pericardium, which may be acute or chronic. Acute pericarditis is caused by infections, MI or cardiac surgery (Dressler's syndrome), uremia, radiation, autoimmune disease, and idiopathic causes. Chronic pericarditis leads to pericardial thickening and fibrosis as well as constriction. Constrictive pericarditis occurs with chronic pericardial inflammation that leads to fibrosis, impeding normal relaxation and filling of the ventricles. It has the same etiologies as acute pericarditis.

Signs and Symptoms

Sharp chest pain that changes with body position, friction rub on auscultation, pericardial effusion, and possibly tamponade. In chronic pericarditis, signs and symptoms of heart failure predominate. **Kussmaul's sign** may be present (observable distension of the jugular vein in the neck with inspiration).

Diagnosis

ECG may be diagnostic if **diffuse ST elevations** are seen with the chest pain, with PR segment depression. Echocardiography is the diagnostic tool of choice, demonstrating thickened pericardium, with or without an effusion. Treatable etiologies must be ruled out.

Treatment

Treat underlying etiologies, and otherwise, provide supportive care. Resolution usually occurs within 6–8 weeks. Corticosteroids and nonsteroidal anti-inflammatory drugs may help the inflammation and pain. Pericardectomy may be necessary in severe cases.

Myocarditis

Myocarditis is acute myocardial inflammation. Causes include infection of the myocardium (mainly viral, **particularly coxsackie**), production of a myocardial toxin (e.g., diphtheria), or an autoimmune inflammatory process (e.g., rheumatic fever). Bacterial infection is rare, but may be due to *Mycoplasma pneumoniae*, *Staphylococcus*, *Streptococcus*, or *Rickettsiae*. Parasites (e.g., trypanosomiasis) may also be the cause. Other causes include hypersensitivity reactions and radiation toxicity.

Signs and Symptoms

Fever, dyspnea, palpitations, and chest pain are common as are typical symptoms of heart failure.

Diagnosis

ECG shows nonspecific ST or T wave changes or arrhythmias with conduction system involvement.

Treatment

Antiarrhythmics if arrhythmias are present, treat the CHF, and give steroids if the etiology is clearly not infectious.

VASCULAR DISEASE AND VASCULITIS

Peripheral Arterial Vascular Disease

Intermittent claudication is a result of stenosis (usually atherosclerosis) of the lower extremities leading to calf pain on exercise and relieved by rest.

Signs and Symptoms

Patients experience leg pain on exertion that is relieved by rest. The amount of walking that precipitates pain is usually reproducible (e.g., five blocks). Patients may also display signs of poor circulation, including pallor, poor pulses, and cool extremities. Patients will also hang their legs over the side of the bed at night to relieve pain.

Diagnosis

Differential BPs in all four limbs: The ankle brachial index (ABI) is an excellent predictor of disease. ABI is the ratio of BP in the ankle to that of the arm. Angiography is the gold standard for diagnosis.

Treatment

Pentoxifylline is a drug that theoretically makes RBC membranes more pliant and thereby improves peripheral blood flow. The definitive treatment is surgical revascularization: Either native vein or synthetic grafts are used to bypass discrete lesions.

Polyarteritis Nodosa

Polyarteritis nodosa (PAN) is the inflammation of medium-sized muscular arteries, leading to ischemia. It is idiopathic but may be related to hypersensitivity reactions to drugs and viruses. Males are afflicted three times more often than females. The kidneys are the organ system most likely involved. A rapidly progressing glomerulonephritis may result. Cardiac involvement can lead to ischemia and MI. The GI, CNS, and skin can also be involved.

Signs and Symptoms

Pain and local ischemia in the affected area.

Diagnosis

Laboratory tests show elevated acute-phase reactants, urinalysis shows proteinuria and RBC casts, and complement may be low (from being depleted). Tissue biopsy is the definitive diagnostic tool. Blood test may be positive for pANCA, but the test is neither sensitive nor specific.

Treatment

Corticosteroids and immunosuppressants.

Granulomatosis with Polyangiitis (formerly Wegener's Granulomatosis)

Wegener's granulomatosis is systemic necrotizing vasculitis, with necrotizing granuloma formation in the upper and lower respiratory tract and involvement of other vascular beds. Incidence peaks in the fourth to fifth decades of life.

Signs and Symptoms

Upper respiratory infections (nasal congestion, sinusitis, mastoiditis, otitis media, etc.), ocular involvement, and skin nodules. Symptoms include cough, dyspnea, and hemoptysis.

Diagnosis

Laboratory tests show elevated acute-phase reactant levels and **positive cytoplasmic antineutrophil cytoplasmic antigen (cANCA)**. CXR demonstrates lung involvement, and definitive diagnosis requires tissue biopsy.

Treatment

Corticosteroids and cytotoxic agents.

Takayasu's Arteritis

Takayasu's arteritis is a vasculitis that favors the branches of the aortic arch. It is common in Asian females and known as **"pulseless disease"** because it results in absent arm pulses. BP is low but rarely symptomatic. The patients may show evidence of transient ischemic attacks (TIAs) and cerebrovascular insufficiency. Diagnosis is made by tissue biopsy, and treatment is with corticosteroids, although many patients do not require treatment.

Giant Cell (Temporal) Arteritis

Temporal arteritis favors small and medium vessels, and patients are usually older than age 50. Onset is usually insidious. Patients may note jaw claudication, headache, fatigue, vision changes, scalp tenderness, fever, weight loss, and malaise. Acute-phase reactants are elevated, and biopsy is required for definitive diagnosis. Treatment is with corticosteroids.

Raynaud's Phenomenon and Disease

Raynaud's phenomenon and disease are characterized by intermittent cyanosis of the fingers and toes caused by exposure to cold or emotional distress. Raynaud's disease is the idiopathic form caused by vasospasm of the digital arteries in a bilateral symmetric manner. Raynaud's phenomenon can be unilateral and limited to only one or two fingers. It can occur in the setting of rheumatoid arthritis, systemic lupus erythematosus, CREST, and mixed connective tissue disease. Young women are disproportionately affected.

Signs and Symptoms

Blue and/or pale fingers (and, less commonly, toes) following exposure to cold or emotional distress. During an attack, the fingers are stiff and painful. The digits can become markedly red and throbbing during recovery, due to compensatory hyperemia. Gangrenous ulcers may form on the fingertips.

Diagnosis

Evidence of other disorders (e.g., SLE, rheumatoid arthritis) on history and physical examination distinguish Raynaud's phenomenon from Raynaud's disease. Raynaud's can be differentiated from thromboangiitis obliterans (see below) because the former affects women and the latter men, and in the latter, peripheral pulses tend to be diminished.

Treatment

Treatment is to keep extremities warm and use calcium channel blockers, although the latter is controversial.

Thromboangiitis Obliterans (Buerger's Disease)

Thromboangiitis obliterans is a disease of **young male smokers**, most commonly in Ashkenazi Jews of Eastern European descent. It is characterized by peripheral ischemia secondary to inflammation and thrombosis of the arteries and veins.

Signs and Symptoms

You should be highly suspicious of the diagnosis of thromboangiitis obliterans if the patient is a male under 40 who smokes and demonstrates signs and symptoms of arterial insufficiency in the limbs: intermittent claudication, loss of distal arterial pulses, ischemic neuropathy, ulcers, or a cold distal foot or toe (often asymmetric). There may be a history of small, red, tender cords that are evidence of migratory superficial segmental thrombophlebitis. The course of the disease is usually intermittent, with flare-ups and remissions.

Diagnosis

History and physical examination. Absent peripheral pulses help differentiate thromboangiitis obliterans from Raynaud's disease and antiphospholipid antibody syndrome. The patient population is younger and may not have an established history of atherosclerosis, thus differentiating thromboangiitis obliterans from cholesterol atheroembolic disease.

Treatment

Smoking cessation is mandatory to prevent disease progression, which can lead to amputation of gangrenous fingers and toes.

Deep Venous Thrombosis

Deep venous thrombosis (DVT) is the development of a blood clot in a vein. **Thrombophlebitis** refers to a secondary inflammation of the clot, resulting in pain, tenderness, and warmth. DVT and thrombophlebitis most often occur in the lower extremities. The risk factors that may predispose to the development of **venous thrombi** are referred to as **Virchow's triad**: injury to the endothelium of the vessel (e.g., trauma), hypercoagulable states (e.g., malignancy, estrogen use), and stasis (e.g., postoperative states).

Varicose Veins

Varicose veins are distended, tortuous veins with incompetent valves. They can be caused by a bout with thrombophlebitis or occur congenitally. Most commonly, they result from conditions associated with increased lower-extremity venous pressure: pregnancy, prolonged standing, and ascites.

Signs and Symptoms

Many patients complain of the cosmetic disfiguration of varicosities in the superficial veins. There can be significant discomfort, relieved by elevation of the legs or elastic stockings. Chronic varicosities lead to venous insufficiency, with edema, hyperpigmentation, and ulcers (known as stasis dermatitis). Lymphatic obstruction must be considered in the differential diagnosis.

Diagnosis

Physical examination, with particular attention to the lower extremities.

Treatment

Compression stockings, with venous stripping or sclerosis of the saphenous vein as a last resort.

NEOPLASMS OF THE CARDIOVASCULAR SYSTEM

Cardiovascular tumors are rare. The most common primary tumor is the myxoma, which is usually benign. It arises from the endocardial surface, mostly in the LA but can be found anywhere. According to the 10/10 rule, 10% of myxomas are from the LA, and 10% of myxomas are malignant. Other malignant tumors include sarcomas (e.g., angiosarcoma and rhabdosarcoma). Metastatic tumors are much more common than primary neoplasms and include hematologic malignancies, melanoma, and lung and breast cancer. They tend to involve the pericardium and cause pericarditis and hemorrhagic effusions.

Signs and Symptoms

The patient may have signs of heart failure, a possible stroke from cancer or clot embolization, or other systemic symptoms (e.g., fever, night sweats, weight loss).

Diagnosis

On examination, a "plop" may sometimes be heard from the pedunculated myxoma falling onto the mitral valve. A murmur is common, and it may change with body position. Echocardiography is the diagnostic tool of choice.

Treatment

Surgical excision

CONGENITAL HEART DISEASE

Congenital defects are broadly classified as cyanotic or acyanotic. Cyanotic lesions are ones that result in a right-to-left shunt, bypassing the lungs and causing deoxygenated blood to be pumped to the body.

Acyanotic Congenital Heart Defects

Atrial septal defect (ASD): Patients are often asymptomatic until adulthood, when prolonged left-to-right shunt leads to pulmonary hypertension and heart failure. Classically diagnosed with a **wide, 'fixed' split S2** and a pulmonary flow murmur.

Ventricular septal defect (VSD): VSD is the most common congenital cardiac defect. A small VSD may be hemodynamically insignificant but produce a loud murmur. On the other hand, a very large VSD may cause significant L to R shunting but no murmur may be heard. Long standing left-to-right shunt decreases as pulmonary vascular resistance increases (compensatory). The ensuing pulmonary hypertension results in a right-to-left shunt and cyanosis **(Eisenmenger's syndrome)**. A holosystolic murmur is heard at the lower left sternal border, radiating to the right, with or without signs of pulmonary hypertension.

Patent ductus arteriosus (PDA): PDA is common in premature infants and more frequent in kids born at higher altitudes. Normally, the ductus begins to close soon after birth but may not completely close until 4 weeks after birth. Classically diagnosed as a **"machinery like"** continuous murmur. If left untreated, Eisenmenger's syndrome may develop and cause R to L shunting in the duct, which causes **differential cyanosis** (pink fingers supplied by the subclavian and blue toes fed by PDA). PDA can by medically closed with indomethacin or kept open with prostaglandins in the cases of cyanotic congenital heart disease.

Pulmonic stenosis (PS): PS can be valvular, subvalvular, or supravalvular. A systolic murmur is heard at the left upper sternal border, and signs of right heart failure are present.

Aortic stenosis: A bicuspid aortic valve is the most common congenital cardiac anomaly seen in adults and is seen in 2% of the population. Congenital aortic stenosis is usually more symptomatic. A systolic murmur is heard at the right upper sternal border with radiation to the carotids. The murmur is louder with squatting and softer with Valsalva or handgrip.

Coarctation of the aorta: This is a narrowing of the aorta that can be located anywhere from the aortic root to the descending aorta. It is usually located "juxtaductal" just opposite of the PDA. **Associated with Turner's Syndrome.**

The rule of **5** for cyanotic heart disease:

1. Truncus has 1 vessel

2. Tansposition has 2 vessels reversed

3. "Tri"cuspid atresia

Situs inversus: Failure of organ rotation during development leads to reversal of organ location along the longitudinal axis of the body. The heart can be displaced to the right (dextroversion) or flipped around its axis so that the apex points to the right (dextrocardia), or both. In the case of situs inversus in **Kartagener's syndrome** (ciliary dysmotility syndrome), there is also bronchiectasis, chronic sinusitis, and infertility.

Cyanotic Lesions

Truncus arteriosus: One big vessel with a bicuspid valve leaves a single ventricle, replacing the normal aorta and pulmonary trunk. Because the lungs and body see the same blood oxygenation and blood pressure, severe cyanosis and pulmonary hypertension result.

Transposition of the great vessels: The great vessels (the aorta and pulmonary artery) exit the wrong ventricle causing the pulmonary and systemic circulations flow in **parallel instead of in series**. There is usually bidirectional shunting, and the more shunting there is, the more likely the patient is to survive.

Tricuspid atresia: The tricuspid valve is absent and so the RA and RV do not connect. The patients survive because there is usually an associated ASD and VSD.

Tetralogy of Fallot: This is the most common cyanotic congenital anomaly seen in adults. It includes: VSD, pulmonic stenosis, an 'overriding' aorta, and RV hypertrophy (a result of the other defects). Patients classically have "spells" of cyanosis, hyperpnea, and syncope as a result of intermittent increases in right-to-left shunting. Without treatment, the pulmonic stenosis worsens gradually, leading to increased cyanosis. Diagnosis is with echocardiography and catheterization, and treatment is surgical. Because of the extensive right heart involvement, postsurgical heart block and other arrhythmias are fairly common.

Total anomalous pulmonary venous return: Oxygenated blood returning from the lungs enters the RA instead of the LA. An ASD is usually present, and so the RA blood (mixed with venous return blood) enters the LA through the ASD. The increased fraction of deoxygenated blood results in cyanosis. Increased pulmonary flow leads to pulmonary hypertension.

PHARMACOLOGY

Adrenergic agonists and antagonists are discussed in chapter 14. Specific applications are discussed in each disease entity.

Direct Vasodilators

Direct vasodilators are used primarily for control of hypertension in the acute situation (ICU, emergency room, OR) (Table 4).

Antihypertensives

The four major classes of antihypertensive drugs are as follows:

- β-Blockers
- Calcium channel blockers
- Diuretics
- ACE inhibitors

β-Blockers are discussed in chapter 4, and diuretics are discussed in chapter 14. Calcium channel blockers are discussed later. The major ACE inhibitors are listed in Table 4.

Drug	Mechanism	Toxicities
Nitroprusside	Similar to nitric oxide; direct smooth musle relaxant	Hypotension; prolonged use leads to cynanide toxicity
Nitrates Nitroglycerin Isosorbide dinitrate	Similar to nitric oxide; direct smooth musle relaxant (used for hypotension and angina)	Hypotension
Hydralazine, minoxidil	Direct smooth muscle relaxant	Hypotension
	α-antagonist	Orthostatic hypotension, loss of sympathetic tone
Clonidine	CNS agonist	Hypotension

Table 3 Vasodilators

Drug	Mechanism	Toxicities
	Blocks ACE, disrupting the renin-angiotensin system	Hypotension; prolonged use leads to cynanide toxicity
Losartan	Angiotensin II receptor inhibitor	Vasodilation, decreased venous return; less cough than ACE inhibitors

Table 4 Angiotensin-Converting-Enzyme (ACE) Inhibitors

Antiarrhythmics

Antiarrhythmics are classified according to four classes (Table 5). Specific antiarrhythmics are listed in Table 6. Antiarrhythmics can be pretty daunting. The following are some high-yield facts:

Lidocaine is the first-line agent for prophylaxis against and treatment of ventricular arrhythmias (ventricular tachycardia and the dreaded ventricular fibrillation). Beware its side effects: tremors, anxiety, seizures, and confusion. Also be aware that lidocaine accidentally given intravenously during administration of local anesthesia can *cause* arrhythmias.

Amiodarone may be the best antiarrhythmic drug, in terms of efficaciousness and proven survival benefits. It is effective in most types of arrhythmias. Important side effects are pulmonary fibrosis, liver dysfunction, and thyroid function abnormalities.

Adenosine is a very short-acting drug that slows AV node conduction. It can be used to aid in diagnosis of a supraventricular tachycardia, and it can also break an AV nodal arrhythmia.

Check **LFTs, PFTs**, and **TFTs** with Amiodarone

Class	Mechanism	Effects
Class IA	Na^+ channel blocker	Prolongs the action potential duration
Class IB	Na^+ channel blocker	Reduces maximum velocity of upstrokes
Class IC	Na^+ channel blocker	Prolongs retractory period
Class II	β-Blockers	Slows conduction through the AV junction
Class III	K^+ channel blockers	Prolongs action potential
Class IV	Ca^{2+} channel blocker	Blocks slow inward current

Table 5 Classes of antiarrhythmics

Digoxin

Digoxin is a drug with multiple effects. It blocks the cell membrane Na^+/K^+ pump, prevents Na^+ extrusion from the cell, which then inhibits the Na^+/Ca^{2+} exchanger, resulting in increased intracellular calcium. The increased intracellular calcium directly increases contractility. The secondary effect of digoxin is a slowing of conduction through the AV node. Uses include the following:

- CHF, for increased contractility

- Supraventricular arrhythmias, including atrial fibrillation

Side effects include premature beats, tachycardia, and fibrillation. Severe digitalis toxicity can cause cardiac arrest. Treatment for digoxin toxicity includes the following:

- K^+: antagonizes effect on Na^+/K^+ pump

- Magnesium: antagonizes calcium

- Digoxin immune Fab: antibodies directed against digoxin

Drug	Mechanism	Uses	Side effects
Quinidine	Class IA	Long term treatment of atrial and ventricular arrhythmias (atrial fibrilation, atrial flutter, SVT)	—
Procainamide	Class IA	Same as quinidine	—
Disopyramide	Class IA	Same as quinidine	Urinary retenion, CHF, constipation, blurred vision, glaucoma
Lidocaine	Class IB	Acute ventricular arrhythmias	Dizziness, paresthesias, confusion, coma
Mexiletine	Class IB	Same as lidocaine	—
Tocainide	Class IB	Ventricular tachyarrhythmias	Similar to lidocaine
Flecainide	Class IC	—	CHF, increased ventricular tachyarrhythmias
Propafenone	Class IC	—	Dizziness, blurred vision
Sotalol		Chronic treatment of ventricular arrhythmias	—
Carvedilol	Class II	Atrial and ventricular arrhythmias in the context of acute MI; affects myocardial remodeling	CHF
Bretylium	Class III	Life-threatening ventricular arrhythmias unresponsive to other agents	Orthostatic hypotension, arrhythmias, and vomiting

Table 6 Class I, II, and III Antiarrhythmics

Thrombolytics

In acute MI, coronary occlusion is thought to involve a combination of mechanical occlusion and local activation of the clotting cascade, leading to thrombus formation within the coronaries. Thrombolytics are often used in acute MI. Thrombolytics and anticoagulants (e.g., warfarin, heparin) are discussed in Chapter 14.

Drug	Mechanism	Uses	Toxicities
Nifedipine	Class IV	Coronary and peripheral vasodilation, hypertension, Prinzmetal's angina	Hypotension; nausea and vomiting, bradycardia, left ventricular failure
Diltiazem	Class IV	Supraventricular tachyarrhythmias	Same as nifedipine
Verapamil	Class IV	Supraventricular tachyarrhythmias	Same as nifedipine
Long-acting agents: Amlodipine Felodipine	Class IV	Long-term treatment of hypertension	Same as nifedipine

Table 7 Calcium channel blockers

Cholesterol- and Lipid-Lowering Agents

Table 8 lists common cholesterol- and lipid lowering agents.

Drug	Mechanism	Uses	Side effects
Cholestyramine	Intraluminal GI lipid-binding resin	Elevated LDL	—
Lovastatin, pravastain, simvastatin	HMG-CoA reductase inhibitor; inhibits mevalonate (cholesterol precursor) synthesis	Elevated LDL, elevated triglycerides	Myopathy, hepatotoxicity (monitor CK levels and LFTs every few months)
Gemfibrozi, clofibrate	Increases the activity of lipoprotein lipase	Elevated LDL,VLDL, or triglycerides	Myalgia, liver dysfunction, rash, nausea and vomiting
Niacin	Decreases cholesterol, VLDL synthesis	Elevated LDL, familial hyperlipidemias	Flushing, rash, liver dysfunction
Probucol	Antioxidant; increases LDL and cholesterol destruction and excretion	Hypercholesterolemia, familial hypercholesterolemias	Arrhythmias

Table 8 Cholesterol- and lipid-lowering agents

CHAPTER 5

CELL BIOLOGY

A cell is the basic structural and functional unit for all known living organisms. Each individual cell is separated and defined from other cells and the external environment by its **plasma membrane**. Plasma membrane acts as a fluid mosaic, semi-permeable barrier and also contains different **organelles**, the structural and functional subunits of a cell.

A thorough understanding of the structure and function of a cell allows a deeper understanding of both normal physiology and abnormal disease processes. In this chapter, we will review basic cell biology, placing special emphasis on the role of each cellular component as it pertains to medical pathology.

PLASMA MEMBRANE

The **plasma membrane** is a fluid mosaic model made up of two major components: *lipids* and *proteins,* which form an asymmetric lipid bilayer. The diversity in structure and function of these lipids and proteins allow the plasma membrane to serve several different functions:

1. Protect the cell

2. Regulate transport of material in and out of the cell

3. Communicate with other cells and the external environment

4. Allow for cellular recognition

Phospholipids are the most common lipid found in the plasma membrane, but **sphingolipids**, **glycolipids**, and **cholesterol** are also present. All of these lipids have one polar hydrophilic ("water-loving") head and a nonpolar hydrophobic ("water-fearing") tail, which allows for the formation of a lipid bilayer. Hydrophilic heads interact with water on the intracellular and extracellular surfaces, while hydrophobic tails remain within the lipid bilayer (Figure 1). It is this lipid bilayer that protects the cell and prevents entry of unwanted materials into the intracellular space.

There are certain lysosomal storage diseases that result in the accumulation of specific sphingolipids, such as sphingomyelin in Niemann-Pick, glucocerebroside in Gaucher's disease, and GM2 ganglioside in Tay-Sachs disease (Table 3).

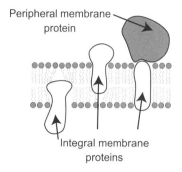

Figure 1 Membrane bilayer
(Adapted from *Biochemistry* 2nd Ed.)

Phospholipids are made of one phosphate group and two fatty acid chains, esterified to a glycerol backbone (Figure 2). Sphingolipids are made of a sphingosine, a fatty acid chain, and an additional moiety group, which determines the subtype of sphingolipid, such as sphingomyelin, cerebroside and ganglioside (Figure 3). The varying lengths and chemical characteristics of the fatty acid chains in lipids affect the fluidity and melting temperature of the overall membrane: longer and more saturated fatty acids result in decreased fluidity and higher melting temperatures.

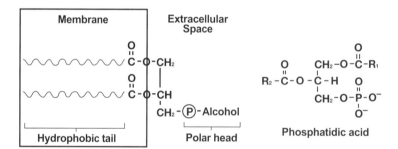

Figure 2 Phospholipid structure

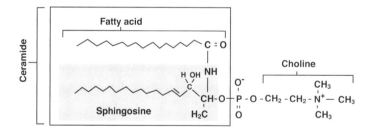

Figure 3 Sphingomyelin structure

Glycolipids are lipids with a carbohydrate group attached. They are located on the extracellular face of the plasma membrane lipid bilayer and may serve as receptors or signals on the surface of the cell, identifying it to other cells and the environment.

Cholesterol functions to enhance the mechanical stability of the membrane and regulates membrane fluidity.

Thus, while the lipid portions of the plasma membranes predominantly act to form the protective barrier for the cell, it is the proteins portion that makes the plasma membrane functionally dynamic. These proteins on plasma membrane may be transmembrane (spanning across the entire lipid bilayer) or peripheral (bound to either the intracellular or extracellular face of the membrane). Carbohydrate groups can also attach to membrane proteins, forming glycoproteins, which like glycolipids, may serve as receptors or signals of the surface of the cell.

Ion Channels and Pumps

Membrane proteins are able to regulate transport of material in and out of the cell by forming channels and pumps.

Simple diffusion describes the movement of particles down an electrochemical gradient with no protein carrier. Gases and small lipophilic molecules typically undergo simple diffusion (e.g. O_2, CO_2, NO, DNP, and steroids).

Facilitated diffusion is the movement of a compound down its electrochemical gradient with help of a carrier protein in the membrane. Larger and polar molecules typically undergo either facilitated diffusion or active transport such as glucose, amino acids, fatty acids, and ions (K^+, Na^+, Ca^{2+}, Cl^-). The channels through which facilitated diffusion occurs are classified into the following categories:

1. **Voltage-gated channels** switch between closed and open conformations with changes in membrane potential. For example, Na^+ and K^+ channels in the plasma membranes of nerve axons and the Ca^{2+} channels found in muscle cells are examples of voltage-gated channels responsible for the initiation of action potentials (Figure 4).

2. **Ligand-gated channels** open and close in response to binding of small molecules, proteins, and covalent modification.

3. **Stretch-activated channels** switch between closed and open forms via mechanical deformation of the plasma membrane.

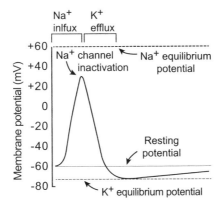

Figure 4 Action Potential

Tetrodoxin, found in the puffer fish, causes respiratory paralysis by binding to Na^+ channel pores and thus blocking nerve impulse conduction.

There are two types of Ca^{2+} channels in cardiac muscle. Dihydropyridine receptors, the target of calcium channel blockers are voltage-gated, while ryanodine receptors, the target of dantrolene, are ligand-gated.

Ouabain, a cardiac glycoside, inhibits the Na$^+$-K$^+$ ATPase by binding to the K$^+$ site.

Digoxin directly inhibits the Na$^+$-K$^+$ ATPase leading to resulting inhibition of Na$^+$/Ca^{2+} exchange and build up of Ca^{2+} in the cell, leading to increased cardiac contractility.

Familial hypercholesterolemia is characterized by defective endocytosis. LDL carry cholesterol in the blood and are taken up into cells by LDL-receptors. Defects in LDL-receptor synthesis leads to elevated serum cholesterol levels and atherosclerosis.

Active transport is the movement of a compound against its concentration gradient using the energy stored in adenosine triphosphate (ATP) (e.g. the Na$^+$-K$^+$ ATPase and Ca^{2+} pumps).

The Na$^+$-K$^+$ ATPase is an integral plasma membrane protein with ATP binding site. For every ATP molecule consumed leading to phosphorylation, 3 Na$^+$ are pumped into the cell and the 2 K$^+$ are pumped out of the cell.

Endocytosis

Endocytosis is another mechanism by which extracellular material may enter the cell. This process is involved in nutrient uptake, receptor internalization, membrane recycling, and antigen presentation. **Receptor-mediated endocytosis** begins when a protein or ligand binds to a receptor on a clathrin-coated pit of cell surface. Once bound, endocytosis is initiated by budding of a clathrin-coated vesicle from the plasma membrane. These vesicles fuse with early endosomes inside the cell and the clathrin-coat is recycled to the plasma membrane. Inside these endosomes, receptors and ligands are allocated to their final destination. Receptors return to the cell surface and ligands are directed for further processing in the lysosomes (Figure 5).

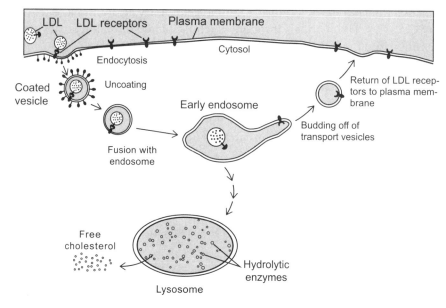

Figure 5 Endocytosis (LDL = low-density lipoprotein). (Adapted from *Molecular Biology of the Cell* 2nd Ed.)

Second Messenger Systems

Plasma membrane proteins can also act as intermediaries between a cell and the outside world, initiating signal transduction cascades by which "messages" to the cell can be amplified and executed. The two major signaling mechanisms occur via: *G protein-coupled receptors* and *phosphorylation cascades*.

G protein-coupled receptors are plasma membrane proteins consisting of 7 transmembrane a-helices that are activated by the binding of a molecule or absorption of a photon on the cell surface. The G protein portion is bound to the intracellular portion of the plasma membrane and are composed of three polypeptide chains: α, β, and γ (Figure 6). When the α subunit is bound to a guanosine triphosphate (GTP) group the G protein is in an active state. Upon hydrolysis of the GTP to guanosine diphosphate (GDP), the G protein complex becomes inactivated.

There are different classes of G proteins, each with different signal cascades, including G_s (stimulatory and activates adenylate cyclase), G_i (inhibitory and inhibits adenylate cyclase), and G_q (activates phospholipase C). Muscarinic acetylcholine (ach) receptors are members of the G protein-coupled receptor family, unlike nicotinic acetylcholine receptors, which are ligand-gated ion channels.

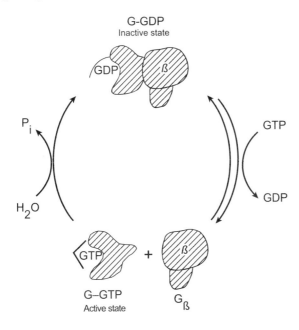

Figure 6 Activation and inactivation of G proteins

Phosphorylation cascades are activated when a ligand binds to a plasma membrane protein with intrinsic tyrosine kinase activity, leading to receptor dimerization and the initiation of a signal transduction cascade.

ORGANELLES

Smooth endoplasmic reticulum

Smooth endoplasmic reticulum (SER) is a lipid bilayer similar in structure to the plasma membrane. Within the cell, it is the site of *steroid synthesis* and *detoxification* of drugs and toxins (Figure 7).

The smooth ER and mitochondria synthesize steroid hormones, such as glucocorticoids, androgens, and estrogen. The SER is specifically involved in the synthesis of cholesterol, a steroid hormone precursor and in the final steps of steroid modification.

Most receptors for growth hormone (GH), prolactin, and cytokines have intrinsic tyrosine kinase activity and activate phosphorylation cascades.

Steroid producing cells in the liver and adrenal cortex are rich with SER.

In neurons, RER consists of Nissl bodies, which synthesize peptide neurotransmitters.

Other cells rich in RER:
Plasma cells: secrete antibodies

Goblet cells in the GI tract: secrete mucus

Pancreatic cells: secrete pancreatic enzymes

In liver cells, enzymes like **cytochrome P-450 oxidase** are located in the SER and enable detoxification of compounds by biochemical modification. Cytochrome P-450 oxidase inactivates and also facilitates clearance of certain drugs and toxins by increasing their solubility through hydroxylation. For USMLE, it is important to know which drugs and toxins induce or inhibit the activity of cytochrome P-450 enzymes (Table 1).

Rough Endoplasmic Reticulum

Rough endoplasmic reticulum (RER) is essentially an SER with ribosomes attached to the lipid bilayer, making the surface appear "rough." Within the ribosome, proteins destined either for the plasma membrane or for secretion are synthesized. Like the SER, the RER also contains P-450 enzymes, which function in protein modification.

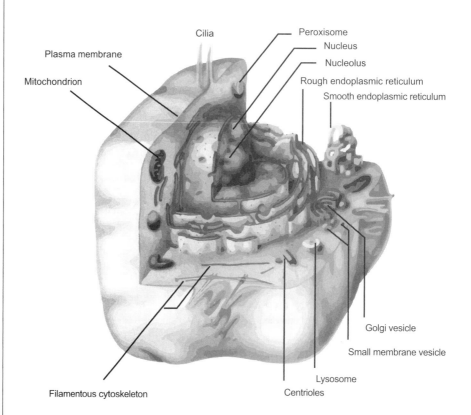

Figure 7 Cell structure and organelles
(Adapted from *Molecular Cell Biology* 2nd Ed.)

Inducers of P-450 enzymes	Inhibitors of P-450 enzymes
Barbituates	Acute alcohol use
Carbamazepine	Cimetidine
Chronic alcohol use	Erythromycin
Griseofulvin	Grapefruit juice
Phenytoin	HIV protease inhibitors: e.g. Indinavir
Quinidine*	Isoniazid
Rifampin	Ketoconazole
St. John's wort	Sulfonamides

Mnemonic: Inducers		Mnemonic: Inhibitors
Cars and **C**hronic **A**lcohol use at	**C**hronic **A**lcohol	I'm **SICK** of **AGE**-ing. I wish I could <u>inhibit</u> the <u>P</u>rocess.
Bars	**B**arbituates	**S**ulfonamides
GReatly	**Gr**iseofulvin	**I**soniazid
STains	**St**. John's wort	**C**imetidine
People's	**P**henytoin	**K**etoconazole
Quiet	**Q**uinidine	**A**cute alcohol
Reputations	**R**ifampin	**G**rapefruit juice
		Erythromycin
		Protease **in**hibitors (HIV medication)

Quinidine may also act to inhibit P-450 enzymes but to a lesser effect.

Table 1 P-450 enzyme interactions

Golgi Apparatus

The **Golgi apparatus** is a group of stacked, flattened sacs with lipid bilayers that acts as the cell's distribution center (Figure 8). Proteins from the RER are modified and sorted in the Golgi apparatus before they are sent to their final destinations (Table 2). There are specific proteins that are responsible for the vesicular transportation of proteins between the Golgi and RER that you need to know for the USMLE:

- COPI (coat protein I) has retrograde function, transporting from the Golgi back to the RER.

- COPII (coat protein II) has anterograde function, transporting from the RER to the cis-Golgi

- Clathrin transports proteins from the trans-Golgi to the lysosomes and plasma membrane.

Clathrin is also involved in receptor-mediated endocytosis, transporting proteins from the plasma membrane to endosomes.

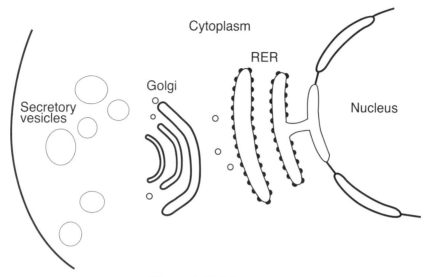

Figure 8 Golgi apparatus
(Adapted from *Cell and Tissue Ultrastructure: A Functional Perspective*)

Function	Location
Modification of N-oligosaccharides	Asparagine amino acid residues
Addition of O-oligosaccharides	Serine and threonine residues
Addition of Mannose-6-Phosphate	On lysosomal proteins (Mannose -6-Phosphate targets those proteins to the lysosome.)
Assembly of Proteoglycans	Non-specific
Sulfation	Sugars on proteoglycans
	Tyrosine residues

Table 2 Specific modifications by the Golgi apparatus

Lysosomes

Lysosomes are the part of the cell in which waste materials and cellular debris are digested by hydrolytic enzymes. ATP-dependent H^+ pumps maintain the acidic interior of lysosomes (pH < 5), which is essential for proper functioning. Membrane vesicles derived from endocytosis or phagocytosis fuse with the lysosomes, allowing their contents to be digested by action of acid hydrolases.

Inclusion cell disease is a genetic condition characterized by empty lysosomes. It is caused by the failure to add mannose-6-phosphate to lysosome proteins, resulting in the expulsion of these proteins out of the cell. Clinical manifestations include coarse facial features, stiff joints, corneal clouding, and mental retardation.

Deficiency in enzymes that lead to lysosomal storage disease is listed in Table 3.

Peroxisomes

Peroxisomes are membrane bound organelles containing oxidases. In the cell, the peroxisome is the site of fatty acid oxidation to acetyl CoA. Some of the oxidative reactions that take place in the peroxisomes generate peroxide (H_2O_2), which is a toxic compound and degraded by catalase into H_2O and O_2.

Zellweger syndrome is an autosomal recessive disease characterized by the lack of peroxisomes in the CNS. Patients accumulate long-chain fatty acids in the cell and are unable to form myelin, resulting in hypotonia, seizures, hepatomegaly, mental retardation, and early death.

Refsum disease is caused by peroxisomal phytanic acid oxidase deficiency. It is milder than Zellweger disease and patients are instructed to avoid chlorophyll, the source of phytanic acid.

Mitochondria

Mitochondria is the site of ATP production and is considered the energy generator of the cell. The inner mitochondrial membrane has many foldings, called cristae, which surrounds the inner matrix. The TCA cycle occurs in the mitochondrial matrix, whereas the electron transport chain and ATP production take place across the inner mitochondrial membrane. The mitochondria also make some of their own proteins as the mitochondria matrix contains its own DNA and ribosomes.

Leber's hereditary optic neuropathy is a mitochondrial disease characterized by central vision loss due to degeneration of the retina and optic nerves.

All mitochondrial diseases are maternally inherited. However, there is variable expression of mitochondrial diseases due to heteroplasmy or the presence of both normal and mutated mitochondrial DNA in each individual. Mitochondrial diseases most commonly affect muscle cells and neurons, where the mitochondria is most metabolically active. The most common mitochondrial diseases are neuromuscular conditions called mitochondrial myopathies, characterized by ragged red muscle fibers.

THE NUCLEUS

Chromosome Structure

Eukaryotic DNA is organized in the form **chromatin**—negatively charged supercoiled DNA wrapped around nucleosome cores (Figure 9). Nucleosomes are composed of positively charged histone octamers: 2 sets of H2A, H2B, H3, and H4 proteins with positively charged lysine and arginine amino acids. An H1 histone links and folds the nucleosomes through a series of successively higher order structures to form a chromosome. This process increases regulatory control for correct gene expression and also greatly condenses the size of DNA.

Chromatins are DNA and proteins that make up the nucleus of a cell. There are two types of chromatin:

1. **Heterochromatin** is methylated but non-acetylated, representing the more condensed form of chromatin. It is transcriptionally inactive.

2. **Euchromatin** is acetylated but non-methylated, representing the less condensed form of chromatin. It is transcriptionally active.

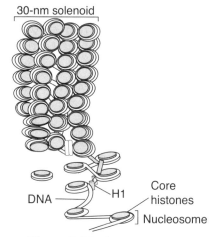

Figure 9 Nucleosome structure

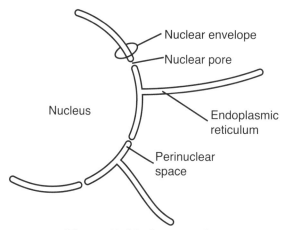

Figure 10 Nuclear membrane
(Adapted from *Cell and Tissue Ultrastructure: A Functional Perspective*)

Nuclear Envelope

The nucleus is separated from the cytoplasm by the nuclear envelope, which consists of a set of parallel membranes enclosing a perinuclear space (Figure 10). The outer membrane of the nuclear envelope is continuous with the ER, and the perinuclear space is rich in proteins. The inner membrane contains proteins called lamins A, B, and C, which facilitate the organization of nuclear pore complexes.

Nucleolus

Ribosomes are produced in the nucleolus, the largest structure in the cell nucleus. The precursor 45S ribosomal RNAs allocated into a 40S small ribosomal subunit and a 60S large ribosomal subunit. Both subunits exit the nucleus via nuclear pores on the nuclear membrane.

CYTOSKELETON

The cytoskeleton of a cell is a dynamic structure, allowing for cell movement, cytokinesis, and the organization of organelles. There are three primary fibers that make up the cytoskeleton. These fibers are listed in order of increasing size:

1. Microfilaments or actin

2. Intermediate filaments

3. Microtubules

Actin

Actin filaments, or **F-actin**, are present in every cell. G-actin is the monomer subunit of the F-actin polymer. These two forms of actin are in constant equilibrium within the cell (Figure 11A).

Lysosomal storage disease	Defective lysosomal enzyme	Accumulated substrate	Characteristics
Sphingolipidoses: accumulation of sphingolipids			
Gaucher's disease* most common -AR	β-glucocere brosidase	Glucocerebro-side	Hepatospleno-megaly, bone pain and frac-tures, Gaucher's cells (macro-phages resem-bling crumpled tissue paper), neuro-dysfunc-tion
Niemann-Pick disease* -AR	Sphingomyelin-ase phingomy-elinase	Sphingomyelin	Cherry-red spot on macula, foam cells (macro-phages in liver and spleen), progressive neu-ro-dysfunction, death usually before age 3

Put a *Hex* on *Sax, so there's NO Hepatospleno-megaly*

Tay-Sachs disease* -AR	Hexosamindase A	GM2 ganglioside	NO hepato-spleno-megaly, cherry-red spot on macula, lysosomes with "onion skin," progressive neuro-dysfunction, developmental delay
Farber disease -AR	Ceramidase	Ceramide	Granulomas and nodules in skin and around joints, neurological deficits
Krabbe's disease -AR	Galactocerebrosidase	Galactocerebroside	Peripheral neuropathy, developmental delay, globoid cells (multi-nucleated macrophages)
Metochromatic leukodystrophy -AR	Arylsulfatase A	Cerebroside sulfate	Central and peripheral neuropathy (demyelination), dementia, hereditary ataxia
Fabry's disease -XR	α-galactosidase A	Ceramide tri-hexoside	Peripheral neuropathy, cardiovascular, renal disease, angiokeratomas
Mucopolysacharidsoses: accumulation of glycosominoglycans (GAGs)			
Hurler's syndrome -AR	α-L-iduronidase	Heparan sulfate, dermatan sulfate	Clouding of corneas, coarse facies (gargoylism), developmental delay
Hunter's syndrome -XR	Iduronate sulfatase	Heparan sulfate, dermatan sulfate	NO clouding of corneas, developmental delay, coarse facies, aggressive behavior

* = more common in Ashkenazi Jews; AR = autosomal recessive; XR = X-linked recessive

Table 3 Lysosomal storage diseases

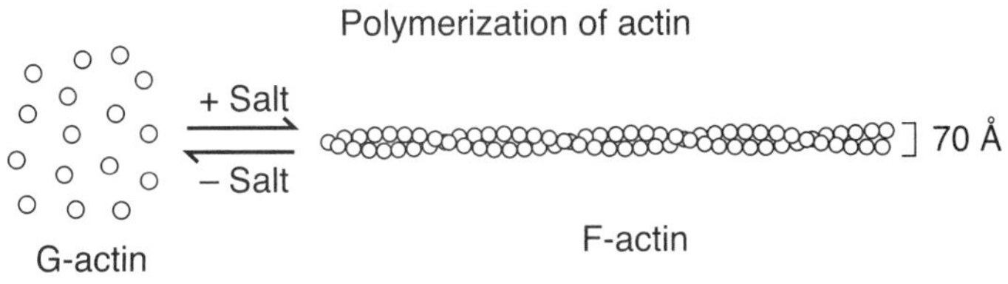

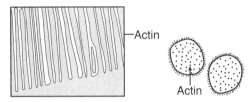

Polymerization of actin

G-actin

+ Salt
− Salt

70 Å

F-actin

Figure 11A Microtubular structure
(Adapted from *Cell and Tissue Ultrastructure: A Functional Perspective*)

—Actin

Actin

Figure 11B Cilia cross-section

Actin has numerous roles in the cell. Actin filaments, such as myosin and tropomyosin, enable muscle contraction by binding to accessory proteins in muscle cells. In the gastrointestinal (GI) tract, actin is a major component of microvilli (Figure 11B). The rapid polymerization and depolymerization of actin chains within the cell enable cellular migration and cytokinesis. In addition, actin filaments are involved in forming zona adherens, or intermediate junctions, between cells.

Intermediate Filaments

Intermediate filaments (IF) are fibrous and stable components that provide tensile strength for the cell. There are five classes of intermediate fibers, each of which has a corresponding immunohistochemical stain:

1. Cytokeratin in epithelial cells

2. Desmin in muscle cells

3. Glial fibrillary acidic protein (GFAP) in neuroglia

4. Neurofilaments in neurons

5. Vimentin in connective tissue fibroblasts

Immunohistochemical staining of these different IF can be useful in identifying abnormal cells or monitoring for disease progression.

Microtubules

Microtubules are large tubular polymers consisting of 13 protofilaments arranged in a circular fashion. Each protofilament is composed of polymerized dimers of α and β **tubulin** monomers (Figure 12A). These polymers grow slowly but are able to collapse very quickly, enabling intracellular and extracellular motion.

Microtubules make up the spindle apparatus and centrioles involved in separating chromosomes during mitosis.

Microtubules have several functions in the cell, one of which is to act as scaffolding and, thus, determine cell shape. This scaffolding may be used as "tracks" within the cell, facilitating intracellular movement. In neurons, kinesin is a protein that binds to microtubules and "carries" vesicles down the axon away from the cell body, resulting in anterograde movement. Dynein moves organelles in the opposite direction, toward the nucleus, resulting in retrograde movement.

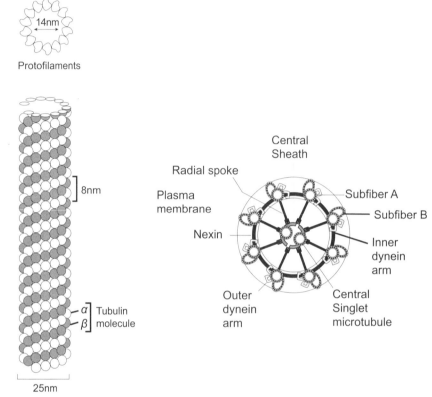

Figure 12A Microtubular structure   **12B** Cilia cross-section
(Adapted from *Cell and Tissue Ultrastructure: A Functional Perspective*)

Microtubules are also found in cilia and sperm flagellae, in a 9+2 arrangement or nine microtubules encircling two microtubules (Figure 12B). Axonemal dyneins are linked to each of the nine peripheral microtubules and function as ATPases, powering the motion of the cilia and flagellae.

Drugs that act on microtubules:

- Colchicine (anti-gout)

- Griseofulvin (antifungal)

- Mebendazole (antihelminthic)

- Paclitaxel (anti-cancer)

- Vincristine and vinblastine (anti-cancer)

Chédiak-Higashi syndrome is an immune deficient condition characterized by microtubule dysfunction, resulting in impaired phagocytosis leading to recurrent infections, peripheral neuropathy, and partial albinism.

Kartagener's syndrome is a condition characterized by immotile cilia due to defective axonemal dyneins, resulting in infertility, bronchiectasis, and recurrent respiratory infections.

SURFACE SPECIALIZATION AND INTERCELLULAR JUNCTIONS

Surface Specialization

Most surfaces in the body are lined with epithelial cells. For example, the lumen of blood vessels, GI tract, kidney tubules, and the epidermal layer of the skin are all lined with epithelial cells. There are different types of epithelial cells: squamous, columnar, and cuboid. Surface cells have specialized structures designed to facilitate and carry out important physiological functions (Table 4).

Surface	Function
Apical	
Microvilli of enterocytes	Increase surface area of absorption
Granules of goblet cells	Secrete mucus to protect the lining of the stomach
Cilia on respiratory mucosa	Transport dust and other foreign material up and out of the bronchioles
Basolateral	
Infolding of the basolateral membrane in the distal tubule of the kidney	Allow increased surface area of ion channels

Table 4 Examples of surface specializations

Junctional Complexes

Junctional complexes are surface specializations located predominantly on the lateral surface of cells. There are five different junctional complexes that join adjacent epithelial cells (Figure 13):

1. **Zona occludens** (tight junctions) form the initial barrier, controlling the movement of molecules from the lumen of the cell through the epithelial layer.

2. **Zona adherens** (intermediate or adherent junctions) are located just basal to the zona occludens, completely encircle the cell, and act to anchor cells together. Zona adherens is also associated with actin filaments within the cell, which allows for apical contraction of the epithelium.

3. **Macula adherens** (desmosomes) are discrete points of attachment located on the lateral surface of cells to the zona adherens. They are associated with intermediate filaments within cells and act to maintain epithelial integrity. Pemphigus vulgaris is a blistering condition characterized by antibodies against desmosomes, resulting in a positive Nikolsky's sign, in which stroking the skin leads to sloughing of the skin.

4. **Hemidesmosomes** are junctional complexes located on the basal surface of the cell that connect cells to the extracellular matrix. Bullous pemphigoid is a blistering condition characterized by antibodies against hemidesmosomes resulting in bullae. It is less severe than pemphigus vulgaris and has a negative Nikolsky's sign.

5. **Gap junctions** are junctional complexes that allow cell-to-cell communication between two neighboring cells. Ions and molecules can readily pass through from one cell to another through gap junctions, allowing electrical and chemical cell coupling.

Cardiac muscle utilizes electrical cell coupling to allow rapid synchronous contraction of the heart. Neurons and smooth muscle cells also use electrical cell coupling via gap junctions.

Mnemonic:
He was overjoyed to have pemphigoid instead of pemphigus vulgaris.

Hemidesmosomes, bullous pemphigoid is less severe than pemphigus vulgaris.

Cilia in the respiratory tract coordinate beating to clear respiratory secretions by means of chemical cell coupling.

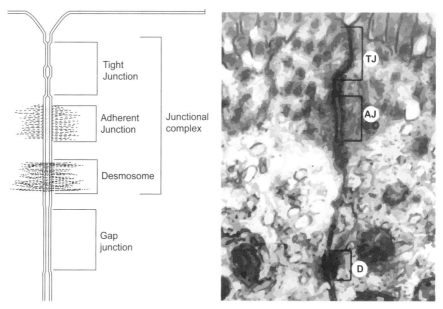

Figure 13 Junctional complexes.
(Adapted from *Functional Histology: A Text and Colour Atlas* Rev. Ed.)

Each type of junctional complex is associated with specific proteins (Table 5).

Some patients with systemic lupus erythematosus have autoreactive antibodies to lamin B.

Junctional complex	Associated proteins	Associated cytoskeletal elements
Zona occludens (tight junctions)	Claudins Occludins	—
Zona adherens (adherent junctions)	Cadherins (Ca²⁺ dependent adhesion molecules)	Actin
Macula adherens (desmosomes)	Cadherins Desmoplakin	Intermediate filaments (e.g. keratin)
Hemidesmosomes	Integrin Laminin and fibronectin (in basement membrane)	—
Gap junctions	Connexon (w. central channel)	—

Table 5 Junctional Complex Proteins

EXTRACELLULAR MATRIX

The **extracellular matrix** is the space between cells filled by **ground substance** and fibers.

Ground Substance

Ground substance is a combination of water, salts, proteoglycans, and glycoproteins that connect cells and fibers, aids in cell-to-cell communication, and provides structural support. Proteoglycans are polysaccharide chains called protein linked glycosaminoglycans (GAGs). Hyaluronic acid is the most common GAG found in the extracellular matrix, whereas chondroitin sulfate is the most common GAG in the body.

Glycoproteins consist mostly of protein with sugar attachments. Fibronectin and laminin are extracellular glycoproteins associated with hemidesmosomes.

Heparan sulfate and dermatan sulfate are GAGs that accumulate in Hurler's and Hunter's lysosomal storage diseases.

Heparin, used clinically as an anticoagulant, is an intracellular GAG found in mast cells.

Fibers

Collagen is the most abundant protein in the body. It is mostly synthesized in the RER of fibroblasts, but also formed in chondroblasts, osteoblasts, and epithelial cells by the following processes:

1. **Preprocollagen**s are α chains that are rich with glycine, proline, hydroxyproline and hydroxylysine amino acids. The hydroxylation of lysine, proline, and the glycosylantion of lysine residues occur in the RER.

2. **Procollagen** is a triple helix of 3 preprocollagen α chains. Hydrogen bonds between the hydroxyprolines stabilize the triple helix. The procollagen molecule is then expelled into the extracellular space.

3. **Tropocollagen** is formed when procollagen peptidases in the extracellular space cleave the water-soluble, disulfide-rich terminal regions to form an insoluble product.

4. **Collagen fibrils** are formed when tropocollagen molecules are crosslinked to one another by lysyl oxidase, covalently linking lysine and hydroxylysine residues.

Collagen acts to strengthen and hold the extracellular matrix together. In tendons and ligaments, collagen provides tensile strength. In blood vessels and organs, collagen provides structural support. There are four different types of collagen with different functions (Table 6).

Mnemonics:
Strong men eat *Fatty T-BONE STeak*

(Type I collagen is the strongest, therefore involved in *Fascia, Tendon, Bone, Skin, and Teeth*)

car*TWO*lage

Type of Collagen	Associated with	
Type I (Strongest and most common form of collagen—90%)	Bone, Skin, Tendon, Dentin, Fascia, Cornea, Late wound repair	Affected in Osteogenesis Imperfecta
Type II	Cartilage, vitreous body, nucleus pulposus	
Type III (reticulin)	Skin, blood vessels, uterus, fetal tissue, granulation tissue	Affected in Ehlers Danlos
Type IV	Basement membrane especially of kidneys, ears and eyes	Affected in Alport's syndrome
Elastin	Skin, large arteries, vocal cords, and lungs	Affected in Marfan's syndrome Affected in Emphysema

Table 6 Types of Collagen

Osteogenesis imperfecta is an autosomal dominant condition characterized by abnormal type I collagen, resulting in "brittle bone disease." It typically presents with **multiple fractures** with minimal trauma, **blue sclera** (defective cornea), hearing loss (defective ossicles), and dental imperfections (defective dentin). Multiple fractures occasionally lead to dwarfism. Type II osteogenesis imperfecta is more severe and results in intrauterine or perinatal death.

Ehlers-Danlos is a genetic condition that can be either autosomal dominant or recessive. It is characterized by defects in lysine hydroxylation. Ehlers-Danlos is characterized by abnormal type III collagen, resulting in increased skin elasticity, hypermobile joints, and easy bruising. Ehlers-Danlos may be associated with berry aneurysms, organ rupture, mitral valve prolapse, and joint dislocation.

Alport's syndrome is an X-linked recessive condition characterized by abnormal type IV collagen, resulting in glomerulonephritis due to fragmented basement membranes. It is also associated deafness and ocular disease.

Elastin fibers are composed of tropoelastin on a scaffolding of **microfibrillar protein, or fibrillin.** While elastic fibers provide structural strength, their primary function is to allow stretch and recoil. **Elastin** contains numerous proline and lysine residues. Lysyl hydroxylase allows cross-linking between lysines in 4 different elastic chains, allowing for increased plasticity.

Marfan's syndrome is an autosomal dominant condition characterized by defective fibrillin. Patients are typically tall and slender with hyperextensible joints, **arachnodactyly** (long fingers and toes), and pectus excavatum. They are at risk for **lens subluxation, mitral valve prolapse,** and **aortic dissection** secondary to cystic medial necrosis of the aorta.

Elastase is the enzyme that breaks down elastin. Elastase is normally inhibited by α-1-antitrypsin. In α**-1-antitrypsin deficiency,** there is increased elastase activity and therefore greater elastin breakdown. α**-1-antitrypsin deficiency** is associated with panacinar emphysema.

NUTRITION

All cells require energy and nutrients. The **basal metabolic rate** is defined as the resting metabolism of energy. For example, basal metabolic rate for a young adult male is approximately 70 kcal/hour. Each day, approximately 25 g of protein is metabolized into amino acids, regardless of whether protein is present in the diet. With increased energy expenditure, such as exercise, additional energy is obtained from different sources within the body (Table 7).

Osteogenesis imperfecta is often mistaken for child abuse.

Both osteogenesis imperfecta and Ehlers Danlos are caused by mutations on chromosome 7.

α-1-antitrypsin deficiency is also associated with liver cirrhosis.

Duration of Exercise	Source of ATP
Seconds	Stored, creatine phosphate, anaerobic glycolysis
Minutes	Above + oxidative phosphorylation
Hours	Glycogen and phosphorylation of free fatty acids

Table 7 Energy use with exercise

Therefore, in order to sustain the life, the daily energy requirement for a human being is approximately 2,500 kilocalories (1 calorie is the amount of heat need to increase the temperature of 1 g of water by 1°C). Different amounts of energy are provided by the consumption of different macromolecules (Table 8). After a meal, the body processes these macromolecules into energy using glycolysis and aerobic respiration. **Insulin** stimulates the storage of remaining lipids, proteins, and glycogen, while **glucagon** and **adrenaline** stimulate the use of these stores.

Macromolecule	Energy
Carbohydrates	4 kcal/g
Proteins	4 kcal/g
Lipids	9 kcal/g
Alcohol	7 kcal/g

Table 8 Calories from macromolecules

Fasting and Starvation

With starvation, glycogen is depleted from hepatic glycogenolysis after 1 day. However, the body is able to maintain homeostasis by hepatic gluconeogenesis and release of free fatty acids (FFA) from adipose tissues. With 1–3 days of starvation, the liver and muscles switch from using glucose as their primary source of energy to using FFAs. After 3 days of starvation, ketone bodies from the metabolism of FFAs become the primary source of energy. When adipose stores are depleted, the body accelerates protein degradation for gluconeogenesis. Low serum albumin and decreased serum proteins often indicate poor nutritional status.

There are two medical conditions that are caused by poor dietary intake:

1. **Kwarshiorkor** is caused by **protein deficiency**. It causes an enlarged fatty liver, edema, and anemia secondary to decreased apolipoprotein synthesis, hypoalbuminemia, and decreased hemoglobin synthesis, respectively. Malabsorption can also occur secondary to decreased synthesis of pancreatic enzymes. Kwarshiokor is commonly seen in poverty stricken areas in young children after weaning of breast milk. It manifests with

Creatine phosphate is stored in skeletal muscle and is a highly mobilizable form of energy made from amino acids. It is liberated by the enzyme creatine kinase, which becomes elevated when muscle is damaged (e.g. in rhabdomyolysis or myocardial infarction).

Mnemonic: C-PAL 4-479

The brain and red blood cells (RBCs) are prioritized to receive glucose.

The body tries to preserve protein, even in starvation states.

RBCs cannot use ketone bodies, only glucose, for energy.

Low protein diets can be indicated in certain conditions like renal failure and cirrhosis to prevent the buildup of excess NH_3 and urea.

weight loss, red hair, and a swollen stomach. Treatment for kwarshiokor is protein supplementation, however, if the protein deficiency is too severe, prognosis is often poor.

2. **Marasmus** is caused by **decreased total calorie intake.** Marasmus results in widespread tissue and muscle wasting without edema, anemia, or other malabsorption syndromes. Treatment is adequate calorie and nutrient intake. Unlike kwarshiokor, marasmus is a reversible condition with a high chance of survival.

Fat-Soluble Vitamin Deficiencies and Toxicities

The **fat-soluble vitamins** are A, D, E, and K (Table 9). Fat-soluble vitamins accumulate in fat and, as a result, achieve toxicity more commonly than water-soluble vitamins. Their absorption is dependent on an intact lining of the digestive tract, adequate release of pancreatic enzymes and bile acids. Therefore, deficiency in fat-soluble vitamins can result from hepatitis, bile duct obstruction, and cirrhosis as well as malabsorptive conditions, such as cystic fibrosis, pancreatic insufficiency, and Celiac sprue.

Vitamin A is an antioxidant, a component of visual pigment, and plays an important role in differentiation of epithelial cells. Vitamin A is found in egg yolk, liver, and leafy vegetables. Deficiency may lead to night blindness and dermatitis. Excess vitamin A can cause elevated intracranial pressure, leading to papilledema and pseudotumor cerebri. When used in acne treatment, patients must be kept on birth control as it is a teratogenic.

There are several sources of **vitamin D**. It can be endogenously synthesized in the skin by photoconversion of 7-dehydrocholesterol from sunlight. Preformed vitamin D from the diet can be absorbed in the small intestine: ergocalciferol (D_2) is ingested from plants and cholecalciferol (D_3) is ingested from milk. Hydroxylation to 25-OH vitamin D occurs in the liver by the cytochrome P450 system. Further hydroxylation to its active form, 1,25-$(OH)_2$ vitamin D, occurs in the kidney (Figure 14).

Mnemonic: A DEcK of fat.

Vitamin A can be used to treat acute myelogenous leukemia M3, measles, and acne.

Vitamin D deficiency can be caused by insufficient intake, inadequate sun exposure, renal failure liver failure, and malabsorption.

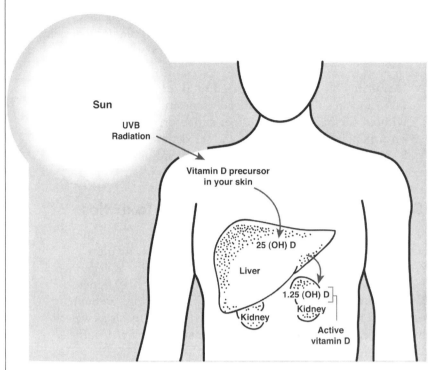

Figure 14 Vitamin D synthesis

Vitamin D increases the absorption of calcium and phosphate in the gastrointestinal tract. Furthermore, vitamin D also increases plasma concentrations of calcium by bone resorption. Excess amounts of vitamin D leads to hypercalcemia, which can manifest with constipation, calcium urinary stones, and delirium.

In **Williams syndrome**, a genetic disorder characterized by elfin facies and mental retardation, there is an increased sensitivity to vitamin D. In **sarcoidosis**, a condition characterized by noncaseating granulomas, there is increased activation of vitamin D due to activity of α-1 hydroxylase in granuloma epithelioid macrophages.

Vitamin D deficiency leads to fragile bones, which manifests as **rickets** in children and **osteomalacia** in adults. Rickets is characterized by bending of the bones, often leading to bow-legged appearance of legs. Vitamin D deficiency also leads to hypocalcemia, which can manifest as tetany.

Vitamin E is an antioxidant that protects erythrocytes and cell membranes from fatty acid oxidation. Deficiency in vitamin E is uncommon, however, deficiency can result in hemolytic anemia due to breakdown of erythrocytes. Vitamin E can also lead to demyelination of the dorsal columns, lateral corticospinal tracts, and spinocerebellar tracts of the spinal cord.

Rickets has the characteristic findings of "pigeon chest" (breastbone pushed forward) and "rachitic rosary" (bumps in the rib cage).

Vitamin B$_{12}$ deficiency and Friedrich's ataxia have patterns of demyelination similar to that of vitamin E, leading to an impaired sense of vibration and proprioception and ataxia.

At toxic levels, vitamin E inhibits the synthesis of vitamin K dependent coagulation factors. **Vitamin K** plays a pivotal role in the carboxylation of coagulation factors II, VII, IX, X, Protein C, and Protein S. It is made by the naturally occurring bacterial flora in the large intestine. Deficiency in vitamin K can lead to hemorrhagic diatheses with elevated partial thromboplastin time (PTT) and prothrombin times (PT). Newborns have immature intestinal flora that do not synthesize vitamin K. Therefore, newborns are injected with vitamin K at birth to prevent intraventricular hemorrhage. Causes of vitamin K deficiency include antibiotics that destroy intestinal flora, malabsorption, and poor dietary intake. Vitamin K toxicity is rare but can lead to hemolytic anemia and jaundice in newborns.

Warfarin is a blood thinner that antagonizes vitamin K.

Vitamin	Deficiency	Toxicity
A (retinol, carotenes)	Night blindness, xerophthalmia (dry eyes), keratomalacia (corneal ulceration), Bitot's spots (corneal keratin plaques), especially metaplasia	Dermatitis, alopecia, vomiting, increased intracranial pressure, hepatomegaly, teratogenic
D	Lack of bone mineralization (rickets or osteomalacia), hypocalcemia (tetany)	Hypercalcemia (constipation, calcium urinary stones, delirium
E	Hemolytic anemia Spinal cord demyelination: 1. Dorsal columns (loss of vibration/proprioception) 2. Corticospinal tract (hyperreflexia, weakness) 3. Spinocerebellar tract (ataxia)	Bleeding
K	Adults: GI bleeding, ecchymoses Newborns: CNS bleed, ecchymoses	Newborns: hemolytic anemia, jaundice

Table 9 Fat-soluble Vitamin Deficiencies and Toxicities

Water-soluble Vitamin Deficiencies and Toxicities

The **water-soluble vitamins** are the B vitamins, folate and vitamin C (Table 10). Many water-soluble vitamins function as cofactors for biochemical reactions. Aside from vitamin B_{12} and folate, which are stored in the liver, water-soluble vitamins are easily cleared from body. Deficiencies in B vitamins manifest with dermatitis, diarrhea, cheilosis, and glossitis.

It is easier to remember the four fat-soluble vitamins (ADEK) and recognize that the rest are water-soluble.

Vitamin B$_1$ (thiamine) is found in liver, eggs, and whole grains. It serves as a cofactor for enzymes involved in ATP synthesis:

- α-ketoglutarate dehydrogenase in citric acid cycle

- Pyruvate dehydrogenase in glycolysis

- Transketolase in HMP shunt/pentose phosphate pathway

Deficiency of thiamine leads to ATP depletion. Tissues with the highest oxygen requirements, such as heart and brain are affected first. Maple syrup disease is caused by decreased levels of α-ketoglutarate dehydrogenase resulting in the build up of α-keto acid, leading to CNS defects.

Wernicke syndrome is a condition caused by thiamine deficiency associated with chronic alcohol abuse. It is characterized by ataxia, opthalmoplegia, and delirium. Wernicke's syndrome is reversible with thiamine repletion. However, Wernicke's syndrome can progress to **Korsakoff's syndrome**, which is characterized by amnesia and confabulation secondary to irreversible damage to the mammillary bodies and medial dorsal nucleus of the thalamus in the limbic system.

Beriberi is another condition caused by thiamine deficiency. Neuromuscular beriberi, or 'dry' beriberi, presents with peripheral neuropathy and muscle wasting. Cardiac beriberi, or 'wet' beriberi, presents with dilated cardiomyopathy, pulmonary, and peripheral edema. Symptoms of both wet and dry beriberi may present simultaneously.

Vitamin B$_2$ (riboflavin, FAD) is found in liver, dairy products, nuts, soybeans, and leafy vegetables. Vitamin B$_2$ has an important role in oxidation and reduction reactions. Deficiency in vitamin B$_2$ is commonly due to insufficient dietary intake and leads to corneal neovascularization. Toxicity has not been documented.

Vitamin B$_3$ (niacin, NAD$^+$) is derived from tryptophan and is found in most animal products, fruits, and vegetables. Like riboflavin, niacin has an important role in oxidation and reduction reactions. Excessive amounts of niacin lead to flushing, cholestasis, hyperglycemia, and hyperuricemia. **Pellagra** is a condition caused by niacin deficiency, characterized by the **3 D's: diarrhea, dermatitis, and dementia.** It is associated with corn-based diet, which is deficient in tryptophan. Hartnup disease, a genetic disorder characterized by an inability to reabsorb tryptophan can also lead to niacin deficiency. In carcinoid syndrome, niacin deficiency can result from excessive tryptophan uptake by excessive serotonin synthesis.

Vitamin B$_4$ (pantothenic acid) is found in most foods and plays an important role in the synthesis of coenzyme-A (CoA) and in the subsequent synthesis and oxidation of fatty acids (acyl-CoA). Deficiency may lead to alopecia and adrenal insufficiency. Toxicity has not been documented.

Vitamin B$_6$ (pyridoxine) is found in most foods and serves as a cofactor in several biochemical reactions:

1. Transamination

2. Decarboxylation reactions

3. Heme synthesis

4. Compound synthesis (niacin from tryptophan; histamine from histidine; cystathione synthesis from homocysteine)

5. Neurotransmitter synthesis (dopamine from L-dopa; GABA from glutamate)

Deficiency in pyridoxine is often caused by chronic alcoholism as well as drug therapy with isoniazid, oral contraceptives, and pencillamine. Pyridoxine deficiency can lead to convulsions, peripheral neuropathy, irritability, and sideroblastic anemia.

Vitamin B$_7$ (biotin) is found in most foods and is a cofactor for carboxylation enzymes such as, pyruvate carboxylase in gluconeogenesis and acetyl-coA carboxylase in fatty acid synthesis. Ingestion of raw eggs or antibiotics can lead to deficiency in biotin. Alopecia is associated with biotin deficiency.

Vitamin B$_{12}$ (cobalamin) is found only in animal products, such as meat, dairy, and eggs, and requires intrinsic factor to be absorbed in the gastrointestinal tract. Intrinsic factor is generated by parietal cells in the stomach. Vitamin B$_{12}$ allows homocysteine methyltransferase to synthesize folate, which is needed for synthesis of the nitrogenous bases in DNA. Vitamin B$_{12}$ is also a cofactor for methylmalonyl-CoA mutase in odd-chain fatty acid metabolism.

Cobalamin deficiency results in macrocytic anemia and demyelination of dorsal columns, lateral corticospinal tracts, and spinocerebellar tracts in the spinal cord, similar to vitamin E deficiency. Fortunately, the liver is able to store several years worth of vitamin B$_{12}$. Therefore, inadequate dietary intake is a rare cause of B$_{12}$ deficiency. However, strict, long-standing vegetarians and vegans who avoid animal products completely can have cobalamin deficiency, despite adequate caloric intake. Chronic malabsorptive disorders, such as Crohn's disease, celiac sprue, and bacterial overgrowth can lead to cobalamin deficiency. Moreover, cobalamin deficiency can be secondary to lack of intrinsic factor or gastric bypass surgery. **Pernicious anemia** is a condition characterized by autoimmune destruction of parietal cells, leading to intrinsic factor deficiency.

The **Schilling test** can elucidate the cause of vitamin B$_{12}$ deficiency. In Schilling test, radioactive B$_{12}$ is orally administered. After the ingestion of radioactive form of B$_{12}$, patient is initially given no treatment and the 24-hour urinary level of radioactive form of B$_{12}$ is measured. If B$_{12}$ is not detected in the 24-hour urine, the test is repeated with radioactive form of B$_{12}$ in combination

Isoniazid, used for treating tuberculosis, is the most common cause of pyridoxine deficiency.

Avidin in egg whites binds to biotin, preventing GI absorption.

The most sensitive test for vitamin B$_{12}$ deficiency is elevated levels of methylmalonic acid.

Diphyllobothrium latum, a tapeworm acquired by consuming undercooked fish, can absorb ~80% of its host's vitamin B$_{12}$.

with intrinsic factor. If urinary B_{12} is detected, pernicious anemia can be diagnosed. Additionally, antibiotics can be given with radioactive form of B_{12} to assess for possible bacterial overgrowth.

Folic acid or **folate** is present in most foods and plays an important role in DNA synthesis. Folate deficiency is the most common vitamin deficiency in the United States and results in macrocytic anemia. Folate deficiency is often confused with cobalamin deficiency. Unlike cobalamin deficiency, folate deficiency does NOT cause neurologic symptoms. Unlike cobalamin, the liver is only able to store 3-month supply of folate in the body. Therefore, inadequate dietary intake is a common cause of folate deficiency, especially in chronic alcoholics and the elderly.

Vitamin C (ascorbic acid) is found in fruits and vegetable and serves several important functions:

1. It is a required cofactor for the hydroxylation of proline and lysine in the synthesis of collagen. Collagen is important for the formation of bone, ground substance, and dentin.

2. It is a required cofactor for β-hydroxylase, an enzyme that converts dopamine to norepinephrine.

3. It is involved in reducing iron to its absorbable form (Fe^{2+}) in the small intestine.

4. It has antioxidant activity and plays a role in regeneration of vitamin E.

Vitamin C deficiency is associated with **scurvy**—a condition characterized by poor wound healing secondary to impaired collagen formation, impaired tooth formation, bleeding gums, easy bruising, corkscrew hairs, and hemarthrosis. Excess amount of vitamin C is usually benign but can lead to the formation of renal uric acid stones and can result in false-negative fecal occult blood tests (FOBT).

Mineral Deficiencies and Toxicities

Many mineral deficiencies and toxicities are due to imbalances in fluids and electrolytes. Summary of toxicities associated with mineral deficiency is provided inTable 11.

In the human body, 40% of calcium is bound to albumin, 13% is bound to phosphorous, and citrate and 47% is free, ionized, and metabolically active. The total serum calcium includes both bound and free calcium.

The most common causes of hypocalcemia include hypoalbuminemia and chronic renal failure and, to a lesser degree, vitamin D deficiency, hypoparathyroidism, decreased calcium intake, diuretics, and acute pancreatitis.

On the other hand, causes of hypercalcemia include hyperparathyroidism, acromegaly, adrenal insufficiency, bone metastases, and thiazide diuretics. Milk-alkali syndrome is metabolic alkalosis caused by the ingestion of large quantities of calcium and vitamin D.

During pregnancy, there is increased utilization of folate for DNA synthesis. Inadequate supplementation may cause neural tube defects in neonates.

Vitamin	Deficiencies	Toxicities
B₁* (Thiamine, TPP)	Wernicke-Korsakoff's syndrome Wet beriberi (neuromuscular) Dry beriberi (cardiac)	—
B₂* (Riboflavin, FAD)	Neovascularization of the cornea	—
B₃* (Niacin, NAD⁺)	Pellagra (dermatitis, diarrhea, dementia)	Flushing, cholestasis, hyperglycemia, hyperuricemia
B₅* (Pantothenate: CoA)	Alopecia, adrenal insufficiency	—
B₆* (Pyridoxine)	Convulsions, peripheral neuropathy, irritability, sideroblastic anemia	—
B₇ (Biotin)	Alopecia	—
B₁₂* (Cobalamin)	Macrocytic anemia Spinal cord demyelination: 1. Dorsal columns (loss of vibration/proprioception) 2. Corticospinal tract (hyperreflexia, weakness) 3. Spinocerebellar tract (ataxia)	—
Folate	Macrocytic anemia, neural tube defects in neonates	—
C (Ascorbic acid)	Scurvy (impaired healing, bruising, bleeding gums, anemia)	Falsely negative FOBT Renal uric acid stones

Table 10 Water-soluble vitamin deficiencies and toxicities

Sodium is the major cation of the extracellular space and plays a key role in maintaining fluid equilibrium. There are many causes of hyponatremia that can be differentiated by the tonicity of body fluid. Isotonic hyponatremia can be due to hyperproteinemia or hyperlipidemia. Hypertonic hyponatremia can result from hyperglycemia. On the other

Deficiencies of B vitamins may all lead to similar symptoms: dermatitis, diarrhea, cheilosis, and glossitis

Rapid correction of hyponatremia can cause central pontine myelinolysis, leading to paralysis, loss of consciousness, and other neurological symptoms.

hand, hypotonic hyponatremia can be due to salt loss, renal loss secondary to diuretics, nephropathy, and mineralocorticoid deficiency. Hypotonic hyponatremia can also be due to extrarenal loss, such as diarrhea and vomiting or polygenic polydipsia, excess sweating, syndrome of inappropriate ADH release, liver disease, and congestive heart failure.

Hypernatremia is usually caused by inadequate water intake and often accompanied by orthostatic hypotension and oliguria. Other potential causes of hypernatremia include diabetes insipidus, osmotic diuresis from uncontrolled diabetes or mannitol, and osmotic diarrhea.

Potassium is the predominant cation of the intracellular space and plays an essential role in the functioning of the heart, kidneys, gastrointestinal system as well as the musculoskeletal system

Shift of potassium into cells by alkalosis, insulin, and β-adrenergic stimulation can lead to hypokalemia. Other potential causes include insufficient potassium intake, mineralocorticoid excess, Bartter's syndrome, Liddle's syndrome, and diuretic use.

Hyperkalemia can be transiently induced shifting of potassium out of cells by tissue injury, acidosis, insulin deficiency, use of β-blockers, or digitalis. Renal failure, adrenocorticoid insufficiency, potassium-sparing diuretics, and excess potassium intakes can also lead to hyperkalemia.

The most common cause of **iron** deficiency in adults is gastrointestinal bleed. Excess blood donation and menorrhagia in women can also lead to iron deficiency anemia.

Phosphorus homeostasis is strongly linked to calcium homeostasis. Hypophosphatemia is often found in chronic alcoholics or patients on corticosteroids and β_2-agonists, which cause increased renal excretion of phosphate. Hyperphosphatemia is most commonly caused by chronic renal failure and hypoparathyroidism.

Magnesium homeostasis is strongly linked to potassium and calcium homeostasis. Hypomagnesemia is often caused by diarrhea, renal insufficiency, alcohol, and diuretic use.

Zinc is needed for the function of numerous enzymes involved in wound healing.

Fluoride is stored in the bones and teeth and is important in preventing tooth decay.

Iodine is required for the synthesis of thyroid hormone.

Hyperkalemia presents on ECGs with peaked T-waves (hyper-T waves).

Copper deficiency is rare. Wilson's disease is a condition characterized by inadequate excretion of copper, leading to build up of copper in the liver, cornea, joints, and brain.

Mineral	Deficiency	Toxicity
Calcium (Ca)	Nerve and muscle excitability (cramps, tetany, laryngospasm, convulsions and paresthesias) Chvostek's sign (contraction of facial muscle when facial nerve is tapped) Trousseau's sign (carpal spasm with occlusion of brachial artery with blood pressure cuff)	Polyuria, renal failure, constipation, neurological symptoms
Sodium (Na)	Nausea, headache, seizures, respiratory arrest, encephalopathy	See hyponatremia
Potassium (K)	Muscle weakness, fatigue, cramps, constipation, ileus, flaccid paralysis, tetany, cardiac arrest	Muscle weakness, fatigue, cramps, diarrhea
Iron (Fe)	Microcytic anemia	GI upset, vomiting, acidosis
Phosphorus (P)	Hypocontractility, impaired tissue oxygenation (due to decreased RBC 2,3-DPG), platelet dysfunction, muscle pain, bone fractures	Symptoms related to underlying disorders (hypoparathyroidism, chronic renal failure)
Magnesium (Mg)	Neuromuscular and CNS hyperirritability (cramps, weakness, tremors)	Muscle weakness, neurologic syndromes-cardiac arrest
Zinc (Zn)	Dysgeusia (altered taste), anosmia (altered smell), impaired wound healing, growth retardation	—
Fluoride (F)	Tooth decay	Tooth mottling
Iodine (I)	Goiter, cretinism	—

Table 11 Mineral and vitamin deficiencies and toxicities

Kayser-Fleischer rings are copper rings around the iris that can be seen in slit lamp examination.

Hypercalcemia= urination, constipation, and poor mentation.

Hypocalcemia = twitching

PATHOLOGY

A good comprehension of the basics of pathology—cell injury and repair, inflammation and cancer—is essential to understanding disease in the organ systems.

Cell Injury

Under normal circumstances, a cell is able to adapt to its physiologic and environmental demands by undergoing different changes. For example, muscle cells may **hypertrophy** (enlarge) with weight lifting or **atrophy** (shrink in size) with disuse, as with patients who have been paralyzed. Other causes of stress to the cell include hypoxia, physical trauma, microbial invasion (viruses, bacteria and parasites), and immunologic reactions. When the demands on a cell exceed its ability to adapt, cell injury occurs.

Reversible cell injury is typically characterized by a decrease in ATP synthesis. This lack of ATP leads to impairment of the Na^+/K^+ pump and build up of sodium within the cell, which leads to swelling of the cell. Clumping of chromatin, fatty change, lactic acid build-up, and decreased protein synthesis occur in reversible cell injury but may all be reversible with the administration of oxygen.

There are a lot of tables containing a lot of information in this section. You do not need to memorize all of the information right away. However, these tables will serve as a good reference for you as you move further along in your studies.

HyperTROPHY is one big cell (like one big trophy) vs. hyperplASIA which is the increase in the number of cells (more than one country is Asia.)

If blood supply is restored soon enough after a heart attack, damage done to the cardiac muscle remains salvageable.

Irreversible cell injury occurs when either the mitochondria or the plasma membrane of the cell has been damaged beyond the reparative ability of the cell. It is characterized by fragmentation of the nucleus and the influx of Ca^{2+} into the cell. The result of irreversible cell injury is cell death—either by apoptosis or necrosis. (Figure 15).

Pro-apoptotic protein: Bax

Anti-apoptotic protein: Bcl-2

Cytochrome c: mitochondrial protein that activates caspases

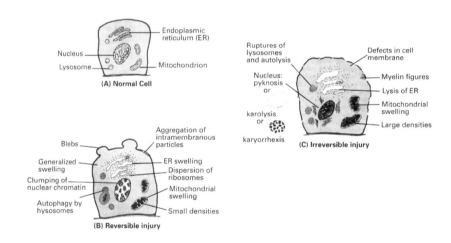

Figure 15 Reversible and irreversible cell injury

Cell Death

Apoptosis is programmed cell death, whereas **necrosis** refers to the biochemical reactions resulting from exogenous damage. There are two pathways by which apoptosis can occur: intrinsic and extrinsic.

The intrinsic pathway is activated by changing levels of intracellular pro- and anti-apoptotic proteins. The varying balance between these proteins causes increased permeability of mitochondria and the release of **cytochrome c**, which stimulates apoptosis. Embryogenesis and endometrial shedding during menstruation utilize apoptosis.

The extrinsic pathway occurs by either ligand-receptor interaction on the cell surface or via the release of enzymes from killer T-cells. Tumor cells can be destroyed by way of the extrinsic apoptotic pathway.

Both pathways ultimately lead to the influx of intracellular calcium and activation of cytosolic **caspase** proteins. Caspase proteins lead to cellular disintegration, which is characterized by blebbing of the plasma membrane, **pyknotic** (shrunken and degenerated) nuclei, and the formation of **apoptotic bodies**. Macrophages then phagocytose the apoptotic bodies, allowing apoptosis to be a tidy process of degradation, where organelle structure is largely preserved and there is little inflammation to surrounding tissue.

On the other hand, **necrosis** is death by inflammatory cells, which results in cellular swelling, rupture of the nucleus and cell membranes, DNA digestion, and loss of organelle structure. There are four different types of necrosis:

1. **Coagulative necrosis** is characterized by intracellular lactic acid building up and destroying the cell from the inside out. The outline of the cell is maintained in coagulative necrosis. It is what occurs in myocardial infarctions or ischemia to solid organs (like the liver or kidney).

2. **Liquefactive necrosis** is caused by neutrophilic degranulation of lysosomal contents leading to the destruction and dissolution of cells. Abscesses are a form of liquefactive necrosis, as is ischemia to the brain.

3. **Granulomatous necrosis** is characterized by macrophages forming granulomas containing a "cheese-like" substance. Tuberculosis and systemic fungi often result in granulomatous necrosis of cells, but not all diseases characterized by the formation of granulomas will exhibit granulomatous necrosis (Table 12).

4. **Fatty necrosis** or **saponification** is essentially enzymatic fat necrosis, where fat is digested into fatty acids and calcium. This commonly occurs with pancreatic trauma or pancreatitis.

Granulomatous Disease
Tuberculosis
Fungal infections
Syphilis
Leprosy
Cat scratch fever
Sarcoidosis
Crohn's disease
Berylliosis
Listeria
Foreign body reaction
Collagen vascular disease: Wegener's
Chronic granulomatous disease

Table 12 Granulomatous diseases

Fas-ligand: released from T-cells and binds to Fas-receptor CD95

Perforins and granzymes: released from killer T-cells (alternate method of activating extrinsic pathway)

Dry gangrene is a form of coagulative necrosis

Wet gangrene is dry gangrene + bacteria leading to liquefactive necrosis.

Sarcoidosis is characterized by non-caseating granulomas.

Calcifications from fatty necrosis can be seen on X-ray.

Interferon-gamma activates macrophages which release TNF-alpha to induce granuloma formation.

Hypoxia

Hypoxia, or deficient oxygen reaching the tissues, is one of the most common causes of cell injury and cell death. Table 13 lists the areas of the body that are most susceptible to hypoxia, like **watershed regions**, the areas supplied by the terminal ends of two separate arteries, leading to the potential for decreased oxygen delivery. Two common watershed regions are:

1. Between the anterior cerebral artery (ACA) and middle cerebral artery (MCA)

2. Between the inferior mesenteric artery (IMA) and superior mesenteric artery (SMA), also known as the **splenic flexure.**

Infarction is the occlusion of blood supply to regions of the body. It is most commonly caused by thrombi (blood clots) or emboli (masses traveling within the bloodstream: blood clots, air, fat, tissue, etc.) Hemorrhagic infarcts occur in tissues with significant collateral blood supply that allow continued perfusion (for example, the liver, lungs, and intestine). Pale infarcts occur in tissues with a single blood supply (for example, the heart and kidneys).

Shock is essentially systemic hypoxia, leading to multi-organ failure and eventually death. There are four different types of shock:

1. **Hypovolemic:** Insufficient intravascular volume, from dehydration or hemorrhage, can lead to insufficient oxygen supply to the tissues. Severe burns can induce hypovolemic shock as the damaged skin becomes unable to retain water in the body.

2. **Cardiogenic:** In patients with cardiac defects, whether secondary to a myocardial infarction, congestive heart failure, or some other form of cardiomyopathy, the heart is unable to pump sufficient amounts of oxygenated blood to the tissues.

3. **Septic:** In patients with overwhelming infection, acute respiratory distress syndrome (ARDS) or disseminated intravascular coagulation (DIC), their vasculature is significantly vasodilated with high cardiac output and high venous return. However, due to the speed at which blood rushes through the dilated vasculature, tissues are still poorly perfused.

4. **Anaphylactic:** Anaphylactic shock is a severe allergic reaction characterized by histamine-mediated systemic vasodilation.

Hypovolemic and cardiogenic shock are forms of low-cardiac-output failure where peripheral vessels are vasoconstricted to maintain blood pressure and patients are cool to the touch. Septic and anaphylactic shock are forms of high-cardiac-output failure where peripheral vessels are vasodilated and patients are hot to the touch.

The Circle of Willis in the brain temporarily maintains perfusion to the brain during shock by distributing blood to the most important areas.

Treat hypovolemic shock with isotonic saline.

Treat anaphylactic shock with epinephrine.

High output failure is characterized by increased mixed venous O_2 content (due to decreased O_2 extraction by tissues).

Locations
Watershed regions
Subendocardium
Renal medulla and proximal tubules
Neurons
Zone III hepatocytes (around the central vein)

Table 13 Areas most susceptible to hypoxia

Some Other Mechanisms of Cell Injury

Free radicals like superoxide (O_2^-) and hydroxyl ion radicals ($\bullet OH$) are extremely unstable and reactive molecules that cause damage to different cellular components (proteins, nucleic acids, and lipids). They can be generated via drug metabolism (like for acetaminophen), redox reactions within our bodies, leukocyte oxidative bursts in immune cells, radiation, chemical toxins, or UV exposure. Hydrogen peroxide (H_2O_2) can also react with transitional metals such as iron to generate hydroxyl ion radicals.

Reperfusion injury is the paradoxical tissue damage that occurs when tissue is reperfused after a period of ischemia. The reintroduction of oxygen to the cells, leads to the formation of free radicals. Other pathologies caused by free radicals include retinopathy of prematurity and G6PD-deficiency hemolytic anemia.

Enzymes that reduce free radical damage by neutralizing them include: **catalase** (in peroxisomes), **superoxide dismutase** and **myeloperoxidase** (in macrophages), and **glutathione peroxidase** (in the liver). Free radicals can also be eliminated either by antioxidants such as vitamins A, C, and E, or by eventual spontaneous decay.

Myeloperoxidase deficiency and chronic granulomatous disease (caused by superoxide dismutase deficiency) are characterized by recurrent bacterial infections.

Excitatory neurotransmitters, such as asparatate and glutamate, are released during central nervous system (CNS) ischemia and can also lead to nerve cell damage due to excessive stimulation (**excitotoxicity**).

There are also a number of toxic environmental products that mediate cell injury and death (Table 14). Some of the toxins mentioned will be discussed further in subsequent chapters.

N-acetylcysteine is the antidote for acetaminophen toxicity because it regenerates glutathione.

Mnemonic: FADE for treatment of methanol/ ethylene glycol overdose

Toxin (common sources)	Symptoms of Toxicity	Antidote
Lead (lead-based paint) (See Hematology)	Anemia, muscle weakness, convulsions, abdominal pain, coma, death	1. Chelators: Editate disodium (EDTA) and pencillamine 2. Increase excretion: Dimercaprol
Methanol (moonshine)	CNS depression, blindness	1. Fomepizole (alcohol dehydro genase antago nist) 2. Activated charcoal 3. Dialysis 4. Ethanol infusion to competitively inhibit formation of toxic metabolites by alcohol dehydro- genase
Ethylene glycol (antifreeze)	CNS depression, oxalate crystalluria, renal failure	Same as methanol
Arsenic (pesticides)	Abdominal pain, diarrhea, vomiting, muscle cramps, dehydration, shock, sensory neuropathy, garlic breath	1. Dimercaprol 2. Penicillamine
Cyanide (smoke inhalation, nitroprusside) (See Chapter 16)	Convulsions, respiratory failure, coma, lactic acidosis (Inhibits mitochondrial cytochrome oxidase)	1. Sodium nitrite to oxidize hemoglobin to Methemoglobin, which binds to cyanide 2. Thiosulfate binds to cyanide for renal excretion

Carbon monoxide (exhaust, smoke inhalation, gas heater) (See Chapter 16)	Headache, dizziness, nausea, vomiting	1. O_2 to promote CO dissociation
Radiation exposure	Dose dependent: 1. < 100 rads: long-term effects including cataracts, cancer 2. 200–300 rads: myelo-suppression 3. > 1000 rads: CNS injury, death	Prophylaxis

Table 14 Common toxic environmental products

Inflammation

Inflammation is the cellular reaction to injury. The classic local signs of inflammation are: **rubor** (redness), **tumor** (swelling), **calor** (heat), **dolor** (pain), and possible loss of function. Inflamed tissue is the result of increased vascular flow, vessel permeability, and leukocyte migration.

The initial phase of an inflammatory response is characterized first by vasoconstriction, then by vasodilation of arterioles and the opening up of new capillary beds to the region. The function of the initial vasoconstriction is to increase vascular permeability. **Histamine, interleukin 1 (IL-1)** and **tumor necrosis factor (TNF)** induce endothelial cell contraction leading to intercellular gaps in the vessel and thus allowing fluid to escape. As fluid escapes, the surrounding interstitial space becomes more edematous or swollen.

Once fluid has left the vasculature, it can be characterized as either transudate or exudate. **Transudate** is essentially plasma ultrafiltrate, with few cells, few proteins, and a specific gravity < 1.012. It is commonly caused by increased hydrostatic pressure, decreased oncotic pressure, and/or sodium retention. **Exudate**, on the other hand, is protein rich, cell rich, and with a specific gravity > 1.020. It is caused by increased vascular permeability secondary to inflammation. In pleural effusions, transudates are characterized by low levels of **lactate dehydrogenase (LDH)**, while exudates have pleural-fluid/serum LDH levels > 0.6 OR 2/3 normal serum LDH.

Leukocyte Migration

Increased vascular flow and permeability are accompanied by increased leukocyte migration to the site of injury. The method by which leukocytes move from the vasculature into the interstitial space is called **extravasation** and it occurs in 4 steps:

IL-1 and TNF are also acute phase reactants.

Transudate causes: nephrotic syndrome, cirrhosis, CHF

Exudate causes: lymphatic obstruction, malignancy, infection, collagen vascular disease.

The process of extravasation is also the method utilized by cancer cells to metastasize to other parts of the body.

1. **Margination**: Increased vascular permeability leads to stasis of blood flow, and leukocytes begin to migrate towards and "roll" along the endothelial lining of the vessels.

2. **Adhesion:** Leukocytes and endothelial cells carry adhesion receptors (see Table 15), which facilitate adhesion of the leukocytes along the endothelium. Pavementing is the term used to describe an endothelium lined with leukocytes.

3. **Diapedesis:** This is the process by which a leukocyte exits between two endothelial cells on a blood vessel. It is also known as **emigration**. Type IV collagenase is used to drill a hole through the basement membrane to allow the cell to pass through.

4. **Chemotaxis:** Once the leukocytes have left the vasculature, they migrate towards the site of injury by following chemotactic signals, which include bacterial products, complements, and cytokines.

Once leukocytes arrive at the site of injury, they act to clear infection and debris by degranulation and phagocytosis.

	Leukocyte	Endothelium
Molecule for initial adhesion	Sialyl-Lewis^x	E-selectin P-selectin
Molecule for tight binding	LFA-1 (integrin)	ICAM-1

Table 15 Adhesion molecules involved in extravasation

Acute and Chronic Inflammation

Acute inflammation, lasting minutes to days, has a rapid onset of seconds to minutes and is mediated by neutrophils, eosinophils, and antibodies (See Table 16). **Leukocytosis** (> 15,000 white cells/mL) is due to bone marrow release of white cells and is often a sign of inflammation, but **leukopenia** (4,000 white cells/mL) can also be associated with certain infections, especially in neonates and the elderly.

Cytokines, like **IL-1, IL-6,** and **TNF** are **acute phase reactants** and induce an acute phase reaction characterized by fever, hypotension, loss of appetite, increased somnolence, and the hepatic synthesis of more acute phase reactants: **C-reactive protein**, complements, and coagulation proteins like **fibrinogen.** In inflammation, these products coat red blood cells (RBCs) leading to increased aggregation. These aggregated RBCs fall faster in a test tube, allowing for a nonspecific laboratory marker of inflammation: an increased **erythrocyte sedimentation rate (ESR).**

Chronic inflammation is predominantly mediated by monocytes, macrophages, lymphocytes, and plasma cells and may persist for weeks to months. Macrophages are the workhorses of chronic inflammation, secreting cytokines, metabolites, and growth factors crucial for successfully sustaining an inflammatory response.

Diabetes, corticosteroid use, and acute ethanol intoxication can cause defects in adhesion.

Diapedesis usually occurs at venules, where vascular flow and, thus, hemodynamic shear forces are lower.

Mnemonic for chemotactic factors: BLICK 485a

Bacterial products, LTB4, IL-8, C5a, Kallikrein

Sialyl-Lewis and **S**electins **S**tart the Adhesion process. (**L** for Lewis and **L**eukocyte)

Leukocyte adhesion deficiency, an immune deficiency characterized by neutrophilia and recurrent bacterial infections, is caused by LFA-1 deficiency.

Leukemoid reaction is an extreme leukocytosis (>50,000 white cells/mL) resembling leukemia, except that in a leukemoid reaction mature leukocytes are present.

Leukocyte Type	Association
Neutrophils	Bacterial infections
Eosinophils	Parasitic infections, asthma, allergies
Lymphocytes	Viral infection, tumors
Basophil/Mast cells	Allergy
Macrophages/Giant cell	Granulomas

Table 16 Cell types in inflammation

Repair and Regeneration

Following cell injury and inflammation, damaged or destroyed tissue is replaced. **Regeneration** occurs when the replacement tissue is similar to the original tissue in structure and function. **Repair** occurs when the replacement tissue is less specialized and less functional, like scar tissue. Cells can be divided into three categories, depending on their healing characteristics:

1. **Labile cells** are able to proliferate throughout life. When damaged they are replaced by identical cells.

2. **Stable cells** do not normally proliferate but can do so when stimulated, like after an injury.

3. **Permanent cells** are unable to regenerate after an injury and are thus replaced by scar tissue.

Regeneration and repair can occur simultaneously, as after a surgical incision: the epidermis regenerates but the dermis and subcutaneous tissue are repaired.

Tissue repair occurs by 4 steps:

1. **Demolition** is the removal of tissue debris, fibrin, blood clots, etc. by inflammatory cells.

2. **Granulation tissue,** which is highly vascular and fibrotic, begins to form as blood vessels and fibroblasts migrate to the site of injury in response to chemotactic factors (**vascular endothelial growth factor or VEGF** and **fibronectin**, respectively). Fibroblasts act to deposit significant amounts of Type III collagen into the extracellular matrix of granulation tissue.

3. **Maturation**: This step involves the maturation of granulation tissue to avascular fibrous tissue. Blood vessels apoptose and atrophy leading to devascularization. **Myofibroblasts** (actin-containing fibroblasts) contract to bring wound edges together.

Increased ESR: infection, malignancy, pregnancy, autoimmune disease, anemia

Decreased ESR: sickle cell anemia, polycythemia, CHF

When there are more immature leukocytes in circulation (e.g,. more neutrophilic band forms), this is referred to as a "left shift" and indicative of active inflammation.

Labile cells: epithelial cells of GI and respiratory tract, bone marrow cells, skin, hair follicles.

Stable cells: hepatocytes, lymphocytes, smooth muscle.

Permanent cells: neurons, cardiac muscle, skeletal muscle, RBC.

Angiogenesis is the development of new blood vessels.

4. **Remodeling** occurs as Type III collagen is digested by **metalloproteinases** and replaced with Type I collagen by fibroblasts to form a stable scar.

Throughout this wound repair process, complications may occur. **Ulceration** results from inadequate vascularization early in the healing process. Insufficient scar tissue formation can lead to **dehiscence** (opening of the wound). Excess scar tissue can lead to the formation of **keloids** (hypertrophic scars characterized by excess amounts of type III collagen). **Abscesses** (collections of pus surrounded by fibrous tissue) and **fistulas** (abnormal communications between hollow organs or with the body surface) are also results of incomplete or faulty wound healing.

The most common cause of poor wound healing is infection.

NEOPLASIA

Carcinogenesis

Carcinogenesis is the course by which the regulatory processes in the cell cycle malfunction and lead to loss of growth control and **tumor** formation.

Tumor cells are characterized by the following:

1. Self-sufficiency in growth signals

2. Insensitivity to anti-growth signals

3. Evasion of apoptosis

4. Limitless growth potential

5. Sustained angiogenesis

6. Tissue invasion and metastasis

In vitro, they demonstrate disordered multilayered growth because unlike normal cells, in which cell-cell contact prevents excess growth, they are **not contact inhibited**. They are also **anchorage independent** and can grow in soft agar. Tumor cells also require less serum than normal cells because they can **secrete growth factors** on their own. When injected into an animal model, tumor cells can cause formation of a tumor in that animal.

There is substantial evidence to suggest that tumors cells are **monoclonal,** meaning that they arise from a single cell. This typically proceeds in several stages:

1. **Hyperplasia** or increase in cell number is the initial response to cellular insult.

2. **Dysplasia** is when cells begin to lose their original size, shape, and orientation. It is essentially a precancerous state of atypical hyperplasia. **Metaplasia** is when one differentiated cell type is replaced

Hyperplasia, dysplasia, and metaplasia are all reversible conditions.

by another type. It is often in response to external irritation (e.g., with Barrett's esophagus) and can be a neoplastic precursor.

3. **Anaplasia** is when cells become undifferentiated and have little semblance to their original cell.

4. Finally, **neoplasia** is the uncontrolled and excessive proliferation of **tumor** cells. It may be accompanied by **desmoplasia**, the formation of fibrous tissue around the tumor.

Anaplasia and neoplasia are irreversible conditions.

There are several conditions that appear to be pre-neoplastic conditions, characterized by dysplasia or metaplasia secondary to external irritation and may but do not always lead to neoplasia:

- **Actinic keratosis** are small rough patches of skin caused by sun damage and may progress to squamous cell carcinoma.

- **Barrett's esophagus** is caused by long-standing gastroesophageal reflux disease (GERD), in which the lining of the esophagus is replaced with intestinal epithelium to protect from the acid.

- **Cirrhosis** is characterized by diffuse fibrosis of the liver and can be induced by alcohol, viruses, or other conditions affecting the liver (like hemochromatosis) and can progress to hepatocellular carcinoma.

- **Chronic gastritis**—either post-surgical, due to autoimmune conditions like pernicious anemia, or medication induced—can lead to gastric adenocarcinoma.

- **Chronic pancreatitis**—secondary to alcohol, gallstones, or other risk factors—predisposes to the development of pancreatic cancer.

Cell Division

A brief review of normal cell division will facilitate understanding the process by which a normal cell may transform into a tumor cell.

The cell cycle has four phases (Figure 16):

1. **S phase (synthesis)** is when DNA is replicated.

2. **G_2 (gap) phase** is a gap phase during which the cell prepares for cell division.

3. **M phase (mitosis)**, the shortest phase, is when the replicated parent cell DNA separates into two daughter copies and cell division occurs. **Mitosis**, producing two diploid daughter cells (46 chromosomes each), is the process by which somatic cells divide, while **meiosis**, producing 4 haploid daughter cells (23 chromosomes each), is the process by which sex cells divide (Figure 15).

The four phases of mitosis are: prophase, metaphase, anaphase, and telophase.

Collectively, G_1, S, and G_2 make up **interphase**.

Drugs that act on various phases of the cell cycle:

- S: alkaloids, methotrexate

- G2: etoposide, bleomycin

- M: griseofulvin, paclitaxel, vincristine, colchicine

4. G_1(gap) is the phase during which the cell grows and organelles, protein, and RNA are synthesized.

From G_1, cells may enter a quiescent phase known as G_0. Depending on cell type, G_1 and G_0 have varying durations. Labile cells have short G_1 phases and almost never enter G_0 because they are dividing too quickly. Stable cells enter G_0 after cell division but may reenter G_1 when stimulated to divide again by growth factors or hormones. Permanent cells remain in G_0 because they no longer undergo cell division.

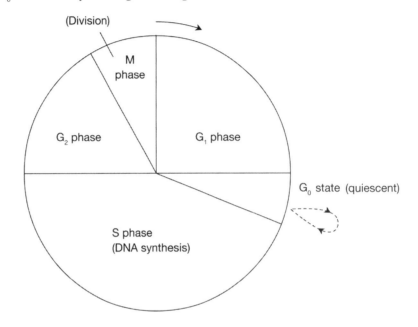

Figure 16 Cell cycle

Tumor cell cycle time is NOT shorter than a normal cell cycle, and a tumor cell does not divide any faster than its normal counterpart. Instead, the **growth fraction**, the fraction of tumor cells that are proliferating is higher than normal. Either a higher percentage of cells is proliferating or a smaller percentage is dying.

Throughout the cell cycle, there are checkpoints in place to ensure proper cell division. Until the cellular requirements for the checkpoints are met, normal cells are unable to proceed into the next phase of the cell cycle. **Cyclins, cyclin-dependent kinases (CDKs),** and **tumor suppressors** are the proteins involved in this regulatory process. CDKs are activated by cyclins to form various cyclin-CDK complexes, which allow progression through different parts of the cell cycle.

Mitosis   Meiosis

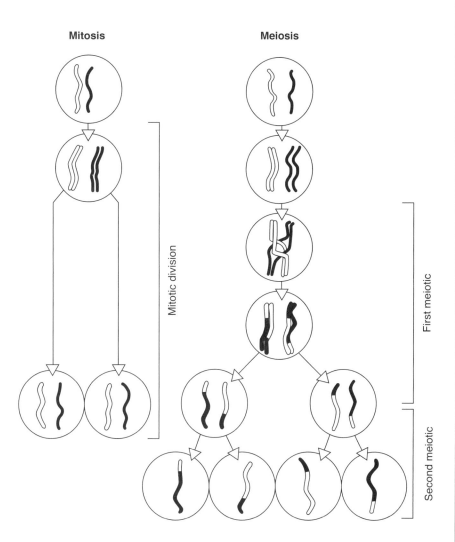

Figure 17 Mitosis and Meiosis

Oncogenes and Tumor Suppressor Genes

Oncogenes arise when **proto-oncogenes** (genes involved in cellular growth) undergo a **gain-of-function**, which leads to uncontrolled cell proliferation. They transform cells in a dominant fashion, meaning only one allele needs to be damaged in order for an oncogene to cause cancer. Proto-oncogene mutations can lead to proteins that are aberrantly functioning or normally functioning but present in abnormally high amounts. **Growth factor receptors, growth factors**, or other signaling molecules involved in cell proliferation can all serve as proto-oncogenes.

One of the most well known oncogenes is the **Philadelphia chromosome (Ph)** or *bcr-abl* in **chronic myelogenous leukemia (CML)**. It is the result of a translocation of part of chromosome 9 to chromosome 22: t(9→22). Although the function of *bcr* is unknown, *abl* is a tyrosine kinase that is normally found in the nucleus. The fusion of *bcr-abl* leads to increased tyrosine kinase activity and the initiation of additional growth signaling cascades. Imatinib is an anti-*bcr-abl* antibody that is used as treatment for CML. Table 17 lists other oncogenes that are important to know for Step 1.

Chromosomal trans-locations can lead to abnormal activation of oncogenes.

Mnemonic: Clean my bling:
CLN-myc BLN

Mnemonic for tyrosine
kinases: ERB: *erb-B2, ret,
bcr-abl*

Oncogene	Gene product	Associated tumor	Clinical correlations
c-myc	Transcription factor	Burkitt's lymphoma	Associated with Epstein-Barr virus (EBV)
l-myc	Transcription factor	Lung cancer	—
n-myc	Transcription factor	Neuroblastoma	—
bcl-2	Anti-apoptotic molecule	Follicular and undifferentiated lymphomas	—
erb-B2 (HER2, neu)	Tyrosine kinase	Breast, ovarian, gastric cancer	Trastuzumab (Herceptin) is an anti-erb-B2 antibody
ret	Tyrosine kinase	Multiple endocrine neoplasia (MEN) types II and III	—
bcr-abl	Tyrosine kinase	Chronic myelogenous leukemia (CML)	Imatinib is an anti-bcr-abl antibody
ras	GTPase	Colon cancer	—
c-kit	Cytokine receptor	Gastrointestinal stromal tumor (GIST)	—
sis	Platelet-derived growth factor (PDGF)	Astrocytoma, osteosarcoma	—

Table 17 Important human oncogenes

Tumor suppressor genes are best thought of as anti-oncogenes. Unlike oncogenes, which behave in a dominant fashion, both copies of tumor suppressor genes must be **inactivated** for neoplastic transformation; this is known as **Knudson's two-hit model** of carcinogenesis. With protective genes that suppress tumor formation, only one actively expressed chromosome is needed to produce a functioning protein. Growth inhibitory factors, cell adhesion molecules, signal transduction molecules, and cell cycle regulators are all within the scope of tumor suppressor genes.

Rb and **p53**, are the most well known tumor suppressor genes and act to inhibit G_1 to S phase cell cycle progression. Rb does this by sequestering transcription factors in an inactive state during the G_1 phase of the cell cycle. It can be overcome by growth factors, which cause a rise in cyclin D and CDK levels, leading to Rb phosphorylation and inactivation by cyclin activated CDK. Once Rb is inactivated, the cell cycle is able to proceed. p53 levels have been shown to rise rapidly in cells experiencing DNA damage. It acts to arrest cells in G_1 phase to allow for DNA repair.

DCC (deleted in colon cancer) and **APC** are two genes associated with colon cancer and thought to encode molecules related to cell adhesion. Loss of normal adhesion can make a cell insensitive to environmental cues that control its growth and proliferation.

Tumor suppressor gene (chromosome)	Associated tumor	Gene product
Rb (13q)	Retinoblastoma, osteosarcoma	Blocks G1S phase
p53 (17p)	Li Fraumeni syndrome, most cancers	Blocks G1 → S phase
p16 (9p)	Melanoma	Blocks G1 → S phase
BRCA1 (17q)	Breast and ovarian cancer	DNA repair protein
BRCA2 (13q)	Breast cancer	DNA repair protein
APC (5q	Colorectal cancer	Decreases expression of cadherin
WT1 (11p)	Wilm's tumor	Regulate nuclear transcription factors
NF1 (17q)	Neurofibromatosis type 1	GTPase: inactivates ras pathway
NF2 (22q)	Neurofibromatosis type 2	Cytoskeleton protein
DCC (18q)	Colon cancer	Transmembrane receptor related to cell adhesion
DPC (18q)	Pancreatic cancer	Little known

Table 18 Important tumor suppressor genes

Carcinogens

Carcinogens, whether chemical, viral, or physical (like radiation) act by causing DNA damage. However, in order for DNA damage to translate to abnormally functioning oncogenes and tumor suppressor genes leading to carcinogenesis, the damage must also (1) escape repair by the cell and (2) be replicated to sustain the mutation. This process of propagating the mutation is called promotion.

Virtually every cancer demonstrates homozygous loss of p53

Li Fraumeni syndrome is the result of inheriting 1 mutated copy of p53, leading to an increased risk of malignancy.

It can be daunting to learn all of the tumor suppressor genes and oncogenes. Focus initially on the gene name and associated tumors.

Certain genetic conditions predispose patients to sustaining DNA mutations.

There are two forms of **chemical carcinogens:** direct and indirect. Compounds such as alkylating agents directly attack DNA, RNA, and proteins, but other compounds, like aromatic amines, are called procarcinogens and require metabolic activation first. Table 19 lists some common chemical carcinogens.

Chemical	Associated tumor
Aflatoxins (produced by *Aspergillus*, may be found in peanut butter)	Liver cancer (hepatocellular carcinoma)
Alkylating agents (e.g., mustard gas, certain anti-neoplastic drugs)	Leukemia
Arsenic	Skin (squamous cell carcinoma), liver cancer (angiosarcoma)
Asbestos	Lung cancer (mesothelioma, bronchogenic carcinoma)
Beryllium	Lung cancer
CCl4 (Carbon tetrachloride) (in cleaning solvents)	Liver cancer
Cigarette smoke	Lung (squamous cell carcinoma), kidney (renal cell carcinoma), bladder cancer
Naphthalene (aniline) dye	Bladder cancer
Nitrosamines (in smoked foods)	Esophageal and stomach cancer
Vinyl chloride	Liver cancer (angiosarcoma)

Table 19 Chemical carcinogens

Acute transforming retroviruses, like the *Rous sarcoma virus*, are RNA viruses that carry oncogenes, usually hyperactive forms of cellular proto-oncogenes. Infection with these viruses leads to the rapid development of cancer, but thus far, acute transforming retroviruses have not been found to be the cause of cancer *in humans*.

DNA tumor viruses, on the other hand, DO cause cancer in humans, but do not appear to use oncogenes. Instead, they are notable for integrating into host genomes. For example, the **human papillomavirus (HPV)** expresses two early viral proteins, E6 and E7, which predispose infected cells to transformation. E6 binds to and inactivates the tumor suppressor gene, p53, while E7 displaces the transcription factors sequestered by Rb. The more carcinogenic HPV strains have E6 and E7 proteins with higher affinity for p53 and Rb.

Cyclophosphamide for lymphoma treatment can also cause bladder cancer. Patients are pre-treated with mesna as a preventative measure.

Mnemonic: A Bath in the Bladder (Napth rhymes with Bath)

Mnemonic: angioVARco-ma: angiosarcomas in Vinylchloride and Arseni

High-risk HPV strains: 16, 18, 31 (associated with cervical cancer)

Low-risk HPV strains: 6, 11 (associated with benign genital warts)

Microbe	RNA retrovirus	Associated Cancer
HTLV-1	RNA retrovirus	T-cell leukemia/lymphoma
HIV	RNA retrovirus	CNS primary lymphoma
HCV	RNA Flavivirus	Hepatocellular cancer
HBV	DNA Hepadnavirus	Hepatocellular cancer
HPV (16, 18, 31)	DNA Papillomavirus	Cervical, penile, anal cancer
EBV	DNA Herpesvirus	Burkitt's lymphoma, nasopharyngeal carcinoma
HHV-8	DNA Herpesvirus	Kaposi's sarcoma, B-cell lymphoma
H. pylori	Gram-negative rod	Gastric cancer and lymphoma
Schistosoma	Helminth/worm	Bladder cancer

Table 20 Common oncogenic microbes

HTLV-1 and HIV are carcinogenic RNA retroviruses but do not contain oncogenes, but act by upregulating transcription factors.

Tumor Immunology and Invasion

There are at least three ways that a tumor escapes immune recognition after transformation and invasion:

1. **Decreased immunogenicity**: Tumors can "look normal" to T-cells because novel proteins expressed by the tumor cell are unable to be presented by major histocompatibility complex (MHC) class I molecules and thus are undetectable by T-cells.

2. **Selection**: Because the immune system attacks tumor cells whose surface markers it recognizes, this process selects for tumor cells lacking these tumor antigens.

3. **Immune suppression**: Tumor cells may secrete factors, such as transforming growth factor-beta (TGF-beta) and interleukin-10 (IL-10) that lead to immune suppression.

When neoplastic cells remain confined to the basement membrane, they are considered **in situ carcinomas**. Once cells invade past the basement membrane using Type IV collagenases, they are able to invade blood or lymphatic vessels and metastasize to different parts of the body by extravasation. There are varying theories about where tumor cells metastasize. The "seed" theory states that tumor cells embolize and travel where they may through the blood and lymphatic systems, whereas the "soil" theory proposes that there are target organs for different types of cancers. With both theories, angiogenesis to the site of metastasis is important for continued tumor survival. (Figure 18)

Approximately 50% of brain tumors are metastases, most commonly from the breast, lung, GI tumors, skin (melanoma), or kidneys. Tumors that metastasize via the lymphatics commonly travel to the liver and lung. These tumors are the colon, stomach, pancreas, breast, and lung. The tumors that most commonly metastasize to bone are the prostate and breast but also the thyroid, testes, lung and kidney. Liver and bone metastases are much more common than primary liver and bone tumors, especially when there are multiple masses present.

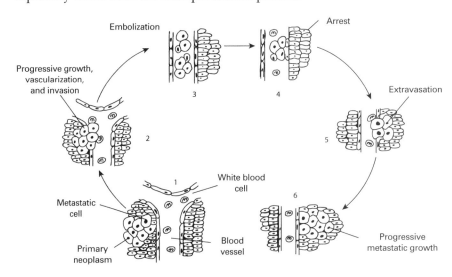

Figure 18 Tissue metastasis

Types of Tumors

It is important to note that tumors can behave differently. **Benign** tumors are usually slower growing, better differentiated, better demarcated, and have lower chance of metastasis, whereas **malignant** tumors tend to grow more quickly, to invade and metastasize. Depending on the degree of differentiation and spread, tumors are classified into various grades and stages.

Grade refers to the degree of differentiation and number of mitoses in the tumor. Tumors of higher grades tend to be more invasive but also more radiosensitive because they are dividing more rapidly and are less likely to be able to repair the DNA damage done by the radiation vs normal cells. **Tumor stage** refers to the degree of spread from the primary lesion. It is designated based on three criteria, known as the **TNM staging system**: <u>T</u>umor size, number of <u>N</u>odes, and number of distant <u>M</u>etastases.

Not only are tumors distinguished by their mitotic characteristics and invasiveness, they are named based on the original cell type involved and whether they are benign or not. For example, a tumor originating from an epithelial cell is called a **carcinoma**, whereas a tumor originating from a mesenchymal cell (like muscle or bone) is called a **sarcoma**. Table 21 further describes how tumors are named.

In addition, **hamartomas** describe a special type of benign tumor characterized by overgrowth of tissue normally found in that region. This is in contrast to **choristomas**, which describe benign tumors found where it is normally absent.

Teratomas are also special tumors that are characterized as having more than one cell type, more specifically more than one of the three germ cell layers. As a result, teratomas are often characterized by bizarre findings such as hair, bones, teeth and occasionally more complex organs like eyes, hands and feet. Teratomas are characterized as either mature or immature. Mature teratomas are named as such because they tend to be well differentiated, encapsulated, and benign. Immature teratomas are less differentiated and more malignant in nature.

Cell type	Benign	Malignant
Epithelial cells	Adenoma (glandular epithelium)	Adenocarcinoma (glandular)
	Papilloma (squamous epithelium)	Papillary carcinoma (squamous)
Blood cells	—	Leukemia, lymphoma
Blood vessels	Hemangioma	Angiosarcoma
Bone cells	Osteoma	Osteosarcoma
Fat cells	Lipoma	Liposarcoma
Muscle cells	Leiomyoma (smooth muscle)	Leiomyosarcoma (smooth)
	Rhabdomyoma (skeletal muscle)	Rhabdomyosarcoma (skeletal)

Table 21 Tumor nomenclature

Leukemia is widespread with tumor cells arising from bone marrow, whereas lymphoma is more discrete with tumor cells arising from lymph nodes.

Neoplastic Associations

Different tumor types secrete different biochemical products, a property which allows clinicians to test for various **tumor markers**. It should be noted that tumor markers are not specific or used for primary diagnosis; instead, they are used more to monitor tumor response to therapy or recurrence. See Table 22 for important tumor markers.

Certain tumors can also cause specific **paraneoplastic effects** which are symptoms secondary to the presence of cancer cells in the body, but not directly due to local tumor presence. Just as certain cancers secrete specific tumor markers, they can also secrete biochemically active products. For example:

- Small cell lung tumors and intracranial tumors can secrete anti-diuretic hormone (ADH) causing a **syndrome of inappropriate ADH secretion (SIADH)**, presenting as hyponatremia and highly concentrated urine.

- Small cell lung cancers can also secrete **adrenocorticotropic hormone (ACTH)** or ACTH-like peptides leading to an increase in adrenal gland stimulation. The result is **Cushing's syndrome,** caused by excess cortisol (an adrenal hormone), presenting with the typical moon facies, buffalo hump, telangiectasias, and central obesity.

- Squamous cell lung cancers, renal carcinomas, and breast cancers can secrete **parathyroid hormone-related peptides (PTH-rP)** leading to the stimulation of PTH receptors, most commonly presenting as **hypercalcemia.**

- Thymomas and small cell lung cancers can secrete antibodies against neuromuscular pre-synaptic Ca^{2+} channels, similar to the pathophysiology of **Lambert-Eaton syndrome**, both of which result in muscle weakness.

- Renal call carcinomas and hemangioblastomas can lead to increased **erythropoietin** secretion causing **polycythemia.**

- Leukemias and lymphomas have such high turnover rates that they can result in **hyperuricemia**, leading to gout and urate nephropathy.

There are also a significant number of conditions that are merely associated with specific neoplasms, some of which are straightforward and some of which are not. For example, patients with **Paget's disease** are predisposed to bone cancer because the condition is already characterized by abnormal activity of bone cells. Similarly, patients with **dyplastic nevus syndrome** tend to develop more moles than the typical patient and are thus predisposed to developing malignant melanoma.

Then there is **acanthosis nigricans**, dark, and poorly defined velvety skin lesions and **migrating thrombophlebitis,** venous inflammation due to clots at multiple sites of the body, which are more signs of visceral malignancy rather than causative conditions.

See Table 23 for a complete list of disease-neoplasm associations.

Tumor Marker	Neoplasm
Alpha-fetoprotein (AFP)	Hepatocellular carcinoma, yolk sac tumors
Alkaline phosphatase (ALP)	Paget's disease of bone, bone metastases
Beta-human chorionic gonadotropin (beta-hCG)	Hydatiform moles, choriocarcinomas, gestational trophoblastic tumors
Bence Jones protein (light chain immunoglobulin)	Multiple myeloma
Bombesin	Neuroblastoma
Calcitonin	Thyroid medullary carcinoma

Calretinin	Mesothelioma
Carcinoembryonic antigen (CEA)	GI tumors: mostly colorectal and pancreatic, but also gastric, breast
CA-125	Ovarian, epithelial tumors
CA-19-9	Pancreatic adenocarcinoma
Prostate-specific antigen (PSA)	Prostate carcinoma, benign prostatic hypertrophy (BPH), prostatitis
S-100	Melanoma, astrocytomas, neural tumors
Tartrate-resistant acid phosphatase (TRAP)	Hairy cell leukemia

Table 22 Tumor markers

Neurocutaneous disorders	Associated Neoplasm
Neurofibromatosis type I (von Recklinhausen's disease)	Neurofibromas in skin, optic gliomas
Sturge-Weber syndrome	Ipsilateral leptomeningeal angiomas
Tuberous Sclerosis	Hamartomas, cardiac rhabdomyomas, renal angiomyolipoma, astrocytoma
Von Hippel Lindau disease	Bilateral renal cell carcinoma, hemangioblastomas, cavernous hemangiomas
Disease	Associated Neoplasm
Acanthosis nigricans	Visceral malignancy
AIDS	Primary CNS lymphoma, Kaposi sarcoma
Dermatomyositis	Leukemia, lymphoma, lung cancer
Down syndrome	Acute lymphocytic leukemia (ALL), acute myelogenous leukemia (AML)
Migrating thrombophlebitis	Visceral malignancy
Myasthenia gravis	Thymoma
Peutz-Jehgers syndrome	Colorectal, breast and gynecological cancer, GI hamartomas
Plummer-Vinson Syndrome	Esophageal squamous carcinoma
Ulcerative colitis	Colonic adenocarcinoma
Dysplastic Nevus syndrome	Malignant melanoma
Paget's disease of bone	Osteosarcoma, fibrosarcoma

Table 23 Diseases associated with neoplasms

Familial Cancer Syndromes

Familial cancers, which are rare, follow a dominant inheritance pattern. Germline inactivation of tumor suppressor genes seems to be the most common cause of familial cancer syndromes.

Retinoblastoma is the most common eye tumor in children, appearing in two forms. The sporadic form of retinoblastoma occurs in one eye and accounts for 60% of the cases. The inherited form of retinoblastoma is autosomal dominant, occurring earlier in life and resulting in multiple tumors.

There are also a number of autosomal dominant familial forms of colon cancer:

- **Li-Fraumeni syndrome,** characterized by p53 mutations, is found in 70% of sporadic colon carcinomas.

- **Familial adenomatous polyposis (FAP)** involves mutation of the APC gene leading to 100% penetrance, meaning all patients with FAP will get thousands of polyps that eventually progress to colon cancer. The definitive treatment for FAP is a total colectomy.

- **Hereditary nonpolyposis colorectal cancer (HNPCC)** or **Lynch syndrome** is a mutation of a DNA mismatch repair gene that leads to 80% of patients with colon cancer.

Chromosomal fragility diseases are rare and tend to follow an autosomal recessive inheritance pattern. They result in a very high incidence of malignancy in young patients. For example:

- **Bloom syndrome** is most common in Ashkenazi Jews, who have lower cellular levels of DNA ligase. Symptoms include growth retardation, skin sensitivity to sun, and immunosuppression.

- **Ataxia telangiectasia** is also common in Jewish individuals and is a chromosomal breakage syndrome causing immune deficiency, cerebellar ataxia, and telangiectasias. Patients also have a heightened sensitivity to radiation and developing abnormalities in the cell cycle.

- **Fanconi anemia** is caused by multiple defective proteins involved in DNA repair. It is marked by aplastic anemia before age 10, skin hyperpigmentation, developmental abnormalities, especially in the limbs and kidneys, and increased rates of hepatic tumors and acute myelogenous leukemias.

Cancer Epidemiology

Cancer is the second leading cause of death in the United States (second to heart disease). Of the different types of cancers, the most lethal in both men and women is lung cancer. The most common cancers in men and women are listed in Table 24. Since the implementation of pap smears to screen for cervical cancer, the most common gynecologic cancer in women is now endometrial cancer, followed by ovarian, then cervical. The most lethal gynecologic cancer is ovarian, followed by cervical, then endometrial. The most common childhood cancer is acute lymphocytic leukemia (ALL).

Male	Female
Most common to least common: • Prostate • Lung • Colorectal	Most common to least common: • Breast • Lung • Colorectal
Most lethal: • Lung • Prostate	Most lethal: • Lung • Breast

Table 24 Cancer prevalence

Gardner's syndrome: FAP + soft tissue and bony tumors
Turcot syndrome: FAP + CNS tumors

Gynecologic: incidence EOC→ lethal OCE (the order remains the same, but the E shifts to the back because the End is lethal)

CHAPTER 6

ENDOCRINE SYSTEM

HYPOTHALAMUS AND PITUITARY GLAND

Embryology

The hypothalamus and pituitary, which sit at the base of the brain, are key players in many of the endocrine functions of the body. The hypothalamus is real brain tissue, arising from the diencephalon (which gives rise to all structures with "thalamus" in their names: epithalamus, thalamus, subthalamus, and hypothalamus).

The pituitary, on the other hand, is made up of two different origins. The posterior pituitary, or neurohypophysis, also arises from neuroectoderm—the infundibulum, to be precise. The anterior pituitary, or adenohypophysis, rises up from the oral ectoderm—known as Rathke's pouch—between weeks 4 and 6 of development. The connection between the pouch and oral cavity degenerates, but if remnants persist, it may later give rise to craniopharyngiomas.

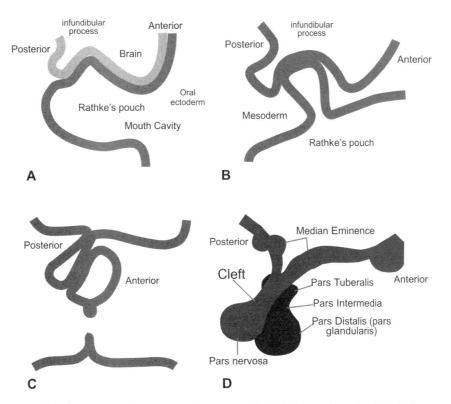

Figure 1 Pituitary development. **A.** Beginning formation of Rathke's pouch and infundibular process. **B.** Neck of Rathke's pouch constricted by growth of mesoderm. **C.** Rathke's pouch pinched off. **D.** Mature form.

Anatomy

The hypothalamus is connected to the pituitary gland in two ways. First, nerve fibers travel directly from the hypothalamus to the **posterior pituitary** (Figure 2). The hormones **vasopressin** (antidiuretic hormone, ADH) and **oxytocin** are synthesized in these nuclei and travel down into the bloodstream of the posterior pituitary.

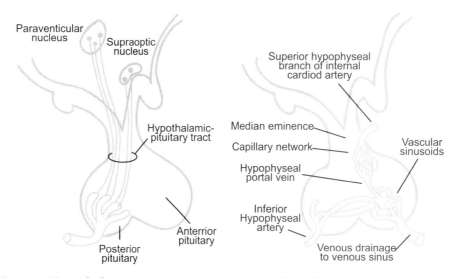

Figure 2 Hypothalamic-pituitary connections. **A.** Hypothalamohypophyseal tract. **B.** Hypophyseal portal system.

The anterior pituitary is connected to the hypothalamus through a portal blood supply, which allows blood to travel between two separate capillary beds before returning to the heart, like the liver portal system. The **superior hypophyseal arteries** descend on each side and divide to become a capillary network within the anterior pituitary. This blood supply carries many released hormones from the hypothalamus, which stimulate secretion in the anterior pituitary. These hormones include **gonadotropin-releasing hormone** (GnRH), **somatostatin**, **growth hormone–releasing hormone** (GHRH), **thyrotropin-releasing hormone** (TRH), **dopamine**, and **corticotropinreleasing hormone** (CRH). The pituitary hormones are listed in Table 1.

Anterior pituitary	Posterior pituitary
FSH	Oxytocin
LH	Vasopressin (ADH)
GH	
TSH	
Prolactin	
ACTH	
MSH	

Table 1 Pituitary Hormones

One way to remember the hormones released by the anterior pituitary is to use a mnemonic based on the histological staining of the cells. "GPa" reminds you of **GH** and **prolactin,** which are produced in acidophilic cells. "b-FLAT" refers to **FSH, LH, ACTH,** and **TSH,** which are produced in basophilic cells. Interestingly, FSH, LH, and TSH have identical a subunits and differentiate themselves through their b subunits. Another useful fact to remember about the anterior pituitary hormones is that ACTH is derived from proopiomelanocortin, or **POMC,** a precursor which also gives rise to MSH, b-lipotropin, and b-endorphin. A disorder which causes elevated ACTH levels will also cause stimulation of melanocytes, a phenomenon which explains the darkening of crural folds seen in **Addison's disease**.

Because the pituitary sits above the optic chiasm, a pituitary tumor may cause visual disturbances.

Panhypopituitarism

If there is a deficiency of all pituitary hormones (panhypopituitarism), whether congenital or acquired (e.g., trauma), FSH and LH are usually the first to decrease, resulting in **menstrual irregularities** and **genital atrophy**. Adrenocorticotropic hormone (ACTH) and thyroid-stimulating hormone (TSH) are the next to fall, leading to **hypoadrenalism, hypotension, hyperkalemia,** and **hypothyroidism**.

Clinical scenarios in which you should suspect panhypopituitarism include patients with the above findings who have a history consistent with pituitary adenomas or brain tumors, trauma, stroke, surgery to the brain, or postpartum pituitary necrosis (**Sheehan's syndrome**). The pituitary tumor may be a component of **multiple endocrine neoplasia (type I)**, discussed later in this chapter. Treatment is with replacement hormones.

VASOPRESSIN

Vasopressin causes the collecting tubules of the kidneys to reabsorb water back from the urine (hence, its other name, antidiuretic hormone). It also acts directly on peripheral arterioles, causing vasoconstriction. Both of these actions serve to increase blood pressure.

Vasopressin release is regulated by osmoreceptors in the **paraventricular** and **supraoptic nuclei** of the hypothalamus. When the hypothalamus detects a rise in plasma osmolality (for example, when a patient is dehydrated), it stimulates the release of vasopressin from the posterior pituitary.

Diabetes Insipidus

Diabetes insipidus (DI) causes the inappropriate production of large amounts of dilute urine, which leads to frequent urination, extreme thirst, and nocturia. **Central DI** is due to a deficient secretion of ADH as a result of trauma, pituitary sugery, or hypoxic or ischemic encephalopathy. **Nephrogenic DI** is characterized by renal resistance to ADH. This can be

GPa: GH and prolactin

b-FLAT: FSH, LH, ACTH, TSH

The Supraoptic nucleus helps you "sop" up water from kidneys.

due to genetics (mutation in ADH receptor or aquaporin), lithium use, hypercalcemia, or an ADH antagonist.

A classic case of central DI would be a patient who begins to produce large amounts of low-osmolality urine after head trauma. The differential diagnosis for large volumes of low-osmolality urine would be central DI, nephrogenic DI, or psychogenic polydipsia (in other words, the patient is drinking extremely excessive amounts of water). The osmolality of the plasma would differentiate polydipsia from DI: if the plasma osmolality is high, then DI is the culprit. If the plasma osmolality is low, the patient is drinking too much water. Another test to differentiate the two entities would be to deprive the patient of water: In patients with DI, the urine osmolality remains unchanged, but in patients with polydipsia, the urine osmolality rises. The next step would be to differentiate central from nephrogenic DI. In central DI, the plasma ADH level is low, and urine osmolality rises following intravenous administration of ADH (or its analogue, desmopressin). If the DI is nephrogenic, on the other hand, the plasma ADH levels may be normal or high, and intravenous ADH would not affect the urine osmolality since the kidneys simply cannot respond to the hormone.

A low solute diet is recommended for both types of DI. For central DI, intranasal desmopressin is a standard therapy. For nephrogenic DI, a thiazide diuretic (hydrocholorothiazide), amiloride, or NSAIDs (indomethacin) is common.

Syndrome of Inappropriate Antidiuretic Hormone Secretion

Too much ADH causes excess free water absorption in the kidneys relative to the body's needs. The results are hyponatremia in the setting of overly concentrated urine. There are many etiologies, including pulmonary disease, cranial lesions, and ectopic ADH production—(oat cell carcinoma of the lung is a classic example). Treatment is water restriction and treatment of the underlying disorder. Demeclocycline blocks the action of ADH on the collecting ducts.

Making the diagnosis of SIADH is not trivial. The patient must have hyponatremia in the presence of plasma hypo-osmolality, since artifactual hyponatremia can arise from disorders like hyperglycemia and hyperlipidemia. The urine must also be inappropriately concentrated, which differentiates SIADH from excessive water intake. Euvolemia must be present; in other words, rule out congestive heart failure, cirrhosis, and nephrotic syndrome. Finally, the patient must not have any renal, adrenal, or thyroid insufficiency, which could cause salt wasting.

GROWTH HORMONE

Growth hormone (GH), or **somatotropin**, acts on the skeletal system to increase linear growth. GH acts on the liver to promote the synthesis of insulin-like growth factor (IGF-1, also known as somatomedin C), which then act on chondrocytes in the bone to increase cell division. Related actions of GH include increased protein synthesis and increased lipolysis. GH is also a counter-regulatory hormone—that is, it counters the actions of insulin on carbohydrate metabolism by increasing glucose release by the liver and decreasing glucose uptake in tissue.

Regulation of GH is varied (Figure 3). Increased secretion of GH is triggered by multiple factors, including secretion of GHRH by the hypothalamus, sleep, stress, hypoglycemia, increased serum amino acids, and dopamine. Decreased secretion occurs during hypothalamic secretion of somatostatin (also known as *growth hormone-inhibiting hormone*), obesity, hyperglycemia, cortisol, and, of course, high levels of GH.

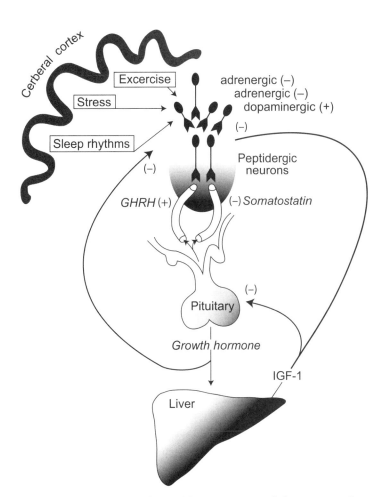

Figure 3 Growth hormone feedback loop. (GHRH = growth hormone-releasing hormone.)

Acromegaly occurs when excess growth hormone is produced by a pituitary tumor in adults (after the epiphyseal plates have fused in bones). Bony overgrowth (jaw) as well as soft tissue overgrowth (heart) are common. Diabetes mellitus due to glucose intolerance can occur, albeit rarely, from excess growth hormone activity. Treatment is via transsphenoidal surgery or local radiation.

Short Stature

The number of non-endocrine and endocrine causes of short stature is rather extensive (Table 2). Common causes of short stature include constitutional short stature, genetic short stature, and malnutrition. A child with constitutional short stature has physiologically but not mentally delayed development and will reach normal or low-normal height after a delayed puberty. In genetic short stature, other family members are also short, and the child does not have a delayed bone age or delay in reaching puberty.

The benefits of GH therapy for short children depends greatly on the cause of short stature. Children with classic growth hormone deficiency (a diagnosis that is difficult to make, as various factors can influence the results of a GH challenge test) have proven benefit. Children with Turner's syndrome and renal failure have some benefit, as do extremely short children with delayed bone age and very slow growth velocities, as defined by a research protocol. For other children with short stature, it is unclear whether GH treatment results in an increase in adult height.

Cause	Associated findings
Non-endocrine	
Constitutional short stature	Familial history of delayed puberty
Genetic short stature	Parents are also short
Prematurity	Will usually catch up by 1–2 years of age
Intrauterine growth retardation (IUGR)	Will usually remain of short stature
Turner's syndrome	45,XO; phenotypic female
Prader-Willi syndrome	Hypotonia, mental retardation, obesity
Achondroplasia	Autosomal dominant, short extremities, and large head
Chronic disease	Diagnosis of chronic disease
Malnutrition	Consider food faddism, anorexia nervosa, poor diet
Drugs (e.g., high-dose methylphenidate)	Known drug use
Endocrine	
Congenital GH deficiency	Obesity, immature facial appearance, immature high-pitched voice, mid-line defects
Acquired GH deficiency	History of tumor
Psychosocial dwarfism	History of abuse (ignored or severely disciplined child)
Hypothyroidism	Low free T4, apathy, bradycardia
Cushing's syndrome	Buffalo hump, moon facies, central obesity
Rickets (Vitamin D deficiency)	Bow-legged, chest deformity

Table 2 Causes of short stature

Tall Stature

Non-endocrine causes of tall stature include constitutional tall stature and genetic tall stature. In constitutional tall stature, the child may be taller than his or her peers throughout childhood but grows at a normal velocity with a moderately advanced bone age. The final height is usually within normal range for the child's family. Genetic tall stature refers to a tall child who comes from a tall family. The child's growth velocity is normal, as is his or her bone age.

Endocrine disorders that can cause tall stature include pituitary gigantism, commonly from a GH-secreting adenoma. The somatic features of acromegaly are present, and the individual also undergoes excessive linear growth becausethe GH excess is present prior to epiphyseal fusion. Tall stature in children from sexual precocity, or early onset of estrogen or androgen secretion, leads to a paradoxically short adult because the bone age is advanced, causing early cessation of growth. Thyrotoxicosis also produces advanced growth and bone age that can lead to decreased adult height.

The causes of tall stature are listed in Table 3.

Cause	Associated findings
Non-endocrine	
Constitutional tall stature	Advanced bone age, no other disorders, possible obesity
Genetic tall stature	Tall parents, normal bone age
Syndromes	
Marfan's syndrome	Long thin fingers, hyperextension of joints, heart murmur, lens subluxation
XYY syndrome	Abnormal karyotype
Klinefelter's syndrome	XXY karyotype, gynecomastia, hypogonadism
Beckwith-Wiedemann syndrome	Overweight, macroglossia, omphalocele, hypoglycemia
Cerebral gigantism	Prominent forehead, high-arched palate, sharp chin, hypertelorism, mental retardation
Homocystinuria	Phenotype similar to Marfan's syndrome, mental retardation, seizures, osteoporosis, thromboembolism
Endocrine	
Pituitary gigantism	Acromegaly, pituitary adenoma
Sexual precocity	Early puberty, short adult height
Thrytoxicosis	Advanced bone age, short adult height

Table 3 Causes of tall stature

THYROID GLAND

Physiology

The thyroid gland secretes hormones that act on the nucleus and mitochondria of cells all over the body. Their main role is activating metabolic activity. Some effects of thyroid hormone include increased synthesis of protein, increased degradation of glycogen and fat, and increased heart rate and contractility.

The release of thyroid hormone is regulated by the hypothalamus and anterior pituitary gland (Figure 4). **TRH** triggers the release of **TSH** from the pituitary. This in turn stimulates the synthesis and release of thyroid hormone from the thyroid gland. Thyroid hormone in the bloodstream then exerts a negative feedback effect on both the pituitary and hypothalamus. In addition, the thyroid gland has some capacity for self-regulation. When iodine is deficient, iodine transport is increased; as iodine becomes overabundant, iodine transport is inhibited. Complete inhibition of iodine transport due to excess iodine is known as a **Wolff-Chaikoff affect**.

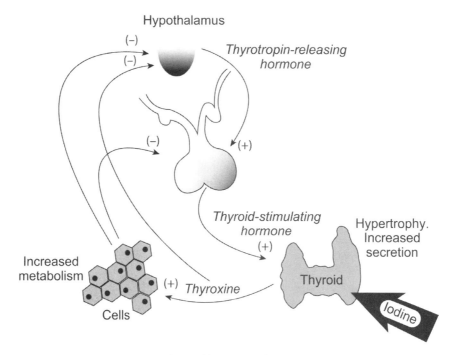

Figure 4 Thyroid hormone feedback loop

Development

The thyroid gland is the first endocrine gland to develop in humans, starting around weeks 3–4. A downgrowth of ectoderm from the floor of the pharynx descends in the neck while maintaining its connection to the tongue by a tube known as the **thyroglossal duct**. Although the thyroglossal duct usually atrophies, remnants may form thyroglossal cysts and sinuses, which present later in life. The site of origin of the thyroglossal duct is known as the **foramen cecum**. In some cases, the thyroid may fail to descend, or may descend incompletely, resulting in a lingual thyroid or an accessory thyroid gland in the tongue or neck.

Anatomy and Histology

The thyroid glands consist of two lobes, connected across the midline by an isthmus across the second to fourth tracheal rings. Blood supply arises primarily from the superior thyroid artery (off the common carotid artery) and inferior thyroid artery (off the subclavian artery); venous drainage is from the superior, middle, and inferior thyroid veins (Figure 5).

Anterior view

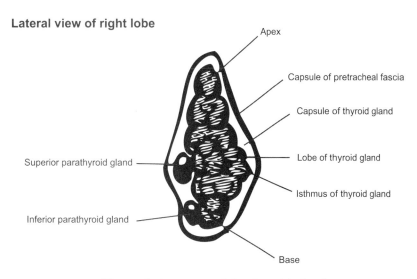

Lateral view of right lobe

Figure 5 Anatomy of the thyroid gland

Histologically, the thyroid gland consists of multiple follicles filled with **colloid**, a gelatinous substance (Figure 6). These follicles are lined by simple cuboidal epithelium, which synthesizes the thyroid hormones thyroxine (T4) and triiodothyronine (T3). **Parafollicular cells** are also present in the follicles and secrete **calcitonin**.

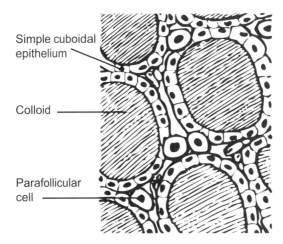

Figure 6 Histology of the thyroid gland

Thyroid Hormone Synthesis

During thyroid hormone synthesis, the thyroid gland takes up iodide, a nutrient rapidly absorbed in the gastrointestinal (GI) tract. Uptake occurs via active transport aided in the thyroid by an Na^+/K^+-adenosine triphosphatase (ATPase). The iodide is then oxidized and attached to thyroglobulin, a glycoprotein synthesized by the thyroid gland. This results in **monoiodotyrosine** (MIT), which subsequently acquires another iodide and becomes **diiodotyrosine** (DIT). Two molecules of DIT are then joined together to form T4, or one molecule of DIT and one MIT can be joined to form T3 (Figure 7). T4 and T3 are released into the bloodstream as required.

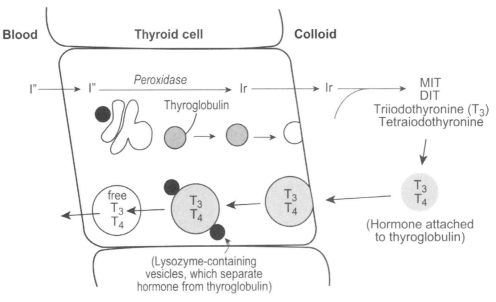

Figure 7 Thyroid hormone synthesis (MIT = monoiodotyrosine; DIT = diiodotyrosine; T4 = thyroxine).

Once T3 and T4 are in the serum, they can remain free or else can be bound to thyroid hormone transport proteins. Only the free forms are biologically active; therefore, variations in the quantity of thyroid-binding proteins can alter total serum T3 and T4 without changing the amount of free forms available. Most T4 is bound to T4-binding globulin (TBG), and the remainder is bound to

T4-binding prealbumin (TBPA) and albumin. T3 is also bound primarily to TBG, although a small amount is found bound to albumin as well.

Although free T4 is found in higher concentrations in the blood than free T3, T3 is about four times more potent than T4. In general, T4 is converted locally to T3 so that tissues have the benefit of the stronger hormone. T4 may also be converted to reverse T3, an inactive form. Most T3 in the blood comes from the metabolism of T4.

Thyroid Function Tests

The first step in assessing thyroid dysfunction (after a history and physical examination) involves checking the status of the pituitary. Levels of TSH are low when the thyroid is hyperactive and high when the thyroid is hypoactive as a result of feedback suppression, assuming that the pituitary is functioning correctly. Assessing the levels of thyroid hormone is done by checking T4 levels because it is much more difficult to check T3 levels. T4 levels vary depending on the amount of free T4 and the binding capacity of proteins in the serum. In conditions such as pregnancy, hepatitis, and cirrhosis, there is an increased thyroid-binding capacity, whereas in situations of protein loss or steroid use, there is a decrease of binding capacity. Therefore, hypo- or hyperthyroidism can be missed by placing too much stock in "normal" total T4 levels.

To determine binding capacity, a resin T3 uptake measurement can be performed. This measure, along with the total T4 level, can provide the **free T4 index**, which is proportional to the amount of free T4 in the serum.

To evaluate thyroid nodules, a **thyroid scan** is performed. A thyroid scan uses small doses of radioactive iodine or technetium, which is taken up by the metabolic activity of the thyroid gland. This makes it possible to visualize the gland and is useful in determining whether a nodule is "hot" (overactive) or "cold" (underactive) relative to the rest of the thyroid. Fine-needle aspiration (FNA), core biopsy, and excision are also used to establish a diagnosis.

Hypothyroidism

Chronic Autoimmune (Hashimoto's) Thyroiditis

Hashimoto's thyroiditis is the most common cause of hypothyroidism in iodine-sufficient areas. It is an autoimmune disorder and presents with high levels of serum antibodies against **thyroglobulin**, **thyroid peroxidase**, or the **TSH receptor**, as well as lymphocytic infiltration of the thyroid. It is characterized by gradual thyroid failure, goiter formation, or both. Thyroid function tests may be normal unless the patient is hypothyroid (20% of cases). Treatment consists of thyroid replacement therapy, even in patients with normal thyroid function tests, because it helps to reduce the size of the thyroid.

Congenital Hypothyroidism (Cretinism)

Congenital deficiency of thyroid hormone is most often due to agenesis or dysgenesis of the thyroid. It may also be transient if the mother has TSH-R blocking antibodies or takes antithyroid drugs. Infants display poor feeding, coarse skin, excessive somnolence, and a hoarse cry. Their appearance is stocky with enlarged tongue and wide-set eyes. These children must be treated with thyroid replacement as soon as possible to avoid the development of mental retardation.

Iatrogenic Hypothyroidism

There are many causes of iatrogenic hypothyroidism, including thyroid surgery, neck irradiation, and chronic lithium therapy. Therapeutic use of iodine-131 for thyrotoxicosis may lead to hypothyroidism.

Iodine

Both iodine deficiency and excess can cause hypothyroidism. Iodine deficiency is the most common cause of hypothyroidism worldwide. Iodine excess causes hypothyroidism by inhibiting iodide organification and T4 and T3 synthesis.

Infiltrative disease

Fibrous thyroiditis (Reidel's thyroiditis), hemochromatosis, scleroderma, leukemia, and cystinosis are rare causes of hypothyroidism.

Secondary or Tertiary Hypothyroidism

Secondary hypothyroidism is that caused by TSH deficiency, and tertiary hypothyroidism is caused by TRH deficiency. Both are rare causes of hypothyroidism.

SIGNS AND SYMPTOMS

Lethargy, cold intolerance, constipation, weight gain despite reduced appetite, and irregular menses. Coarse hair and dry skin with nonpitting edema (myxedema) and slowed relaxation phase of deep tendon reflexes are noted. Women may experience menorrhagia.

DIAGNOSIS

Serum T4 is decreased. TSH is high in primary hypothyroidism.

TREATMENT

Treatment consists of thyroid replacement therapy and regular TSH monitoring.

Hyperthyroidism

Graves' Disease

Graves' disease is an autoimmune disorder that is the most common cause of hyperthyroidism. Patients develop antibodies that bind to the thyroid's TSH receptors and stimulate thyroid hormone synthesis.

SIGNS AND SYMPTOMS

Tremors, anxiety, weight loss despite increased appetite, diarrhea, palpitations, heat hypersensitivity, insomnia, and occasionally exophthalmos (big, bulging eyeballs like Marty Feldman). Signs include tachycardia, widened pulse pressure, tremor, warm skin, and occasional atrial fibrillation.

DIAGNOSIS

Elevated T3, T4, and the presence of anti-TSH receptor antibodies. Antimicrosomal antibodies are also seen.

TREATMENT

Surgery, radioactive iodine, or antithyroid medications, such as propylthiouracil (PTU) and methimazole. A thyroidectomy would leave the patient hypothyroid and requiring lifelong thyroid replacement therapy. Also, remember that the recurrent laryngeal nerve runs through the thyroid gland and may be damaged during surgery, resulting in vocal cord paralysis on the affected side.

Symptomatic relief can be given with propranolol.

Subacute Thyroiditis

Subacute thyroiditis (also known as de Quervin's thyroiditis) is most likely viral in etiology, leading to inflammation of the thyroid. The ensuing damage to thyroid follicles and proteolysis of the thyrogobulin stored within the follicles causes unregulated release of T4 and T3, resulting in mild hyperthyroidism and fever.

SIGNS AND SYMPTOMS

Patients are often asymptomatic or have a tender, enlarged thyroid gland with neck pain.

DIAGNOSIS

Diagnosis is made based on symptoms, but laboratory tests show decreased radioactive iodine uptake and elevated sedimentation rate.

TREATMENT

Anti-inflammatory agents, including glucocorticoids are used, and β-blockers are used for cardiovascular symptom control. Patients may need temporary thyroid replacement therapy for periods of hypothyroidism which follow the hyperthyroidism.

Toxic Adenoma and Toxic Multinodular Goiter

Toxic adenoma and toxic multinodular goiter are the result of hyperplasia of thyroid follicular cells that begin to function independent of TSH regulation. Mutations of the TSH-receptor are most common.

DIAGNOSIS

In toxic adenoma, hyperthyroid patients will present with a palpable thyroid nodule that corresponds to increased radioiodine uptake while the surrounding tissue will show decreased uptake.

In toxic multinodular goiter, there will be multiple areas of increased radioiodide uptake.

TREATMENT

Treated with a thionamide (PTU or methimazole), radioiodine therapy, or if indicated, surgery.

Struma ovarii

Ovarian teratomas may contain thyroid tissue. The tissue may hyperfunction independently due to a toxic nodule, or it may secrete excess hormone in parallel with the thyroid in Grave's disease or toxic multinodular goiter.

DIAGNOSIS

Excess T3 and T4 are noted, along with depressed pituitary TSH production. Thyroid scan shows one or more "hot spots" with a hypoactive background.

TREATMENT

Treatment is with surgery or radioiodine.

Thyrotoxicosis Factitia

Thyrotoxicosis factitia is caused by ingestion of excessive quantities of thyroid hormone, sometimes done for weight loss. The treatment is obvious (to stop taking the hormone!), and the patient may need to be referred for psychiatric evaluation.

Thyroid Storm

Thyroid storm is a medical emergency in which patients present with extreme manifestations of thyrotoxicosis, resulting in an exaggeration of the usual symptoms of hyperthyroidism. Patients present with tachycardia, arrhythmia, heart failure, fever, delirium, seizures, coma, vomiting, diarrhea, and jaundice. This condition can be triggered by surgery, trauma, infection, or an acute iodine load in patients with baseline thyroid abnormalities.

β-Blockers, PTU, or methimazole are given to control symptoms, and glucocorticoids may inhibit the conversion of T4 to T3. Intravenous sodium iodide also blocks hormone release via the Wolff-Chaikoff effect. Definitive treatment by surgery or radioactive iodine postponed until the patient is euthyroid.

Thyroid Nodules and Goiters

Any enlargement of the thyroid gland that is *not* the result of a neoplasm is termed a **goiter**. It can be associated with hyperthyroidism (Graves' disease, toxic nodular goiter), euthyroidism (iodine deficiency), or hypothyroidism (Hashimoto's thyroiditis). Thyroid enlargement may result from overstimulation with TSH or a TSH-like substance or may be due to inflammation. **Endemic goiter** is present when a large proportion of a population has a goiter, and it is usually due to iodine deficiency.

Approximately 5% of people in the United States have thyroid nodules. The majority of thyroid nodules are benign, although malignancy must always be considered in the workup. If benign, a nodule may produce appropriate or excessive amounts of thyroid hormone. Malignant tumors typically do not produce hormone and are therefore "cold" on thyroid scan. Risk of malignancy is increased in the following:

- Young, male patients

- Previous history of head or neck irradiation

- "Cold" nodule on radionuclide scan

- Solid nodule rather than cystic

Evaluation usually includes a thyroid scan, ultrasound, and FNA. Benign nodules require treatment (surgery or iodine-131) if symptoms of hyperthyroidism are present. Treatment for malignant nodules is discussed later.

Thyroid Carcinoma

Thyroid cancer is the most common endocrine cancer, with four types of malignancy.

Papillary Carcinoma

Papillary carcinoma is the most common thyroid malignancy, with the best prognosis. This slow-growing tumor often metastasizes to local cervical nodes. It is strongly associated with previous irradiation and is often found in women under age 40. On microscopic examination, the tumor consists of papillary structures covered with glandular epithelium. Small, calcified bodies known as psammoma bodies are often present. The cells are large with a "ground glass" looking cytoplasm. The large nuclei have "holes" (cyoplasmic incusions) that look like "Orphan Annie eyes".

Follicular Carcinoma

Follicular carcinoma is more common in older patients, with a poorer prognosis than papillary. Spread occurs via blood to bone, lung, brain, and liver. The follicular pattern may be difficult to distinguish from benign adenomas. Follicles are uniform and the characteristics of papillary cancer should be absent.

Anaplastic Carcinoma

Anaplastic carcinoma, which occurs in the elderly, is the least common type of thyroid cancer and has the poorest prognosis. These undifferentiated tumors can invade the neck and trachea to cause dyspnea, dysphagia, hoarseness, and cough. On microscopic examination, sheets of poorly differentiated cells are seen.

Medullary Carcinoma

Medullary carcinoma is a malignancy of the parafollicular C cells, which produce calcitonin, thus an elevated serum calcitonin is characteristic. Prognosis is poor. This tumor often occurs as a component of familial multiple endocrine neoplasia, type II (MEN II).

SIGNS AND SYMPTOMS

The most common presentation of thyroid malignancy is an asymptomatic nodule noted by the patient or physician.

DIAGNOSIS

Diagnosis is by thyroid scan, ultrasound, and biopsy.

TREATMENT

Surgery, with subsequent ablation of remaining thyroid tissue using radioactive iodine, is the usual treatment. Thyroid hormone–replacement therapy is necessary after surgery.

PARATHYROID GLANDS AND CALCIUM REGULATION

Physiology

The parathyroid glands secrete the parathyroid hormone (PTH). PTH is responsible for elevating serum calcium. It mobilizes calcium stores by:

- Stimulating osteoclasts in bone

- Increasing reabsorption of calcium in the kidney

- Increasing the production of 1,25-dihydroxycholecalciferol (the active form of vitamin D), which increases calcium absorption from the GI tract.

PTH also decreases phosphate reabsorption in the renal tubules, lowering serum phosphate. PTH levels are regulated directly by serum calcium levels. Increased serum calcium results in decreased PTH secretion, whereas decreased serum calcium triggers increased PTH secretion.

Calcitonin, a hormone synthesized by the parafollicular cells of the thyroid gland, also plays a role in calcium regulation. Calcitonin decreases serum calcium by inhibiting bone resorption and by increasing urinary excretion of calcium and phosphate.

PTH works in concert with calcitonin and vitamin D to regulate the body's calcium balance (Table 4). Calcitonin is a hormone synthesized by the parafollicular cells of the thyroid gland. It decreases serum calcium by inhibiting bone resorption and by increasing urinary excretion of calcium and phosphate. Vitamin D, on the other hand, is a sterol hormone that assists in increasing serum calcium concentrations by increasing uptake of calcium from the jejunum and ileum through direct action on enterocytes. It also enhances calcium and phosphate reabsorption from the kidney. Its action on the bone includes stimulation of both osteoblast and osteoclast activity.

	Serum Calcium	Serum Phosphate	Bone	Kidney	Intestine	Stimulus for Activity
PTH	Increase	Decrease	Increased resorption	Increased calcium reuptake, decreased phosphate reuptake	Increased calcium update (indirect through vitamin D)	Decreased serum calcium
Vitamin D	Increase	Increase	Stimulates osteoclasts and osteoblasts; increased resorption in vitamin D intoxication	Increased calcium reuptake, increased phosphate reuptake	Increased calcium update	Decreased serum calcium, increased PTH, decreased serum phosphate
Calcitonin	Decrease	—	Decreased resorption	—	—	Increased serum calcium

Table 4 Calcium regulation

The influence of PTH on the production of 1,25-dihydroxycholecalciferol [1,25-(OH)2D], the most active form of vitamin D, links vitamin D activity to the regulation of calcium homeostasis. Endogenous vitamin D_3, or cholecalciferol, is synthesized in the skin by the action of ultraviolet rays on 7-dehydrocholesterol. (Vitamin D_2, or ergocalciferol, is taken in through fortified milk. It is equipotent to cholecalciferol and undergoes an identical metabolic pathway.) The next step is hydroxylation in the liver to produce 25-hydroxycholecalciferol [25-(OH)D]. 25-(OH)D can be stored in fat as a reservoir of vitamin D. The final activation step is conversion of 25-(OH)D to 1,25-(OH)2D in the proximal tubule of the kidney by the enzyme 1a-hydroxylase. Factors that boost 1a-hydroxylase activity include decreased serum calcium, increased PTH levels (which also arise from decreased serum calcium), and decreased serum phosphate levels (which can be secondary to increased PTH activity). Large amounts of dietary phosphate can depress 1a-hydroxylase activity.

Development

The parathyroid glands derive from the third and fourth pharyngeal pouches (Figure 8). Paradoxically, the glands from the third pouch travel further downward than those of the fourth pouch, which remain superior.

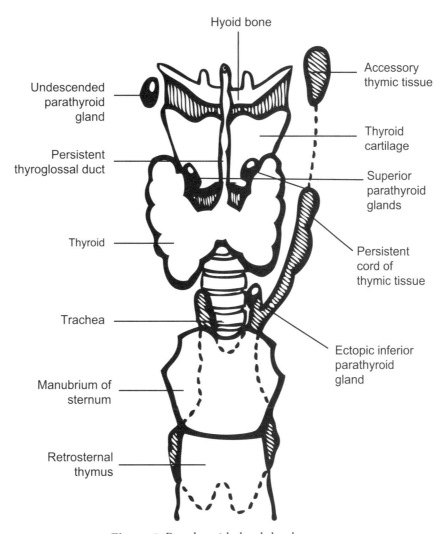

Figure 8 Parathyroid gland development

Anatomy and Histology

The parathyroid glands are located within the fascia of the thyroid gland, usually along the posterior border. Typically, there are four parathyroid glands, which share the thyroid's blood supply. Histologically, the parathyroid is composed of chief cells, which secrete PTH, and oxyphil cells, whose function is unknown.

Primary Hyperparathyroidism

Primary hyperparathyroidism occurs when excess PTH is secreted by the parathyroid gland. A single, benign adenoma is responsible in 80% of cases. Hyperplasia of all four glands accounts for most of the other cases. Parathyroid cancer is rare, comprising less than 2% of primary hyperparathyroidism. Patients with primary hyperparathyroidism are usually older women.

Signs and Symptoms

The disorder is often asymptomatic, but evidence of hypercalcemia (GI disturbances, muscle weakness, emotional lability), osteitis fibrosa cystica (demineralized bone due to excess PTH, bone pain, "salt and pepper" appearance, bone cysts, and brown tumors), or renal stones may be present.

Diagnosis

Laboratory tests reveal high PTH, which results in high calcium and low phosphorus.

Treatment

Treatment is surgical. Beware of postoperative hypocalcemia, as "hungry bones", freed from the power of PTH, take up the available calcium.

Secondary Hyperparathyroidism

Secondary hyperparathyroidism is parathyroid hypertrophy that develops in response to low serum calcium. Common causes of low serum calcium are vitamin D deficiency or malabsorption, renal tubular problems causing calcium loss (renal tubular acidosis, Fanconi syndrome), and certain antiseizure medications that interfere with vitamin D metabolism (phenytoin, phenobarbital). Serum phosphorus is low, unless there is renal insufficiency, which results in phosphorus retention. The underlying disorder is treated.

Hypoparathyroidism

Hypoparathyroidism occurs when parathyroid glands fail to develop (DiGeorge syndrome), when they are removed by surgery, or when target tissues are not responsive (pseudohypoparathyroidism).

Signs and Symptoms

The ensuing hypocalcemia causes tingling of the lips and fingers and can lead to tetany. A positive Chvostek's sign occurs when a tap on the cheek causes facial muscle spasms. Trousseau's sign is present when a blood pressure cuff inflated on the arm induces carpal spasm.

Diagnosis

Low levels of PTH causing low calcium and high phosphorus.

Treatment

Calcium and vitamin D supplementation.

Hypercalcemia

Hyperparathyroidism and malignancy are the most common causes of hypercalcemia. Bony metastases and osteolytic tumors (multiple myeloma, lymphoma, leukemia) may raise calcium levels by increasing bone resorption. Certain cancers (e.g., bronchogenic tumors) can also secrete a parathyroid hormone-related protein that results in hypercalcemia, low serum phosphate, and bone resorption in the presence of low serum PTH (a paraneoplastic syndrome). Prolonged bed rest may aggravate hypercalcemia in cancer patients. Other causes include:

- Increased intestinal absorption (sarcoidosis, hypervitaminosis A or D)

- Increased renal reabsorption (thiazide diuretics, Addison's disease)

- Ingestion of large amounts of calcium carbonate and milk (**milk-alkali syndrome**)

Signs and Symptoms

"Stones, bones, abdominal groans, and psychic moans." Renal stones may result in acute urinary tract obstruction. Polyuria occurs because the excess calcium blocks ADH receptor sites in the distal convoluted tubules. Also, potentiation of digoxin may occur, resulting in arrhythmias.

Diagnosis

Serum calcium should be corrected for albumin. A large proportion of calcium is bound to albumin in the serum. Patients with low albumin levels have low total calcium levels, although their free calcium level may be normal. To adjust for the effect of low albumin, the lower limit of normal for calcium should be shifted down by 0.8 mg/dl for every 1 g/dl of albumin below normal. For example, if the normal albumin level is 4.0, and the patient's albumin level is 3.0, a total calcium level of 7.6 mg/dl (0.8 mg/dl below normal) would still be considered normal.

Treatment

In severe cases, administration of saline (hydration), along with calcitonin and a bisphosphanate. Glucocorticoids can be effective depending on underlying cause of hypercalcemia (lymphoma, sarcoid).

Hypocalcemia

Etiologies include hypoparathyroidism, vitamin D abnormalities (deficiency, malabsorption, or impaired metabolism), renal tubular defects, and acute pancreatitis (the released fats chelate calcium).

Magnesium deficiency (common in alcoholics) causes hypocalcemia by decreasing PTH secretion and decreasing PTH's effect on target organs. In this case, magnesium supplementation must be added to calcium and vitamin D.

Signs and Symptoms

Tetany in severe cases. Chvostek's sign and Trousseau's sign may be present.

Diagnosis

Serum phosphate is high in hypoparathyroidism and renal failure but not in vitamin D deficiency.

Symptoms of hyper-parathyroidism: "Bones, stones, abdominal groans, and psychic moans."

Treatment

Calcium and magnesium supplementation.

ADRENAL GLANDS

Physiology

The adrenal gland consists of two types of endocrine tissue. The adrenal **cortex** secretes steroid hormones, specifically **aldosterone**, **cortisol**, and **androgens**, whereas the adrenal **medulla** secretes **catecholamines**, such as epinephrine (Figure 9). The adrenal cortex is further subdivided into three zones, the **glomerulosa**, the **fasciculata**, and the **reticularis**, each of which is responsible for the synthesis of a particular class of steroids (Figure 10).

Adrenal cortex zones, out to in: GFR—glomerulosa, fasiculata, reticularis

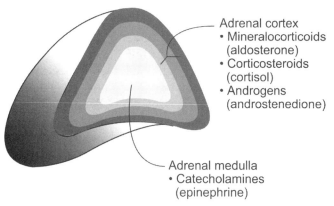

Figure 9 Adrenal gland: cortex and medulla

Hormone production, out to in: Salt, sugar, sex— aldosterone, glucocorticoids, androgens

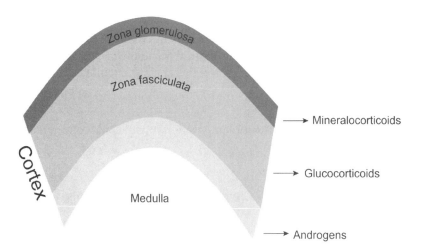

Figure 10 Zones of the adrenal cortex

Aldosterone

Aldosterone acts on the distal tubules and collecting ducts of the kidney to increase the absorption of sodium, exchanging it for potassium and hydrogen ions. As sodium is reabsorbed, more water molecules are retained as well. This leads to increased volume of water and increased blood pressure.

Aldosterone is regulated by the renin-angiotensin system. In the juxtaglomerular apparatus of the kidney, the hormone renin is secreted when fluid volumes drop, as in dehydration or hemorrhage. In the bloodstream, renin converts **angiotensinogen** (a hormone precursor secreted by the liver) into **angiotensin I**. Angiotensin I is then converted to **angiotensin II** by **angiotensin-converting enzyme** (ACE) in the lungs (Figure 11). Angiotensin II then stimulates the release of aldosterone from the adrenal cortex. Angiotensin II is also a potent vasoconstrictor that also stimulates thirst and increases blood pressure centrally.

Aldosterone phones a "collect" call to the connecting ducts.

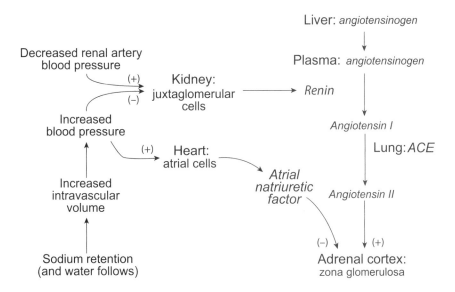

Figure 11 Aldosterone actions

Cortisol

Cortisol is a glucocorticoid hormone that is responsible for a wide range of physiologic effects concerned with immediate response to stress. Cortisol, along with growth hormone and epinephrine, is known as a **counter-regulatory hormone** because it acts to counter the regulatory effects of insulin by increasing blood glucose. The effects of cortisol are as follows:

• Increased serum glucose (through hepatic gluconeogenesis)

• Increased serum amino acids (through protein catabolism)

• Increased plasma lipids and ketone bodies (through lipolysis)

- Increased concentration of neutrophils

- Decreased concentration and migration of other white blood cells (through inhibition of IL-2 production)

- Decreased synthesis of inflammatory mediators, such as prostaglandins and histamine

Cortisol is regulated by the secretion of corticotropin-releasing hormone (CRH) from the hypothalamus and ACTH from the anterior pituitary (Figure 12). Levels of cortisol rise and fall through the day in a circadian rhythm, with the highest levels just before waking and the lowest levels in the late evening. Cortisol is bound to corticosteroid-binding globulin (CBG) and albumin in the blood; just like T4, only free cortisol is biologically active. Free cortisol levels provide negative feedback to the hypothalamus and pituitary, acting to decrease the secretion of CRH and ACTH.

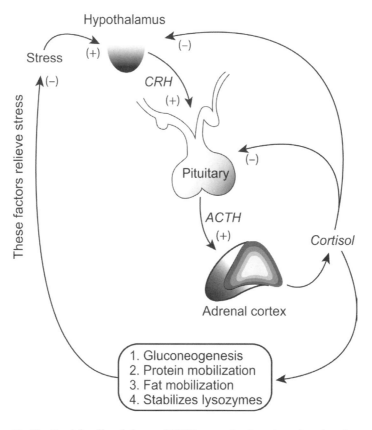

Figure 12 Cortisol feedback loop. (CRH = corticotropin-releasing hormone; ACTH = adrenocorticotropic hormone)

Adrenal Androgens

Adrenal androgens are generally present in tiny amounts when compared to the amounts secreted by the gonads. The two most significant androgens, **dehydroepiandrosterone** (DHEA) and **androstenedione**, are weak androgens and are converted to more potent androgens peripherally.

Development

The adrenal cortex and the adrenal medulla develop from different sources. The adrenal cortex arises from **mesoderm**. The adrenal medulla arises from **neural crest cells** from adjacent sympathetic ganglia.

Zonal differentiation occurs late in fetal life. The zona glomerulosa and zona fasciculata are present at birth, but the zona reticularis does not develop until later in childhood.

Congenital adrenal hyperplasia is a genetic deficiency of the enzymes of adrenal hormone synthesis. 95% of cases are caused by a defective 21-hydroxlyase (CYP21A2 gene), which converts 17-hydroxyprogesterone to 11-deoxycortisol. Because cortisol cannot be produced, there's no negative feedback on the pituitary, so ACTH levels increase. Increased ACTH then causes adrenal hyperplasia and the shunting of steroid precursors down the paths that produce androgens.

Classic 21-hydroxylase deficiency presents as either a salt-losing form or a simple virilizing form. With either forms, girls present as nenonates with ambiguous genitalia. Boys present as neonates with hyponatremia, hyperkalemia, and failure to thrive with the salt-losing form or as toddlers with early puberty (pubic hair, growth spurt, adult body odor) in the simple virilizing form.

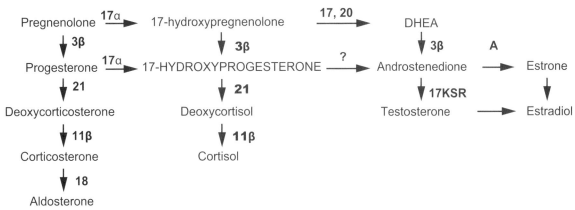

Figure 13 Pathways of adrenal steroid synthesis

Anatomy and Histology

The adrenal glands lie above the kidneys and are enclosed within the renal fascia. Normal adrenal cortex tissue consists of steroid-secreting cells. In the adrenal medulla, brown-colored cells that store catecholamines are known as **chromaffin cells**.

Disorders of the Adrenal Gland

Chronic Primary Corticoadrenal Insufficiency (Addison's Disease)

Destruction of both adrenal glands results in a deficiency of mineralocorticoids (most significantly aldosterone), glucocorticoids (most significantly cortisol), and androgen (women).

Etiology is usually autoimmune, infectious (tuberculosis, fungal), or hemorrhagic.

SIGNS AND SYMPTOMS

Symptoms are nonspecific, including malaise, lassitude, fatigue, weakness, anorexia, weight loss, nausea, and vomiting. A notable feature is hyperpigmentation of the skin (acanthosis nigricans), which develops because ACTH and melanocyte-stimulating hormone are made from the same precursor. When ACTH increases in an attempt to stimulate cortisol production, melanocyte-stimulating hormone increases as well, causing darkening, especially of the folds of the skin (e.g., armpits, crural folds, back of the neck).

DIAGNOSIS

Loss of aldosterone causes hyponatremia, with associated dehydration, orthostatic hypotension, and hyperkalemia. Eosinophilia is also characteristic, although the etiology of this is unknown.

An ACTH stimulation test assesses serum cortisol before and after ACTH is given. No increase in cortisol, along with a high serum ACTH, is diagnostic because the adrenals are already nonfunctioning and more ACTH doesn't help to increase cortisol production.

TREATMENT

Glucocorticoid and mineralocorticoid replacement. Glucocorticoid doses should be increased in times of stress and illness. If they aren't, patients may develop an "addisonian crisis," which can cause profound weakness, shock, fever, and even coma.

Secondary Corticoadrenal Insufficiency

This adrenal hypofunction is due to a lack of ACTH. It most commonly occurs in patients who have received corticosteroids for more than 4 weeks. Exogenous steroids suppress ACTH, thus allowing the adrenal glands to atrophy. If steroid use is abruptly discontinued, the adrenals are not able to produce a sufficient supply of endogenous steroid. Because of this phenomenon, patients should be tapered off steroid medications. Symptoms are similar to those of primary disease, except that hyperpigmentation and hyperkalmia are not present. Corticosteroid taper is sufficient treatment.

Cushing's Syndrome

Many things can lead to excess glucocorticoids:

- Cushing's disease refers specifically to Cushing's syndrome caused by a pituitary adenoma. Usually microadenomas, they produce ACTH, which causes adrenal hyperplasia. ACTH levels may be normal or elevated. (Either is inappropriate because the high levels of cortisol in blood should suppress ACTH secretion.) High doses of glucocorticoids do suppress cortisol levels somewhat because the pituitary still has some feedback regulation intact. Treatment is transsphenoidal removal of the pituitary tumor.

- Ectopic ATCH production is usually associated with a lung tumor. This nonpituitary tumor secretes ACTH, which causes bilateral adrenocortical hyperplasia and hyperfunction. If the tumor is not resectable for cure, treatment is symptomatic. This ACTH production is not suppressible, even with high-dose glucocorticoids.

- An adrenal cortical tumor may produce high levels of cortisol. ACTH levels are suppressed, and cortisol production is not suppressible with glucocorticoids. Treatment is with surgical resection of the tumor. Glucocorticoids must be given postsurgically, while the remaining atrophied adrenal gland tissue recovers.

- Chronic glucocorticoid therapy is the most common cause but the least reported. It is required for a number of diseases, from asthma to lupus. The problem is that prolonged steroid use can have many negative consequences. Besides the signs and symptoms discussed below, these patients may develop cataracts, glaucoma, hypertension, and osteoporosis, to name a few.

DIAGNOSIS

The dexamethasone suppression test is performed. Dexamethasone is a potent glucocorticoid analogue. In normal people, 1–2 mg dexamethasone, given at night, feeds back to inhibit ACTH release from the pituitary and results in lower serum cortisol levels the next morning. This serum cortisol suppression does not occur in people with Cushing's syndrome. A salivary cortisol and urinary cortisol test can also be done (levels should be clearly elevated).

Adrenogenital Syndrome

Adrenogenital syndrome includes any condition in which high levels of adrenal androgens cause virilization. Effects are more obvious in women and can include hirsutism, baldness, acne, voice changes, amenorrhea, and clitoral hypertrophy. The condition can be congenital, in which an enzyme defect causes precursors of cortisol and aldosterone synthesis to be shunted to androgen synthesis. Later in life, adrenal hyperplasia, adenoma, or adenocarcinoma can increase androgen production and cause symptoms.

Hyperaldosteronism

Primary hyperaldosteronism (**Conn's syndrome**) is caused by adrenal hyperplasia or adrenal adenoma. Patients have hypertension and hypokalemia. Treatment is with the aldosterone antagonist, spironolactone. Adenomas are surgically resected.

Secondary aldosteronism is caused by increased activity of the reninangiotensin system. The most common cause is a decrease in the blood pressure perceived by the juxtaglomerular cells, as in congestive heart failure, cirrhosis, and nephrotic syndrome. The underlying disorder is treated.

Pheochromocytoma

This rare tumor of the adrenal medulla or sympathetic ganglion secretes bursts of catecholamines, mostly epinephrine, NE, or dopamine.

- It is associated with VHL, MEN2, and neurofibromatosis type 1.

- In association with hypertension, the increased sympathetic activity causes the classic triad of episodic symptoms: headache, sweating and tachycardia.

- Diagnosis is confirmed with elevated levels of catecholamines and their metabolites in the urine or plasma.

- Treatment involves preoperatively administering an α-blocker (phenoxybenzamine usually) followed by β-blockers before the tumor is surgically removed.

ENDOCRINE PANCREAS

Physiology

Insulin's job is to store energy for our bodies from the foods we eat in the form of glucose, amino acids, and lipids. Insulin is synthesized in the pancreas and acts on almost all tissues, except the brain and red blood cells. When blood sugar or amino acids levels rise, insulin secretion is triggered. Fat intake does not trigger insulin secretion. The functions of insulin include:

- Increased synthesis of glycogen, lipids, and proteins in the liver

- Increased synthesis of fatty acids from glucose and decreased lipolysis in peripheral adipose tissues

- Increased glucose and amino acid uptake in skeletal muscle

Glucagon is a catabolic hormone that works to oppose the actions of insulin and provides energy to your body when there isn't a meal in sight. It acts mainly on the liver to degrade and release glucose, lipids, and ketones into the bloodstream. It also stimulates gluconeogenesis.

Somatostatin is secreted by the pancreas and appears to play a local regulatory role in the secretion of insulin and glucagon, as well as some role in GI function.

Development

During development of the pancreas (described in more detail in chapter 7), **endocrine cells** form groupings amidst the **exocrine pancreas** glandular tissue. These groups of cells, known as the islets of Langerhans, contain three hormone-secreting types of cells. The first, known as **alpha cells**, secretes glucagon. **Beta cells**, the most numerous endocrine cell in the islets, secrete insulin. **Delta cells** secrete somatostatin.

Diabetes Mellitus (Type I)

Type I diabetes is also called *juvenile-onset diabetes* or *insulin-dependent diabetes*. Patients lose their ability to produce endogenous insulin. The mechanism is unknown, but it is thought to be autoimmune, as patients generally have anti–islet cell antibodies. Type I diabetes is associated with the MHC class II molecules HLADR3, HLA-DR4, and HLA-DQw3.2 and it may run in families. The average age of onset is 11–13 years.

Signs and Symptoms

The classic triad of symptoms is **polyuria** (caused by osmotic diuresis from glucose dumping in the urine), **polydipsia** (to replenish water loss), and **polyphagia** (in a futile effort to increase available energy). Weight loss occurs because energy from glucose cannot get into the tissues. Accelerated fat breakdown, in an effort to provide energy to the body's cells, leads to ketoacidosis, and patients may present with nausea and vomiting, air hunger (known as **Kussmaul's respirations**), or coma. In general, the onset of symptoms is rapid.

Diagnosis

One of the following is present:

- Hemoglobin A1c levels > 6.5%

- Fasting plasma glucose > 126 mg/100 ml on two separate days

- Positive oral glucose tolerance test on more than one occasion (plasma glucose > 200 mg/100 ml two hours after an oral glucose load)

Treatment

Insulin injections are required. Insulin doses and combinations must be titrated to maintain optimal blood glucose levels. Patients must be taught how to monitor their glucose level at home (fingerstick monitoring) and how to adjust diet and insulin accordingly.

Type I diabetics often have a "honeymoon" period shortly after their diabetes is diagnosed, during which endogenous insulin levels rise. Therapy may not be needed for several months, but symptoms and insulin requirements inevitably return.

Diabetes Mellitus (Type II)

Type II diabetes is also called *adult-onset diabetes* or *non–insulin dependent diabetes*. This type of diabetes arises when the body's response to insulin decreases, and the tissues become increasingly resistant to insulin. Initially, the pancreas responds by increasing insulin production, but the beta cells' capacity to produce insulin may wane later in the disease. Thus, depending on the stage of disease at the time of diagnosis, insulin levels may be low, normal, or even high. Although patients may need insulin therapy (insulin-requiring non–insulin dependent diabetes), endogenous insulin production is usually sufficient to protect against diabetic ketoacidosis (discussed later). Obesity and a positive family history for type II diabetes are common, but there is no association with any HLA type. Typical onset occurs after age 40, and it is diagnosed the same way that type I diabetes is.

Signs and Symptoms

Although the classic symptoms are the same as in type I, onset is more insidious, and ketoacidosis does not occur. Patients may complain of blurry vision due to osmotic changes in the lens.

Treatment

- Diet should be low in concentrated sugar to minimize serum glucose fluctuations.

- The patient should be taught to monitor serum glucose with fingersticks.

- Weight loss and exercise may increase insulin sensitivity in the tissues.

- Oral hypoglycemic agents, called sulfonylureas, stimulate insulin secretion.

- Insulin injections are required in type II patients who do not respond to more conservative measures.

- A newer class of medications, called biguanides, may increase peripheral glucose uptake by increasing the effects of insulin on muscle cells.

Ketoacidosis

Insulin normally inhibits peripheral lipolysis. When insulin is extremely low, triglycerides are degraded into free fatty acids, which are then converted to ketoacids by the liver. The three types of ketones seen are acetone, acetoacetate, and b-hydroxybutyrate. Diabetic ketoacidosis (DKA) occurs most commonly in type I diabetics who do not take their insulin. It also occurs when infection or myocardial infarction has increased the body's insulin requirements. Type II diabetics usually produce enough insulin of their own to protect against DKA.

Signs and Symptoms

The prodrome involves 12–24 hours of weakness, polyuria, and polydipsia. The patient may hyperventilate and take deep, rapid breaths (Kussmaul's respirations) in an attempt to compensate for the metabolic acidosis caused by ketone bodies. A fruity, acetone odor may be smelled on the breath. Abdominal pain and vomiting are also common, but care must be taken to determine if GI complaints are due to ketoacidosis or to a precipitating infection. As dehydration worsens, mental status changes can occur.

Diagnosis

Serum glucose is 300–800 mg/dl.

Treatment

Hydration and insulin. Potassium must also be given and monitored carefully. The diuresis leads to depletion of the body's K^+ stores. Then, with treatment, insulin causes potassium to enter cells, and if it is not replaced, hypokalemia can cause fatal cardiac arrhythmias.

Hyperosmolar Coma

This complication of type II diabetes usually occurs after many days of infection or other illness.

Signs and Symptoms

The symptoms of polyuria, polydipsia, and dehydration are similar to those of ketoacidosis; however, because some insulin is present, lipolysis and ketoacidosis do not occur. Therefore, there is no hyperventilation or acetone smell to the breath, but dehydration is profound and causes significant mental status changes. Dehydration may not be immediately apparent, because urine output remains normal due to osmotic diuresis. Hemoconcentration may lead to stroke.

Diagnosis

Serum glucose is 600–2,000 mg/dl, much higher than in DKA.

Treatment

Treatment is similar to that of DKA.

Hypoglycemia/Hyperinsulinism

Several clinical entities can cause hypoglycemia. **Reactive hypoglycemia,** also known as postprandial hypoglycemia, is lowered blood glucose that occurs 2–4 hours after eating. A pancreatic islet cell tumor, or insulinoma, can produce excess insulin, causing hypoglycemia. Iatrogenic hypoglycemia can result from administration of too much insulin (remember Klaus von Bulow?) or, less frequently, from excessive oral hypoglycemics.

Signs and Symptoms

The symptoms of hypoglycemia fall into two categories. Faintness, weakness, tremulousness, palpitations, sweating, and hunger are the symptoms of a hypercatecholamine state, as epinephrine induces glycogen mobilization. The other type of symptoms are CNS-related: headache, confusion, and personality changes.

Diagnosis

Reactive hypoglycemia is diagnosed if hypoglycemia coincides with the occurrence of typical symptoms and are relieved by carbohydrate ingestion. Elevated insulin in the presence of hypoglycemia indicates insulinoma or an exogenous insulin source. A favorite board question is hypoglycemia in the presence of high levels of insulin, particularly in a patient with access to exogenous insulin (for example, the family member of a diabetic). If the plasma C peptide (the non-functional portion of insulin that is clipped off when the body produces endogenous insulin) is low, then the insulin must have been administered exogenously.

Treatment

Eating frequent small meals improves reactive hypoglycemia. Surgery is required to treat insulinoma. For iatrogenic hypoglycemia, increased care should be used in monitoring glucose and administering insulin.

Chronic Complications of Diabetes

Most chronic complications are due to microvascular disease. Development of complications is more severe in patients with poorly controlled diabetes and seems to be associated with chronic exposure to high levels of glucose, although the mechanism is unknown.

- **Retinopathy**: In background retinopathy, effects include microaneurysms, blot hemorrhages, infarcts, hard exudates, and macular edema. Changes are seen early and do not usually cause visual loss until macular edema develops. In proliferative retinopathy, new vessels grow on the retinal surface (**neovascularization**). These vessels are fragile and prone to hemorrhage. Fibrosis occurs during healing and may put traction on the retina, leading to retinal detachment and visual loss. Laser therapy can slow the progression of proliferative retinopathy.

- **Renal disease**: The first sign is proteinuria, with a subsequent decrease in creatinine clearance after 1–3 years. End-stage renal disease, requiring dialysis or transplant, typically occurs 3 years after that. Preventative measures include keeping strict control of plasma glucose, eating a low-protein diet, controlling hypertension (especially with ACE inhibitors), avoiding contrast dye, and aggressively treating urinary tract infections.

- **Atherosclerosis**: Coronary artery disease, stroke, and peripheral vascular disease are more common in diabetics. Peripheral vascular disease presents as intermittent claudication (leg pain with exercise due to ischemia) or nonhealing foot ulcers. Diabetics are also prone to having "silent" heart attacks (only detected by electrocardiography later) and may not have anginal symptoms because they often have a concomitant neuropathy.

- **Neuropathy**: Bilateral symmetric sensory impairment usually begins in the feet and progresses proximally. Patients may complain of pain or numbness. Foot ulcers may develop and become infected without patients' noticing, so diabetic patients should be trained to examine their feet regularly for ulcerations. Autonomic dysfunction can include impotence, orthostatic hypotension, constipation or diarrhea, and silent myocardial infarction. Finally, mononeuropathies may be caused by infarction of a single nerve, frequently a cranial nerve. Pain is followed by a palsy, which usually resolves in several months.

MULTIPLE ENDOCRINE DYSFUNCTION

This group of autosomal dominant syndromes involves hyperplasia or neoplasms in more than one endocrine gland. All patients who have hyperplasia or neoplasms in one endocrine gland should be evaluated for these syndromes, and the family history should be thoroughly reviewed. The features of MEN syndromes are listed in Table 5.

Syndrome	Characteristics
MEN 1 (Wermer's syndrome)	Parathyroid adenomas
	Pancreatic adenomas
	Pituitary adenomas
MEN 2A (Sipple's syndrome)	Parathyroid adenomas
	Pheochromocytomas
	Medullary thyroid carcinoma
MEN 2B	Medullary Thyroid carcinoma
	Pheochromocytoma
	Neuromas

1 and 2A: Parathyroid adenoma

2A and 2B: Pheochromocytoma

Table 5 Multiple endocrine neoplasias (MEN)

PHARMACOLOGY

See Tables 6 through 9 for a description of the drugs used to treat the disorders that were discussed in this chapter.

Agent	Mechanism	Uses	Toxicities
Levothyroxine (T_4)	Acts directly at thyroid R (converted to T_3)	Thyroid replacement therapy	Periodic TSH checks; T_4 levels not accurate in assessing thyroid function if taking levothyroxine; large doses cause thyrotoxicosis
Propylthiouracil	Prevents iodine metabolism and T_4 to T_3 conversion	Hyperthyroidism	Teratogenic to fetal thyroid
Iodine	Inhibits T_4 release	Thyrotoxicosis	—
Methimazole	Prevents iodine metabolism	Hyperthyroidism	Teratogenic to fetal thyroid

T_3 = triiodothyronine; TSH = thyroid-stimulating hormone.

Table 6 Thyroid-related drugs

Agent	Mechanism	Uses	Toxicities
Calcium carbonate	↑ serum calcium	Osteoporosis Renal failure Hypocalcemia	Renal stones Hypercalcemia
Vitamin D (calcitriol)	↑ calcium absorption	Renal failure Hypocalcemia Hypoparathyroidism	Renal stones Hypercalcemia
Calcitonin	Inhibition of bone resorption	Paget's disease Osteoporosis Hypercalcemia	—
Mithramycin Bisphosphonates (e.g., etidronate)	Cytotoxic antibiotic that inhibits osteoclasts	Paget's disease Hypercalcemia	Hepatic and renal toxicity Thrombocytopenia
Bisphosphonates (e.g., etidronate)	↓ bone turnover by reducing osteoclasts	Hypercalcemia Osteoporosis Paget's disease	EKG changes Renal failure

Table 7 Calcium-related drugs

Agent	Mechanism	Uses	Toxicities
Prednisone	Acts at cortisol receptor; weakly active at mineralocorticold receptors	Asthma, autoimmune disorders	4 times more potent than cortisol
Hydrocortisone	Acts at cortisol receptor; weakly active at mineralocorticold receptors	Addison's disease, Inflammatory bowel disease (enemas)	As potent as cortisol
Dexamethasone	Acts at cortisol receptor	Adrenal evaluation, high intracranial pressure	Rapid action
Triamcinolone	Acts at cortisol receptor; no mineralocorticold effect	Adrenal hormone replacement, Dermatitis	30 times more potent than cortisol
Beclomethasone	Acts at cortisol receptor	Allergic rhinitis (spray)	Few systemic effects
Spironolactone	Antagonist at mineralocorticoid receptor; acts as diuretic	Hyperaldosteronism Hirsutism	Hyperkalemia
Aminoglutethimide	Blocks steroid synthesis by blocking conversion of cholesterol to pregnenolone	Cushing's disease ACTH tumors, hormone-sensitive tumors	—
Fludrocortisone	Acts at mineralocorticoid receptor	Addison's disease	Hypertension Hypokalemia

ACTH = adrenocorticotropic hormone.

Table 8 Corticosteroids

Type 1 DM: Managed diet, exercise, and insulin replacement

Type 2 DM: 3 major components of nonpharmacologic therapy: Dietary modification, exercise, weight reduction

Exenatide, Liraglutide	Glucagon levels		
Alpha-glucosidase inhibitors: acarbose, miglitol	Inhibit alphaglucosidase (Glenzyme) that converts complex polysaccharide carbohydrates into mono-saccharides, which slows absorption of glucose. Leads to slower rise in postpran-dial blood glucose	Type 2 DM	Diarrhea, abdomi-nal pain, flatulence
Mimetics: Pramlintide	Analog of amylin (cose-creted with insulin by beta cells); posprandial glucose increase	Type 2 DM	Type 2 DM

Agent	Mechanism	Uses	Toxicities
Insulin: Lispro (rapid-acting) Aspart (rapid-acting) Glulisine (rapid-acting) Regular (rapid acting) NPR (intermediate) Glargine (long-acting) Detemir (long-acting)	Binds insuline receptor	Type 1 and 2 DM	Hypoglycemia, weight gain
Biguanides: Metformin	↑Gluconeogenesis, ↓intestinal absorption of glucose, ↑insulin sensitivity (↑peripheral glucose uptake and utilization)	First drug of choice when diet/excersise isn't enough. May also be administered in combination with other diabetes drugs	Diarrhea nausea/vomiting, flatulence, weakness; contraindicated in renal dysfunction or abnormal creatinine clearance
Sulfonylureas: 1st gen: tolbutamide, tolazamide, chlorpropamide 2nd gen: glipizide, glyburide, gliclazide, glimepiride	Binds to and inhibits potassium channel in pancreatic beta cell, leading to altered resting potential, calcium influx, and finally ↑insulin secretion	1st gen rarely used now; type 2 DM; first choice of drug if intolerant of metformin; not useful for type 1 DM	Hypoglycemia
Meglitinides: repaglinide, nateglinide	Different structure, but acts similar to sulfonylurea	Type 2 DM; not useful for type 1 DM	Headace, hypoglycemia, upper respiratory tract infection
Thiazolidinediones: rosiglitazone, pioglitazone	↑Insulin sensitivity; mechanism unclear but they bind and activate PPARs, which regulate gene expression	Type 2 DM	Hypoglycemia, weight gain, fluid retention/heart failure, hepatotoxicity
DPP-IV inhibitors: Sitagliptin, saxagliptin	Inhibit DPP-IV, an enzyme that deactivates GIP and GLP-1; has effects on glucose homeostasis	Type 2 DM	Nasopharyngitis, UTI headache
Glucagon-like peptide: 1 analog	Bind to GLP-1 receptor; ↑insulin secretion	Type 2 DM	Gastrointestinal, hypoglycemia

Table 9 Diabetic agents

CHAPTER 7

GASTROINTESTINAL SYSTEM

EMBRYOLOGY

The gastrointestinal system develops from the foregut, midgut, and hindgut, with its individual autonomic innervation and blood supply (Figure 1).

The foregut develops into the esophagus, trachea and lungs, stomach, and proximal duodenum. The liver, pancreas, liver, and biliary system also arise from outpouchings of the endoderm. Of note, the tracheoesophageal septum divides the trachea and lung buds anteriorly and the esophagus posteriorly. Deviation of this septum can lead to esophageal atresia or tracheoesophageal fistula.

The midgut is the primary intestinal loop. During the 6th week, it rapidly lengthens and protrudes into the umbilical cord (physiologic herniation) but returns into the abdominal cavity during the 10th week. While this is occurring, the midgut loop undergoes a 270 counterclockwise rotation bringing the cecum to its final position in the right lower quadrant. The midgut is connected to the yolk sac through the vitelline duct, which acts as a pivot point for this rotation (Figure 2). Abnormalities at any point during this process may lead to congenital malformations. Failure to complete the 270 counterclockwise rotation leads to malrotation, resulting in a misplaced left-sided colon for example, or volvulus, twisting of the intestine and its blood supply with risk of infarction. Incomplete obliteration of the vitelline duct causes an outpouching of the ileum, which is also known as a Meckel's diverticulum (ileal diverticulum, Figure 3). An omphalocele (Figure 4) results from failure of the intestinal contents to return to the abdominal cavity. In contrast, gastroschisis (Figure 5) is a similar looking herniation caused by an abdominal wall muscle defect and is unrelated to the vitelline stalk herniation. In an omphalocele, a two-layered sac of amnion and peritoneum covers the abdominal contents whereas in gastroschisis the abdominal contents are not covered. This is further discussed in the small bowel disease section.

The hindgut develops into the distal third of the transverse colon up to the upper part of the anal canal. Abnormalities in the hindgut include imperforate anus (anal membrane fails to breakdown) and Hirshsprung disease (parasympathetic ganglion fails to migrate into the bowel wall). This is further discussed in the large bowel disease section.

	Foregut	Midgut	Hindgut
Structural derivatives	Esophagus Lungs Stomach Duodenum (1st and 2nd portion) Liver Pancreas Gallbladder Spleen	Duodenum (2nd, 3rd, 4th portion) Jejunum Ilieum Ascending colon Transverse colon (proximal 2/3)	Transverse colon (distal 1/3) Descending colon Sigmoid colon Rectum Anus (above pectinate line)
Blood Supply	Celiac artery	Superior mesenteric artery	Inferior mesenteric artery
Congenital disorders	Esophageal atresia Tracheoesophageal fistula Pyloric stenosis Annular pancreas Hiatal hernia	Meckel's diverticulum Volvulus Malrotation Omphalocele	Imperforate anus Hirshsprung disease

Hirshsprung disease = failure of parasympathetic ganglion to migrate into the bowel wall

Also known as congenital megacolon

Gastroschisis— the abdominal contents are not covered

Table 1 Development of the gastrointestinal tract

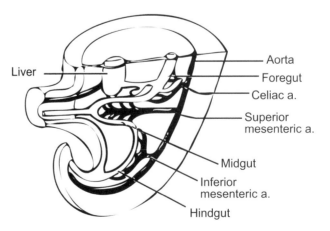

Figure 1 Development of the gastrointestinal tract (Adapted from *The Big Picture: Gross Anatomy*)

Three germ layers contribute to the formation of the digestive system. Both endoderm and mesoderm contribute to the formation of organs.

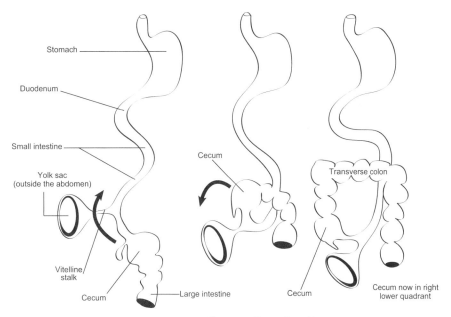

Figure 2 Vitelline stalk and yolk sac

Endoderm	Epithelial lining and glands of the digestive tract
Mesoderm	Connective tissue, smooth muscle, vasculature, and mesentery
Ectoderm	Meissner plexus (Submucosal plexus) Auerbach plexus (Myenteric plexus)

Table 2 Germ Layers of the Gastrointestinal Tract

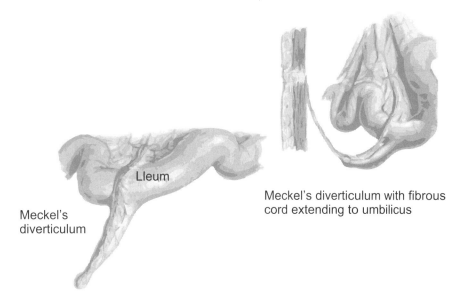

Figure 3 Meckel's diverticulum
(Adapted from *Netter's Clinical Anatomy*, 2nd Ed.)

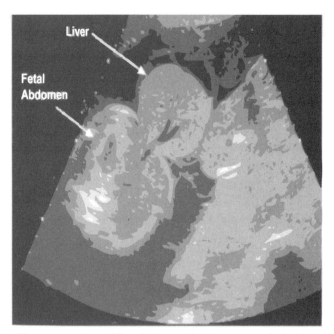

Transverse view of the abdomen showing an omphalocele
as a large abdominal wall defect with exteriorized liver
covered by a thin membrane.

Figure 4 Omphalocele

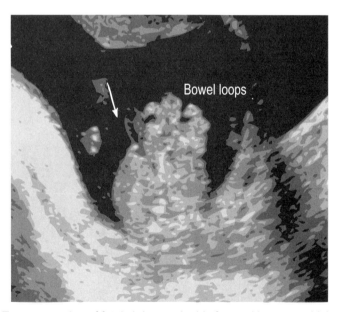

Transverse view of fetal abdomen. In this fetus with gastroschisis,
extruded bowl loops are floating in the amnionic fluid to the right
of the normal umbilical cord insertion site (arrow).

Figure 5 Gastrochisis
(Adapted from *Williams Obstetrics*, 23rd Edition)

HISTOLOGY

Location	Histologic Features
Esophagus	Mucosa is comprised of nonkeratinized stratified squamous epithelium Upper 1/3 is composed of skeletal muscle only Middle 1/3 is composed of both skeletal and smooth muscle Last 1/3 is composed of smooth muscle only
Stomach	Mucosa is comprised of columnar epithelium, which secretes mucus to form a protective layer against gastric acid Parietal cells secrete HCl and intrinsic factor Chief cells secrete pepsinogen D cells secrete somatostatin G cells secrete gastrin
Small intestine	Entire small intestinal mucosa is comprised of columnar epithelium
Duodenum	Only segment with Brunner's submucosal glands, which secrete bicarbonate to neutralize stomach acid Goblet cells secrete mucus Villi and crypts
Jejunum	Goblet cells secrete mucus Villi and crypts
Ileum	Goblet cells secrete mucus Peyer's patches (lymphoid nodules) Villi and crypts
Colon	Entire large intestinal mucosa is comprised of columnar epithelium Many goblet cells Only crypts, lack villi

Table 3 Histological features of the gastrointestinal tract

The mucosa from the stomach to the colon consists of columnar epithelium

Brunner's submucosal glands secrete bicarbonate in the duodenum Peyer's patches are lymphoid nodules in the ileum

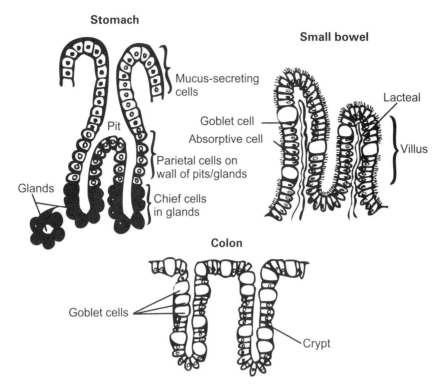

Figure 6 Mucosa of the stomach, small bowel, and colon.

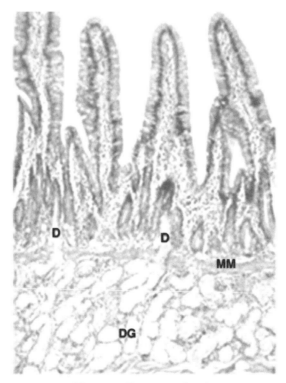

Figure 7 Brunner glands
(Adapted from *Junqueira's Basic Histology: Text and Atlas*, 12th Edition)

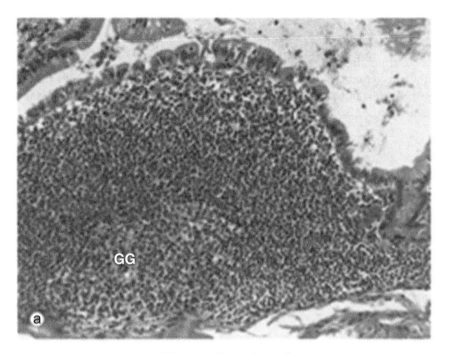

Figure 8 Peyer's patches
(Adapted from *Wheater's Functional Histology*, 5th Ed.)

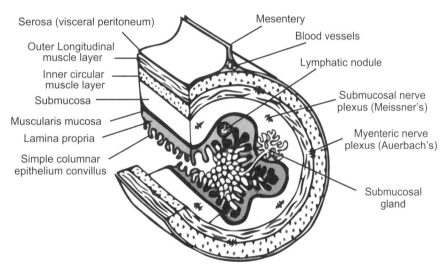

Serosa (visceral peritoneum)
Outer Longitudinal muscle layer
Inner circular muscle layer
Submucosa
Muscularis mucosa
Lamina propria
Simple columnar epithelium convillus

Mesentery
Blood vessels
Lymphatic nodule
Submucosal nerve plexus (Meissner's)
Myenteric nerve plexus (Auerbach's)
Submucosal gland

Figure 9 The entire gastrointestinal tract has the same four layers:
mucosa, submucoa, muscularis, and serosa.

GROSS ANATOMY

The gastrointestinal tract can be viewed as a long, continuous, and muscular tube beginning at the mouth and terminating at the anus. At different points along its length, various glands and organs empty their secretions into the gut lumen: salivary glands, pancreas, liver, and gallbladder. The physiology, function, and pathology of each gland and organ will be discussed in its respective subsections below.

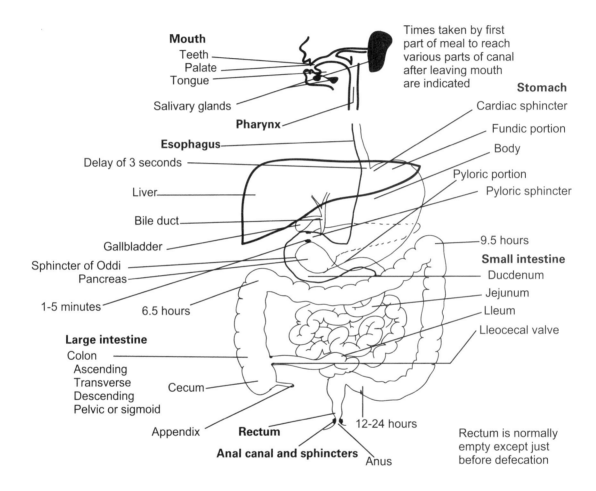

Figure 10 Overview of the gastrointestinal tract
(Adapted from *Pathophysiology of Disease: an Introduction to Clinical Medicine*)

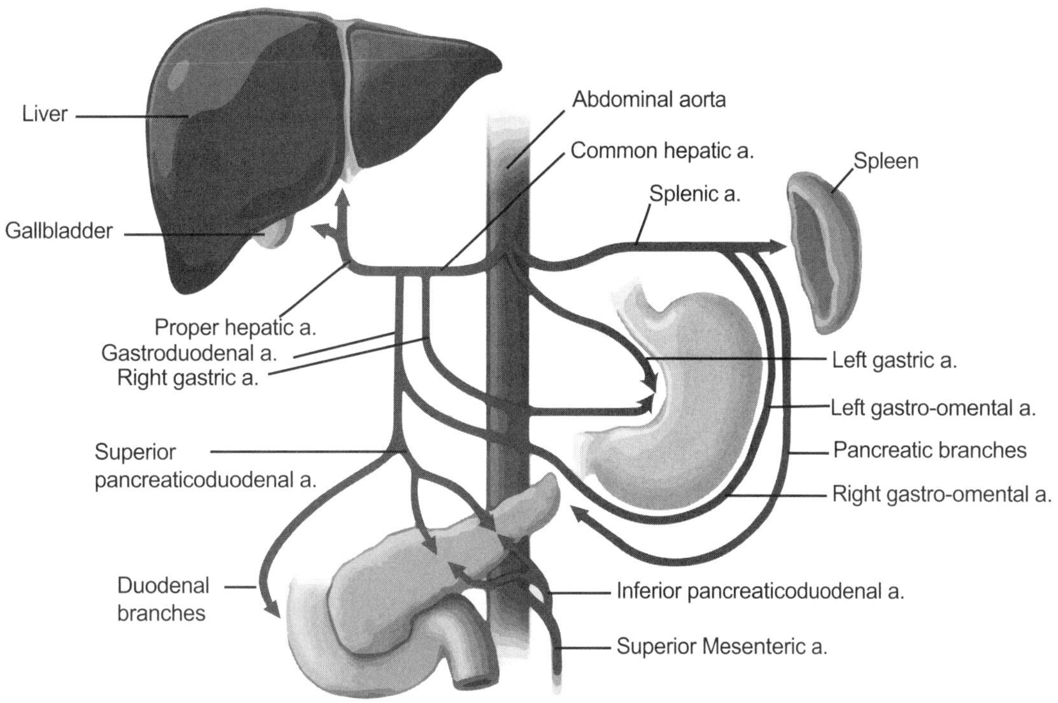

Liver

Gallbladder

Abdominal aorta

Common hepatic a.

Splenic a.

Spleen

Proper hepatic a.
Gastroduodenal a.
Right gastric a.

Left gastric a.

Left gastro-omental a.

Pancreatic branches

Right gastro-omental a.

Superior
pancreaticoduodenal a.

Duodenal
branches

Inferior pancreaticoduodenal a.

Superior Mesenteric a.

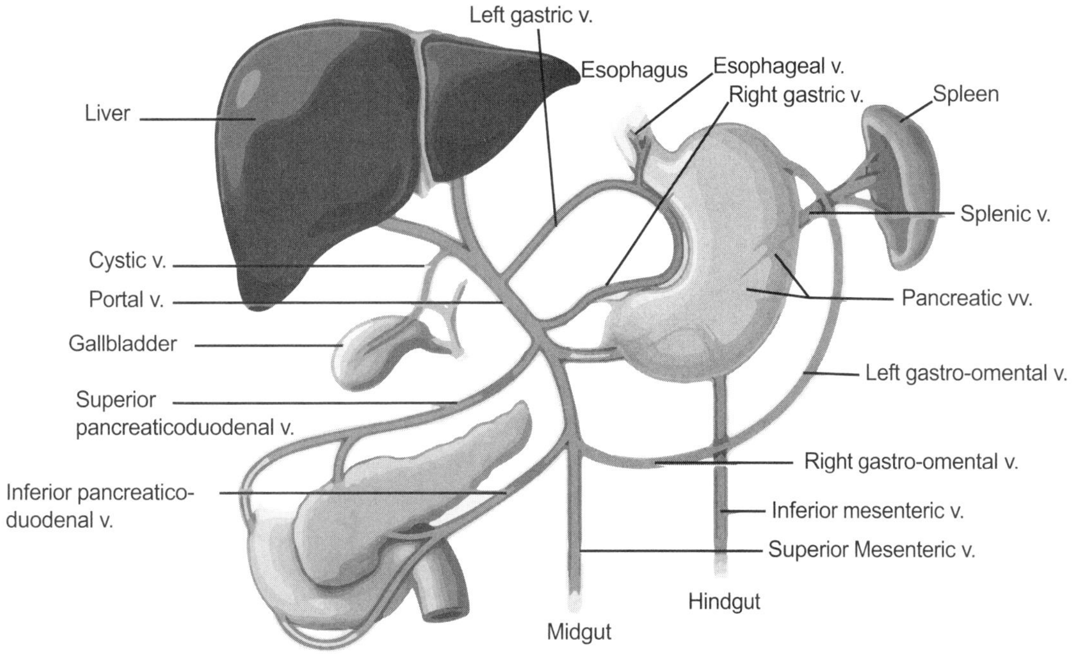

Left gastric v.

Esophagus

Esophageal v.

Right gastric v.

Spleen

Liver

Cystic v.

Portal v.

Gallbladder

Superior
pancreaticoduodenal v.

Inferior pancreatico-
duodenal v.

Splenic v.

Pancreatic vv.

Left gastro-omental v.

Right gastro-omental v.

Inferior mesenteric v.

Superior Mesenteric v.

Hindgut

Midgut

A. Arterial supply to the foregut supplied principally by the celiac trunck.
B. Venous drainage of the foregut supplied principally by the portal vein.

Figure 11 Vasculature of the foregut
(Adapted from *The Big Picture: Gross Anatomy*)

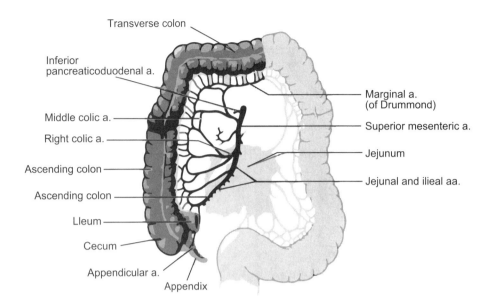

Figure 12 Vasculature of the midgut
(Adapted from *The Big Picture: Gross Anatomy*)

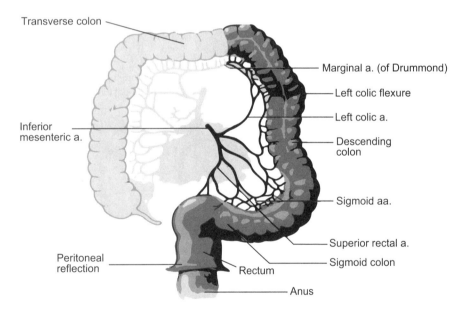

Figure 13 Vasculature of the hindgut
(Adapted from *The Big Picture: Gross Anatomy*)

Salivary Glands

Saliva is important for initiating the digestion of starches (α-amylase) and lipids (lingual lipase), lubricating food with mucus, and buffering the mucosa from toxins. There are three paired salivary glands: the parotids, submandibulars, and sublinguals. Saliva is made mainly of water, electrolytes, kallikrein, mucus, α-amylase, and lingual lipase.

Saliva is made in the acinar cells and modified in the ductal cells by sodium and chloride reabsorption as well as potassium and bicarbonate secretion. Aldosterone acts on duct cells to increase sodium reabsorption and potassium secretion.

Interestingly, there are several unique characteristics in the regulation of salivary secretion:

1. Salivary secretion is completely under neural control.

2. Salivary secretion is stimulated by both the parasympathetic and sympathetic nervous system.

3. Increased by food, smell, and nausea; it is decreased by anticholinergic drugs, sleep, and fear.

	Pathology	Clinical Findings
Salivary stones	Usually occurs in submandibular and sublingual glands since their secretions are more mucinous (secretions from the parotid's tend to be more serous)	Swelling and pain of the cheek
Sjögren's Syndrome	Autoimmune destruction of salivary and lacrimal glands Usually possess antibodies to the Ro/SSA or La/SSB antigens	Dry eyes and mouth Associated with other autoimmune conditions (rheumatoid arthritis)
Salivary tumors	Tumors most commonly arise in the parotid glands and are usually benign (80-85%) Most common type of benign salivary gland tumor = pleomorphic adenoma Other benign salivary gland tumors: Warthin tumor, basal cell adenoma, and canalicular adenoma. Most common malignant salivary gland tumors: mucoepidermoid carcinoma and adenoid cystic carcinoma	Painless mass or swelling of the parotid, submandibular, or sublingual gland

Table 4 Diseases of the salivary glands

Sjögren's Syndrome
Dry eyes and mouth
Usually possess antibodies to the Ro/SSA or La/SSB antigens

Most tumors occur in the parotid gland

Most common type of benign salivary gland tumor = pleomorphic adenoma

Esophagus

The role of the esophagus is to propel food from the oral pharynx to the stomach through sequential phasic contractions known as peristalsis (Figure 14). When the peristaltic wave and food bolus reaches the lower esophageal sphincter, the smooth muscle of the sphincter relaxes to facilitate transit of the food bolus into the stomach. This process is mediated by the vagus nerve, which releases VIP.

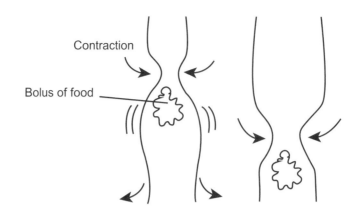

Figure 14 Peristalsis

Achalasia
Lack of myenteric (Aeurbach's) plexus → impaired LES relaxation and ↑ LES pressure

Barium swallow: bird beak

Esophagitis
1. GERD
2. Infection
3. Drugs

Achalasia → bird beak on barium swallow

	Pathology	**Clinical Findings**
Esophagitis	Most commonly caused by gastroesophageal re-flux disease (GERD) Can also be caused by infection: CMV, candida, HSV-1, disseminated bac-teremia or viremia Can also be caused by drugs: NSAIDS, antibiotics, caustic agents (acids, bases), alcohol	Heartburn or regurgita-tion is common May have odynophagia or painful swallowing
Achalasia	Either idiopathic or acquired Acquired cause include Chagas disease, which is caused by infection with the protozoan parasite Trypanosoma cruzi Impaired relaxation of the lower esophageal sphinc-ter (LES) due to lack of the myenteric (Aeurbach's) plexus Elevated LES pressure leads to proximal dilata-tion	Dysphagia to both liquids and solids, regurgitation Barium swallow (Figure 15): "bird beak" Increases risk of esopha-geal cancer May be associated with esophageal ulcers

Barrett's esophagus	Intestinal columnar epithelium replaces squamous epithelium in the distal esophagus due to GERD (glandular metaplasia)	Progresses to adenocarcinoma ~10 % Diagnosed by endoscopy and biopsy
Boerhaave syndrome	Complete perforation of the esophagus from vomiting and retching Other etiologies of perforation include caustic ingestion, pill esophagitis, Barrett's ulcer, infectious ulcers, and post dilatation of esophageal strictures	Odynophagia, tachypnea, dyspnea, cyanosis, fever, and shock
Esophageal carcinoma	Majority are adenocarcinomas Associated risk factors include: alcohol, smoking, Barrett's esophagus, achalasia, cigarettes Squamous cell carcinoma affects the upper 2/3 of the esophagus Adenocarcinoma affects the lower 1/3 of the esophagus	Dysphagia (first to solids then liquids) Poor prognosis
Esophageal varices	Dilatation of the esophageal venous plexus from portal hypertension (discussed further in the liver section)	Hematemesis
Hernias	2 types (Figure 16): Sliding: gastroesophageal junction (GE) moves above the diaphragm Paraesophageal: GE junction does not move but the adjacent stomach herniates through the diaphragm	GERD from loss of diaphragmatic anchoring

Most important risk factor for Barrett's esophagus is chronic GERD

Boerhaave syndrome = complete esophageal perforation

Esophageal Cancer
Squamous cell carcinoma affects the upper 2/3 of the esophagus

Adenocarcinoma affects the lower 1/3 of the esophagus

Mallory Weiss tear—commonly seen in alcoholics and bulimics

Only causes mucosal laceration

Plummer-Vinson Syndrome
1. Dysphagia,
2. Iron deficiency anemia
3. Glossitis

Mallory-Weiss tear	Forceful vomiting/retching causes mucosal laceration (not transmural perforation like Boerhaave syndrome)	Hematemesis Commonly associated with alcoholics or bulimics
Plummer-Vinson Syndrome	Mucosal folds or webs that protrudes into the lumen	Triad of dysphagia, iron deficiency anemia, glossitis
Schatzki rings	Mucosal rings at the GE junction (Figure 17)	Dysphagia (solid) Treat with dilatation
Zenker diverticula	A sac-like protrusion at the junction of the pharynx and esophagus	Dysphagia Regurgitation of undigested food shortly after meal

Table 5 Diseases of the esophagus

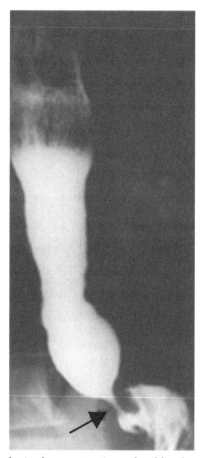

Figure 15 Achalasia demonstrating a bird beak on barium swallow

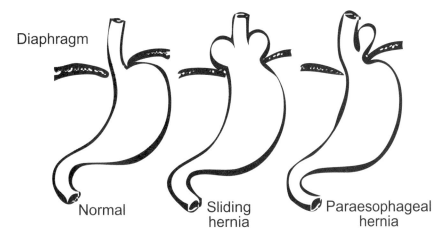

Diaphragm

Normal

Sliding
hernia

Paraesophageal
hernia

Figure 16 Types of diaphragmatic hernias

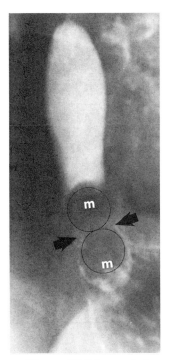

Figure 17 Mucosal ring

GI Hormone	Origin	Action	Regulation
Cholecystokinin (CCK)	I cells of small bowel	↓ gastric emptying to help digestion ↑ pancreatic secretions to help digestion ↑ gallbladder contraction for bile production	↑ fat- or protein-rich chyme ↓ by somatostatin
Gastrin	G cells of stomach	↑ acid production and gastric motility ↑ Zollinger-Ellision Syndrome	↑ by amino acids (esp. tryptophan and phenylalanine) ↑ vagal stimulation by VIP ↓ stomach distention and acid in the stomach
Gastric inhibitory peptide (GIP)	K cells of small bowel	↑ insulin release ↓ acid secretion by parietal cells	↑ by protein, fat, carbohydrate
Motilin	Enterochromaffin cells of small bowel	Promotes migrating motor complexes (MMC) in the stomach and intestine	↑ during fasting states
Secretin	S cells of small bowel	Role is to decrease acidity in the lumen of small bowel ↑ pancreatic bicarbonate secretion ↓ bile secretion ↓ acid production by parietal cells	↑ by fatty acids and acid in lumen
Somatostatin	D cells of stomach, small bowel, and pancreas	↓ release of other GI hormones: CCK, gastrin, GIP, motilin, VIP ↓ gallbladder contraction ↓ pancreatic hormones: insulin, glucagon, secretin	↑ by acid secretion in GI lumen ↓ by vagal stimulation
Vasoactive intestinal polypeptide (VIP)	Parasympathetic ganglion of the GI tract	Stimulates relaxation of GI smooth muscle and lower esophageal sphincter ↑ bicarbonate secretion from pancreas ↓ acid release from stomach	↑ by gastric distention and parasympathetic stimulation ↓ by sympathetic stimulation

Table 6 Hormones of the gastrointestinal tract

Stomach

The role of the stomach is to receive the food bolus from the esophagus, begin digestion of the food bolus with gastric acid, and propel the resulting chyme into the small intestine. Gastric emptying is hormonally regulated for the optimal digestion and absorption of food contents. Both fat and low duodenal pH slows gastric emptying. Fat slows gastric emptying via CCK while the presence of acid in the duodenum initiates a local enteric nervous system reflex.

There are three layers of muscle in the stomach: an outer longitudinal layer, a middle circular layer, and an inner oblique layer. Three anatomic divisions are present in the stomach: the fundus, the body, and the antrum (Figure 18).

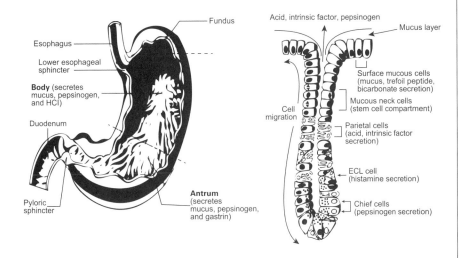

Figure 18 Anatomic divisions of the stomach and associated cell types (Adapted from *Ganong's Review of Medical Physiology*, 24th Edition)

Gastric juice is made of four components, secreted by cells located in different regions of the stomach: hydrochloric acid, pepsinogen, intrinsic factor, and mucus. Synergistically, HCl and pepsinogen starts the protein digestion process. Intrinsic factor mediates the absorption of vitamin B12 in the ileum. Mucus forms a protective barrier on the gastric mucosa from gastric acid.

Cell Type	Location	Secretory Product
Chief cells	Body	Pepsinogen
Parietal cells	Body	HCl Intrinsic factor
G cells	Antrum	Gastrin
Mucous cells	Antrum	Mucus

Table 7

Gastric emptying is delayed by
1. Fat via CCK
2. Low pH in the duodenum

Chief cells: pepsinogen

Parietal cells: HCl, intrinsic factor

G cells: gastrin

Gastric secretion is mediated by the H^+/K^+ adenosine triphosphatase (ATPase) pump, which secrets H+ in the lumen of the stomach in exchange for K^+. Proton pump inhibitors (ex. omeprazole) block this process.

Acid secretion is stimulated by

- Gastrin

- Parasympathetic nervous system

- Histamine binding to H_2 receptors (which is why cimetidine, ranitidine, and all the other H_2 blockers decreases acid secretion)

Acid secretion is inhibited by the following:

- Gastric pH less than 3.0 (via negative feedback on gastrin)

- Secretin released from the duodenum in response to acid

- Prostaglandins (aspirin blocks the production of prostaglandins and can lead to gastritis)

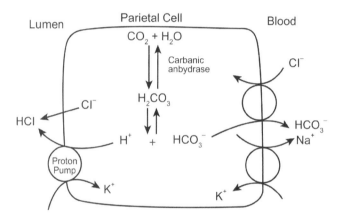

Figure 19 Proton pump

Diseases of the Stomach

	Pathology	Clinical Findings
Acute gastritis (erosive)	Mucosal inflammation causes disruption of mucous barrier → erosions Etiologies include NSAIDs, alcohol, tobacco, steroids, burns (Curling ulcers), brain injury (Cushing ulcers)	Acute or erosive gastritis is remarkable for its tendency to cause upper GI bleeding Epigastric pain, nausea, vomiting, hematemesis, anemia, melena

Acute or erosive gastritis
- NSAIDs
- Alcohol
- Tobacco
- Steroids
- Burns (Curling ulcers)
- Brain injury (Cushing ulcers)

Chronic gastritis (nonerosive)	2 types: Fundal (type A): Autoimmune Pernicious anemia, intrinsic factor deficiency, achlorhydia (antibodies against parietal cells and intrinsic factor) Antral (type B): chronic infection with H. pylori	Same as acute gastritis Antral (type B) caused by H. pylori increases risk of MALT lymphoma	Chronic or nonerosive gastritis: Autoimmune 1. Pernicious anemia 2. Achorhydia 3. Intrinsic factor deficiency H. pylori infection
Gastric adeno-carcino-ma	Risk factors: nitrosamines (smoked foods), H. pylori infection, pernicious anemia, alcohol, smoking, achlorhydia Histology: signet ring cells (Figure 20)	Late presentation, anorexia, epigastric pain, weight loss, anemia Can be associated with acanthosis nigricans Several common sites of metastasis: 1. Krukenberg's tumor-bilateral ovaries 2. Sister Mary Joseph's nodule-periumbilical metastasis 3. Virchow's node-left supraclavicular node	Gastric adenocarcinoma 1. Krukenberg's tumor-bilateral ovaries 2. Sister Mary Joseph's nodule-periumbilical metastasis 3. Virchow's node-left supraclavicular node
Peptic ulcer disease	Focal breakdown in the mucosa extending through the muscularis mucosa (Figure 21) due to decrease mucosal protection against acid or increased acid production (Zollinger-Ellison syndrome) Appear as "punched out" lesion with a smooth, clean floor and without a raised edge Common locations: esophagus, stomach, duodenum	High association with H. pylori with positive urease test Epigastric pain, nausea, vomiting, hematemesis, anemia, melena, possible perforation Complications include perforation, bleeding, and erosion into the pancreas Gastric ulcer: worse with food, possible malignant transformation Duodenal ulcer: better with food, no malignant transformation	PUD **Gastric ulcer**: worse with food, possible malignant transformation **Duodenal ulcer**: better with food, no malignant transformation
Pyloric stenosis	Congenital hypertrophy of the gastric outflow tract muscle	Projectile nonbilious vomiting in an infant within the first 2 months of life Olive-like mass in the epigastrium, which represents the hypertrophied muscular pylorus	**Pyloric stenosis** • Nonbilious projectile vomiting • Olive-like mass in epigastrum

Table 8 Diseases of the stomach

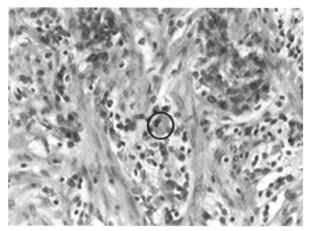

Figure 20 Signet cell of gastric carcinoma

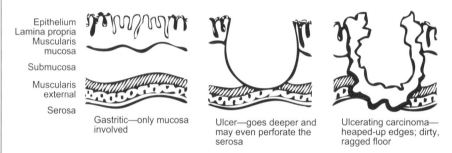

Epithelium
Lamina propria
Muscularis
mucosa

Submucosa

Muscularis
external

Serosa

Gastritic—only mucosa involved

Ulcer—goes deeper and may even perforate the serosa

Ulcerating carcinoma—heaped-up edges; dirty, ragged floor

Figure 21 Gastritis, ulcer, and ulcerating carcinoma

Gallbladder

The role of the gallbladder is to store, concentrate, and secrete bile into the small intestinal tract. The major stimulus for gallbladder contraction is CCK, which is produced by the I cells of the small intestine in response to fatty acids and amino acids. In addition, CCK causes relaxation of the sphincter of Oddi to allow bile to be expelled into the small intestinal tract.

Diseases of the Gallbladder

	Pathology	Clinical Findings

Cholelithiasis	Usually caused by 3 types of stones:
	
	1. Pigment stones
	  • Multiple small, black radiolucent stones
	  • Occur with hemolytic disease (ex. sickle cell disease, hereditary spherocytosis)
	
	2. Cholesterol stones (majority of stones)
	  • Usually solitary yellow stone
	  • Radiolucent
	
	3. Mixed stones
	  • Majority are associated with acute cholecystitis
	  • Consist of calcium bilirubinate and cholesterol
	
	Inflammation of the gallbladder due to gallstones
	
	Other infrequent causes include infection or ischemia
		Can lead to cholecystitis, pancreatitis, cholangitis (Charcot's triad):
		
		1. Jaundice
		2. Fever
		3. Right upper quadrant pain
		
		Risk factors include the 4Fs:
		  • Forty
		  • Fertile
		  • Female
		  • Fat

Risk factors for cholelithiasis include the 4Fs:
1. Forty
2. Fertile
3. Female
4. Fat

Cholecystitis
+ Murphy's sign-ultrasonic examination in the right upper quadrant causes pain

Acalculous cholecystitis usually occurs in very ill patients (ICU patients)

Cholecystitis	Right upper quadrant pain, fever + Murphy's sign-ultrasonic examination in the right upper quadrant causes pain	Complications: • Gangrene-most common complication • Perforation-occurs after the development of gangrene • Cholecystoenteric fistula-perforation of the gallbladder directly into the duodenum/jejunum • Gallstone ileus- gallstone moves through a cholecystoenteric fistula and causes mechanical bowel obstruction, usually in the terminal ileum • Emphysematous cholecystitis-secondary infection of gallbladder wall with gas-forming microbes
Acalculous cholecystitis	Clinically identical to acute cholecystitis but is not associated with gallstones Generally occurs in critically ill patients	Associated with a high mortality
Cholangiocarcinoma	Carcinoma of the bile ducts Not associated with gallstone disease Associated with ulcerative colitis, chronic inflammation, cholangitis	Obstructive jaundice

Table 9 Diseases of the gallbladder

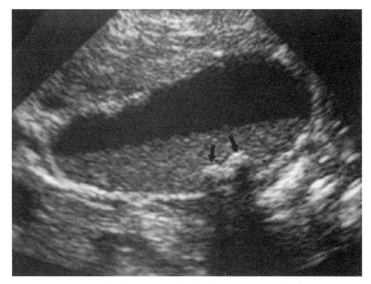

Figure 22 Gallstone and sludge in acute cholecystitis

Liver

The liver is involved with:

- The processing of absorbed substances such as carbohydrates, lipids, and proteins

- Production and secretion of bile acids

- Detoxification

- Production and excretion of bilirubin derived from heme products

Heme Metabolism

During heme metabolism, hemoglobin is converted to biliverdin (green-colored), which is then converted to bilirubin (yellow-colored) by the reticuloendothelial system. This bilirubin travels in the blood bound to albumin towards the liver, where it is conjugated to glucoronic acid via the UDP-glucuronyl transferase enzyme. The resulting conjugated bilirubin is water-soluble and is either excreted in the urine or bile. When bile reaches the terminal ileum and colon, it is deconjugated by bacterial enzymes into urobilinogen. Urobilinogen can be absorbed via the enterohepatic circulation and returned to the liver or converted to urobilin and stercobilin, which are eliminated in feces.

Detoxification

The liver receives blood from the stomach, intestines, pancreas, and spleen (portal circulation) and modifies its content through "first pass metabolism." Bacteria are filtered from the blood through Kupffer cells, a hepatic macrophage. Toxins are converted to water-soluble substances to be excreted in bile or urine (Phase I and II reactions).

Physiologic neonatal jaundice
Suboptimal functioning of UDP-glucuronyl transferase enzyme at birth leads to unconjugated bilirubinemia → jaundice/kernicterus

Tx: phototherapy

Carbohydrate metabolism

The liver is involved with gluconeogenesis, the production of glucose, and glycogenolysis, the degradation of glycogen to release glucose, to maintain a normal blood sugar range.

Protein metabolism

The liver produces all plasma proteins, such as albumin and clotting factors. It manufactures non-essential amino acids and deaminates existing amino acids for use in other metabolic pathways (ex. carbohydrate synthesis). Ammonia is transformed into urea for excretion in urine.

Lipid metabolism

The liver is responsible for synthesizing lipoproteins, phospholipids, and cholesterol. The lipoproteins are used to carry fats in the circulation. Cholesterol and phospholipids are used in bile and cell membranes. It also oxidizes fatty acids to generate energy.

Bile acids

Bile acids are made from cholesterol. Once conjugated to a polar group (glycine or taurine), the bile acids are converted into bile salts, which are stored in the gallbladder. CCK promotes gallbladder contraction and expulsion of bile salts into the intestinal lumen. This facilitates digestion and absorption of dietary lipids. It is then recycled from the terminal ileum back to the liver through the enterohepatic circulation (Figure 23).

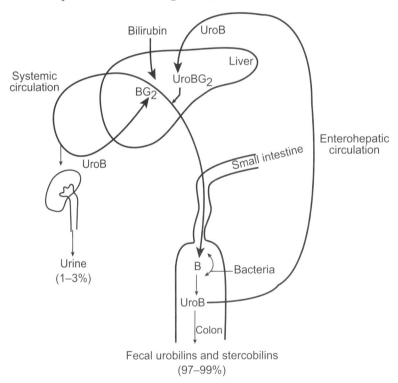

Figure 23 Enterohepatic circulation
(Adapted from *Gastrointestinal Physiology*)

Diseases of the Liver

PORTAL HYPERTENSION

Portal hypertension is characterized by a portal venous pressure gradient greater than 5 mmHg and results from an increase in intrahepatic vascular resistance. The cirrhotic liver loses the physiologic characteristic of a low-pressure circuit for blood flow seen in the normal liver. The increased blood pressure within the sinusoids is transmitted back to the portal vein. Because the portal vein lacks valves, this elevated pressure is transmitted back to other vascular beds (Figure 24), resulting in splenomegaly, portosystemic shunting, and many of the complications of cirrhosis discussed later.

The portal vein is comprised of the adjoining splenic and superior mesenteric vein. Passive congestion of the splenic vein leads to splenomegaly. In cirrhosis, portosystemic collateral vessels develop in order to shunt blood between the portal and systemic veins. This allows for an alternative route for blood to reach the inferior vena cava to return to the heart, as the portal circulation is a relatively high-pressure circuit for blood flow in cirrhosis. Thus, the portosystemic collaterals that are often evident include:

- Esophageal, paraesophageal, and gastric veins (varices)

- Paraumbilical veins (caput medusa)

- Inferior rectal veins (hemorrhoids)

Cirrhosis also leads to alteration of the estradiol to testosterone ratio. Essentially, there is more estradiol circulating in the body, and this leads to physical manifestations such as spider angiomas (spider telangiectasias), gynecomastia, loss of sexual hair, testicular atrophy, and palmar erythema. Ascites only occurs in patients with both cirrhosis and portal hypertension. It is not simply a consequence of mechanical obstruction but is hypothesized to involve the complex interaction between circulatory, vascular, and biochemical abnormalities. Asterixis (flapping of the hands at the wrists) is observed in patients with hepatic encephalopathy and is thought to occur secondary to defective processing of toxic metabolites. Congestive splenomegaly leads to anemia (along with possible gastrointestinal bleeding), leukopenia, and thrombocytopenia through sequestration. Most of the proteins involved in the coagulation cascade are made in the liver and thus, worsening hepatic dysfunction leads to more severe coagulopathy.

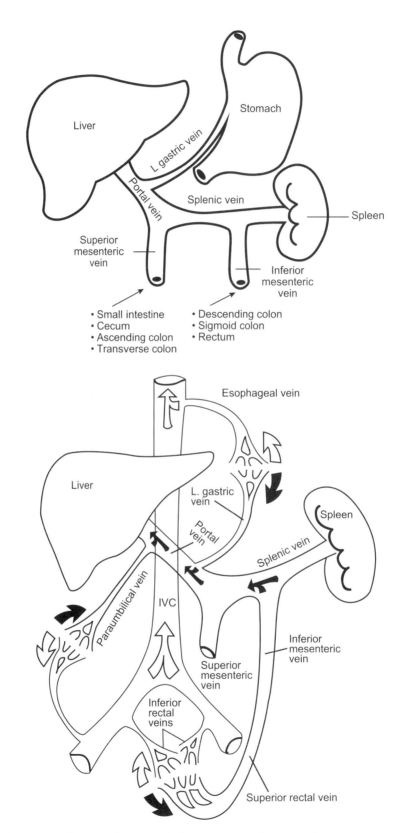

Figure 24 The portal vein and shunts in portal venous hypertension

Lab findings	↑ AST, ALT, GGT (gamma-glutamyl transferase) ↑ Bilirubin ↓ Albumin ↑ PT
Clinical manifestations	Spider nevus Hepatic encephalopathy Jandice Esophageal varices and hematemesis Gynecomastia Splenomegaly Ascites Melena Palmar Erythema Tremor and asterixis Edema Hepatorenal syndrome

Table 10 Manifestations of cirrhosis

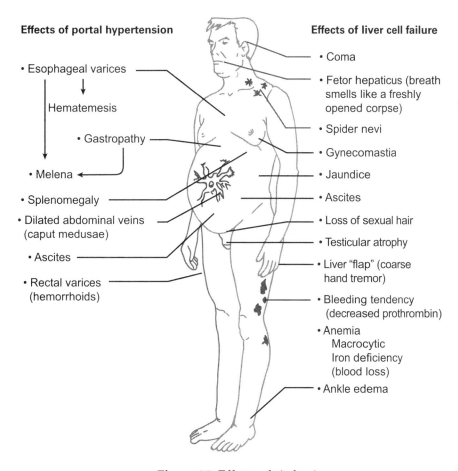

Figure 25 Effects of cirrhosis
(Adapted from *Pathophysiology of Disease: an Introduction to Clinical Medicine*)

HYPERBILIRUBINEMIA

Unconjugated
bilirubinemia

1. Overproduction of
bilirubin

2. Impaired bilirubin
uptake

3. Impaired bilirubin
conjugation

Hyperbilirubinemia can be classified into two major categories: unconjugated bilirubinemia versus conjugated bilirubinemia. It is important to distinguish between the two in order to define the mechanism of disease. Unconjugated hyperbilirubenima is generally caused by the overproduction of bilirubin, impaired bilirubin uptake, or impaired bilirubin conjugation. In contrast, conjugated bilirubinemia is generally caused by intrahepatic or extrahepatic cholestasis. The color of the urine can provide a clue to the diagnosis. An increase in urinary bilirubin, which imparts a brown color, is almost entirely due to the conjugated compound (Figure 26).

Initial laboratory tests include serum total and unconjugated (indirect) bilirubin, alkaline phosphatase, aminotransferases, prothrombin time, and albumin. Normal liver enzymes usually indicate that the jaundice is probably not from hepatic injury. A normal alkaline phosphatase suggests that it is not from biliary tract disease. For these patients, hemolysis or genetic disorders of bilirubin metabolism are more likely to play a role in the hyperbilirubinemia. For example, genetic disorders of isolated unconjugated hyperbilirubinemia include Gilbert's and Crigler-Najjar syndrome. In contrast, causes of isolated conjugated hyperbilirubinemia include Rotor and Dubin-Johnson syndrome.

Biliary Obstruction

Serum alkaline
phosphatase level >
aminotransferases (AST
and ALT) suggests biliary
obstruction or intrahe-
patic cholestasis.

Alcoholic hepatitis

AST/ALT > 2

An alkaline phosphatase level that is significantly elevated in comparison to aminotransferases (AST and ALT) suggests biliary obstruction or intrahepatic cholestasis. The present of acholic stools (pale stools) also points to an obstructive cause. Normally, the color of stool is derived from bilirubin breakdown products, namely urobilin and stercobilin. However, alkaline phosphatase is not specific to the liver, as it may arise from bone. If there is doubt about the origin of the alkaline phosphatase, levels of gamma-glutamyl transpeptidase can be obtained to determine its origin.

Primary abnormalities in transaminases implicate that the jaundice is caused by intrinsic hepatocellular disease, for example, due to viral or alcohol hepatitis. Of note, alcohol hepatitis is remarkable for the significant elevation of AST compared to ALT (ratio is usually greater than 2). Other clues of more severe liver dysfunction include impaired synthetic function, which is manifested by hypoalbuminemia or a prolonged prothrombin time that is not responsive to vitamin K.

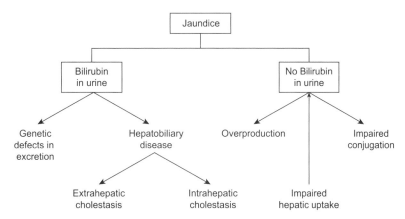

Figure 26 Differential diagnosis of jaundice
(Adapted from *Gastrointestinal Physiology*)

Cause of unconjugated bilirubinemia	Causes of conjugated bilirubinemia
1. Impaired bilirubin conjugation • Gilbert's syndrome • Crigler-Najjar syndrome type I and II • Hyperthyroidism • Infants (physiologic jaundice)	1. Intrahepatic cholestasis • Hepatitis (infectious, alcohol, nonalcoholic steatohepatitis) • Primary biliary cirrhosis • Drugs (ex. chlorpromazine)
2. Overproduction of bilirubin • Intravascular or extravascular hemolysis	2. Extrahepatic cholestasis • Choledocholithiasis (stones in the common bile duct) • Tumor compression of the bile ducts
3. Impaired bilirubin uptake • Inhibited by certain drugs (ex. rifampin) • Heart failure	—

Table 11 Causes of unconjugated and conjugated bilirubenima

Syndrome	Pathology	Clinical Findings
Gilbert	Deficiency of UDP-glucuronyl transference causes an increase in unconjugated bilirubin	Asymptomatic but bilirubinemia occurs with stress and fasting
Crigler-Najjar type I	Absent UDP-glucuronyl transference causes an increase in unconjugated bilirubin Autosomal recessive	Severe jaundice and kernicterus Death within a few years
Crigler-Najjar type II	Less severe than type I Autosomal dominant	No kernicterus
Dubin-Johnson	Impaired bilirubin transport leads to conjugated hyperbilirubinemia	Dark liver Asymptomatic
Rotor	Similar to Dubin-Johnson but milder	Lacks dark liver Asymptomatic

Table 12 Disease of bilirubin metabolism

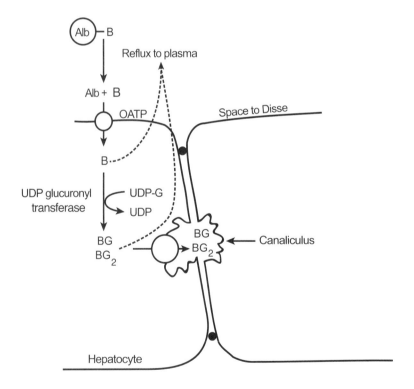

Figure 27 Bilirubin metabolism pathway
(Adapted from *Gastrointestinal Physiology*)

Disease	Pathology	Clinical Findings/Notes
Alcoholic liver disease	Alcohol causes inflammation, fatty changes, fibrosis, and eventual cirrhosis	Cirrhosis (see section above)
α-1-antitrypsin deficiency	Deficiency of enzyme Autosomal recessive	Emphysema and cirrhosis
Cirrhosis	Most commonly due to alcohol and hepatitis C	See above section on cirrhosis GI: portal hypertension, hemorrhoids, varices, caput medusa, ascites CNS: encephalopathy, asterixis Endocrine: gynecomastia, palmar erythema Skin: jaundice, scleral icterus, spider nevi Hematology: coagulopathy
Hemochromatosis	Two forms: 1. Inherited: autosomal recessive 2. Acquired: multiple transfusions (ex. thalassemia major) Iron deposits in multiple organs	Classic triad: 1. Diabetes mellitus 2. Skin pigmentation → "Bronze diabetes" 3. Cirrhosis High risk of hepatocellular carcinoma Treat with phlebotomy or deferoxamine
Primary biliary cirrhosis	Autoimmune: antimitochondrial antibody Associated with other autoimmune conditions (ex. CREST, celiac)	Commonly affects middle-aged women Pruritis , fatigue, jaundice, dark urine, hepatosplenomegaly
Reye syndrome	Unclear etiology May be due to viral syndrome (ex. upper respiratory infection, varicella) and aspirin Fatty liver changes	Edematous encephalopathy: altered mental status, coma, death

Sclerosing cholangitis	Chronic fibrosing inflammation of bile ducts → alternating dilation and strictures leading to "beading" appearance of bile ducts (Figure 28)\n\nAssociated with inflammatory bowel disease (ulcerative colitis)\n\nHigher risk of cholangiocarcinoma	Pruritis , fatigue, jaundice, dark urine, hepatosplenomegaly
Wilson's (hepatolenticular degeneration)	Autosomal recessive\n\nDecreased ability to excrete copper, deposits in multiple organs (joints, liver, kidneys, brain) → cirrhosis, hepatolenticular degeneration\n\nDecreased ceruloplasmin levels\n\nIncreased urinary copper excretion	Kayser-Fleischer ring on cornea\n\nCirrhosis: portal hypertension, weakness, jaundice, fever\n\nCNS: dementia, chorea, asterixis\nTreat with penicillamine

Table 13 Disease of the liver

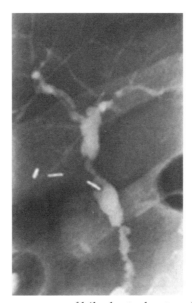

Figure 28 Beaded appearance of bile ducts due to sclerosing cholangitis

HEPATIC INFECTIONS

The clinical manifestations of acute viral hepatitis generally occur in three phases: the prodrome, the icteric phase, and the convalescent phase.

Prodrome (3–4 days):

- Nonspecific constitutional symptoms/signs: malaise, fatigue, and fever

- GI symptoms and signs: anorexia, nausea, vomiting, right upper quadrant pain

- Other symptom/signs: headache, photophobia, cough, coryza, myalgias, urticarial skin rash, arthralgias

Icteric phase (1–4 weeks):

- Improvement of constitutional symptoms

- Right upper quadrant abdominal pain persists

- Possible splenomegaly in some patients

- Possible pruritus due to cholestasis

Convalescent phase:

- Resolution of constitutional symptoms but persistent abnormalities in liver function tests

Chronic hepatitis is defined as continued evidence of hepatic injury (elevated hepatic enzyme) past 6 months. Usually acute hepatitis resolves in 3–6 months.

	Hepatitis A	Hepatitis B	Hepatitis C	Hepatitis D	Hepatitis E
Transmission	**Fecal-oral** route, raw food (oysters, clams, mussels) International travel is most common risk factor in US	**Parenteral**, transfusion, personal contact, needle sticks/sharing, male homosexuals	**Parenteral**, transfusion, personal contact	**Parenteral**, personal contact Dependent on HBV for replication	**Waterborne Pregnant woman**
Onset	Abrupt	Insidious	Insidious	Insidious	Abrupt
Type of virus	RNA Picornavirus	DNA Hepadnavirus	RNA Flavivirus	RNA Defective virus	RNA Unknown

Diagnosis	Anti-HAV antibodies	Window period: +IgM anti-HBc +HBV DNA Acute infection: +HBsAg +HBeAg +IgM anti-HBc +HBV DNA Chronic infection: +HBsAg +IgG anti-HBc Variable HBV DNA Note: +HBeAg = high infectivity +Anti- HBe = low infectivity	Anti-HCV	Anti-HDV, HBsAg, IgM anti-HBc	Anti-HEV
Treatment	Usually supportive, disease is usually self-limited	Usually supportive, low progression to chronic state However, if severe disease can treat with nucleoside/tide therapy	Genotype 1: triple therapy (peginterferon, ribavirin, and a protease inhibitor) Genotype 2: peginterferon and ribavirin	Optimal treatment of HDV is uncertain	Usually supportive
Increased risk of HCC	No	Yes	Yes	Yes	No
Evolves to chronic hepatitis	No	Yes, but less than HVC	Yes, high rate	Yes	No
Vaccination available	Yes	Yes	No	No	No

Table 14 Types of Hepatitis

Pancreas

The exocrine pancreas secretes ~ 1 L of fluid into the duodenum each day, which consists mainly of HCO_3 and enzymatic juices. The HCO_3 element neutralizes the acidity of partially digested food from the stomach. The enzymatic juice assists with digesting carbohydrates, proteins, and lipids into smaller, absorbable components. Acinar cells produce the enzymatic component of pancreatic secretion while centroacinar and ductal cells work synergistically to produce the aqueous component consisting of HCO_3, Na^+, K^+, and Cl. Pancreatic amylase and lipase are secreted in their active forms. In contrast, pancreatic proteases are secreted in inactive forms and converted to their active forms in the lumen of the duodenum. In cystic fibrosis, there is a defect in the chloride channel, which results in thickened secretions that eventually clogs the ducts and lead to autodigestion of the pancreas. Pancreatic secretion is promoted by secretin, CCK, and the parasympathetic nervous system.

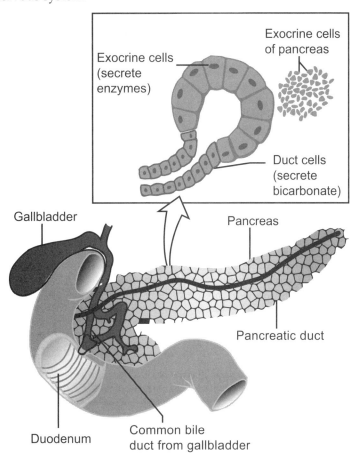

Figure 29 Pancreatic anatomy
(Adapted from *Ganong's Review of Medical Physiology*, 24th Edition)

	Pathology	Clinical Findings
Pancreatitis	Activation of pancreatic enzymes (autodigestion) leads to fat necrosis, pseudocyst formation, abscess Associated with gallstones, alcohol, steroids, mumps, ERCP, hyperlipidemia, hypercalcemia, biliary tract disease, drugs (ex. sulfa)	Severe abdominal pain often radiating to the back, fever, ecchymosis of flank (Grey Turner sign), ecchymosis of periumbilical area (Cullen sign), anorexia, nausea DIC, ARDS, hypocalcemia, hemorrhage, infection, multi-organ failure Elevated lipase, amylase
Adenocarcinoma	Commonly develop in the pancreatic head → obstructive jaundice with palpable gallbladder (Courvoisier's sign) Risk factors include alcohol, smoking	Abdominal pain radiating to the back, jaundice, migratory thrombophlebitis (Trousseau's syndrome), weight loss, anorexia Aggressive and leads to rapid death (prognosis < 6 months) Most useful serum marker: CA-19-9
Cystic Fibrosis	Aberrant chloride transport caused by mutations in the cystic fibrosis transmembrane conductance regulator gene (CFTR) located on chromosome 7 Mutations lead to production of abnormally thick mucus → lungs, gut, pancreas, and hepatobiliary system → lumens of these organs become obstructed	Malabsorption of fat causes steatorrhea (if severe enough can lead to vitamin A, D, E, and K deficiency) Failure to thrive is a common manifestation

Table 15 Diseases of the pancreas

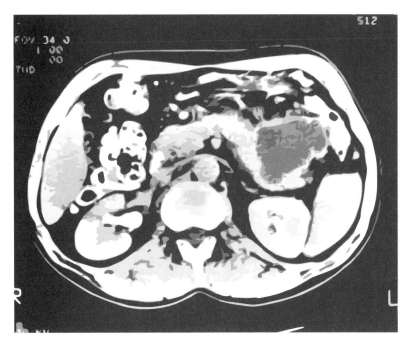

Figure 30 Pseudocyst of the pancreas

Small Bowel

Digestion of Carbohydrates

Only monosaccharides are absorbed by the intestinal epithelium and thus, all ingested carbohydrates need to be broken down into monosaccharides, which can either be glucose, galactose, or fructose. Starch is initially digested by salivary α-amylase in the mouth but is inactivated by low gastric pH. Starch digestion continues, however, in the small bowel by the action of pancreatic amylase yielding three disaccharides, α-limit dextrins, maltose, and maltotriose. These disaccharides are eventually converted into the monosaccharide glucose by the intestinal brush-border enzymes, α-dextrinase, maltase, and sucrase.

Three disaccharides exist in food contents: trehalose, lactose, and sucrose. These disaccharides do not need amylase, as they are already in the disaccharide form. They are digested respectively by the enzymes trehalase, lactase, and sucrase.

trehalose (trehalase) $\rightarrow$ 2 molecules of glucose

lactose (lactase) $\rightarrow$ glucose and galactose

sucrose (sucrase) $\rightarrow$ glucose and fructose

maltose (maltase) $\rightarrow$ 2 molecules of glucose

To simplify, carbohydrate digestion yields 3 end point monosaccharides (glucose, galactose, and fructose), which is then absorbed across the epithelium.

Glucose and galactose are transported across the apical membrane by Na^+-dependent cotransport (SGLT1). Glucose and galactose moves across the basolateral membrane by facilitated diffusion (GLUT 2).

Fructose is transported across the apical membrane by facilitated diffusion (GLUT 5) and in the basolateral membrane by GLUT 2.

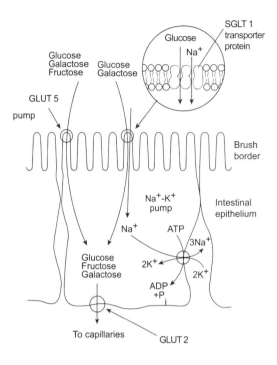

Figure 31 Monosaccharide transport
(Adapted from *Harper's Illustrated Biochemistry*, 29th Edition)

Disorders of carbohydrate absorption are usually secondary to the failure of completely digesting carbohydrates into monosaccharides. If undigested carbohydrates remain in the gastrointestinal lumen, they draw in water and cause an osmotic diarrhea. A classic example is lactose intolerance due to lactase deficiency. Here, lactose is not digested to glucose and galactose and remains undigested in the lumen of the intestine.

Digestion of Proteins

Proteins are metabolized into absorbable forms by proteases in the stomach and small intestine. Protein digestion initially starts in the stomach by the action of pepsin and then is completed in the small bowel by the synergistic actions of brush-border and pancreatic proteases. In the stomach, gastric chief cells secrete pepsinogen, which is cleaved into active pepsin at low gastric pH. It is then denatured and inactivated at higher pH in the duodenum. In the duodenum, 5 major pancreatic enzymes are released in its inactive forms: trypsinogen, chymotrypsinogen, proelastase, procarboxypeptidase A, and procarboxypeptidase. These precursors are activated by trypsin, which is activated by the brush-border enzyme enterokinase and its own intrinsic autocatalytic activity. Only amino acids, dipeptides, and tripeptides are absorbable by the intestinal epithelium. The amino acids cross the lumen into the cell by Na^+-amino acid cotransporters in the apical membrane (4 separate cotransporters exist for neutral, acidic, basic, and imino amino acids). The dipeptides and tripeptides are transported from the lumen into the intestinal epithelium through separate H^+-dependent cotransporters that again, exist for each type of amino acid (4 separate cotransporters exist for neutral, acidic, basic, and imino amino acids).

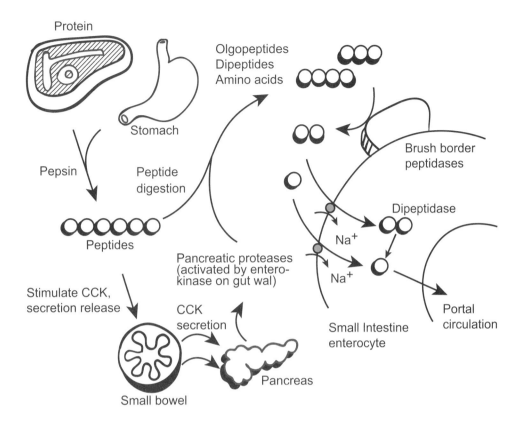

Figure 32 Protein digestion
(Adapted from *Ganong's Review of Medical Physiology*, 24th Edition)

Digestion of Lipids

Dietary lipids consist of triglycerides, cholesterol, and phospholipids, which are quite insoluble in the aqueous solution of the gastrointestinal tract due to their hydrophobicity. Lipids are initially digested in the mouth and stomach by lingual and gastric lipases, respectively. It is completed in the small intestine through the following pancreatic enzymes: pancreatic lipase, cholesterol ester hydrolase, and phospholipase A2.

The end products of lipid breakdown (ex. cholesterol, monoglycerides, lysolecithin, and free fatty acids) are solubilized in the intestinal lumen in mixed micelles. These micelles diffuse to the apical membrane and release their lipids. The bile salts are consequently left behind in the intestinal lumen to be absorbed and recycled in the ileum. Within the epithelial cells, the products of lipid digestion are reconstituted into their original ingested lipids, triglycerides, cholesterol ester, and phospholipids and packaged in lipid-carrying particles known as chylomicrons. Chylomicrons are absorbed in the lymphatic circulation.

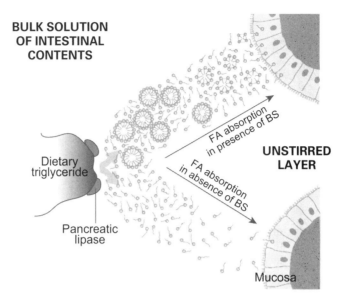

Figure 33 Micelle assisted fat absorption

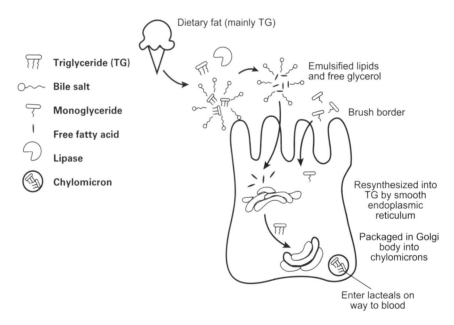

Figure 34 Fat digestion

Congenital Anomaly	Pathology	Clinical Findings
Omphalocele	Midgut fails to return into the abdominal cavity	Loops of bowel is found in a shiny sac outside the abdomen

Meckel's diverticulum	Persistent ophalomesenteric vitelline duct, which may contain pancreatic or gastric tissue that can cause ulceration	Abdominal pain
		
		GI bleeding
		
		Intussusception, volvulus, or obstruction
		
		Five 2's:
		  2 inches long
		  2 feet from the ileocecal valve
		  2% of population
		  First 2 years of life
		  2 types of tissue

Viteline fistula	Persistent vitelline duct, which connects the intestinal lumen to the umbilicus	Drainage of meconium from the umbilicus

Table 16 Congenital Anomalies

Disease of the small bowel	Pathology	Clinical Findings
Celiac	Sensitivity to the gliadin portion of gluten (ex. wheat, barley, rye, oats) T-cell mediated response to gliadin leads to mucosal inflammation and villous atrophy in jejunum (intestinal biopsy) Presence of anti-gliadin and anti-endomysial Ab	Chronic diarrhea Rash (dermatitis herpetiformis) Failure to thrive Weakness Steatorrhea
Intussusception	Telescoping of proximal bowel into distal bowel leading to obstruction Lead point usually an intraluminal mass including hypertrophy of Peyer's patches or Meckel's diverticulum	More common in infants and children Abdominal pain GI bleeding (currant jelly stool) May be reduced with barium enema "Target" sign on cross section with CT or US due to loops of bowels within each other (Figure 35)

Volvulus	Twisting of the bowel around its mesentry → obstruction or infarction Associated with maltrotation of the midgut	Abdominal pain Obstruction symptoms: nausea, vomiting, and lack of stool or flatus
Whipple's	Caused by Tropheryma whippelii (gram + bacilli) Periodic acid-Schiff (PAS)-positive macrophages in the lamina propria	More common in older men Abdominal pain, diarrhea, fever, weight loss and arthralgias Cardiac: endocarditis CNS: AMS, headaches, seizures

Table 17 Diseases of the small bowel

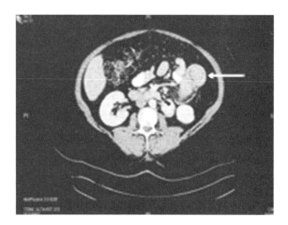

A

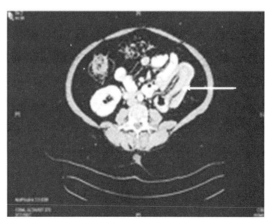

B

Figure 35 Intussusception

Colon

The colon consists of the cecum, ascending, transverse, descending, sigmoid colon, and rectum. It is mainly involved with absorption of water and electrolytes, secretion of mucus, and formation of feces. The colon can absorb up to five liters of water a day. Under the influence of aldosterone, there is increased sodium reabsorption in the setting of volume depletion. Colonic intestinal microbes are important for digestion. For example, they generate short chain fatty acids from dietary fiber, which is an important source of energy, to maintain the health of the colonic epithelium. The major secretory product of the colon is mucin. It serves two purposes: lubrication and formation of a protective barrier.

	Pathology	Clinical Findings
Appendicitis	Obstruction by a fecalith or lymphoid hyperplasia (after an acute illness) Figure 36	Fever Periumbilical pain that migrates to the right lower quadrant (McBurney's point) Nausea and vomiting Rovsing's sign: palpation of the left lower quadrant results in more pain in the right lower quadrant Psoas sign: flexion of hip causes pain Obturator sign: flexion and internal rotation of the hip causes pain
Angiodysplasia	Dilated tortuous veins in the mucosa/submucosa	Most commonly in cecum and right colon GI bleeding
Diverticular disease	Multiple outpouchings of the colon due to prolonged intraluminal pressure (ex. constipation) leading to focal weakness in the muscular wall	More common in elderly patients Asymptomatic if no superimpose infection If infected, fever, pain, possible perforation, peritonitis, and abscess formation May cause GI bleeding May be referred to as left-sided appendicitis
Hirschsprung	Lack of Meissner and Auerbach plexus in distal colon due to impaired neural crest cell migration Common in ileum, cecum, and ascending colon	Proximal distention of colon before abnormal segment Failure to pass meconium, nausea, vomiting, abdominal distention Chronic constipation
Irritable bowel syndrome	No organic abnormalities	Chronic abdominal pain and altered bowel habits (constipation, diarrhea)

Table 18 Diseases of the colon

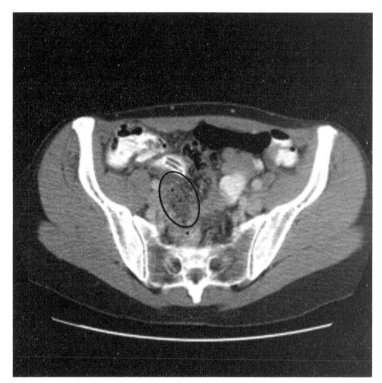

Figure 36 Acute appendicitis

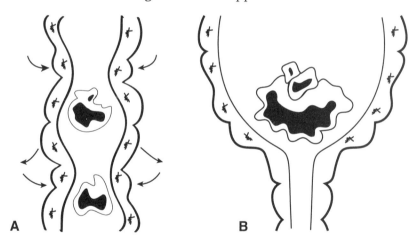

Figure 37 Normal peristalsis (A) versus Hirschsprung's disease (B)

Inflammatory Bowel Disease

There are two forms of chronic inflammatory bowel disease: Crohn's disease and ulcerative colitis.

	Ulcerative Colitis	Crohn's disease
Pathology	Mucosal and submucosal inflammation of rectum to colon	Transmural inflammation of any part of the GI tract (mouth to anus)
Most common location	Rectum	Ileum
Distribution	Continuous	Skip lesions
Gross morphology	Extensive ulcerations, pseudopolyps, "lead pipe" appearance (loss of haustra)	Linear mucosal fissures, thickened bowel walls, creeping fat, cobblestone appearance, "string sign"
Microscopic morphology	Crypt abscesses	Noncaseating granulomas
Complications	Toxic megacolon (Figure 38), malnutrition, colorectal cancer (higher in ulcerative colitis than crohn)	Obstruction, abscesses, fistulas, sinus tracts, malnutrition, colorectal cancer
Gastrointestinal symptoms	Bloody diarrhea	Non bloody or bloody diarrhea
Extra-gastrointestinal symptoms	Both diseases share similar extra-gastrointestinal symptoms due to disease activity: Skin: pyoderma gangrenosum, eryth ema nodosum Arthritis: sacroiliitis, ankylosing spondylitis Eye: uveitis, iritis, episcleritis Biliary: primary sclerosing cholangitis	
Treatment	Oral 5-aminosalicylates (eg, sulfasalazine, mesalamine) Antibiotics (eg, ciprofloxacin, metronidazole) Conventional glucocorticoids (eg, prednisone) Non-systemic glucocorticoids (eg, budesonide) Immunomodulators (eg, azathioprine, 6-mercaptopurine, methotrexate) Biologic therapies (eg, infliximab, adalimumab)	

Table 19 Inflamatory bowel diseases

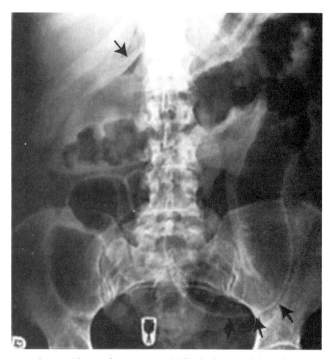

Figure 38 Toxic megacolon with perforation in UC. Colon is dilated with free air underneath the diaphragm.

Colonic Polyps

There are three types of colonic polyps. Their malignant potential increases with size and villous elements.

Tubular adenoma	Most common Pedunculated polyps Sporadic or familial
Villous adenoma	Least common Sessile Highest malignant potential
Tubulovillous adenoma	Contain both tubular and villous components Malignant potential increases with villous component

Table 20 Colonic polyps

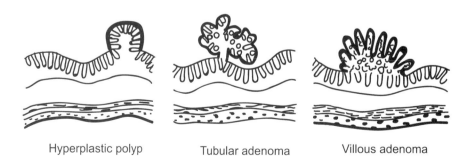

Hyperplastic polyp   Tubular adenoma   Villous adenoma

Figure 39 Colonic polyps

Polyposis Syndromes

Polyposis syndromes	Pathology	Clinical Findings
Familial adenomatous polyposis (FAP)	Autosomal dominant APC gene mutations Presence of more than 100 adenomatous colorectal polyps	Majority of patients develop colorectal cancer Prophylactic colectomy
Hereditary nonpolyposis colorectal cancer (HNPCC) or Lynch syndrome	Autosomal dominant DNA mismatch repair gene mutations	High risk of colorectal cancer Associated with endometrial cancer and several other cancers including ovarian, upper urologic tract, gastric, small bowel, biliary, pancreatic, skin, brain cancers Manage with serial colonoscopies and colectomy
Turcot's syndrome	FAP + brain tumors	Commonly associated with medulloblastomas
Gardner's syndrome	FAP + bone/soft tissue tumors	Associated with desmoid tumors, sebaceous or epidermoid cysts, lipomas, osteomas, supernumerary teeth
Peutz-Jeghers	Autosomal dominant Multiple hamartomas throughout the entire GI tract	Associated with melanin pigmentation of the buccal mucosa, lips, genitalia, hands, feet Small bowel intussusception, obstruction, and bleeding Associated with colorectal cancer and nongastrointestinal cancers (breast, ovarian, cervical, testicular, pancreatic)
Juvenile polyposis syndrome/familial juvenile polyposis	Autosomal dominant with high penetrance Defined as the occurrence of 10 or more juvenile polyps	Rectal bleeding and/or anemia Also rectal prolapse of polyps, abdominal pain, or intestinal obstruction Increased risk of colorectal cancer

Table 21 Polyposis syndromes

Malignant Tumors of the Small and Large Intestine

Adenocarcinoma	Comprise majority of colonic cancers
	Most common sites: rectum, sigmoid
	Left-sided cancers: obstruction, annular constriction, may lead to frank bright red blood per rectum
	Right-sided cancers: anemia, obstruction is less likely because fecal matter is still liquid on the right side, melena and anemia due to slow bleeding
Carcinoid tumor	Neuroendocrine tumors that arise from the gastrointestinal tract
	Most common sites: appendix, ileum, rectum
	Many secretory products have been identified (~40), most prominently serotonin, histamine, tachykinins, kallikrein and prostaglandins
	Liver inactivates tumor products secreted into portal circulation, carcinoid syndrome only develops with hepatic metastases when tumor products are released into systemic circulation
	Clinical findings include flushing, venous telangiectasia (purple skin lesions), diarrhea, bronchospasm, cardiac valvular lesions
Colorectal cancer	Associated with FAP, Gardner's syndrome, Turcot's syndrome, Lynch syndrome
	"apple core" sign (Figure 40)
	CEA is elevated
Squamous cell tumor	Common site: anal region
	Associated with HPV
	Increase incidence in HIV and homosexual men

Table 22 Malignant tumors of the small and large intestine

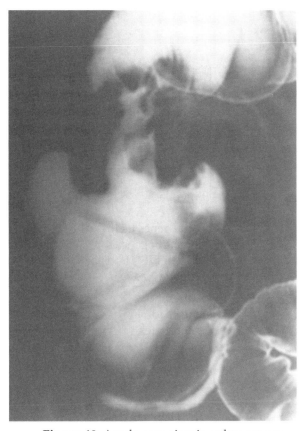

Figure 40 Apple core sign in colon cancer

Gastrointestinal Infections

Organism	Source	Pathogenesis	Treatment	Clinical Notes
Bacillus cereus	Fried rice	Heat stable toxin	Supportive therapy	Vomiting and diarrhea
Campybacter jejuni	Poultry, domestic animals Infection by consumption of raw meat or food cross contaminated with raw meat	Invades epithelium	First line agents for treatment fluoroquinolones (if sensitive) or azithromycin	Reactive arthritis or Guillain-Barré syndrome (GBS)
C. diff	Can be intestinal colonizer	Previous antibiotic use can lead to over colonization	Vancomycin or metronidazole	Severe disease treat with vancomycin initially Can lead to toxic megacolon

Enterohemor-rhagic E. coli (EHEC, O157:H7)	Fecal-oral, food (undercooked hamburger)	Shiga toxins	Mainly supportive therapy Antibiotic therapy is not beneficial in patients with EHEC and may increase hemolytic uremic syndrome	Hemolytic uremic syndrome Bloody diarrhea
Enteroinvasive E. coli (EIEC)	Fecal-oral, food, water	Similar to Shigella Same genes facilitate pathogenesis of both EIEC and Shigella	Supportive therapy	EIEC may be differentiated from Shigella principally by fermentation of glucose and xylose
Enteropathogenic E. coli (EPEC)	Fecal-oral, food, water	Adherence factors to enterocytes	Mainly supportive therapy	Diarrhea outbreaks, most commonly among children < 6 months in developing countries
Enterotoxigenic E. coli (ETEC)	Food, water	Heat labile toxins (LTs) Heat stable toxins (STs)	Mainly supportive therapy	Common diarrheal illness in children < 2 years of age in developing regions
Giardia lambia	Fecal-oral, food, water, day care, travelers	There are two morphological forms: cysts and trophozoites The cysts are the infectious form	Metronidazole	Boiling or heating water eliminates Giardia cysts
Shigella	Fecal-oral, food, water	Invasion of colonic mucosal cells leading to ulcerations and abscesses	Azithromycin or trimethoprim-sulfamethoxazole	30–100 organisms can cause disease
Salmonella	Poultry, eggs, reptiles	Adherence to and invasion of the gastrointestinal tract and submucosal lymphoid system	Mainly supportive therapy	Severe disease can be treated with fluoroquinolone, trimethoprim-sulfamethoxazole, or amoxicillin

Vibrio cholera	Fecal-oral, food, water	Stimulation of adenylate cyclase	Mainly supportive with rehydration	Rice water diarrhea
Vibrio parahae-molyticus	Contaminated seafood	Production of thermostable direct hemolysis responsible for the beta-hemolysis	Mainly supportive with rehydration	Disease can be severe with underlying liver disease→sepsis

Table 23 Gastrointestinal infections

Hernias

INDIRECT

Abdominal contents protrude through the internal inguinal ring, external inguinal ring, and finally into the scrotum. It occurs **lateral** to the inferior epigastric artery.

DIRECT

Abdominal contents protrude directly through an area of the abdominal wall denoted as Hesselbach's triangle, which only involves the external inguinal ring. It occurs **medial** to the inferior epigastric artery.

FEMORAL

Abdominal contents protrude through the femoral canal underneath the inguinal ligament. It is the **most common** cause of bowel incarceration.

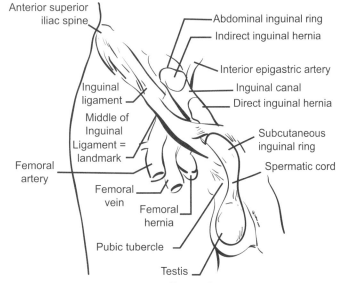

Figure 41 Different hernias
(Adapted from *DeGowin's Diagnostic Examination*, 9th Edition)

PHARMACOLOGY

	Mechanisms	Side effects	Clinical Notes
Proton pump inhibitors	Irreversibly block H^+/K^+ —ATPase by parietal cells	Can lead to bacterial overgrowth	Omeprazole, lansoprazole
Histamine blockers ("dine")	Reversible block of histamine H2 receptors → decrease acid secretion by parietal cells	Cimetidine is a potent inhibitor of P-450 → slows metabolism of drugs (warfarin, diazepam, phenytoin) Cimetidine has antiandrogenic effects (gynecomastia, impotence) Penetrate blood-brain barrier to cause CNS symptoms (confusion, headaches)	Cimetidine, ranitidine, famotidine
Antacids: Aluminum hydroxide Magnesium hydroxide Calcium carbonate	Neutralize stomach acid	Aluminum hydroxide —constipation Magnesium hydroxide —diarrhea Calcium carbonate —hypercalcemia	Can be toxic in renal failure patients because of their inability to clear the ions in these solutions

Table 24 Antacid and antisecretory medications

Drugs	Mechanism
Diphenoxylate	Opioid derivatives, which inhibit ACh release in the enteric nervous system
Loperamide	

Table 25 Antidiarrheals

Drug	Mechanism
Metoclopramide	Cholinergic stimulation, dopamine antagonist Can be used for gastroparesis

Table 26 Motility agents

Drug	Mechanism
Promethazine	Block dopamine receptors
Prochlorperazine	
Metoclopramide	
Odansetron	Block serotonin receptors

Table 27 Antiemetics

Drug Type	Mechanism	Examples
Stimulant, irritant	Stimulate or irritate the bowel	Castor oil Senna Bisacody
Bulking	Indigestible and causes osmotic retention of water making stool bulky → reflex bowel contraction	Psyllium, fiber Lactulose Saline enemas
Stool softener/ emollient	Either softens stool or lubricates stool for easier passage	Mineral oil Docusate Glycerin

Table 28 Laxatives

Infections of the Gastrointestinal Tract

Disease	Treatment
H. pylori	Triple therapy: Metronidazole Amoxicillin (or Tetracycline) Bismuth.
C. diff	Metronidazole or vancomycin (used in more severe cases)
Traveler's diarrhea	Usually fluoroquinolones (ciprofloxacin) or trimethoprim-sulfa-methoxazole (Bactrim)
Giardia lambia	Metronidazole
Entamoeba histolytica	Metronidazole

Table 29 Infections of the gastrointestinal tract

Oncology

Disease	Treatment	Mechanism
Gastrointestinal stromal tumor	Imatinib	Inhibits Bcr-Abl tyrosine kinase

Also used for the abnormal gene product of the Philadelphia chromosome in chronic myeloid leukemia (CML) |

Table 30 Oncology

Inflammatory Bowel Disease

Ulcerative colitis	Oral 5-aminosalicylates (eg, sulfasalazine, mesalamine)
Crohn's disease	Antibiotics (eg, ciprofloxacin, metronidazole)
	Conventional glucocorticoids (eg, prednisone)
	Non-systemic glucocorticoids (eg, budesonide)
	Immunomodulators (eg, azathioprine, 6-mercaptopurine, methotrexate)
	Biologic therapies (eg, infliximab, adalimumab)

Table 31 Inflammatory bowel diseases

CHAPTER 8

GENETICS

PEDIGREE ANALYSIS AND MODES OF INHERITANCE

Useful definitions and concepts related to pedigree analysis:

- All somatic cells (non-germ cells) have one pair of sex chromosomes (XX or XY) and 22 pairs of autosomes for a total of 46 chromosomes.

- XX individuals are female, and XY individuals are male.

- There are approximately 150 million base pairs per chromosome; each chromosome has "bands" that can be identified by cytogenetic studies. Each "band" contains several thousand genes (see Figure 1).

- One copy of every autosomal chromosome is inherited by each offspring from parents.

- A **locus** is defined by its position along the chromosome

- A **gene** is defined by its product. For example, phosphofructokinase (PFK) is produced by the PFK gene.

- Alleles are slight variations of the gene that are caused, for example, by a single base change. A given gene can have one or more alleles. Alleles can cause variations in phenotype and do not necessarily cause expression of a mutant phenotype.

- An individual is a **homozygote** at a locus if both alleles are the same.

- An individual is a **heterozygote** at a locus if the two alleles are different.

- In **Pedigree analysis**, family history is examined to deduce patterns of inheritance—an integral part of genetic counseling. Some common symbols are listed in Figure 2.

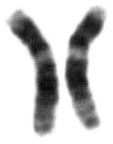

Figure 1 Chromosome banding

Autosomal Dominant Inheritance

Autosomal Dominant

Only need one copy
of disease gene to
be affected.

Risk of passing on the
disease if one parent is
affected is 50%.

On a pedigree, at least
one person will be
affected in each genera-
tion if the family is still
carrying the disease.

- Carrying a dominant genetic mutation predisposes an individual to the disorder even if the normal gene is present (i.e. the individual is a heterozygote).

- The risk of a child inheriting the gene is 50%.

- Males and females have an equal chance of transmitting the mutant gene.

- Affected individuals typically also have affected parents who carry an existing mutation. However, many autosomal dominant diseases arise by new mutations.

- Selected examples of Autosomal Dominant diseases are included in Table 1.

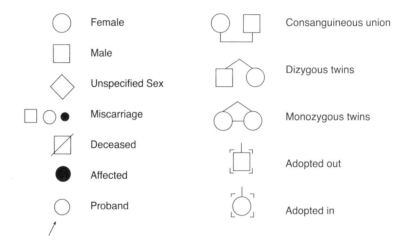

Figure 2 Symbols used in pedigree analysis

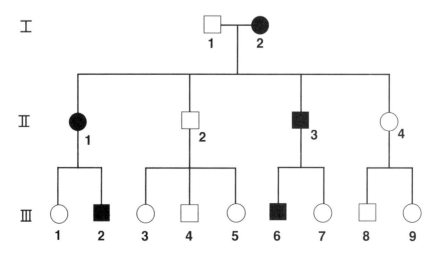

Figure 3 Autosomal dominant inheritance

Disease	Mutation	Characteristics
Achondroplasia	Fibroblast Growth Factor Receptor 3	Dwarfism. Associated with advanced paternal age. Normal-sized head, short limbs.
Autosomal dominant polycystic kidney disease (ADPKD)	PKD1	Bilateral, massive, cystic enlargement of kidneys. Features include flank pain, hematuria, renal failure, cerebral/berry aneurysms, mitral valve prolapse, and polysistic liver disease. Presents during adulthood. There is a recessive form that presents during infancy.
Familial adenomatous polyposis	APC gene (chromosome 5)	Multiple adenomatous colonic polyps. Colon resection is needed to prevent advancement to colon cancer.
Familial hypercholesterolemia	LDL receptor	Marked elevation in LDL. Heterozygotes have cholesterol of 300+, homozygotes with cholesterol 700+. Associated with tendon xanthomas (often Achilles), and early MI.
Hereditary hemorrhagic telangiectasia (Osler-Weber-Rendu syndrome)	Endoglin (ENG)	Most common genetic vascular disease associated with telangiectasias, recurrent epistaxis, arteriovenous malformations (AVMs).
Huntington's disease	CAG trinucleotide repeat	Decreased levels of GABA and ACh in the brain and atrophy of the caudate nucleus lead to findings of dementia and depression in 30–50 year old individuals.
Hereditary spherocytosis	Spectrin or ankyrin defect	Spectrin or ankyrin defect causes spheroid erythrocytes, hemolytic anemia, increased MCHC. Cured by splenectomy.
Marfan syndrome	Fibrillin	Fibrillin mutation causes a connective tissue disorder. Characteristic long extremities, tall stature, hyperextensive joints, pectus excavatum, arachnodactyly, cystic medial necrosis of the aorta causing dissecting aortic aneurysms, lens subluxation and mitral valve prolapse.
Multiple endocrine neoplasias (MEN)	Ret gene (MEN 2A and 2B)	Tumors of the pancreas, parathyroid, thyroid, adrenal medulla, and pituitary glands.
Neurofibromatosis type I	NF1	Café au lait spots, neural tumors, Lisch nodules, scoliosis, optic gliomas, pheochromocytomas. Chromosome 17.
Neurofibromatosis type II	NF2 (merlin)	Bilateral acoustic neuroma. Chromosome 22.
Osteogenesis imperfecta	Type I collagen	Easily fractured bones with minimal trauma, blue sclerae, deafness, and tooth defects. Can be confused with child abuse
Tuberous sclerosis	TSC	Seizures, mental retardation, renal failure. Hamartomas ("tubers") in multiple organ systems, including the brain, retina, kidneys, and heart.
Von Hippel Lindau disease	VHL	Hemangioblastomas of the central nervous system, bilateral renal cell carcinomas, pheochromocytomas. Caused by a gene deletion in a tumor suppressor gene (VHL) on chromosome 3.

Table 1 Select autosomal dominant diseases

Autosomal Recessive Inheritance

- Horizontal transmission: when a phenotype is seen in siblings rather than offspring or parents.

- New mutations are rare (unlike autosomal dominant inheritance).

- 25% of children are affected if both parents are carriers, 50% of children are affected if one parent is a carrier and one parent is affected. Both parents must either be a carrier or affected for a child to be 100% of children are affected if both parents are affected.

- **Cystic Fibrosis**

  ○ CFTR gene on chromosome 7, most often mutation of phe508

  ○ CFTR channel secretes Cl^- in lungs and GI tract and absorbs Na^+ from sweat glands

  ○ Thick mucus plug secretion in lungs, pancreas, and liver resulting in recurrent pneumonias (often *pseudomonas* and *S. aureus*), bronchitis, bronchiectasis, pancreatic insufficiency, and meconium ileus (characteristic first finding in newborns)

  ○ CF is the most common fatal autosomal recessive disorder in the US. The most common cause of death is pneumonia.

  ○ Male infertility due to bilateral absence of vas deferens

  ○ Test: elevated Cl^- in eccrine sweat glands

  ○ Treatment: n-acetylcystine to loosen mucous plugs

  ○ Additional examples of autosomal recessive diseases, prevention and control of lung infections, nutritional support, prevent dehydration, lung transplantation are included in Table 2.

Disease	Mutation	Characteristics
Albinism	Tyrosinase	Lack of melanin, increased skin cancer risk.
Alkaptonuria	Homogentisic oxidase	Dark urine, ochronosis, brittle articular cartilage.
Childhood polycystic kidney disease	PKHD1 gene	Collecting duct dilation, progressive renal insufficiency early in life
Cystic fibrosis	Cystic fibrosis transmembrane conductance regulation gene (CFTR)	Thick secretions, pneumonia, pancreatic insufficiency. Diagnosis by sweat electrolyte test. Defective Na/Cl pump.
Gaucher disease	Glucocerebrosidase deficiency	Accumulation of glucocerebroside in macrophages (leading to Gaucher's cells), hepatosplenomegaly.

Hurler syndrome	Lysosomal alpha-L-iduronidase (leading to accumulation of glycosoaminoglycans)	Developmental delay, abnormal facies (gargoylism, coarse facial features), cloudy corneas, deafness, claw hand, hepatosplenomegaly, heart valve abnormalities.
Krabbe disease	Galactocerebrosidase (GALC)	Accumulation of cerebroside sulfate, leading to peripheral neuropathy and developmental delay, along with severe seizures, vision loss, and hearing loss.
Metachromatic leukodystrophy	Arylsulfatase A	Central and peripheral demyelination, seizures, developmental delay and behavioral problems, dementia.
Niemann-Pick disease	Shingomyelinase	Hepatosplenomegaly, "cherry-red" spot on macula, foam cells, progressive intellectual decline, seizures, tremors
Phenylketonuria	Phenylalanine hydroxylase	Mousy odor, mental retardation, eczema, convulsions.
Tay-Sachs disease	Hexosaminidase A deficiency	Mental deficiencies, blindness, "cherry-red" spot on macula.

Table 2 Select autosomal recessive diseases

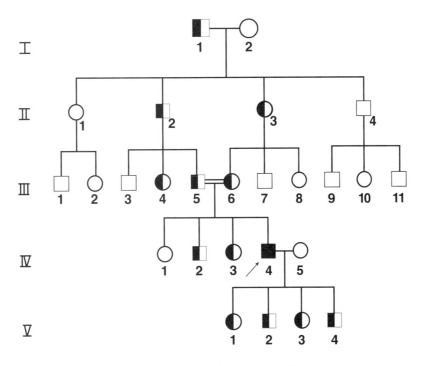

Figure 4 Autosomal recessive inheritance

X-linked Recessive Inheritance

- Phenotypes are expressed in males because the Y chromosome lacks the normal allele counterpart.

- Transmission rate is 50% for both daughters and sons if the mother is a carrier. Sons are affected; daughters are carriers.

- Transmission rate is 100% for daughters and 0% for sons if the father is affected. Daughters are carriers only.

- If the condition is lethal, there is a 33% chance that the phenotype arises as a result of a new mutation.

- Examples:

  ○ Duchenne's muscular dystrophy: frameshift mutation with deleted dystrophin gene (protective to muscle) causing muscle breakdown. Presents with pelvic girdle weakness which spreads superiorly and calf muscle pseudohypertrophy, cardiac Myopathy.

    ○ Test: Gower maneuver—use of upper extremities to stand up. Onset before age 5.

  ○ Becker's muscular dystrophy: caused by a mutated dystrophin gene. Onset occurs in adolescence/adulthood. Diagnosis of muscular dystrophies is with CPK and muscle biopsy.

  ○ Fragile X Syndrome: Caused by a defect in FMR-1 transcription, leads to mental retardation, oversized jaws and ears, and enlarged testes.

  ○ Other diseases: Hunter syndrome, Hemophilia A (Factor VIII), Hemophilia B (Factor IX), Lesch-Nyhan syndrome, Ocular albinism, Fabry disease, G6PD deficiency, Burton agammaglobulinemia, Wiskott-Aldrich syndrome.

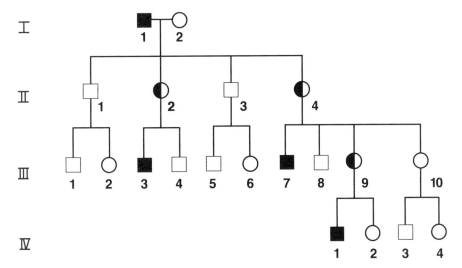

Figure 5 X-linked recessive inheritance

X-linked Dominant Inheritance

- Heterozygous females (unlike X-linked recessive patients) are also affected.

- Transmission rate is 50% for both daughters and sons if the mother is a carrier.

- Transmission rate is 100% for daughters and 0% for sons if the father is affected.

- If the condition is lethal, there is a 33% chance that the phenotype is a result of a new mutation.

- Example: ornithine decarboxylase deficiency.

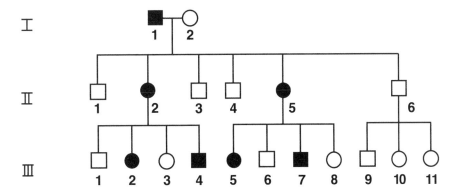

Figure 6 X-linked dominant inheritance

LINKAGE ANALYSIS

Linkage analysis may be used if direct methods for detecting mutant alleles are not available. In linkage analysis, the mutant allele is indirectly detected by its association with a polymorphic marker locus.

Figure 7 illustrates the importance of an informative marker locus in detection of an autosomal dominant disease. In figure 7A, both the disease allele and the normal allele are associated with marker A in the affected parent because the parent is homozygous for marker A, so we can't tell whether the offspring (Aa) inherited the disease allele. In Figure 7B, however, we can see that, barring any recombination, the disease allele and marker A are linked. In other words, we know the phase of the alleles. Hence, we can guess with a good probability that the child will get the disease. The requirements for linkage analysis are as follows:

- An informative marker locus: The marker locus can't be homozygous in the affected parent, and the parents and offspring can't all be heterozygous for the marker alleles.

- A known phase: Marker locus and mutant allele are on the same chromosome.

It is important to note that recombination rates between the marker allele and the disease allele must be counted in estimating the likelihood of a child developing the disease. For instance, if linkage analysis indicates a 100% chance of a child being affected without recombination, a 10% recombination reduces the chance of being affected to 90%. Recombination frequency is measure in centiMorgans (cM); one cM is roughly equal to a recombination frequency of 1%.

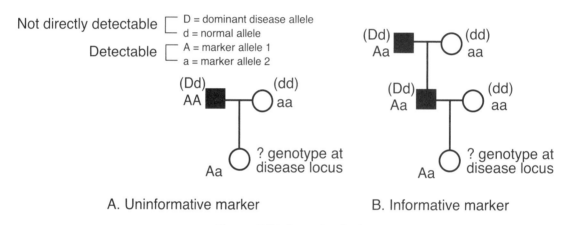

Figure 7 Linkage Analysis

CONGENITAL ABNORMALITIES

Congenital abnormalities are present at birth and can be classified as follows:

- *Malformations*: present at birth as a result of abnormal development in early embryogenesis. Examples: spina bifidia and polydactyly.

- *Disruptions*: the result of intervention in the natural development process by agents such as teratogens.

- *Deformations*: the result from nondisruptive mechanical forces. Some causal agents are the mother's small pelvis and unusual positioning of the fetus. Most deformations occur in the last 4 months of pregnancy.

- *Dysplasia*: abnormal development of a group of cells. Unlike deformations and disruptions, dysplasia is often a result of abnormal gene expression. Example: hemangiomas.

PATTERNS OF ANOMALIES

- Sequences: anomalies that can be traced to one mechanical or structural defect.

  - **Oligohydramnios sequence.** The common effect of this sequence is a limited amount of amniotic fluid which leads to pulmonary hypoplasia, limb deformities, and Potter facies (when insufficient amniotic fluid causes compression of the fetus's body and face).

- Syndromes: groups of anomalies that are a result of genetic mutations or chromosomal abnormalities.

  - Down syndrome (trisomy 21):
    - Flat facies, mental retardation, prominent epicanthal folds, simian crease, endocardial cushion defects, early Alzheimer disease
    - Most commonly due to meiotic disjunction associated with advanced maternal age, also due to robertsonian translocation or down's mosaicism (no maternal association)
    - **Quad Screening**: decreased alphafetoprotein (AFP), increased beta-hCG, decreased estriol, increased inhibin A

  - Edward syndrome (trisomy 18)
    - Severe mental retardation, small jaw (micrognathia), rocker bottom feet, overlapping fingers in closed hands, prominent occiput, low set ears
    - Death usually within 1 year of birth
    - **Triple screening**: decreased beta-hCG, decreased AFP, decreased estriol

  - Patau syndrome (trisomy 13)
    - Microphthalmia, microcephaly, cleft lip/palate, holoprosencephaly (single eye), polydactyly
    - Death usually occurs within one year of birth

  - Sex chromosome aneuploidies:
    - **Klinefelter Syndrome** (47, XXY): Tall and thin body habitus, small male genitalia, infertile, gynecomastia. Low IQ. Barr bodies present.
    - **Trisomy X** (47, XXX): Phenotypically female, risk of infertility and/or menstrual abnormalities, mild mental retardation
    - **Double Y** (47 XYY): Male, tall stature, acne, mild mental retardation. Frequent antisocial/aggressive behavior. Normal fertility.

Trisomies

D = Drinking age
(21, Down Syndrome)
E = Election age
(18, Edward Syndrome)
P = Puberty
(13, Patau Syndrome)

AFP levels

Decreased in trisomies 18 and 21

Increased in twin pregnancies and with neural tube defects

- **Turner Syndrome** (45, XO): Short stature, ovarian dysgenesis (infertile), webbed neck, shield chest, cardiac defects (coarctation of the aorta), horseshoe kidney, no Barr body.

- **Microdeletions** (deletion of several million bases—about 100 genes).

- **22q11** deletion syndrome leads to dominant inheritance of **c**left palate, **a**bnormal facies, **t**hymic aplasia, **c**ardiac defects, and **h**ypocalcemia (CATCH -22). DiGeorge Syndrome is a type of 22q11 deletion syndrome.

- **Cri-du-chat** (*"cry of the cat"*) **syndrome** caused by congenital microdeletion of short arm (*p*) of chromosome 5 (46,XX or XY 5p-). Children have a characteristic high pitched cry which resembles a cat's "meow" along with epicanthal folds, microcephaly, and cardiac defects.

- **Williams Syndrome** caused by microdeletion of long arm of chromosome 7. Findings are well-developed verbal skills, excessive friendliness, mental retardation, elfin facies, and cardiac problems.

- **Associations** of abnormalities occur together more often than would be predicated by chance. Some associations are expected to be reclassified into one of the above categories as more is learned about the underlying causes

ENVIRONMENTAL CAUSES OF ANOMALIES

Teratogens—environmental factors which the fetus can be exposed to during development which can lead to congenital abnormalities. See Table 3.

Drug	Risks to Fetus
ACE inhibitors	Renal dysfunction, oligohydramnios, growth retardation, fetal death
Aminoglycosides	CN VIII toxicity, renal defects
Carbamazepine	Mental retardation, facial and cranial abnormalities, neural tube defects.
Chemotherapeutics	Antineoplastic agents can cause severe birth defects, including risk of spontaneous abortion, growth restriction, mental retardation.
Diazepam	Cleft palate, renal defects
Diethylstilbestrol (DES)	Vaginal clear cell carcinoma
Fluoroquinolones	Cartilage damage
Heparin	Prematurity, low risk of fetal demise (much safer than warfarin)

Isotretinoin or Vitamin A excess	Spontaneous abortion, cleft palate, cardiac defects
Lithium	Ebstein's anomaly, atrialized right ventricle
Phenytoin	Craniofacial dysmorphism, limb and cardiac defects, intrauterine growth restriction, mental retardation.
Quinine	Deafness
Radiation	Increased mutations
Streptomycin	Deafness
Sulfonamides	Kernicterus
Tetracycline	Tooth and bone abnormalities
Thalidomide	Total or partial absence of long bones in the limbs ("flapper limbs")
Valproic acid	Neural tube defects (due to inhibition of maternal folate absorption)
Warfarin	Fetal hemorrhage, abortion, bone defects.
Drugs of Abuse	
Cocaine	Fetal heart defects, fetal addiction, abruptio placentae, small/premature or stillbirth
Alcohol	Leading cause of birth defects and MR, fetal alcohol syndrome
Tobacco	Preterm labor, IUGR, ADHD
LSD	Limb and CNS malformations in high doses

Table 3 Common teratogens

Maternal Illness

- Diabetes

  o 3 fold increase in risk of congenital abnormalities such as neural tube defects and congenital heart disease

  o Strict glucose control with insulin reduces risk of malformations

  o Must avoid hypoglycemia which is also teratogenic

  o Elevated glucose in the mother results in elevated insulin in the fetus which acts as a growth factor and causes overgrowth syndromes

- Phenylketonuria (PKU):

  o Buildup of phenylalanine and lack of tyrosine causes decreased synthesis and increased degradation of myelin sheaths and competitive inhibition of transport of amino acids across the blood brain barrier

  o Mental retardation

- Microcephaly

- Congenital heart defects

- Hypopigmentation

- Risk significantly reduced in women who maintain low phenylalanine diets prior to conception

- Treatment: low phenylalanine diet and tyrosine supplements

- **Maternal Malnutrition** (e.g., iodine deficiency is most common cause of **cretinism**)

  - Definition: hypothyroidism in utero, infancy, or early childhood

  - Cause: maternal hypothyroidism before fetal thyroid development

  - Manifestations: mental retardation—the brain requires thyroid hormone for proper development; short stature; increased weight (pituitary dwarfism)

- **Infectious agents** (TORCHeS infections) identified as teratogens which can cross the placenta

  - **T**oxoplasmosis: chorioretinitis, hydrocephalus and intracranial infection

  - **O**ther (varicella-zoster, group B streptococcus, chlamydia, gonorrhea): varied effects on fetus, not necessarily teratogenic but can cause harmful congenital infections.

  - **R**ubella: PDA, cataracts, deafness +/- blueberry muffin rash

  - **C**ytomegalovirus (CMV): unilateral hearing loss, seizures

  - **H**IV: recurrent infections, diarrhea, prevent with zidovudine in 3rd trimester

  - **He**rpes simplex (HSV): temporal lobe encephalitis

  - **S**yphilis: stillbirth/hydrops fetalis, facial abnormalities (notched teeth, saddle nose), saber shins

  - Parvovirus B19: hydrops fetalis in utero

GENETIC FACTORS IN HUMAN DISEASE

Types of Mutations

- *Missense* mutation: a base pair point mutation that affects the protein coding sequence.

- *Nonsense* mutation: causes early termination of translation by creating a stop codon. The result is a shortened, often nonfunctioning protein.

- *Frameshift* mutation: deletion or insertion of nucleotides which changes the reading frame of the mutation and often results in a nonsense mutation.

- *Pleiotropy:* Pleiotropy: when one gene affects multiple different phenotypic traits.

Genetic Anticipation and Unstable/Dynamic Mutation

Mutations not transmitted by the rules of classical Mendelian genetics:

- **Fragile X syndrome**—transmitted by "premutation" by asymptomatic individuals (unstable mutation)

- **Genetic Anticipation**: Disease onset occurs earlier in life with more severe symptoms with each successive generation. This has been shown to be related to trinucleotide repeat expansions (TREs) -- intragenetic expansions of triplet repeats in DNA which localize in an untranslated region (loss of function) or localize in the translated region (gain of function). Examples:

  - Huntington's Disease
    - CAG trinucleotide repeats on chromosome 4
    - Caudate and putamen atrophy
    - GABA deficiency in striatum
    - Symptoms: aggression, flat affect, depression/anxiety, decreased memory/concentration, psychosis
    - 4 Cs: crazy, chorea, CAG, Caudate
    - Treatment: dopamine antagonism (haloperidol)

  - Freidrich's Ataxia
    - Autosomal recessive trinucleotide repeats of GAA in the frataxin gene
    - Impaired mitochondrial function
    - Degradation of posterior columns and spinocerebellar tracts causing loss of position and vibration sense
    - Symptoms: unsteady gait, falls, dysarthria, hypertrophic cardiomyopathy, high plantar arch, kyphoscoliosis

  - Myotonic Dystrophy
    - Trinucleotide repeats of CTG in the DMPK gene on chromosome 19
    - Symptoms: muscle degradation, defective heart conduction, cataracts, changes in endocrine function

Chromosomal Abnormalities

Chromosomal abnormalities in which the number of chromosomes has changed are classified as *numeric abnormalities*:

- *Triploidy:* three sets of the haploid genome (69, XXX, XXY, or XYY).

- *Aneuploidy:* The number of chromosomes is increased or decreased from the normal 46, XX or 46, XY complement.

Huntington's Disease

Hunting 4 food with a CAGe—CAG repeat on chromosome 4.

4 C's = crazy, chorea, CAG, caudate

- *Monosomy:* An aneuploid condition in which a chromosome is present in only one copy, resulting in a total of 45 chromosomes (Table 4). Autosomal monosomies are almost always incompatible with survival.

- *Trisomy:* An aneuploid condition in which there is an extra copy of one chromosome, resulting in a total of 47 chromosomes (Table 5).

Abnormality	Frequency	Characteristics
Turner Syndrome (45, X)	1 in 3,000	Hypogonadism, gonadal streak (remnant tissue), no estrogen or menses, no secondary sex characteristics, webbed neck, short stature, coarctation of aorta, infertility
45,Y	Unknown	Lethal

Table 4 Monosomy-associated diseases

Abnormality	Frequency	Characteristics
Trisomy X (47,XXX)	1 in 1,200	Usually benign, sometimes sterility or mild mental retardation
Down syndrome (trisomy 21)	1 in 800	Mental retardation, cardiac malformations, close-set, slanted eyes, palmar simian creases, poor immunity
Patau Syndrome (trisomy 13)	1 in 10,000	Mental retardation, cleft lip and palate, microphthalmia, postaxial polydactyly
Edward Syndrome (trisomy 18)	1 in 6,000	Mental retardation, "rocker-bottom" feet, micrognathia

Table 5 Trisomy-associated diseases

Structural Chromosomal Abnormalities refer to deletions, translocations, and inversions of chromatid parts. For example:

Deletions

- See Prader-Willi and Angelman Syndromes below

- *Cri-du-chat ("cry of the cat") syndrome*

- *22q11 deletion syndromes*

- *Williams Syndrome*

Translocations

- *Down Syndrome:* up to 4% of Down Syndrome cases are caused by Robertsonian translocation (long arms of Chromosomes 14 and 21 are joined).

Penetrance and Variable Expressibility

- *Penetrance:* not all individuals inheriting the disease-causing allele express the disorder. Example: polydactyly, Huntington's disease.

- *Variable expressivity:* some diseases are expressed in different degrees in different individuals carrying the responsible allele. Example: osteogenesis imperfecta

Imprinting

- Also called *parent-of-origin effect*, imprinted genes are differentially expressed in offspring depending on the parent they are inherited from.

- During gametogenesis, the functional allele from one parent is inactivated via methylation. If the allele inherited from one parent is mutated, then the disease phenotype is expressed due to inactivation of the normal allele.

- Examples of imprinting are **Prader-Willi** and **Angelman syndromes**. The cytogenetic changes in both syndromes are the same: a small deletion on chromosome 15. However, inheritance of this deletion from the father results in Prader-Willi syndrome and inheritance from the mother results in Angelman syndrome (think "Pater"-Willi and Angel-"mom").

- *Prader-Willi Syndrome*: hyperphagia and obesity, mental retardation, hypotonia, behavioral problems, hypogonadism, fluent speech.

- *Angelman Syndrome*: inappropriate laughter, hypotonia, and ataxia: *"Happy Puppet."* Also, mental retardation, seizures, microcephaly, and complete absence of speech.

Mosaicism

This phenomenon occurs *when different cells in the body have different genotypes* or even different numbers of chromosomes. Usually, the mosaicism is due to one normal and one abnormal cell line. This can occur, for example, due to mitotic errors in the very early stages in embyogenesis, leading to genetic abnormalities in the abnormal cell line that are not present in either parent. An important clinical example of this is mosaic trisomy 21. It is estimated that 1–2% of individuals suffering from Down syndrome are mosaics. Mosaic Turner syndrome (45, X) and trisomies 8, 13, and 18 are also possible.

Multifactorial Diseases

Unlike single gene disorders, most human diseases are caused by a combination of genetic and environmental factors. New genomic technologies are increasing our understanding of the genetics of these diseases, with numerous risk alleles being identified for a wide variety of such conditions.

- Diabetes Mellitus

  ○ **Type I (juvenile onset, insulin dependent)** is strongly linked to the major histocompatibility complex genes HLA-DR3/4 and results from autoimmune destruction of pancreatic islet cells.

Imprinting

"Pater"-Willi (paternal) and Angel-"mom" (maternal) Syndromes are caused by a deletion at the same locus.

Epigenetic modifications inhibit expression of the healthy allele on the chromosome from the other parent, causing the two different syndromes.

However, monozygotic twin studies (50% concordance rates) also indicate that environmental causes also play a role.

- ○ **Type II (adult onset, non-insulin dependent)** has a near 100% concordance rate in monozygous twin studies. The strong genetic predisposition is tempered by environmental factors, such as obesity, which can accelerate the disease manifestations. Hence, controlling obesity can help prevent type II diabetes even if an individual is predisposed.

- **Coronary Artery Disease** has a 65% concordance rate among monozygotic twins. Genetic predisposition is particularly important in patients with premature coronary artery disease (defined as angina or heart attack before age 45 in men and 55 in women). Low-density lipoprotein–receptor gene mutations, as in familial hyperlipidemia, can be one factor contributing to atherosclerosis and premature coronary artery disease.

- **Schizophrenia** affects about 0.5% of the U.S. population, and twin and family studies indicate a multifactorial genetic basis.

- **Bipolar disorder (formerly known as "Manic-Depressive" disorder)** affects about 1% of the population. There is a 20% risk among first-degree relatives of affected individuals. The concordance rate among monozygotic twins is 70%.

POPULATION GENETICS AND THE HARDY-WEINBERG LAW

Population genetics describes genetic variations in human populations. It has great implications regarding diagnosis and therapy of human diseases, evolution, and forensics.

Hardy-Weinberg Law

For any single DNA locus with two alleles, we can describe the frequencies of those alleles in a population by measuring it in each individual. For example:

Genotypes

AA = 60 people

Aa = 30 people

aa = 10 people

$p = f(A)$ = Allele frequency of A allele = $(60 + 60 + 30)/200 = 150/200 = 0.75$

$q = f(a)$ = Allele frequency of a allele = $(30 + 10 + 10)/200 = 50/200 = 0.25$

The sum of frequencies of all alleles at a locus must add up to 1, so $p + q = 1$. The Hardy-Weinberg Equilibrium Principle states that as long as the allele frequencies in a population are stable, the genotype frequencies can be calculated:

$f(AA) = p^2 = (0.75)^2 = 0.5625$

$f(Aa) = 2pq = 2(0.75)(0.25) = 0.375$

$f(aa) = q^2 = (0.25)^2 = 0.0625$

These quantities represent all possible frequencies in a probability distribution, and $p^2 + 2pq + q^2 = 1$.

This law has several assumptions:

- No selection for either allele at the locus

- No mutation at the locus

- No migration into or out of the population

- Mating is completely random

Hardy-Weinberg equilibrium allows us to predict the frequency of heterozygous carriers if the frequency of the disorder (mutant homozygotes) is known. For example, if it is known that the prevalence of an autosomal recessive disease is 0.5%, we can calculate that

$f(aa) = q^2 = 0.005$

Thus $q = \sqrt{(0.005)} = 0.07$

and $p = 1 - q = 0.93$

So the prevalence of heterozygous carriers in the population is $2pq = 2(0.07)(0.93) = 0.13 = 13\%$.

Note that in the case of an X-linked recessive disease with an allele on the X-chromosome occurring with frequency q in a population, the frequency of the disease in the population will be q for males (only 1 X chromosome) and q^2 for females (2 X chromosomes).

HUMAN GENETICS IN CLINICAL PRACTICE

Genetic Screening

One of the important motivations behind genetic screening is *patient management*. For example, PKU screening of newborns allows for dietary management to prevent mental retardation. Likewise, testing of pregnant women via serum quad and triple marker screening and amniocentesis (Table 6) provides the women who test positive with information so that the parents may choose to either abort the fetus or to prepare for a child with potentially severe congenital diseases.

Genetic Testing

When family history of a certain disease is present, genetic testing can inform an asymptomatic member of the family whether or not he or she carries the mutation. Hence, this form of testing can allow an individual to plan for what he or she might face and seek preventive treatment if possible. An example in which preventive treatment is not possible is Huntington's Disease, which is an autosomal dominant condition that causes dementia and early death with a variable age of onset (though the average is 40 years).

Genetic Counseling

The goal of genetic counseling is to provide families and individuals with risk assessment for a genetic disease as well as alternatives for dealing with the disease. A recurrence risk is also included in this assessment. Family history is the first step of genetic counseling, followed by clinical examinations and laboratory tests. At the very least, family history should include first-degree relatives, family ethnicity, disease history, and consanguinity information.

Prenatal Diagnosis

One of the objectives of prenatal diagnosis is to allow parents at high risk to have a normal child (Table 6). Reproductive options for high-risk parents can include adoption, in vitro fertilization, and artificial insemination. Prenatal diagnosis also gives parents options if the fetus is found to be abnormal (termination of pregnancy or preparation for the child). It is important to note, however, that prenatal diagnosis can't guarantee a normal child because many abnormalities cannot be detected. Nevertheless, prenatal diagnosis should be strongly considered if any of the following factors are present:

- Family history of a disorder that is testable

- Previous children with chromosomal abnormalities or serious birth defects

- Advanced maternal age

Diagnostic test	When performed	Risks and other comments	Detected
Ultrasonography	Throughout pregnancy	Minimal	Structural defects
Amniocentesis	At 14–18 weeks of gestation	Risk of spontaneous abortion is 1 in 200	Chromosome abnormalities, neural tube defects, select metabolic diseases
Chorionic villus sampling	At 9–12 weeks of gestation	Risk of spontaneous abortion is < 1%	Chromosome gestation abnormalities, select metabolic diseases
Cordocentesis	After 18 weeks of gestation	Risk of fetal loss is 1–2%	Chromosome abnormalities, hematologic and immune disordershia

Table 6 Prenatal diagnosis

Methods of Gene Therapy

Many methods of gene therapy are being explored.

- **Transplantation** seems to be a promising strategy for treatment of certain genetic disorders. For instance, bone marrow transplantation is one way to circumvent the immunodeficiency caused by **adenosine deaminase deficiency**.

- **Somatic gene therapy** attempts to correct the genetic defect by delivering a normal copy of the diseased gene via some vector (e.g. adenoviruses, transposons). Excessive gene expression can be blocked, for example, by small interfering RNA.

- **Targeted mutagenesis** may eventually be used to correct a genetic mutation. Whereas somatic gene therapy treats the patient only, germline therapy can correct the defect in future generations if successful.

Pharmacogenetics

An individual's genetic background can affect his or her response to medications. Genes controlling drug metabolism can have dramatic effects on therapy. **Acetylation**, for instance, is important for removal of many drugs from the body, and the rate of acetylation can affect the dosage needed for effective treatment. For example, an individual whose genes dictate a high rate of acetylation need more of a drug for treatment. In addition, there are polymorphisms for genes involved in the **cytochrome P-450 system**, which is also essential for drug metabolism. Numerous groups have specific genetic polymorphisms in the P-450 system that directly impact the clearance of certain drugs from the body. As such, these individuals have high rates of drug side effects at regular doses. Polymorphisms in the **acetaldehyde dehydrogenase gene** cause individuals of East Asian descent who lack this gene to be more susceptible to the effects of ethanol.

CHAPTER 9

HEMATOLOGY-ONCOLOGY

HEMATOLOGY

Erythropoiesis

Age	Location
1st Trimester	Yolk sack mesoderm
2nd Trimester	Mostly liver, also spleen
3rd Trimester	Bone marrow
Adulthood	Mostly axial skeleton, also proximal femur and humerus

Table 1 Erythropoeisis

Hematopoetic pleuripotent stem cells initially allocate into the myeloid line and the lymphoid line. The myeloid line gives rise to RBCs, platelets, eosinophils, basophils, neutrophils, and monocytes. The lymphoid line gives rise to B-cells and T-cells (Figure 1). RBCs begin as proerythroblasts and, with exposure to erythropoietin (EPO), proerythroblasts spits out its nucleus and becomes a reticulocyte. Reticulocytes are distinguishable from mature RBCs by their slightly blue color in a peripheral blood smear. Secretion of EPO by the juxtaglomerular apparatus of the kidney is stimulated by hypoxia, anemia, cardiopulmonary diseases, and high altitudes. The site of erythropoiesis changes throughout life (Table 1).

Blood Groups

Blood groups are generated by differences in antigens on the cell surface of RBCs. Two of the 30+ blood groups are of daily clinical importance: ABO and Rh (+ vs. –). People with blood group A express A antigens on their RBCs and have antibodies against B antigens. The inverse is true for people who are B. Thus, the universal recipient is AB+; the universal donor is O–; and persons with type O– may only receive transfusions from O– donors.

Patients with Type O blood show reduced incidence to cancer, especially pancreatic.

Hemoglobin

Normal adult hemoglobin is a tetramer of two α-globin chains and two β-globin chains. Two copies of the α-globin gene are inherited from each parent, making a total of 4 α-globin genes. We receive one copy of the β-globin gene from each parent, making a total of 2β-globin genes. Normal fetal hemoglobin can be distinguished by its two γ-chains instead of the β-chains. By 6 months of age, all of the fetal hemoglobin will be converted to adult hemoglobin.

Oxyhemoglobin Dissociation Curves

Causes of a Right shift:
"CADET, right-face!"
CO_2 **A**cid 2,3-**D**PG
(aka 2,3 BPG)
Exercise **T**emperature

The primary purpose of red blood cells is the delivery of oxygen to tissues. There are several physiologic situations that require more oxygen to be delivered, hence shifting the oxyhemoglobin dissociation curve to the RIGHT. On the other hand, when less oxygen is delivered, the oxyhemoglobin dissociation curve will shift to the LEFT. Think **L**eft = **L**ess O_2 (Figure 1).

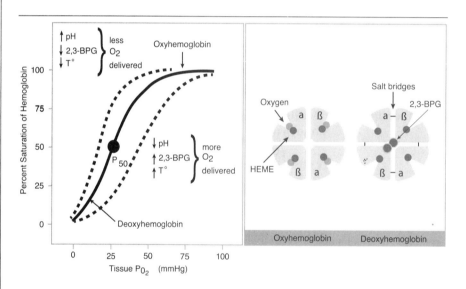

Figure 1 Oxyhemoglobin dissociation

RED CELL DISORDERS

Red cell disorders can be divided into two simple categories. Red cells can have too little functionality due to defective red blood cells or not having enough red blood cells. Let us start with too few red cells, otherwise known as anemia.

Anemia is defined as a deficiency in RBCs or hemoglobin. Anemic patients classically present with weakness, fatigue, and dyspnea on exertion. Red cell disorders often occur in three general situations:

- Decreased RBC production occurs in setting of iron, vitamin B_{12}, and folate deficiencies, as well as anemia of chronic disease (ACD).

- Increased RBC destruction occurs in hemolytic anemias and other genetic abnormalities.

- Blood loss occurs in young women, commonly due to menstrual blood loss. In older women and men, gastrointestinal (GI) tract blood loss is often suspected.

Laboratory Evaluation

In clinical practice, the following parameters are routinely evaluated:

Parameter	Unit	Clinical Utility	Note
Hemoglobin (Hgb)	gm/dL	Is this patient anemic?	Can be used as a validity check.
Hematocrit (Hct)	%	An alternative to Hgb. Can be used to verify the accuracy of the Hgb value.	Hct should be roughly 3x the Hgb.
Mean corpuscular volume (MCV)	femtoliters	Is this anemia macrocytic or microcytic?	< 80 = microcytic > 100 = macrocytic May appear falsely normal if there are equal sizes of large and small cells.
Mean corpuscular hemoglobin concentration (MCHC)	gm/dL	How much hemoglobin is in each RBC?	—
Red cell distribution width (RDW)	—	How much variability is there in the size of red cells relative to the mean size?	Can be used in conjunction with MCV to determine if there is a mixed macrocytic and microcytic anemia.

Table 2 Clinical parameters

The most important values to interpret when evaluating a patient with anemia are the Hgb, MCV, RDW, and reticulocyte count. First step of anemia workup is the assessment of Hbg or Hct. If the patient has a low Hgb or Hct, he or she has an anemia of unknown etiology. Next step is to determine the MCV. MCV of less than 80 is microcytic anemia, while greater than 100 is macrocytic anemia. The reticulocyte count is a measure of erythropoesis. If there are more than > 100,000 reticulocyte cells/microliter, it suggests that there is an appropriate erythropoietic response to the anemia. If reticulocyte count is < 75,000, it indicates that there is a hypoproliferative process.

The clinical utility of the Hgb value in the setting of acute blood loss is somewhat limited because the concentration Hgb during acute hemorrhage remains same as that in the intravascular space.

Morphologic characteristics of RBCs on a peripheral blood smear are also used to determine the etiology of anemia. The table below presents descriptive terms that are commonly tested in USMLE.

Term	Definition
Poikilocytosis	Differences in RBC shape
Anisocytosis	Differences in RBC size
Spherocytosis	Lack of central pallor; seen as a congenital defect or in autoimmune hemolytic anemia
Elliptocytosis	More oval than round; seen in macrocytic anemia
Teardrop cells	May indicate bone marrow abnormalities
Acanthocytes	RBCs with spikes sticking out; seen after splenectomy or with liver disease due to lack of sequestration of abnormal cells
Target cells	With darkening in the center, rather than pallor; seen in thalassemias
Schistocytes (e.g., helmet cells, triangles)	Fragments of cells; cell damage usually caused by hemolytic anemia or prosthetic heart valves; also seen in platelet disorders)

Table 3 Descriptive terms

Acquired Anemias

Iron-Deficiency Anemia

Iron deficiency anemia is the most common cause of anemia worldwide. Aside from menstruating women, pregnant women and babies are also at increased risk of developing iron deficiency. In men, the GI tract is the primary site of blood loss in absence of traumatic injury. Duodenal crypt cells regulate iron absorption. Therefore, disruptions in duodenal absorption, such as short gut syndrome, can also result in iron deficiency anemia despite adequate intake. Furthermore, there is no method for actively excreting iron in human body and increased consumption of iron can be harmful.

Hepcidin is the major regulator of iron hemostasis. Hepcidin is produced in the liver and decreases plasma iron-transferrin complexes. Production of hepcidin is facilitated by increased inflammatory cytokines and hypoxia. The paradoxical decrease in iron carrying capacity in setting off inflammation and hypoxemia is due to the fact that bacteria thrive with iron. By decreasing iron in plasma, hepcidin plays a novel antimicrobial role in the immune system.

Hepcidin DECREASES physiologically active iron, MOA by (1) prevent absorption at the duodenum (2) decrease iron release from macrophages and hepatocytes.

Signs and Symptoms

If anemia is not severe, patients may be asymptomatic. Iron deficiency, anemia is also associated with brittle fingernails, smooth tongue, stomatitis and pica.

DIAGNOSIS

Iron deficiency anemia has the characteristic microcytic RBCs with increased central pallor on peripheral blood smear. Serum iron, transferrin saturation, and ferritin are low due to deficiency in iron. In contrast, TIBC is high because there are plenty of empty irons binding sites due to lack of iron. Bone marrow smears show no hemosiderin due to depleted iron storage.

TREATMENT

Ferrous sulfate supplementation is used to correct the anemia and rebuild iron stores. Side effects of iron supplementation include constipation and GI distress, making patient compliance an issue. Postpartum women should continue to take prenatal vitamins to restore blood losses during delivery. Breast-fed babies require iron supplementation as breast milk lacks iron.

Lead poisoning

This heavy metal causes anemia by disrupting the porphyrin aspect of heme synthesis. Specifically it blocks two steps.

1. Conversion of δ-Aminolevulinate (δ-ALA) to porphobilinogen via inhibition of δ-ALA dehydratase.

2. Conversion of protoporphyrin IX to heme via inhibition of ferrochelatase

Ferrochelatase's dependence on iron as a cofactor is why lead poisoning acts synergistically with iron deficiency. Of note blood lead level reflects recent exposure, however use of K X-ray fluorescence (KXRF) reflects cumulative exposure. For female patients contemplating children with significant cumulative exposure, 1200 mg of daily calcium supplementation has been shown in a randomized trial to decrease mobilization to the blood stream.

SIGNS AND SYMPTOMS

In adults, peripheral motor neuropathy, anemia, constipation, and abdominal pain are common. More severe cases may include nephropathy. In children, the major neurologic symptom is acute encephalopathy.

DIAGNOSIS

Primarily done by blood lead level. "Lead lines" or bands of increased density and long bone metaphysis may be seen on X-ray. Peripheral blood smear will show basophilic stippling of red cells.

TREATMENT

Primary prevention is the best strategy for addressing lead poisoning. Secondary treatment strategies include EDTA, penicillamine, and dimercaprol (British anti-lewisite aka BAL).

Sideroblastic Anemia

Sideroblastic anemia results from a defect in metabolism or synthesis of the porphyrin ring, resulting in iron accumulation in the mitochondria. Sideroblastic anemia is associated with nutritional deficiency in setting of chronic alcoholism, or toxicity from isoniazid, chloramphenicol, and cycloserine.

SIGNS AND SYMPTOMS

Sideroblastic anemia presents in a similar manner to other forms of anemia.

DIAGNOSIS

Prussian blue staining of bone marrow aspirates show large erythrocyte precursor cells with perinuclear rings of bluish green iron.

TREATMENT

Treatments include removal of the toxin and pyridoxine supplementation for alcohol related nutritional deficiencies. Transfusion of RBCs and erythropoietin may also be utilized.

Anemia of Chronic Disease (ACD)

ACD is the most common anemia in hospitalized patients and the second most common cause of anemia, overall. The mechanism of ACD is related to chronic inflammatory state secondary to (1) iron sequestration, leading to low serum iron with normal serum ferritin, (2) up-regulation of hepcidin, leading to decreased iron in plasma, and (3) down-regulation of erythropoietin.

SIGNS AND SYMPTOMS

ACD is usually asymptomatic. Patient may present with variety of symptoms secondary to his or her underlying chronic illness.

DIAGNOSIS

Anemia is usually mild. The best test for ACD is low serum ferritin.

TREATMENT

Treatment of the underlying disease is the key to ACD treatment. Iron replacement can be used judiciously as transferrin saturation > 20% is associated with increased risk of bacteremia. Erythropoietin is only approved for cancer patients undergoing myelosuppressive chemotherapy, HIV infection, and chronic renal failure.

Megaloblastic Anemias

Megaloblastic anemias develop when DNA synthesis is disrupted in the bone marrow. The most common causes of megaloblastic anemia are nutritional deficiency and medication toxicity. Vitamin B12 and folate deficiency play a key role in megaloblastic anemia. Common drugs associated with megaloblastic anemia are methotrexate, a folate antagonist, sulfasalazine, proton-pump inhibitors, metformin, and colchicine. Megaloblastic anemias are characterized by the following:

- Macrocytic cells, known as macro-ovalocytes

- Pancytopenia, due to effects on DNA of all three cell lines

- Hypersegmented neutrophils, presenting with nucleus with > 5 lobes

- Decreased reticulocyte count

Folate deficiency is the most common cause of megaloblastic anemia, as humans typically carry only a few months of folate stores. Folate is present in green, leafy vegetables, and deficiency in folate commonly occurs in chronic alcohol abusers and people with poor GI absorption, such as Crohn's patients. The hepatic stores of folate can be depleted in 3–4 months with prolonged negative folate balance. Pregnant women require folate supplementation, as folate deficiency is associated with neural tube defects.

Vitamin B_{12} deficiency develops over 3–4 years. Therefore, vitamin B_{12} deficiency is usually caused by problematic GI absorption rather than poor intake. Vitamin B_{12} binds to intrinsic factor (IF), which is produced by gastric parietal cells. The complex is then taken up by the terminal ileum. The most common cause of vitamin B_{12} deficiency is pernicious anemia, an autoimmune disorder in which patients have antibodies to IF and parietal cells, resulting in atrophic gastritis and achlorhydria. Other less common causes of vitamin B_{12} deficiency include bacterial overgrowth and infection with the fish tapeworm, Diphyllobothrium latum.

Signs and Symptoms

In addition to the anemia, folate deficiency is characterized by mouth sores and smooth, beefy red tongue. It is also common to present with "blunted mask-like facies". Vitamin B_{12} deficiency presents in a similar manner as folate deficiency. However, the key differentiation between folate and vitamin B_{12} deficiency is the association of vitamin B_{12} and neurologic defects, such as ataxia, paresthesias, loss of vibration sense, and proprioception. These neurologic symptoms may become permanent if vitamin B_{12} stores are not replenished.

Diagnosis

Serum folate level is the most useful and cost-effective initial laboratory test for folate deficiency. Serum vitamin B_{12} levels can be checked for vitamin B_{12} deficiency. For cases where serum cobalamin and folate levels are borderline, methylmalonic acid (MMA) and homocysteine levels can also be utilized. Once the diagnosis of vitamin B_{12} deficiency is made, a Schilling test can be performed to determine the etiology. First, the patient is given an intramuscular injection of high-dose vitamin B_{12} to saturate the B_{12} carrier protein, transcobalamin. Then, the patient is given an oral dose of radiolabeled B_{12}. The radiolabeled B_{12} has no available carrier proteins and is excreted by the kidney. Therefore, if the urine has low levels of B_{12}, vitamin B_{12} is not being absorbed from the gut; if there's presence of radiolabeled B_{12} in the urine, absorption is normal.

If GI absorption of vitamin B_{12} is poor, the test can be repeated with a dose of IF. If urinary excretion of vitamin B_{12} is then normal, the patient has an IF deficiency. If B_{12} urinary excretion is still low, other causes, such as bacterial overgrowth or fish tapeworm must be considered.

Treatment

Supplementation with folate or vitamin B_{12} is adequate. Folate deficiency is corrected in several weeks. Prophylaxis with folate is indicated for (1) all women who are pregnant, contemplating pregnancy, or lactating; (2) patients on methotrexate, an anti-folate metabolite, and (3) patients with hemolytic anemias or hyper-proliferative hematologic states. Depending on the cause, patients with vitamin B_{12} deficiency usually need daily, weekly, and then monthly injections to replenish stores and avoid recurrence. Prophylaxis with vitamin B_{12} is indicated for patients undergoing total gastrectomy, those with vegetarian diets, or for infants of mothers with pernicious anemia.

INHERITED DEFECTS IN RED CELL FUNCTION

Hemoglobinopathies

α-Thalassemia occurs from the deletion of one or more copies of the α-globin gene. β-Thalassemia occurs from defective β-globin chains, rather than gene deletion. Both diagnoses are made via electrophoresis.

Thalassemias

Thalas-semias	Loci Involved	Lab Abnormalities	Treatment	Comments
Alpha				
Silent carrier	Mutation/deletion of 1 α-locus	Normal Hb/Hct	No Tx necessary	—
Trait	Mutation/deletion of 2 α-loci	Mild microcytic hypo-chronic anemia	No Tx necessary	Common in African-Americans
Hb-H Disease	Mutation/deletion of 3 α-loci	Significant microcyctic, hypochronic anemia Hb electrophoresis shows HbH	Frequent PRBC transfusions splenectomy helpful	—
—	Mutation/deletion of all 4 α-loci	Fatal at birth (hydrops fetalis) or shortly after birth	—	—
Beta				
Minor	One defective β-chain	Mild microcytic hypo-chromic anemia	Usually not necessary; Not transfusion dependent	—
Major	Two defective β-chains	Severe microcytic hypo-chromic anemia, massive hepatospleno-megaly expansion, of marrow space/distor-tion of bones, elevated HbF	Frequent PRBC transfusions	Homozy-gous β-chain thalassemia, AKA Cooley's anemia. Can cause failure to thrive

Table 4 Thalassemias

Sickle Cell Anemia

Sickle cell anemia is an autosomal recessive disease due to a structural defect in the β-globin gene causing RBCs to change shape from normal biconcave discs to irregular, sickle-shaped discs. A single base change from GAG to GTG results in a change of the sixth amino acid from glutamic acid to valine. This produces hemoglobin that becomes insoluble and polymerizes in hypoxic or low pH states. Sickle cell anemia is seen predominantly in people of African descent. However, it is also prevalent in people of Middle-Eastern or Mediterranean descent.

If patients carry only one copy of the sickle gene, they have sickle cell trait and are usually asymptomatic. Those with sickle cell trait have a normal life expectancy and have a genetic advantage of being more resistant to contracting malaria.

If patients carry two copies of the sickle gene, full-blown sickle cell disease is present, which is manifested by the following:

- **Hemolytic anemia**: Sickle cell patients can present with jaundice and scleral icterus due to hemolysis of sickled RBCs. There is also an excess of unconjugated bilirubin, which leads to hyperpigmented gallstones. They may present with concomitant folate deficiency, due to high-production of RBCs and iron overload from frequent Hb breakdown.

- **Destruction of the spleen and increased risk of infection**: Spleen becomes enlarged from sickled RBCs becoming trapped in splenic vessels. Parts of the spleen can become ischemic, leading to autosplenectomy. Poor splenic function places sickle cell patients at greater risk for infection from encapsulated bacteria, such as Streptococcus pneumonia, as well as Salmonella osteomyelitis

- **Aplastic Crisis**: Aplastic crisis can be provoked by a viral infection, most notably Parvovirus B19, which can suppress the bone marrow's ability to compensate.

- **Painful sickle crisis**: Sickle crisis occur secondary to vaso-occlusion, in settings of dehydration, stress, or illness. These crises can cause excruciating bone pains. Patients can also develop dactylitis of hands and feet caused by avascular necrosis of the metacarpal and metatarsal bones. Pain crises can also manifest as acute chest syndrome, which is caused by pulmonary infarctions. Symptoms include chest pain, dyspnea, hypoxia, and may present similar to pneumonia. Chest X-ray may show pulmonary infiltrates.

DIAGNOSIS

Diagnosis is made by findings of sickle-shaped RBCs in peripheral blood smear. However, hemoglobin electrophoresis is the gold standard.

TREATMENT

There is a three-fold approach to treatment of sickle cell disease: 1) prophylaxis, 2) avoidance of stressors, and 3) symptomatic management. Prophylactically, sickle cell patients should get vaccinated against S. pneumoniae, H. influenzae, and Neisseria meningitis, due to their poor splenic sequestration of capsulated bacteria. Folic acid supplements are also recommended for the folate deficiency secondary to hemolysis as well as frequent transfusions.

Patients are also advised to maintain hydration and avoid areas of low oxygenation, such as high altitudes. Hydroxyurea have been shown to increase HbF levels, which hinders the sickling process and lead to a decreased incidence of pain crisis. Patients may require multiple blood transfusions throughout their life.

Glucose-6-Phosphate Dehydrogenase (G6PD) Deficiency

G6PD is part of the pentose phosphate pathway and used to create the reduced form of NADPH. G6PD deficiency leads to poor defense against oxidative damage. The hemoglobin in the RBCs become easily oxidized and denatures, causing it to precipitate and form **Heinz bodies**, which damage the cell membrane. The damaged cells are sequestered by the spleen, leading to hemolytic anemia. There are many different G6PD deficiency variants. Often, G6PD deficiency is X-linked and affects people of Mediterranean and African descent. Offending substances include quinine derivatives, sulfa drugs, dapsone, aspirin, isoniazid, and fava beans.

SIGNS AND SYMPTOMS

Hemolysis occurs 1–3 days after ingesting the offending substance. The patient may present with jaundice and report dark urine.

DIAGNOSIS

G6PD enzyme assay can be used for diagnosis. Spherocytes and bite cells are seen on peripheral smears. Heinz bodies may be seen on crystal violet stain.

TREATMENT

Patients must avoid the offending substances. Patients undergoing a hemolytic episode should receive hydration, supportive care, and transfusions.

Hemolytic Anemias

Hemolytic anemias can be congenital or acquired and result from three basic defects:

1. Defects in the hemoglobin and enzymes, such as G6PD deficiency

2. Defects in the RBC membrane

3. Defects in the circulating environment

Patients with hemolytic anemia may develop jaundice, scleral icterus, dark urine, and gallstones from increased serum levels of unconjugated bilirubin secondary to heme breakdown. Patients also present with splenomegaly as a result of erythrocyte sequestration. Serum LDH is elevated and free plasma haptoglobin level is low.

Hereditary Spherocytosis

Hereditary spherocytosis is an autosomal dominant disorder of cell membrane proteins, spectrin, and ankyrin. Altered RBC membranes results in dysfunctional and fragile RBC surfaces that are prone to destruction.

Signs and Symptoms

Patients are often asymptomatic. Hereditary spherocytosis can lead to hemolysis with jaundice, scleral icterus, and gallstones.

Diagnosis

In addition to a blood smear, an osmotic fragility test can be diagnostic.

TREATMENT

Splenectomy is often the last resort for hereditary spherocytosis. Patients should receive folic acid supplementation.

Pyruvate Kinase Deficiency

This enzyme defect is the second most common cause of hemolytic anemia behind spherocytosis. Most PK patients have two different heterozygous missense mutations. Like the sickle mutation, PK deficiency confers protection against malaria.

SIGNS AND SYMPTOMS

Usually presents as persistent neonatal jaundice with significant reticulocytosis. The associated anemia ranges from mild to severe. In mild cases, it is often subject to delayed diagnosis because of increased 2,3-DPG causing better oxygen delivery to tissues.

DIAGNOSIS

Blood tests for enzymatic activity of RBC pyruvate kinase.

TREATMENT

Supportive, folic acid, transfusions, and iron chelation.

Porphyrias

Porphyrias are a collection of acquired and inherited disorders caused by enzyme defects in the biosynthesis of the heme molecule and/or porphyrins. They typically present with neurological and/or dermatological abnormalities. It is suspected that the neurological symptoms are secondary to the build up of porphyria precursors. Dermatological symptoms are secondary to the buildup of porphyrins which, with exposure to light, cause the release of oxygen radicals which damage the skin.

Cutaneous Porphyria

This is the most common form of porphyrias, especially porphyria cutanea tarda, which is the most common form. This is caused by a deficiency of uroporphyrinogen decarboxylase, and causes iron overload. This disorder is usually acquired, from alcohol, estrogen, or certain drugs, but can also be inherited.

SYMPTOMS

Most common symptoms include blister formation in areas of skin with sun exposure. These blisters can range from small vesicles to fragile bullae. Areas with the blister can become scarred and hyperpigmented. Some may also develop increased hair growth on the cheeks and eyebrows.

TREATMENT

Preventative treatment includes avoiding sunlight, alcohol, or estrogens, however the mainstay of therapy is decreasing iron saturation in the blood. This may involve phlebotomy or treatment with deferoxamine.

Acute Intermittent Porphyria

This disorder is caused by a deficiency in the enzyme porphinobillinogen deaminase. It is a genetic condition that is autosomal dominant. Just as with cutaneous porphyria, drugs may exacerbate symptoms of acute intermittent porphyria. Other factors that may lead to worsening symptoms include infection and starvation.

SYMPTOMS

The most common symptom is abdominal pain, however complaints of dysuria, numbness and paresthesias, and some complaints of hallucinations or anxiety. During an acute attack, the patient's urine may be red due to the presence of porphyrins. However, unlike other porphyrias, there are no dermatological manifestations.

TREATMENT

Preventative treatment includes avoiding the inciting drug, preventing starvation, and keeping well hydrated with a high carbohydrate solution. Treatment also involves the prevention of infections. During acute attacks, hematin and heme arginate can be given. They help to decrease duration of symptoms.

Microangiopathic hemolytic anemia

Microangiopathic hemolytic anemia is due to external defects in the circulatory system. Prosthetic valves and endothelial abnormalities, such as aneurysms, can cause RBC damage from trauma. These patients develop the typical signs of hemolytic anemia. Treatment is aimed at eliminating the underlying cause and includes the use of vitamin supplements and transfusions.

Autoimmune hemolytic anemia

Autoimmune hemolytic anemia occurs when antibodies and complements bind to the RBC membrane causing erroneous self-destruction of RBCs. Autoimmune hemolytic anemia can be caused by the following:

- Warm-reacting antibodies, which cling to RBCs at warmer temperature. It is associated with 90% of autoimmune hemolytic anemias and seen in patients with systemic lupus erythematosus and malignancy. It is treated with steroids and splenectomy.

- Cold-reacting antibodies, which cling to RBC at temperatures between 0 and 5 C. Symptoms occur when the extremities become cold, resulting in vaso-occlusion and cyanosis in the fingers, toes, nose, and ears. It is treated by keeping extremities warm, in addition to steroids.

- Drug-induced hemolysis. Some drugs, such as penicillin, can act as haptens. Quinidine can form immune complexes leading to hemolysis. L-dopa can induce antibodies long after the drug has been cleared.

DIAGNOSIS

Coombs' test is used to diagnose autoimmune hemolytic anemia. It is performed by mixing complement and antibodies to human immunoglobulins with the patient's RBCs. If agglutination occurs, the test is positive.

TREATMENT

Treatment for severe cases of autoimmune hemolysis includes cytotoxic drugs and plasmapheresis.

Aplastic anemia

Aplastic anemia is a life-threatening condition characterized by bone marrow's failure to produce all hematopoietic cell lines. Aplastic anemia can be caused by:

- Drugs such as chloramphenicol, chlorpromazine, thiouracil, gold compounds, sulfonamides, and chemotherapeutic agents

- Chemicals such as solvent benzene

- Radiation

- Infections such as hepatitis C and Epstein-Barr virus

- Congenital anomalies such as fanconi's aplastic anemia, Diamond-Blackfan Syndrome, and dyskeratosis congenita

- Autoimmune disorders

- Pregnancy

SIGNS AND SYMPTOMS

Anemia causes fatigue, dyspnea, and syncope. Neutropenia results in increased infections, particularly bacterial. Thrombocytopenia causes easy bleeding, bruising, and petechiae. Fanconi's aplastic anemia is associated with other congenital anomalies, such as skeletal malformation and hyperpigmentation. Hepatosplenomegaly or lymphadenopathy is absent in aplastic anemia as there is no blood product to sequester. Presence of hepatomegaly or lymphadenopathy in setting of pancytopenia can occur in leukemia, lymphoma, or myeloid metaplasia.

DIAGNOSIS

Complete blood count (CBC) with peripheral blood smear is diagnostic. Bone marrow biopsy will reveal hypocellularity with fatty replacement.

TREATMENT

If the cause of pancytopenia is drug induced, removal of the offending agent is the first line of treatment. If severe, patients will likely require irradiation of RBCs and platelet transfusions.

Red Cell Aplasia

Unlike aplastic anemia, RBC aplasia is characterized by reticulocytopenia and normocytic anemia in the presence of normal levels of leukocytes and platelets. Causes of red cell aplasia include:

- Parvovirus B19 infection of individuals with chronic hemolytic anemia (e.g., sickle cell anemia, hereditary spherocytosis, acquired immune hemolytic anemia) or with immunodeficiency (primary or secondary to AIDS or chemotherapy)

- Transient erythroblastopenia of childhood (TEC)

- Diamond-Blackfan syndrome

- Acquired pure red cell aplasia (PRCA) in adults, associated with hematologic malignancy, autoimmune diseases, and various drugs

SIGNS AND SYMPTOMS

In addition to symptoms of anemia, patients may have symptoms of their underlying disease process. TEC is often preceded by a viral infection in children up to 4 years of age. Patients with Diamond-Blackfan syndrome may have other anomalies, such as a malformed thumb or short stature.

DIAGNOSIS

Bone marrow reveals normal myelopoiesis, normal thrombocytopoiesis, and a markedly reduced presence of erythroid precursors. Diamond-Blackfan syndrome can be differentiated from TEC by markedly elevated erythropoietin levels, macrocytic anemia presenting in the first six months of life, "i" antigen, and increased fetal hemoglobin content.

TREATMENT

Parvovirus B19-associated erythroid aplasia in patients with chronic hemolytic anemia and resolves on its own after a few days. Likewise, spontaneous recovery from TEC occurs over a few weeks, and no treatment is required other than a single RBC transfusion. Intravenous gamma globulin containing anti-B19 antibodies may be helpful in immunodeficiency-associated red cell aplasia.

Diamond-Blackfan syndrome is treated with corticosteroids, RBC transfusions, and bone marrow transplantation. Removal of possible instigating drugs, evaluation for thymoma, and treatment of underlying disease is the primary course of action for patients with PRCA. Immunosuppression with steroids may help achieve remission.

Intravascular Hemolysis vs. Extravascular Hemolysis (Sequestration)

Generally speaking, intravascular hemolysis is due cell membrane damage. There are a variety of causes including toxins, mechanical destruction (e.g., artificial heart valves). In contrast, extravascular hemolysis (sequestration) should be conceptualized as premature phagocytosis by the liver or spleen. The sequestration is triggered by abnormal shape (e.g. sickle cell disease) or abnormal inclusions (e.g., Heinz bodies seen in G6PD deficiency). Below are laboratory features of the two processes.

Hepatomegally and/or splenomegaly is a tip-off for an extravascular sequestration.

Intravascular Hemolysis	Extravascular Sequestration
Hemoglobinemia (free heme in circulation)	Spherocytes on peripheral blood smear
Hemoglobinuria (if severe)	No hemoglobinemia since no distruction of RBCs
Increased LDH	
Decreased haptoglobin	Normal LDH and haptoglobin

Table 5 Intravascular vs Exravascular Hemolysis

CYTHEMIA

Polycythemia

Polycythemia, or increase in RBCs, can occur secondary to:

- Spurious polycythemia occurs when a patient is dehydrated and the CBC looks as if the RBC count is too high. It is corrected with fluids.

- Blood doping, or induced erythrocythemia, refers to intentional transfusion of packed red blood cells or whole blood. Athletes induce erythrocythemia in order to increased oxygen-carrying capacity for greater endurance. This practice is illegal and banned by both the International Olympic Committee and the National College Athletic Association. Alternatively, athletes might use recombinant erythropoietin to increase oxygen-carrying capacity. Blood doping can result in thrombosis, infarction, and pulmonary embolism.

- Secondary polycythemia is caused by increased EPO secretion. Aside from EPO secreting renal tumors, EPO release is most seen in hypoxic conditions, such as smokers with chronic obstructive pulmonary disease and people at high altitudes. Cardiac shunting and pulmonary hypertension can also cause polycythemia.

Polycythemia Vera

Polycythemia vera is a neoplastic disorder seen in elderly patients, leading to increased number of blood cells. Polycythemia vera leads to hyper-viscosity related complications, such as stroke, pulmonary embolism, and deep vein thrombosis.

Signs and Symptoms

Signs and symptoms of polycythemia vera include headache, weakness, and dizziness. There is a characteristic generalized itching, particularly after taking a warm shower or bath. Nosebleeds and splenomegaly are common in setting off weight loss, shortness of breath, and joint problems.

Diagnosis

Diagnosis is made by CBC, which shows an elevated hematocrit with normal red blood cell morphology. Often, increased WBCs and thrombocythemia are also present. EPO level is decreased due to feedback inhibition. Arterial oxygen saturation is normal.

Treatment

Treatments for polycythemia include phlebotomy and chemotherapy. Despite treatment, 15% of polycythemia vera patients go on to develop acute myeloblastic leukemia (AML).

Myelofibrosis

Myelofibrosis is the fibrous replacement of bone marrow tissue. The cause is unknown. Fetal sites of erythropoiesis, such as liver and spleen are reactivated.

Diagnosis

On blood smear, patients have teardrop-shaped RBCs and giant platelets. Immature WBCs are also seen. Bone marrow aspirate is usually dry.

Treatment

Transfusions, splenectomy, and bone marrow transplantation.

PLATELETS

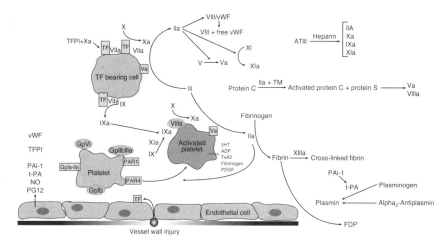

Figure 2 Normal Coagulation and Platelet Function

Overview of hemostasis. 5-HT = Serotonin; ADP = Adenosine Diphosphate; ATIII = Antithrombin III; GP = Glycoprotein; NO = Nitric Oxide; PAI-1 = Plasminogen Activator Inhibitor-1; PAR = Protease-Activated Receptor; PDGF = Platelet-Derived Growth Factor; PGI2 = Prostaglandin I2; TF = Tissue Factor; TFPI = Tissue Factor Pathway Inhibitor; t-PA = Tissue Plasminogen Activator; TxA2 = Thromboxane A2; vWF = von Willebrand Factor.

Platelet plug formation

This is the first step in primary hemostasis. Plug formation may be divided into three phases (1) adhesion, (2) activation, and (3) aggregation.

Adhesion

The key process in this step is "tethering" whereby circulating von Willebrand factor (vWF) reversibly binds to exposed collagen at the site of injury, and then to the GPIb-alpha receptor on non-activated platelets. vWF is found in 4 places.

> Collagen types I and III are the most thrombogenic mediators of platelet adhesion in the plasma matrix.

1. Free in plasma

2. The subendothelial matrix

3. Inside α-granules of platelets

4. Inside Weibel-Palade bodies of endothelial cells

GP1b-α is the only receptor on non-activated platelets that has a significant affinity for vWF.

Activation

Utilizes a tyrosine kinase signal transduction pathway to cause an influx of calcium into the cytoplasm. In turn, this increase in intracellular calcium activates platelets causing exposure of binding sites for clotting factors. The signal is then amplified via Thromboxane A2 (TxA2) and adenosine diphosphate (ADP).

The activation stage is where two important initial interactions between the coagulation cascade and platelets occurs.

1. Ca^{2+} activated platelets bind strongly to vitamin K-dependent clotting factors.

2. Thrombin (the main inducer of coagulation) is also a potent stimulator of platelets, further accelerating plug formation

Aggregation

Occurs via cross-linking of fibrinogen and glycoprotein (GP) IIB/IIIA between the surfaces of adjacent platelets.

The interactions between the platelet, complement, and coagulation systems are shown schematically below.

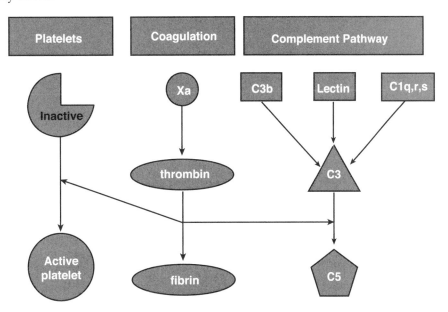

Figure 3 Platelet, complement, and coagulation systems

Test	Mechanism	Clinical Utility
CBC	Gives platelet count	Absolute count without information on function
PT/INR	Time to clot formation AFTER addition of calcium and tissue factor	Test of extrinsic pathway function
PTT	Time to clot formation AFTER adding calcium, phospholipids, and koalin	Test of intrinsic and common pathway function
Mixing Study	Mixing normal plasma with patient's plasma	If it gets better, then this suggests a factor deficiency, if PT or PTT is still prolonged, then suggests use an inhibitor
Incubated Mixing Study	Same as above, but done 1 hour after mixing	Differentiate a lupus anticoagulant from clotting factor inhibitors
Bleed Time	Test of time it takes a standard incision on the volar aspect of the arm to stop bleeding	Will almost never be the right answer

Table 6 Diagnostic modalities

Platelet Disorders

Thrombocytopenia

Thrombocytopenia is a decrease in the number of platelets. Treatment is typically aimed at the underlying cause of thrombocytopenia. Platelet transfusions are not helpful in consumptive processes and should not be given in setting of disseminated intravascular coagulation.

Idiopathic Thrombocytopenia Purpura

Idiopathic thrombocytopenia purpura (ITP) is an autoimmune disorder characterized by IgG antibodies to platelets, leading to platelet destruction. ITP in children typically has an abrupt onset after a viral infection and is self-limited.

SIGNS AND SYMPTOMS

Patients experience poor clotting due to lack of platelets, leading to nosebleeds, menorrhagia, bruising, and mucosal bleeding. Splenomegaly is seen in children.

DIAGNOSIS

Platelet counts are usually less than 10,000/ml. Platelets appear enlarged on blood smear. Platelet-associated IgG assay is often diagnostic.

TREATMENT

Steroids, splenectomy, and other immunosuppressives are used. Platelet transfusions are not helpful due to destruction of donor platelets by the IgG antibodies.

Thrombotic Thrombocytopenia Purpura

Thrombotic thrombocytopenia purpura (TTP) is a rare disease with five major characteristics:

1. Fever

2. Thrombocytopenia

3. Microangiopathic hemolytic anemia

4. Neurologic abnormalities, such as headaches and aphasia

5. Renal insufficiency

DIAGNOSIS

In addition to the characteristics presentation of TTP, patients may also present with anemia and reticulocytosis. On blood smear, schistocytes are present.

TREATMENT

Treatments of TTP include plasmapheresis and steroids. Splenectomy can be performed if plasmapheresis is ineffective. The disease course is waxing and waning with spontaneous remissions.

Hemolytic-Uremic Syndrome

Hemolytic-uremic syndrome is seen in infants and children after Salmonella, Shigella, or Escherichia coli 0157:H7 infection. It has most of the same characteristics as TTP, with concomitant diarrhea. The syndrome is usually self-limiting and requires supportive care.

Other Platelet Dysfunctions

- Glanzmann's thrombasthenia is a rare, autosomal recessive disease with abnormal platelets that are unable to aggregate due to lack of GPIIb–IIIa. Laboratory tests show normal platelet numbers and morphology. Treatment is platelet transfusions.

- Bernard-Soulier disease is a rare, autosomal recessive disease in which platelets lack receptors for von Willebrand's factor (vWF). On smear, platelets appear large. Treatment is platelet transfusions.

- Storage pool disease is an autosomal dominant disease seen primarily in women. Platelets are normal in size and shape, but have decreased d-granule content. Symptoms are usually mild and treatable with platelet transfusions.

- Aspirin and other nonsteroidal anti-inflammatory drugs affect platelets through acetylation of cyclooxygenase, a factor in platelet aggregation. Platelets become dysfunctional throughout their entire life span, leading to increased bleeding risk for approximately 10 days, until new platelets are made.

- Uremia affects platelet aggregation, although the mechanism is not well understood. Platelet transfusions are not helpful. Treatment includes dialysis and cryoprecipitate.

- Heparin induced thrombocytopenia (HIT).

Thrombocytopenia Differential	Thrombocytosis Differential
"HIT SHOCK"	"MAKE MAPS"
HIT or HUS	M yeloproliferative disorders (e.g., PRV or CML)
I TP	A cute hemorrhage
T TP or Treatment (medications)	K awasaki syndrome
S plenomegaly	E ssential thrombocytosis
H ereditary (e.g., Wiskott-Aldrich syndrome)	M alignancy
O ther causes (e.g., malignancy)	A cute or chronic inflammation
C hemotherapy	P ost operative
K asabach hemangioma	S plenectomy

Table 7 Thrombocytopenia and Thrombocytosis differentials

Coagulopathies

Hemophilia A and B

Hemophilia A is an X-linked recessive deficiency in factor VIII that affects about 1 in 10,000 males. Hemophilia B is an X-linked recessive deficiency of factor IX that is less common than hemophilia A, affecting 1 in 100,000 people.

SIGNS AND SYMPTOMS

Patients begin experiencing spontaneous bleeding shortly after birth. A newborn may have serious bleeding after circumcision. Bleeding often occurs in the joints and soft tissues but can occur anywhere, including the urinary tract, GI tract, and central nervous system.

DIAGNOSIS

Prolonged PTT is characteristic, however, definitive diagnosis is made with a factor VIII or IX assay. Bleeding time is normal, as hemophilia is a disorder of coagulation, not platelet plug formation.

TREATMENT

Treatment for hemophilia includes coagulation factor and plasma replacement. The antidiuretic hormone analogue deamino-8-D-arginine vasopressin (ddAVP) may increase factor VIII production.

von Willebrand's Disease

von Willebrand's disease is an autosomal dominant disease with deficiency of von Willebrand's Factor (vWF). vWF is needed for platelet adhesion to endothelial tissue. There is also a functional deficiency of factor VIII activity, since vWF is a carrier protein for factor VIII.

SIGNS AND SYMPTOMS

Bleeding from the skin and mucous membranes is common with easy bruising, nosebleeds, and menorrhagia. Bleeding into the joints is uncommon.

DIAGNOSIS

Bleeding time is prolonged due to poor platelet plug formation. Prolonged PTT also occurs due to the loss of factor VIII function. Factor VIII and vWF assay is diagnostic.

TREATMENT

Replacement of factor VIII and vWF.

Protein C and Protein S Deficiencies

Protein C and protein S are vitamin K–dependent proteases that degrade factors V and VIII. Deficiency of one or both of these proteins is usually autosomal dominant and increases risk of thrombotic events. Protein C and S deficient patients who are started on warfarin may experience hypercoagulability and skin necrosis.

Liver Dysfunction

The liver synthesizes all clotting factors EXCEPT for vWF and t-PA. In liver disease, PT is usually affected before PTT.

DIAGNOSIS

The first step is a good history and physical to diagnose hepatic dysfunction.

TREATMENT

Supplementation of vitamin K and fresh, frozen plasma.

PTT	PT	Both
Factor VIII, IX, XI, or XII deficiency/inhibitor	Factor VII deficiency/inhibitor	Combined Deficiency
	Vitamin K deficiency	DIC
Heparin	Liver disease	Direct thrombin inhibitor
vWF inhibitor	Warfarin	Combined heparin and warfarin use
Antiphospholipid ab		Overdose of heparin or warfarin alone
Liver disease		Liver disease

Table 8 Causes of prolonged PTT and PT

Hypercoagulable States

Antithrombin III Deficiency

Antithrombin III (ATIII) deficiency is autosomal dominant and has clinical presentation similar to patients with protein C and protein S deficiency. Thrombosis is treated with heparin with or without ATIII supplementation. Life-long warfarin therapy can be required.

Factor V Leiden

Factor V Leiden is caused by a single amino acid substitution at the activated protein C cleavage site of factor V. The amino acid substitution decreases degradation of factor V by protein C. Heterozygotes have a ten-fold greater risk of venous thrombosis, while homozygotes have a 50- to 100-fold greater risk. Factor V Leiden has a high prevalence in the Caucasian population and is the most commonly inherited hypercoagulable state.

Disseminated Intravascular Coagulation

Disseminated intravascular coagulation (DIC) occurs when the coagulation system becomes hyperactive. Increased activation of the entire clotting system occurs, resulting in microthrombi and infarction. Overconsumption of platelets and clotting factors lead to uncontrolled bleeding. The cause of DIC is multifactorial and can be secondary to obstetric complications, severe infections, and massive, traumatic injury.

SIGNS AND SYMPTOMS

Patients may experience bleeding, infarction, or both. Organs that are often affected include the kidneys, lungs, and brain. Convulsions and coma are seen in the final stages.

DIAGNOSIS

Laboratory tests show low fibrinogen, low platelets, and elevated D-dimer and other fibrin split products.

TREATMENT

Heparin is given for infarctions, and fresh frozen plasma is given for bleeding. Treatment of the underlying disease is crucial.

ONCOLOGY

Chemotherapeutics and the Cell Cycle

Broadly speaking, chemotherapy drugs are divided into non-cycle dependent and cycle dependent medications. Non-cycle dependent agents work at all points of neoplastic cell division. Cycle-dependent agents work most effectively only during certain cycles.

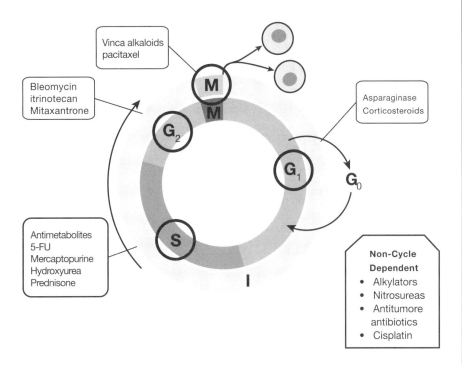

Figure 4 Chemotherapeutics and the cell cycle

LEUKEMIA

Leukemia is an abnormal proliferation of white blood cells. Generally, it is divided into an acute and chronic form, primarily effecting either the myeloid or the lymphoid cell lines. Ionizing radiation is known to increase the risk of the acute leukemias and chronic myelogenous leukemia (CML) but not CLL.

Benzene increases the risk of AML.

Symptoms

Symptoms reflect failure of hematopoetic cell lines. Patients can present with bone pain from infiltration of the periosteum and lymphadenopathy with hepatosplenomegally. Think of leukemia in patients who are HIV negative and prone to opportunistic infections.

Cell line	Signs and Symptoms	Frequency
Red cells	Anemia—lethargy, headache, heart failure	Most patients
White cells	Immune compromise—life-threatening bacterial infections	33%
Platelets	Thrombocytopenia—bleeding gums, petechiae, epistaxis, refractory hemorrhage	33%

Table 9 Leukemia symptoms

Diagnosis

WBC can be misleading since patients can have leukopenia or leukocytosis.

Parameter	Finding
HGB	Anemia in most patients
WBC	Leukocytosis in 50%; leukopenia in 25%
PLT	Mild thrombocytopenia in most; severe (< 20K) in 25%

Table 10 Leukemia diagnosis

ACUTE LYMPHOCYTIC LEUKEMIA (ALL)

Acute lymphocytic leukemia, acute lymphoblastic leukemia, and acute lymphoid leukemia are synonyms. The overwhelming majority of ALL (85%) are B-cell leukemia with a peak incidence at 4 years of age. In fact, ALL is the most common cancer in pre-adolescent children. Adults are subject to developing ALL as a result of viral infection. The two viruses associated with leukemia are type-1 of the Human T-cell lymphotropic virus (HLTLV-1) and the Epstein-Bar virus (EBV), which causes both Burkett's lymphoma and mature B-cell ALL (also known as FAB L3 or Burkitt-like ALL).

Treatment

Treatment of ALL can be divided into three phases (1) induction of remission, (2) post-remission therapy consisting of consolidation and maintenance, and (3) CNS prophylaxis. After induction, complete remission is achieved in 90% of children and almost as many adults within 1 month. Therapies are included in the table below:

Induction	Prednisone, vincristine, and L-asparaginase with daunorubicin
Consolidation	Methotrexate, cyclophosphamide, cytarabine, and others
Maintenance	Low dose, outpatient therapy with 6-mercaptopurine and methotrexate **M**aintenance = 6-**MP**, **MTX** at ho**Me**
CNS Prophy-laxis	High dose methotrexate and cytarabine; or intrathecal methotrexate and radiation

Table 11 ALL treatment

Two important subtypes to consider are mature B-cell ALL (Burkitt-like ALL) and Philadelphia chromosome (translocation 9;22) positive ALL. Both show decreased responsiveness to chemotherapy and require additional therapies that are given after the first remission.

Subtype	Additional Therapy
Mature B-cell ALL	Rituximab
Ph+ ALL	Bone marrow transplantation; imatinib mesylate (tyrosine kinase inhibitor) has shown some promise

Table 12 ALL subtype additional therapy

ACUTE MYELOGENOUS LEUKEMIA

AML is a disease of adults with mean age of diagnosis around 60 years old. AML is also known as acute non-lymphocytic leukemia. AML is distinguished from a leukemoid reaction by analyzing the number of blasts in a bone marrow sample or a peripheral blood smear. Leukemoid reactions never produce > 20% blasts.

Treatment

Chemotherapy for AML carries a very high incidence of bone marrow suppression.

Purpose	Medication
Induction	Idarubicin or high dose daunorubicin
Consolidation	High-dose daunorubicin and cytarabine if patient < 60
Maintenance	No evidence of benefit
CNS Prophylaxis	No evidence of benefit

Table 13 Acute Myelogenous Leukemia treametment

Prognostic Pearls

All of the following are associated with INCREASED survival.

High Yield

Presence of a "Philadelphia Chromosome" t(9;22), or prior EBV infection suggests B-cell lymphoma/leukemia.

t(9;22) = fusion of the ABL tyrosine kinase gene on chromosome 9 with the BCR gene on chromosome 22. With any bone marrow transplantation, a matched sibling donor is always the most optimal choice, followed by matched unrelated donor.

Both ALL and AML	ALL Specific	AML Specific
Younger age of onset	Presence of t(12;21)	Presence of t(9;21)
Low WBC count at diagnosis	Mature T-cell (vs. pre-t-cell)	Presence of inv(16)
		Absence of t(6;9)
		Absence of inv(3)
		Absence of MDR1 (multi-drug resistance gene)

Table 14 Prognostic Pearls

Note that all of the "good" chromosome abnormalities have at least one double-digit, some times bigger is better.

CHRONIC LEUKEMIAS

Chronic Lymphocytic Leukemia

CLL is the most common leukemia in United States and twice as common as CML. CLL has been linked to use of pesticides and exposure to Agent Orange.

Symptoms

Initial symptoms are nonspecific and include fatigue, loss of appetite, and unintentional weight loss. Symptoms often progress to fevers, night sweats, and opportunistic infections. Physical exam shows lymphadenopathy.

Diagnosis

The most sensitive diagnostic test is FISH, AKA fluorescence in situ hybridization. Standard cytogenetic analysis identifies only 40–50% of cases.

Chronic Myelogenous Leukemia

CML is also known as chronic myelocytic leukemia and chronic granulocytic leukemia. CML results in overproduction of the myeloid cell line.

Symptoms

Approximately half of CML patients are asymptomatic until disease is found on physical exam or routine laboratory tests. Marked splenomegaly is the most common initial presentation. Hepatomegaly is found in < 20% of patients. The hallmark of CML is its propensity to enter accelerated phase with increased blasts, increased anemia, and increase size of lymphoid organs. Accelerated phase can deteriorate into a blastic phase once > 30% blasts are seen in peripheral blood or bone marrow. Blastic phase is characterized by worsening of symptoms and a decrease in survival to about 1 year.

Diagnosis

Marked leukocytosis (10,000 to 500,000) of predominantly neutrophils and blasts in peripheral blood smear is diagnostic. CML can be distinguished from leukemoid reactions due to presence of WBC < 50,000, toxic granulocytic vacuolation, Dohle's bodies in granulocytes, no basophilia, and normal or increased LAP. Philadelphia chromosome t(9;22) is present in 90% of cases. Eosinophila and basophilia are more common in Ph-negative CML. The amount of leucocytosis is positively correlated with splenic tumor burden.

Treatment

First line therapy for CML is imatinib mesylate, a selective BCR-ABL tyrosine kinase inhibitor. More potent tyrosine kinase inhibitors may be added as needed. Treatment failure of second line medications can necessitate a bone marrow transplant.

LYMPHOMA

Lymphomas are the solid tumor equivalent of leukemias. They are divided into non-Hodgkins lymphoma and Hodgkins lymphoma.

Non-Hodgkins lymphoma

Non-Hodgkins lymphoma has many associated risk factors listed below. Non-Hodgkins lymphoma is associated with gastric mucosal associated lymphatic tissue (MALT) lymphoma and is one of the only cancers with a bacterial cause secondary to H. pylori. Other etiologies can generally be broken down as shown below:

Inherited Immune Dysfunction	Acquired Immune Disorders	Infections	Exposures
Severe combined	Solid organ transplantation	EBV	Herbicides
Common variable	AIDS	HTLV	Organic solvents
Wiskot-Aldrich	Methotrexate therapy for autoimmune disorders	HHV-8	Hair dyes
Ataxia-telangiectasia		HCV	Ultraviolet light
X-linked lymphoproliferative	Rheumatoid arthritis	Helicobacter pylori	Diet
	Systemic lupus erythematosus	Borrelia Burgdorferi	Smoking
	Sjögren's syndrome	Chlamydia psittaci	
	Hashimoto's thyroiditis	Campylobacter jejuni	

Table 15 Risk factors of Non-Hodgkins lymphoma

Adverse Effects of Bone Marrow Transplant

graft-versus-host disease

cataracts

infertility

secondary cancers

immune-mediated complications

1-yr mortality of 5-40%

Signs and Symptoms

Non-hodgkins lymphoma often presents with cervical, axillary, or inguinal lymphadenopathy. Patients may also present with symptoms of compression from mediastinal nodes, such as cough, chest pain, superior vena cava syndrome. Retroperitoneal node compression symptoms can include back pain, spinal cord compression, and renal insufficiency.

Diagnosis

t(8;14) and enlarged lymph nodes = Burkitt's lymphoma

Diagnosis of non-Hodgkin's lymphoma requires immunophenotyping. Once the diagnosis has been established, lymphoma is staged clinically by multiple factors including age, LDH levels and extranodal involvement.

Treatment (by specific type)

Subtype	Treatment
Precursor (B and T-cell)	Cytarabine and methotrexate +/- intracranial radiation
Mature B-cell	Fludarabine + rituximab
Mycosis fungoides (cutaneous T-cell)	Interferon, retinoids, monoclonal antibodies, histone deacetylase inhibitors (vorinostat, depsipeptide), the fusion toxin denileukin diftitox, and traditional cytotoxic chemotherapeutic agents
MALT	Surgery or radiation, eradication of H. pylori, rituximab
Diffuse large B-cell	CHOP + rituximab, then radiation
Burkitt's lymphoma	Specialized high-intensity regimens + rituximab

Table 16 Non-Hodgkins lymphoma treatment

Hodgkin's Lymphoma

Hodgkin's lymphoma accounts for 40% of all lymphomas and has a bimodal age distribution of younger and older adults. Patients with immune deficiency are at greater risk of developing Hodgkin's lymphoma.

Classic signs include painless, rubbery lymph nodes. Hodgkin's lymphoma is known for its contiguous spread from one group of lymph nodes to adjacent lymph nodes. It is also known to cause systemic symptoms, such as weight loss and night sweats.

Diagnosis is made by a lymph node biopsy revealing Reed-Sternberg cells that looks like a pair of owl eyes on the pathology slide. There are 4 types of Hodgkin's lymphoma.

Type	Demographics	Histology	Prognosis
Nodular sclerosing (60–70%)	F > M Adolescents and young adults	Fibroblastic response with collagen production around Reed-Sternberg cells	Slowly progressive and good prognosis
Mixed cellularity (20%)	No specific predominance	Plasma cells and granulocytes mixed with RS cells	Can be localized or widespread; Intermediate prognosis
Lymphocyte predominant (5–10%)	Occurs in younger individuals (< 35 years old)	Few RS cells with abundant lymphocytes (B cells)	Excellent prognosis
Lymphocyte depleted (< 1%)	Occurs in older patients	Mostly RS cells, lacking inflammatory cells	Asymptomatic and widespread involvement; Poor prognosis

Table 17 Hodgkin's lymphoma

Stage I: Single lymph node

Stage II: Two or more lymph node s on same side of diaphragm

Stage III: Lymph nodes on both sides of diaphragm

Stage IV: Involvement outside of lymphatic system

Treatment

Radiation and/or chemotherapy, depending on particular lymph nodes involved and staging

Plasma Cell Dysfunction

A neoplastic clonal proliferation of plasma cells may be malignant or non-malignant. Benign monoclonal gammopathy of undetermined significance (MGUS) requires no treatment, while multiple myeloma (MM) is a malignant disease with poor prognosis. Waldenström's macroglobulinemia involves proliferation of both lymphocytes and plasma cells.

Signs and Symptoms

MGUS is usually asymptomatic and picked upon routine laboratory studies. The major clinical symptoms of multiple myeloma are bone pain and pathologic fractures, anemia, renal failure, and amyloidosis. In contrast, Waldenström's macroglobulinemia presents with weakness, fatigue, bleeding, and recurrent infections.

Diagnosis

All varieties are diagnosed with characteristic monoclonal proteins on electrophoresis. Of note, Bence-Jones protein with monoclonal light chain is difficult to pick up on serology, but is easily seen in urine specimens. The diagnostic criteria are in the table below.

Disease	Diagnostic Criteria
MGUS	Both criteria must be met: 1. Clonal bone marrow plasma cells < 10% 2. Absence of end-organ damage (lytic bone lesions, renal failure, hypercalcemia, and anemia)
Multiple myeloma	All 3 criteria must be met: 1. Clonal bone marrow plasma cells > 10% 2. Presence of serum and/or urinary monoclonal protein 3. Evidence of end-organ damage attributable to plasma cell proliferative disorder (hypercalcemia, renal failure, anemia, or bone lesions)
Walden-ström's macroglob-ulinemia	Both criteria must be met: 1. IgM monoclonal gammopathy (regardless of the size of the M protein) 2. >10% bone marrow lymphoplasmacytic infiltration (usually intertrabecular) by small lymphocytes that exhibit plasmacytoid or plasma cell differentiation and a typical immunophenotype (surface IgM+, CD5+/–, CD10–, CD19+, CD20+, CD23–) that satisfactorily excludes other lymphoproliferative disorders, including chronic lymphocytic leukemia and mantle cell lymphoma

Table 18 Diagnosis of plasma cell dysfunction

Treatment

MGUS requires no treatment. For newly diagnosed MM, symptomatic patients can receive steroids, thalidomide, and melphalan. Bone marrow transplant can be considered for appropriate candidates after treatment with dexamethasone and lenalidomide or bortezomib. Asymptomatic MM does not require treatment. Initial therapy for Waldenström's macroglobulinemia is rituximab, an anti-CD20 monoclonal antibody.

Langerhans Cell Histiocytosis

This entity has been formerly known as histiocytosis-X, Abt-Letterer-Siwe disease, Hand-Schüller-Christian disease, and eosinophilic granuloma. The etiology is unknown, but presents broadly in two fashions—multi system disease, single-site disease.

Signs and Symptoms

In neonates, the most striking feature is skin lesions which are often mistaken for cradle cap. In children, it most frequently presents as lytic lesions of the skull bones. Multisystem disease is divided into high risk, intermediate, and low risk sites with manifestations related to which particular organ is compromised. Of note CNS disease often presents with *diabetes inspidus*.

In adults, isolated lung disease is associated with smoking. Additionally, adults have significantly more mandibular disease and significantly less skull disease.

High Risk	Intermediate Risk	Low Risk
Spleen and liver	CNS	Skin
Lung		Lymph nodes
Marrow		Endocrine
		GI

Table 19 Signs and symptoms of Langerhans cell histiocytosis

Diagnosis

Biopsy of suspected organ with staining for CD1a or CD207. Lytic lesions may be present on imaging.

Treatment

Lesions at risk for CNS involvement (bones of the face). In this setting, the purpose of treatment is to prevent *diabetes insipidus*.	Vinblastine, prednisone
Lesions of spleen, liver, marrow, lung.	Vinblastine, prednisone, 6-mercaptopurine

	ALL	AML	CLL	CML
WBC Count	50% with moderate leucocytosis; 25% with either leucopenia or extreme leucocytosis		5,000–600,000	10,000–500,000
WBC Differential	Blasts	Blasts and bone marrow fibrosis or necrosis	No shift	Neutrophilia with left shift
Lymphadenopathy	Common	Common	Present in 2/3 of patients	Uncommon
Splenomegaly	Common	Common	Less common at time of diagnosis, more common with disease progression	Marked at diagnosis
Thrombocytopenia	Mild	Mild	10%	Rare
Peak incidence	Childhood	6th Decade	Rare before age 30	Young adult

Table 20 How to differentiate among leukemias

KEY POINTS OF PHARMACOLOGY

Agent	Mechanism	Uses	Toxicity
Heparin and low molecular weight heparin	Potentiates Anti-thrombin III (AT III)	IV anticoagulant of choice; Subcutaneous pharmacoprophylaxis for DVT/PE	Thrombocytopenia
Warfarin	Blocks vitamin K dependent clotting factors (II, VII, IX, X, protein C, protein S)	Prevention of DVT/PE; prevention of embolization in patients with atrial fibrillation	Bleeding, birth defects, skin necrosis
Fondaparinux	Factor Xa inhibitor	—	—
Lepirudin, Desirudin	Direct thrombin inhibitor	—	Accumulates in patients with renal insufficiency
Argatroban	Competitive antagonist to thrombin	Anticoagulation for patients with heparin induced thrombocytopenia	Accumulates in patients with hepatic insufficiency

Table 21 Anticoagulants

Agent	Mechanism	Uses	Toxicity
Aspirin	Irreversible binding to cyclooxygenase, preventing thromboxane formation and platelet aggregation	Stroke prophylaxism, myocardial infarction prophylaxis	GI upset, peptic ulcer
Ticlopidine and Clopidogrel	Inhibition of ADP (prevents platelet aggregation)	Stroke prophylaxis, for people who can't tolerate aspirin	Neutropenia, gastrointestinal upset
Dipyrimidimole	ADP reuptake inhibitor	Thrombosis prevention in patients with heart valve replacements	Angina pectoris, EKG changes
Abciximab	Glycoprotein IIB/IIIA inhibitors	Antithrombotic agent in high risk patients undergoing coronary artery balloon angioplasty (PCTA)	Bleeding, hypertension, thrombocytopenia
Clopidogrel	Irreversible inhibitor of ADP	—	—

Table 22 Antiplatelet Agents

Agent	Mechanism	Uses	Toxicity
t-PA	Binds to fibrin and converts plasminogen to plasmin, which digests fibrin clots	Emergency treatment of coronary artery and treatment of multiple pulmonary emboli	Bleeding, downstream emboli
Streptokinase	Converts plasminogen to plasmin (derived from bacterial cultures)	Emergency treatment of coronary artery thrombosis (acute myocardial infraction), treatment of multiple pulmonary emboli and deep venous thrombosis	Bleeding, downstream emboli, fever, usually avoid giving to patients twice because antibodies may form after first administration
Urokinase	Derived from cultured, human kidney cells, converts plasminogen to plasmin	Treatment of multiple pulmonary emboli, injected for local thrombolysis	Bleeding, downstream emboli

Table 23 Thrombolytics

HISTOLOGY

Picture	Description
Figure 5	**ERYTHROCYTE**. The large red cells are erythrocytes. The smaller bluish cells are reticulocytes.
Figure 6	**NEUTROPHIL**. Multilobed nucleus with fine, light pink granules in the cytoplasm.
Figure 7	**EOSINOPHIL**. Bilobed nucleus with pink/orange granules on HandE staining.

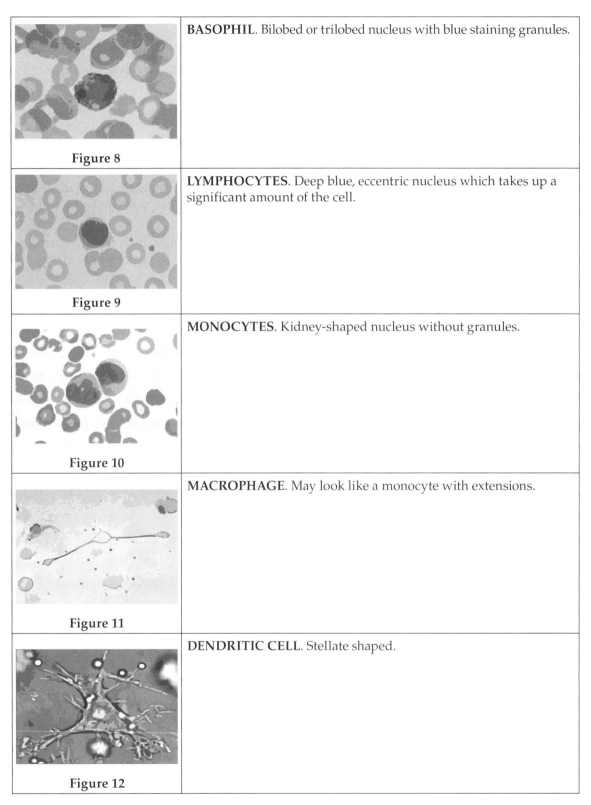

Figure 8	**BASOPHIL**. Bilobed or trilobed nucleus with blue staining granules.
Figure 9	**LYMPHOCYTES**. Deep blue, eccentric nucleus which takes up a significant amount of the cell.
Figure 10	**MONOCYTES**. Kidney-shaped nucleus without granules.
Figure 11	**MACROPHAGE**. May look like a monocyte with extensions.
Figure 12	**DENDRITIC CELL**. Stellate shaped.

Table 24 Normal Blood Constituents

Picture	Description
Figure 13	**REED-STERNBERG CELL**. Seen in Hodgkin's Disease.
Figure 14	**SICKLE CELLS**. Note the sickled shape.
Figure 15	**BASOPHILIC STIPPLING**. Seen in lead-poisoning.
Figure 16	**TARGET CELLS and SPHEROCYTES.** Target cells are named for their bulls-eye shape. They are seen in a variety of conditions including hemoglobin C disease, asplenia, liver disease, thalassemia, and iron-deficiency anemia. Spherocytes are often difficult to distinguish from regular RBCs. The key indicator is that there is no area of central palor.
Figure 17	**SCHIZOCYTES**. Also known as fragmented red cells or helmet cells. Seen in a variety of conditions including TTP, DIC, mechanical destruction of RBCs (e.g. by artificial heart valves), and severe burns.

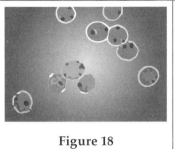 **Figure 18**	**HEINZ BODIES.** Small round cytoplasmic inclusions seen with G6PD deficiency.
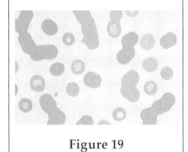 **Figure 19**	**ROULEAUX FORMATION.** Red blood cells stack like coins. Seen with a variety of conditions including diabetes mellitus, multiple myeloma, infections, and some cancers.

Table 25 Commonly tested abnormal pathology

CHAPTER 10

IMMUNOLOGY

INTRODUCTION

Immunity is the ability of the body to limit or block infections. It can be subdivided into two categories: **innate immunity** and **acquired immunity**.

- Innate immunity is non-specific and does not require prior contact with an antigen. It includes barrier defenses (skin, mucous membranes, cilia, normal microbial flora), cells (Natural Killer cells, phagocytes), and proteins (lysozymes in secretions, interferons, complement).

- Acquired immunity is specific and requires contact with foreign antigens. This can be further classified into two types, depending on whether it is B- or T-cell mediated.

Cell-mediated Immunity

Cell-mediated immunity relies on the activation of T-cells. Cell-mediated responses (e.g., delayed hypersensitivity, lymphokine production, cytotoxicity) are directed against the following:

- Viruses

- Fungi

- Parasites

- Tumors

- Organ transplants

Humoral Immunity

Humoral immunity is mediated by antibody-producing B-cells. These antibodies **opsonize** (cover) microorganisms to target them for phagocytosis and neutralize antigens by binding to bacterial and viral receptors. Humoral immunity is directed primarily against the following:

- Toxin-induced diseases, such as toxic shock syndrome

- Polysaccharide-encapsulated microorganisms, such as pneumococci

- Some viruses

Clinical uses of
preformed antibodies
(passive immunity):

Post-exposure to tetanus
& botulinum toxins,
rabies virus,
hepatitis B, RSV.

Humoral immunity can be **active**, in which the host actively produces an immune response, or **passive**, in which preformed antibodies are transferred to the host. Passive immunity can occur naturally (transplacental transfer of maternal IgG to the fetus; IgA through colostrum/breast milk) or through injections of preformed antibodies. The advantage of active immunity (i.e., vaccinations) is that resistance is long term, but the onset is slow. Passive immunity confers fast availability of antibodies, but these are short lived.

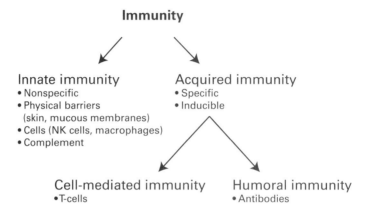

Figure 1 Overview of immunity

CELLS OF THE IMMUNE SYSTEM

All blood cells differentiate from pluripotent hematopoietic stem cells, guided by cytokines that stimulate differentiation into the **lymphoid lineage** (lymphocytes, natural killer cells) or the **myeloid lineage** (erythrocytes, platelets, granulocytes, and monocytes).

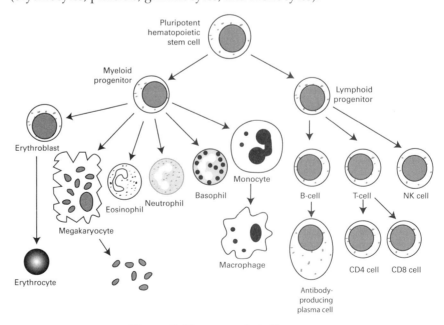

Figure 2 Hematopoietic lineages

Under the influence of colony-stimulating factors (CSF) and other cytokines, the process of differentiation takes place in the bone marrow. The resulting mature cells are released into the bloodstream in order to travel to their site of action. Notably, progenitor cells of what will eventually become T-cells are produced in the marrow; however, they must migrate to the thymus for further differentiation.

In the peripheral blood, white blood cells (WBCs or "leukocytes") make up a relatively small proportion. The absolute value of a white blood cell count is commonly between 4,500–10,000 cells/microliter. Of this, the normal WBC differential lists the following cell types from greatest to least:

- Neutrophils (40–60%)

- Lymphocytes (20–40%)

- Monocytes (2–8%)

- Eosinophils (1–4%)

- Basophils (0.5–1%)

> Neutrophils, eosinophils, and basophils are collectively known as "granulocytes" or "polymorphonuclear cells."

Cells of Innate Immunity

Granulocytes (Polymorphonuclear Leukocytes) contain abundant lysosomes and cytoplasmic granules of collagenases, proteases, nucleases, lipases, and gelatinases, which facilitate the killing of microorganisms. These cells are also referred to as *inflammatory cells* because they play important roles in inflammation and innate immunity.

- **Neutrophils** respond rapidly to chemotactic factors during acute inflammation and migrate to the site of infection. They can be activated by cytokines to phagocytize and destroy bacterial cells and other opsonized (often foreign) particles.

- **Eosinophils** leave the circulation and reside in areas exposed to the external environment, such as skin, mucosa of the bronchi and gastrointestinal (GI) tract. They express IgE receptors and bind avidly to IgE-coated particles. Eosinophils are particularly effective at destroying infectious agents, such as helminthic parasites that stimulate the production of IgE.

- **Basophils** also express high-affinity receptors for IgE. When IgE-antigen complexes are bound, the basophilic granules release heparin, histamine, platelet-activating factor, and other allergic mediators.

Monocytes (Mononuclear Phagocytes) have a single nucleus, and their primary function is phagocytosis (i.e., they engulf foreign particles). Mononuclear phagocytes first differentiate into **monocytes,** which travel through the blood and migrate into tissues to become **macrophages.**

Macrophages in specialized tissues:

Liver	Kupffer cells
Lung	Alveolar macrophages
CNS	Microglia
Connective tissue	Histiocytes

Macrophages function as the principal "scavenger cells" of the body. They have three important functions:

- Phagocytosis

- Antigen presentation

- Cytokine production

Interdigitating dendritic cells are thought to arise from marrow precursors and are related in lineage to mononuclear phagocytes. They are present in the interstitium of most organs, abundant in T-cell rich areas (lymph nodes and spleen), and scattered throughout the epidermis of the skin, where they are then called **Langerhans' cells.** Like the other mononuclear phagocytes, they are extremely efficient in presenting antigens (bacterial, viral, or other foreign particles) to CD4 T-cells through MHC class II proteins located on the membranes of dendritic cells.

Leukocyte Diapedesis and Chemotaxis

So far, we have discussed both the acute mediators of innate cellular immunity (neutrophils and other granulocytes), as well as chronic mediators (macrophages and related antigen-presenting cells). Now, it is important to understand the general mechanism behind these responses.

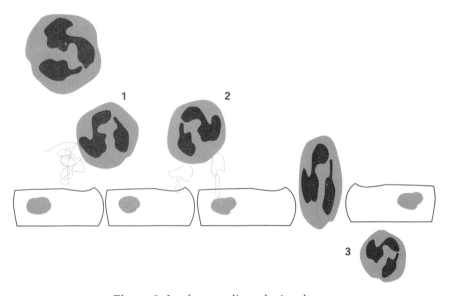

Figure 3 Leukocyte diapedesis scheme

1. **Margination and "rolling":**

   - Cells flow to the periphery of post-capillary venules.

   - Sialyl Lewis X of leukocytes interact with selectin molecules of endothelial cells.

2. **Adhesion:**

   - Cell adhesion molecules (CAMs) on endothelial cells interact with integrins of leukocytes forming a more stable association.

3. Transmigration and chemotaxis:

- After forming a tight association, contraction of endothelial cells allows leukocytes to migrate into the extravascular space.

- Leukocytes follow a trail of chemical attractants to the site of inflammation (e.g., IL-8, C5a, and LTB4)

Natural Killer (NK) cells develop from a lymphoid progenitor, but lack the specific cell surface markers of T- or B- lymphocytes. They are large granular lymphocytes that play an important role in innate immunity by killing tumor cells and virus-infected cells. They may also have an important role in recognition of "self" cells. NK cells are nonspecific, noninducible and have no immunologic memory. They kill their target cells in a manner similar to that of cytotoxic T-cells: by secreting cytotoxins such as perforins or by inducing apoptosis of target cells through FAS ligands. Unlike T-cells, however, NK cells do not require simultaneous recognition of self MHC proteins for killing. They are also able to destroy antibody-coated target cells by a process called antibody-dependent T-cellular cytotoxicity.

Development of Acquired Immunity

T-cell progenitors wander from the bone marrow to the thymus, where T-cells are produced throughout life. Tolerance and clonal deletion are processes involved in T-cell maturation, which occurs in the thymus:

- T-cells, which are capable of recognizing self MHC proteins, are allowed to continue differentiating. Others that do not recognize self MHC proteins are identified by *positive selection* and are killed.

- T-cells that react too strongly with self-proteins are identified by *negative selection* and killed by a system of clonal deletion.

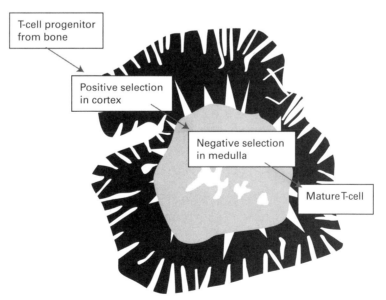

Figure 4 T-cell differentiation and thymus histology

These positive and negative clonal deletion processes produce mature T-cells that are selected for their ability to react to foreign antigens and also to interact with self MHC proteins (*human leukocyte antigen*). This requirement for double recognition is known as **MHC restriction.** T-cells must become activated by T-cell receptors (TCR).

The TCR is formed by somatic gene rearrangement to produce a diverse range of receptors, such that each T-cell has a unique receptor on its surface. Through the use of their TCRs, T-cells recognize foreign protein antigens associated with MHC molecules. Activated T-cells are capable of initiating their own replication, yielding large numbers of cells specific to a particular antigen.

Mature T-cells can be divided into two main categories based on the expression of CD4 or CD8 surface molecules. Regulatory functions, such as IL production, are mediated primarily by **helper T-cells,** which express the CD4 surface molecule. CD4 cells predominate in the thymic medulla, tonsils, and blood.

Other functions—such as the killing of virus-infected cells, tumor cells, and allografts— are carried out primarily by **cytotoxic T-cells,** which express the CD8 surface molecule. CD8 lymphocytes kill either by the release of perforins and granzymes, which poke holes in cell membranes, or by the induction of programmed cell death (apoptosis) via FAS-ligand.

B-cell progenitors mature in the bone marrow before migrating to peripheral lymphoid tissue, where they develop into antibody-producing plasma cells.

The surface receptor of a B-cell has a unique immunoglobulin (either IgM or IgD) that is able to bind different types of foreign antigens. Antigen binding stimulates B-cell proliferation and differentiation into clones of plasma cells, which synthesize and secrete antibody with the same antigenic specificity as that carried by the selected B-cell. Plasma cells secrete thousands of antibody molecules per second for a few days and then die. Some of these stimulated B-cells form memory cells, which can hibernate for long periods, but respond rapidly on re-exposure to the same antigen. That is why antibodies appear so quickly in the secondary response.

B-cells also have an important separate function as antigen-presenting cells. Processed peptide antigens bind to class I and class II histocompatibility proteins (HLAs) and are presented to the TCRs of CD8+ and CD4+ T-cells respectively.

Like T-cells, the pool of B lymphocytes also becomes tolerant to itself by clonal deletion of B-cells, which bear surface immunoglobulins reactive against self-proteins. Such self-reactive B-cells are deleted before being able to form antibody-secreting plasma cells. However, tolerance in B-cells is less complete than in T-cell—an observation supported by the finding that many autoimmune diseases are antibody mediated.

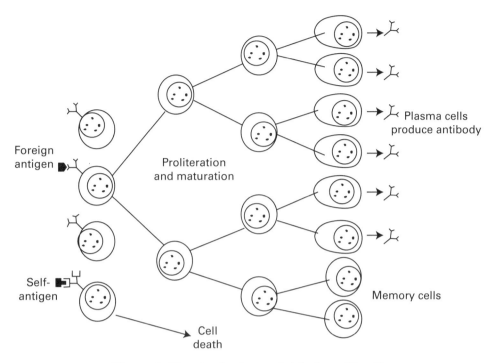

Figure 5 Clonal selection and deletion of B-cells

HUMORAL IMMUNE RESPONSE

The kinetics of humoral immunity occur in two phases: **primary** and **secondary** immune responses (Figure 7). The first encounter with an antigen initiates the primary response, which is characterized by a rise in serum IgM, and is detectable within 7–10 days. The serum antibody concentration (usually IgG) continues to rise for several weeks. At this point, the concentration declines and may drop to very low levels. In addition, there is a formation of a small clone of B-cells and plasma cells specific for the antigen.

After a second encounter with the same antigen, a rapid response occurs within 3–5 days. This rapid response is attributed to the persistence of antigen-specific **memory cells** produced during the primary response. These memory cells proliferate to form a large clone of specific B-cells and plasma cells which mediate the secondary antibody response. Antibodies produced in the secondary response display **higher avidity**, or chemical attraction, for the antigen.

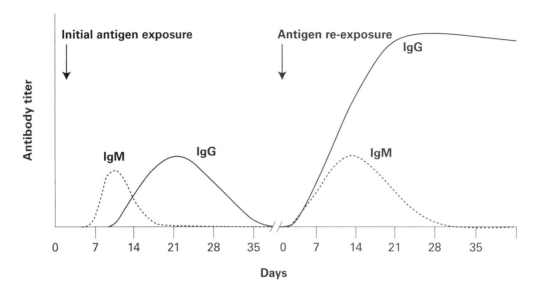

Figure 6 The humoral immune response

With each succeeding exposure to the same antigen, the antibodies tend to bind more firmly, in a process called **affinity maturation.** Affinity maturation occurs by mutations in DNA encoding the antigen-binding site. The mutations can result in stronger or weaker binding to antigen. The key is that B-cells with mutations that code for higher-affinity antibodies bind more readily to antigens and, consequently, receive more stimulation to proliferate and produce antibodies. Those with mutations that code for weaker-affinity antibodies receive less stimulation and may eventually die off.

ANTIGENICITY AND IMMUNOGENICITY

Antigens are molecules that react with antibodies, whereas **immunogens** are molecules that induce an immune response. Immunogenic substances are always antigenic, whereas antigenic substances are not necessarily immunogenic. The principal immunogens are proteins and polysaccharides. **Immunogenicity** of a molecule is determined by:

- Foreignness (nonself)

- Molecular size (most potent immunogens are large proteins)

- Chemical structural complexity (a minimum amount is needed)

- Number of epitopes (described below)

- Administration (dosage, route, timing)

Adjuvants are chemically unrelated to immunogens but can stimulate immunoreactive cells and enhance the immune response to a given antigen. Pertussis toxin, for example, acts as an adjuvant for tetanus and diphtheria toxoids in the DTP vaccine.

Epitopes are antigenic determinant sites. They are small chemical groups on the antigen molecule that can react with an antibody. An antigen can have one or more epitopes but usually has many.

Haptens are nonprotein, antigenic molecules that may become immunogenic only when coupled with a carrier protein. They are usually small molecules containing a limited number of epitopes. Many drugs, such as penicillin, act as haptens.

Idiotopes are the antigen binding areas formed by the hypervariable regions of an antibody molecule. This distinguishes immunoglobulins synthesized from each clone of B lymphocytes. The collection of idiotopes on a given immunoglobulin constitutes the **idiotype** of the antibody. An **anti-idiotype** antibody reacts only with the hypervariable region of the specific immunoglobulin that induced it. Idiotype vaccines comprise antibodies that mimic antigens—that is, the antigen and the anti-idiotype have similar shapes. These vaccines induce immunity specific to the antigens they mimic.

Immunoglobulins, or antibodies, are glycoproteins produced by B-cells. They consist of two light (L) polypeptide chains linked by disulfide bonds to two heavy (H) polypeptide chains (Figure 7). Light and heavy chains are subdivided into **variable** and **constant** regions. The variable regions are responsible for antigen binding, whereas the constant regions are responsible for biological functions, such as complement activation and binding to cell surface receptors. DNA re-arrangement and RNA splicing of variable and constant gene segments produce the large number of different immunoglobulin molecules.

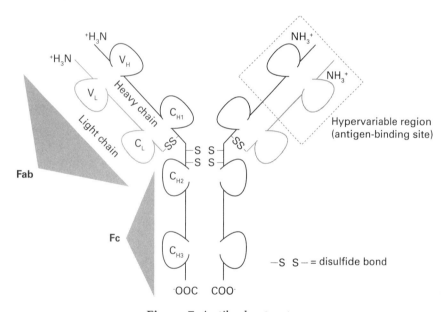

Figure 7 Antibody structure

Monoclonal antibodies are antibodies that arise from a clone of cells, which originated from a single cell. A laboratory trick for making practically unlimited quantities of a monoclonal antibody involves fusing a myeloma cell (an immortal B-cell) with the antibody-producing cell to produce a "hybridoma."

Antibodies are remarkably specific, thanks to **hypervariable regions** in both the light and heavy chains. The hypervariable regions form the antigen-binding site. The Y-shaped antibody can be cleaved below the branch-point so that the V-fork forms the **Fab fragment,** which carries the antigen-binding sites ("ab" stands for antigen-binding). The remaining vertical portion forms the **Fc fragment,** which is involved in placental transfer, complement fixation, attachment sites for various cells, and other biological activities ("c" stands for constant region). Antibody diversity depends on:

- Multiple gene segments

- Rearrangement of DNA into different sequences

- Combining of different L and H chains

- Mutations required for affinity maturation

Figure 8 summarizes the process in the context of B-cell development.

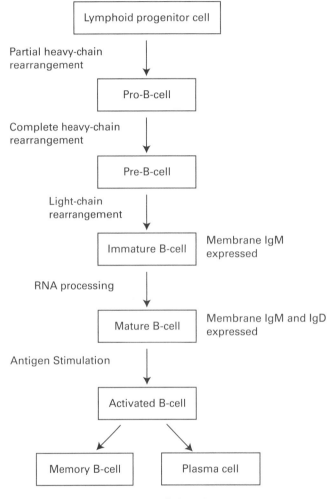

Figure 8 B-cell development

IMMUNOGLOBULINS

There are five major classes, or **isotypes,** of immunoglobulins: IgG, IgE, IgM, IgA, and IgD (Figure 9). The constant region of the H chain determines the isotype. All B-cells initially carry the IgM isotype. When exposed to their specific antigen, they first produce more IgM antibody. Later, gene re-arrangement permits antibody formation of the same antigenic specificity but of different immunoglobulin classes in a phenomenon called **isotype (class) switching.** The same heavy-chain variable region can have different heavy-chain constant regions cut and pasted onto it, so that the immunoglobulins produced later (IgG, IgA, or IgE) are specific for the same antigen as the original IgM but have different biological characteristics.

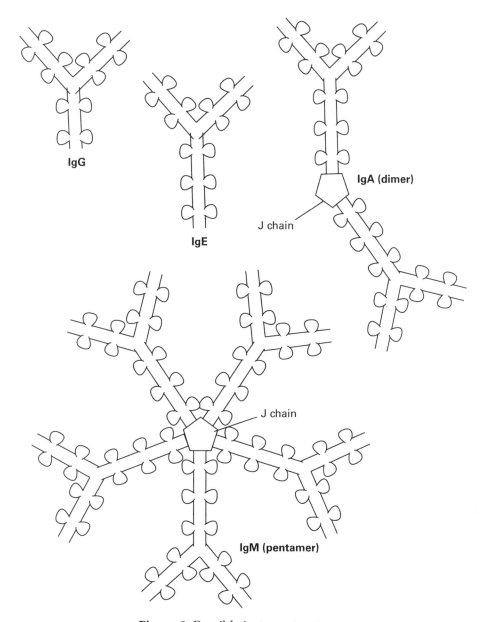

Figure 9 Possible isotype structures

Isotype-switching to IgD can occur through splicing on the mRNA level, without requiring DNA re-arrangement. Isotype-switching to IgG, IgA, or IgE, however, requires a DNA splicing event that permanently removes the section coding for the IgM constant region, thus preventing the cell from ever being able to make IgM again.

Immunoglobulin G

IgG comprises approximately 85% of the serum immunoglobulin in adults and has a major role in the secondary humoral immune response. IgG fixes complement, neutralizes bacterial toxins and viruses, and can opsonize bacteria. IgG is the only antibody able to **cross the placenta** and, therefore, is the most abundant immunoglobulin in newborns.

Immunoglobulin A

IgA comprises 5–15% of the serum antibody pool. In addition to two heavy and two light chains, IgA has a J chain and a secretory component that enables passage to the mucosal surface, where the immunoglobulin dimer is **secreted by mucous membranes.** IgA is present mainly in secretions—such as saliva, tears, and colostrum—and in respiratory, intestinal, and genital tract secretions.

Immunoglobulin M

IgM comprises 5–10% of the antibodies produced by B-cells. It is present in monomeric form on the surface of B-cells and has a major role in the primary humoral immune response. In the serum, it takes the form of a **pentamer,** composed of two heavy and two light chains, plus a J chain. The IgM pentamer is the most efficient immunoglobulin in **agglutination** and **complement fixation.** IgM is also the major antibody produced by the fetus.

Immunoglobulin D

IgD has no known function. It is present in small amounts in the serum and on the surface of B-cells. IgD and IgE together comprise less than 1% of the total serum immunoglobulins.

Immunoglobulin E

IgE is present in trace amounts in the serum, but its level becomes elevated in response to infection with certain parasites and in immediate **hypersensitivity** reactions. The Fc portion of IgE binds to mast-cells and basophils. After cross-linking with an antigen (known as an **allergen**), these cells degranulate and release mediators, causing allergic responses.

ERYTHROCYTE ANTIGENS

All human red blood cells express antigens that vary among individual members of a species. **ABO** and the **Rh (Rhesus)** blood group antigens are the two most important erythrocyte antigen systems.

ABO

The **ABO system** is the basis for blood typing and transfusions. It is based on a glycosphingolipid on the surface of RBCs. Everyone synthesizes the O antigen, which is a sphingolipid attached to a common core glycan. A single genetic locus encoding glycosyltransferase enzymes determines ABO blood type. People with type A and type B blood express enzymes that attach an additional sugar residue—an additional N-acetylgalactosamine on A cells and an additional galactose on B-cells—to the O antigen. People with type O blood lack that enzymatic activity and express only the basic O antigen scaffold on their RBCs.

Erythrocytes are typed for their surface antigens, and all blood for transfusions is matched. This is because individuals produce IgM antibodies against whichever ABO antigens they do not express (probably because gut flora bear similar antigens that sensitize the immune system). Thus, anti-A is carried by group B individuals, anti-B is carried by group A individuals, and anti-A and anti-B are carried by group O individuals (Table 1). As you can imagine, **transfusion reactions** result when incompatible donor red blood cells are transfused, in which immune complexes are formed causing red blood cells to agglutinate.

Individuals with blood group O have no A or B antigens on their red cells and are termed **universal donors** because they can donate blood to all recipients. No one should make antibodies against the O antigen on the transfused RBCs. Donor type O blood does contain anti-A and anti-B antibodies, but a clinically detectable reaction does not occur in the type A or type B recipient because the donor antibody is rapidly diluted below a significant concentration. Individuals with group AB blood have neither anti-A nor anti-B antibodies, and thus, are known as **universal recipients**. Red blood cells containing any of the ABO antigens may be transfused to them without inducing a hemolytic transfusion reaction.

Blood type	Antigen on surface of RBC	Antibody in serum	Reaction with type A donor	Reaction with type B donor	Reaction with type AB donor	Reaction with type O donor
A	A	Anti-B	Normal	Agglutination	Agglutination	Normal
B	B	Anti-A	Agglutination	Normal	Agglutination	Normal
AB	AB	No antibody	Normal	Normal	Normal	Normal
O	No antigens	Anti-A and anti-B	Agglutination	Agglutination	Agglutination	Normal

RBC = red blood cell

Table 1 ABO blood group

Rh Factor

The Rh system is complex, and not all of the Rh alloantigens have been characterized biochemically. The **RhD antigen**, expressed on the erythrocytes of approximately 85% of the human population, is the one of most clinical concern. Unlike the ABO system, anti-Rh antibodies do not occur naturally in the serum. If a RhD– individual is transfused with RhD+ blood, or if a RhD– female has a RhD+ fetus (the D gene being inherited from the father), the RhD antigen stimulates the development of anti-RhD antibodies, which can lead to severe reactions with further transfusions of RhD+ blood. This occurs most often when RhD+ erythrocytes of the fetus leak into the maternal circulation during delivery of an RhD+ child. Subsequent RhD+ pregnancies are likely to be affected by the mother's anti-RhD IgG antibody crossing the placenta and attacking the fetus's RBCs, which can result in hemolytic disease of the newborn (erythroblastosis fetalis). Erythroblastosis fetalis can be prevented by administering high doses of anti-RhD antibodies (Rhogam) to the RhD– mother immediately on delivery of her first RhD+ child. These antibodies bind to contaminating RhD+ fetal erythrocytes and prevent the mother from producing her own antibodies (Figure 10).

Anti-RhD Ab's are IgG and therefore cross the placenta.

Anti-ABO Abs are IgM and cannot cross the placenta. In fact, these may be protective in cases where the fetus is both ABO and Rh incompatible with the mother.

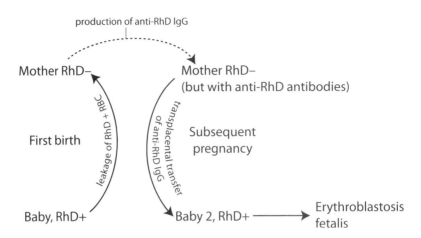

Figure 10 Antibody feedback mechanisms in hemolytic disease of the newborn

Transfusion Reactions

Transfusion refers to the transplantation of circulating blood cells or plasma from one individual to another. **Transfusion reactions** may occur if there are differences between the antigens of the donor and the recipient. Antigens, such as the ABO blood group antigens, which cause an immune response if injected into a genetically dissimilar member of the same species, are called **isoantigens**. Transfusion reactions due to ABO incompatibility result in antigen-antibody binding, complement-dependent lysis of the foreign red blood cells, and anaphylaxis. Symptoms include fever, back pain, nausea, and hypotension.

T-CELL ACTIVATION AND CELL-MEDIATED RESPONSE

Major Histocompatibility Complex

The **major histocompatibility complex (MHC)** is key in the development of acquired immunity. The principal products of the MHC are the **human leukocyte antigens (HLAs)**, which are glycoproteins found on the surface of most T-cells of the body. T-lymphocytes recognize foreign polypeptide antigens only when they are stuck to a HLA of a self-antigen presenting cell (e.g., macrophage)—a phenomenon known as **MHC restriction.**

The human MHC locus is on the short arm of chromosome 6. There are three genes at the class I locus (HLA-A, -B, -C) and three genes at the class II locus (HLA-DP, -DQ, -DR). Between the class I and class II gene loci is a third locus, called class III, which contains genes for complement components and cytokines expressed during severe illness. The HLA genes are **codominantly** expressed. Therefore, each cell expresses genes from both the paternal and the maternal chromosomes, leading to a maximum of six different class I and at least six different class II proteins. (Because class II proteins are made of separate "a" and "b" chains, and because

HLA Associations

DR3, B8	Myasthenia Gravis, Graves disease
DR3, DR4	Type I DM
DR4, DR1	Rheumatoid arthritis
DR2, DR3	SLE
DR3	Sjögren's syndrome

a maternal "a" chain in some cases could pair with a paternal "b" chain and vice versa, the number of MHC class II proteins is probably greater.) The combination of HLA genes inherited from each parent is known as a **HLA haplotype.** There are different alleles of the class I and II genes in the population, which encode unique HLA molecules that can bind just about any antigen. The HLA system then helps to present these antigens to the T-cell receptor (TCR). Transplant donors and recipients must be matched for their HLA antigens to avoid cell-mediated rejection, which is caused by the recipients' T-cells' recognition of the donors' HLA antigens as foreign. Some HLA molecules are strongly associated with certain autoimmune diseases. CD8 T-cells are HLA class I restricted, and CD4 T-cells are HLA class II restricted. (Figure 11)

Class I Major Histocompatibility Complex

Class I molecules consist of a heavy chain covalently linked to b2-microglobulin. Class I HLA molecules are expressed on the surface of all nucleated cells (i.e., all cells except red blood cells). Endogenously derived foreign antigens (e.g., viral proteins), as well as other intracellular proteins, are processed and bind to the class I molecule within the cell. The class I antigen complex is then transported to the cell surface, where it is recognized by the TCR of CD8 T-cells.

Class II Major Histocompatibility Complex

Class II proteins consist of an a chain and a b chain. Class II HLA molecules are expressed on the surface of specialized antigen-presenting cells: macrophages, B-cells, dendritic cells in the spleen, and Langerhans cells in the skin. Foreign antigens derived from extracellular microorganisms that have been phagocytized by the antigen-presenting cell (e.g., bacterial proteins) are processed and bind to the class II molecule within the cell. The class II–antigen complex is then transported to the cell surface, where it is recognized by the TCR of CD4 T-cells.

MHC × CD = 8

MHC I × CD8 = 8

MHC II × CD4 = 8

Class I: On all nucleated cells (not RBCs)

Class II: Antigen-presenting cells (e.g., macrophages and B-cells

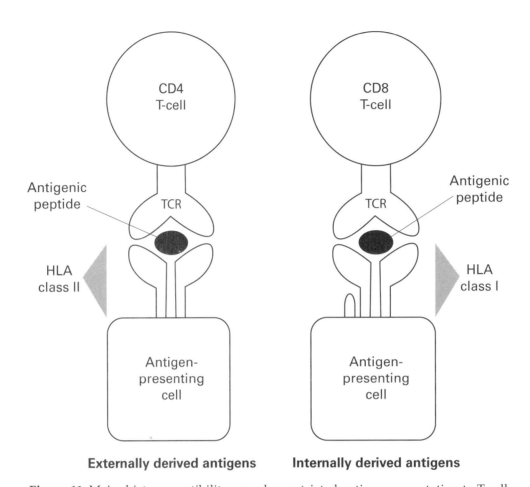

Figure 11 Major histocompatibility complex-restricted antigen presentation to T-cells

The timing of the T-cell response in cell-mediated immunity follows the same pattern as the antibody response in humoral immunity. Primary exposure to an antigen takes place through a three-part interaction between MHC of the antigen-presenting cells, T-cell receptor, and co-stimulatory molecules. The co-stimulatory molecules that act during the time of antigen presentation include the B-cell membrane protein, C7, and its receptor on T-cells, CD28. During this activation, certain factors can influence differentiation into one of two different helper cell phenotypes, Th1 or Th2, each with their own unique cytokine profile.

- **Th1** cells are implicated in initiating cell-mediated responses.

  ○ IL-2: T-cell replication and differentiation.

  ○ Interferon-gamma: stimulation of mononuclear phagocytes.

- **Th2** cells are involved in humoral immunity.

  ○ IL-4: B-cell growth and class-switching for IgE production.

  ○ IL-5: growth and activation of eosinophils.

  ○ IL-10: inhibition of Th1 differentiation and cell-mediated response.

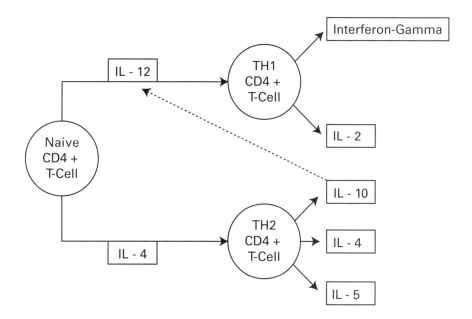

Figure 12 Regulation of CD4+ T-cell proliferation

IMMUNOLOGIC MEDIATORS

Cytokines are immune system proteins that amplify immune reactivity and coordinate antibody and T-cell immune system interactions (Table 2).

Lymphokines refer to cytokines, such as interleukins, IFN-gamma, granulocyte-macrophage colony-stimulating factor (GM-CSF), and lymphotoxin (that are produced mainly by activated T-cells and NK cells).

Monokines are produced by mononuclear phagocytes and include IL-1, TNF, IFN-a, IFN-b, and colony-stimulating factors. Adhesion molecules, which facilitate the interaction of T-cells with other cells, and signal-transducing molecules, which help activate T-cells, are classified as **accessory molecules.**

Name	Produced by	Function
Interleukin 1 (**IL-1**; lymphocyte-activating factor)	Activated mononuclear phagocytes	Similar properties to tumor necrosis factor (TNF) Immunoregulatory effects at low concentrations, activation of CD4 cells, and B-cell growth and differentiation At high systemic concentrations, causes fever, induces synthesis of acute phase plasma proteins by the liver, and initiates metabolic wasting (cachexia)

IL-2 (T-cell growth factor)	CD4+ T-cells	Major autocrine growth factor for T-cells Amount of IL-2 produced by CD4+ T-cells is a principal factor in determining the strength of an immune response Stimulates the growth of NK cells and stimulates their cytolytic function Acts on B-cells as a growth factor and a stimulus for antibody production
IL-3 (multilineage colony-stimulating factor)	CD4+ T-cells	Stimulates growth and differentiation of bone marrow stem cells
IL-4 (B-cell growth factor)	CD4+ T-cells	Regulates allergic reactions by switching B-cells to lgE synthesis and enhancing lgE production Inhibits macrophage activation and stimulates CD4+ cells
IL-5 (B-cell differentiation factor/ B-cell-stimulating factor II)	CD4+ T-cells and mast cells	Facilitates B-cell growth and differentiation Stimulates growth and activation of eosinophils
IL-6 (B-cell differentiation factor/ B-cell-stimulating factor II)	Mononuclear phagocytes, vascular endothelial cells, fibroblasts, activated T-cells, and other cells	Synthesized in response to IL-1 or TNF Serves as a growth factor for activated B-cells late in the sequence of B-cell differentiation Induces hepatocytes to synthesize acute-phrase proteins, such as fibrinogen
IL-7	Bone marrow stromal cells	Facilitates lymphoid stem cell differentiation into progenitor B-cells
IL-8 (neutrophil-activating protein 1)	Macrophages and endothelial cells	Powerful chemo-attractant for T-cells and neutrophils
IL-10	T-cells, activated B	Inhibits T-cell-mediated immune inflammation Also inhibits cytokine production and development of TH1 cells and drives the system toward a humoral immune response
IL-12	Activated monocytes and B-cells	Potent stimulator of NK cells, stimulates the differentiation of CD8+ T-cells into functionally active CTLs Regulates the balance between TH1 and TH2 cells by stimulating the differentiation of naïve CD4+ T-cells to the TH1 subset

IL-13	Produced by activated T-cells	Has a pleiotropic action on mononuclear phagocytes, neutrophils, and B-cells, which produces an anti-inflammatory response and suppresses cell-mediated immunity
Interferon g (IFN-g)	CD4+ T-cells, CD8+ T-cells, and NK cells	A potent activator of mononuclear phagocytes Facilitates differentiation of T- and B-cells, activates cascular endothelial cells and neutrophils, stimulates the cytolytic activity of NK cells, up-regulates HLA class I expression, and induces many cell types to express HLA class II molecules
TNF-a	Mainly, macrophases stimulated with bacterial endotoxin but also activated T-cells, NK cells, and other cell types	Principal mediator of the host response to gram-negative bacteria At low concentrations, it stimulates leukocytes, mononuclear phagocytes, and vascular endothelial cells At high concentrations, it induces fever, cachexia, and septic shock
TNF-b	Activated T-cells	Has similar actions to TNF-a and binds to the same cell surface receptors, although it is usually a locally acting paracrine factor and not a mediator of systemic injury Like TNF-a, a potent activator of neutrophils and an important regulator of acute inflammatory reactions
Transforming growth factor b (TGF-b)	Activated T-cells and endotoxin-activated mononuclear phagocytes	Acts as an "anticytokine," which antagonizes many responses of lymphocytes Inhibits T-cell proliferation and maturation of macrophage activation Acts on other cells, such as polymorphonuclear leukocytes and endothelial cells, to counteract the effects of proinflammatory cytokines Promotes wound healing, synthesis of collagens, bone formation, and angiogenesis
Granulocyte-macrophage colony stimulating factor (GM-CSF)	Produced by activated T-cells, activated mononuclear phagocytes, vascular endothelial cells, and fibroblasts	Promotes growth of undifferentiated hematopoietic cells and activates mature leukocytes Recombinant GM-CSF is administered clinically to promote hermatopoesis

Table 2 Cytokines

Histamine

Histamine is synthesized and stored in mast T-cells and basophils by decarboxylation of histidine. It is the principal pharmacological mediator of **immediate (type I) hypersensitivity** in humans and acts by binding to H1 or H2 receptors on target cells. Its release by degranulation causes the following:

- Vasodilation

- Increased capillary permeability

- Smooth-muscle contraction

- Increased secretion by the mucous glands of the nose and bronchial tree

Antihistamines block histamine receptor sites and inhibit the "wheal and flare" response to intradermal allergen or anti-IgE antibody.

Arachidonic Acid Metabolites

Arachidonic acid derivatives are not stored in the cell but, rather, are synthesized after antigen contact. Membrane phospholipids are broken down to release arachidonic acid—which is converted by enzyme cascades into prostaglandins, thromboxanes, and leukotrienes—by either the cyclooxygenase or lipoxygenase pathways (Figure 13).

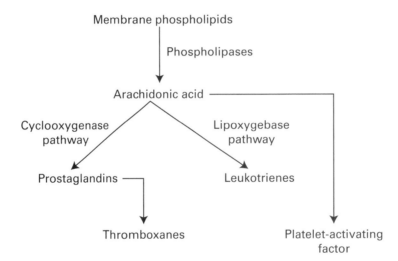

Figure 13 Arachidonic acid metabolites

Prostaglandins and Thromboxanes

Prostaglandins (PGs) and **thromboxanes** (TXs) are made from the cyclooxygenase pathway. Prostaglandins are a family of biologically active lipids that are grouped according to their five-membered ring structure. **PGD2** is released during anaphylactic reactions mediated by IgE on mast cells, producing small blood vessel dilation and constriction of bronchial and pulmonary blood vessels. PGD2 and **PGE2** prevent platelet aggregation. Thromboxanes are formed from prostaglandins PGG2 and PGH2. The term thromboxane refers to thrombus-forming potential. **TXA2** increases after injury to vessels and stimulates a primary hemostatic response. It is a potent inducer of platelet aggregation, in addition to causing vasoconstriction and smooth muscle contraction. Anti-inflammatory agents, such as aspirin, block prostaglandin and thromboxane synthesis.

Leukotrienes

Leukotrienes (LTs) are formed from arachidonic acid by the lipoxygenase pathway. The name derives from their discovery on leukocytes and their triene chemical structure. The three main mast cells–derived leukotrienes are **LTC4**, **LTD4**, and **LTE4**, which cause increased vascular permeability and smooth muscle contraction. They are the principal mediators in the bronchoconstriction of asthma and are not influenced by antihistamines.

Platelet-Activating Factor

Platelet-activating factor (PAF) forms the third class of lipid mediators (along with prostaglandins, thromboxanes, and leukotrienes). It is also produced from fatty acids released by degradation of membrane phospholipids. PAF performs the following actions:

- Accompanies anaphylactic shock

- Direct broncho-constricting actions

- Transient reduction in blood platelets

- Hypotension and vascular permeability

- *No* effects on contracting smooth muscle

- *No* chemotactic activity

Nitric Oxide

Nitric oxide (NO) is an important mediator made by macrophages in response to the presence of endotoxin, a lipopolysaccharide found in the cell wall of gram-negative bacteria. It is toxic to parasites, fungi, tumor cells, and some bacteria. An inducible form of **NO synthase** is stimulated by IFN-g and TNF to convert molecular oxygen and L-arginine to NO. In addition to its bactericidal and tumoricidal effects, release of NO causes vasodilation through the activation of guanylate cyclase. Therefore, overproduction of NO has been implicated in septic shock–induced hypotension in humans. Inhibitors of NO synthase show the most promise for clinical use to prevent the hypotension associated with septic shock.

Complement

Complement proteins are nonspecific mediators of humoral immunity that assist, or complement, the effects of other components of the immune system. The main biological functions of complement are as follows (Figure 14):

- Cell lysis

- Opsonization to promote phagocytosis

- Generation of anaphylatoxins and inflammatory mediators

- Solubilization of immune complexes

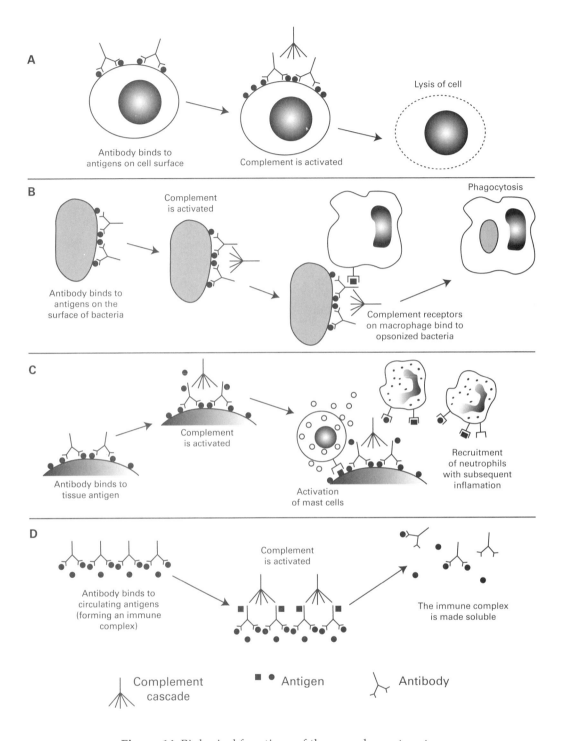

Figure 14 Biological functions of the complement system

The complement system consists of approximately 20 proteins that are present in normal human serum. Complement is synthesized mainly in the liver, although several complement components are proenzymes, which must be cleaved to form active enzymes. Activation of the complement cascade can be initiated either by antigen-antibody complexes via the **classic pathway**, or by a variety of nonimmunologic molecules, such as endotoxin, in the **alternative pathway**. Both pathways lead to the production of C3, which is the central component of the complement system. The proteolytic cleavage products of **C3** have two important functions: opsonization of bacteria and generation of **C5** convertase, the enzyme that leads to the production of the **membrane attack complex (MAC)**. The classic and alternative pathways include distinct protein components that are activated in different ways to generate the C3 convertases. The cleavage of C3 produces C3b, which binds to the C3 convertase enzymes, changing them to C5 convertases. Once C5 is cleaved, both pathways share the same terminal steps (Figure 15).

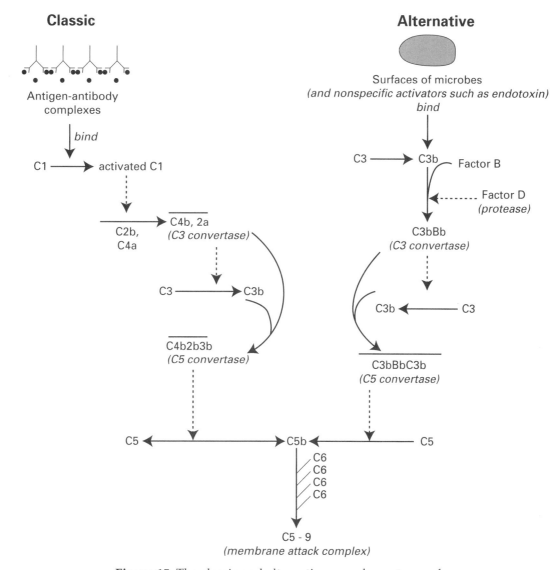

Figure 15 The classic and alternative complement cascades

Alterations in Immunologic Function

Defects in the immune system lead to immunodeficiency diseases, which can be primary (congenital) or secondary (acquired) immunodeficiencies. The principal consequences of immunodeficiency are an increased susceptibility to infections and certain cancers. Deficiencies of B-cells result predominantly in bacterial infections, particularly encapsulated organisms. T-cell defects result mostly in viral, protozoal, and fungal infections (Figure 16).

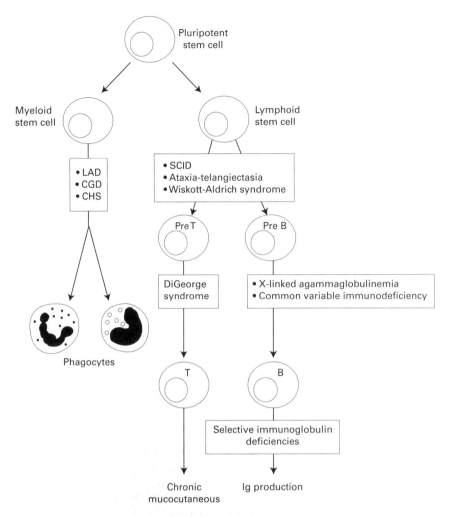

Figure 16 Immunodeficiency diseases caused by congenital defects in lymphocyte and phagocyte development (CGD = chronic granulomatous disease; CHS = Chediak-Higashi syndrome; LAD = leukocyte adhesion deficiency; SCID = severe combined immunodeficiency).

COMBINED B- AND T-CELL IMMUNODEFICIENCIES

Inheritance	Deficiency	Mechanism	Signs/Symptoms	Treatment
Severe Combined Immunodeficiency (SCID)				
X-linked recessive (Most common)	IL-2 receptor	Decreased activation of T-cells, non-functioning B-cells	Failure to thrive, death in the first 2 years of life from overwhelming infections by all types of microorganisms.	Bone marrow transplant. "Living in a bubble"
Autosomal recessive	Adenosine deaminase	Buildup of adenosine results in negative feedback of nucleotide synthesis		

Ataxia Telangiectasia				
Autosomal recessive	ATM gene mutation.	Inability to repair double-strand DNA breaks, which are required for V(D)J rearrangements in lymphocytes.	Abnormal gait, vascular malformations, increased incidence of neoplasia. Frequent mucosal infections from lack of IgA.	—
Wiskott-Aldrich Syndrome				
X-linked recessive	WASP gene mutation	Unclear: a failure of actin polymerization implicated in decreased survival of lymphocytes. Platelets also affected.	Thrombocytopenia, truncal eczema, recurrent infections (particularly of encapsulated bacteria due to lack of IgM production).	Bone marrow transplant

Table 3 Combined B- and T-cell immunodeficiencies

B-Cell Deficiencies

Inheritance	Deficiency	Mechanism	Signs/Symptoms	Treatment
Common Variable Immunodeficiency (CVID)				
Variable	~150 different subtypes	Decreased activation of B-cells and/or antibody production.	Increased susceptibility to pyogenic bacterial infections, enterovirus, and *giardia lamblia*. Presents in late childhood to early adulthood.	Intravenous immunoglobulin (IVIG)
Bruton's Agammaglobulinemia				
X-linked recessive	Btk gene	Loss of a specific tyrosine kinase responsible for differentiation of pre-B-cells to immature B-cells. Therefore absence of mature B-cells and antibodies	Recurrent bacterial infections after 6 months of age (due to disappearance of maternal IgG).	Intravenous immunoglobulin (IVIG) Avoidance of live attenuated vaccines (i.e., polio, MMR)

Selective Immunoglobulin Deficiencies				
—	—	Insufficient quantity of IgA (most common), IgG or IgM	Common in individuals of Caucasian descent. Usually asymptomatic. Associated with atopy, autoimmune disorders, respiratory, and GI infections.	*Avoid IVIG for risk of anaphylaxis.
Hyper-IgM Syndrome				
Autosomal/X-linked dominant	CD40L (T-cell membrane protein) or CD40 (receptor on B-cells)	Decreased interaction with helper T-cell results in inability for B-cells to class-switch.	Serological findings of increased IgM, decreased IgA & IgG. Increased susceptibility to *pneumocystis jirovecii*	—

Table 4 B-Cell deficiencies

T-Cell Deficiencies

Deficiency	Mechanism	Signs/Symptoms	Treatment
DiGeorge Syndrome			
Thymic aplasia Associated with 22q11 deletion	Failure of 3rd and 4th pharyngeal pouches to develop: thymus and parathyroid.	Tetany due to hypocalcemia. Impaired cell-mediated immunity and delayed-type hypersensitivity.	Fetal thymic transplant
Chronic Mucocutaneous Candidiasis			
Variable	Decreased cell-mediated immunity. Decreased expression of Th1 cytokine profile.	Increased susceptibility of skin and mucosal membranes by *Candida albicans.* May be associated with endocrine dysfunction, particularly Addison's disease.	Systemic antifungal therapy

Table 5 T-cell deficiencies

Deficiencies of Phagocytic Cells

Inheritance	Deficiency	Mechanism	Signs/Symptoms
Chronic Granulomatous Disease			
X-linked/ autosomal recessive	NADPH oxidase	Decreased intracellular microbial killing.	Increased susceptibility to catalase positive organisms, including normally nonpathogenic types (*s. epidermis*, etc).
Chédiak-Higashi Syndrome			
Autosomal recessive	Microtubule polymerization	Failure of lysosomal emptying.	Recurrent pyogenic bacterial infection, association with albinism
Leukocyte Adhesion Deficiency			
Autosomal recessive	LFA-1 integrin	Neutrophils are unable to adhere to vessel walls and extravasate to participate in acute inflammation	Recurrent bacterial and fungal infections. Associated with delayed separation of the umbilicus.

Table 6 Deficiencies of phagocytic cells

Complement Deficiencies

- Deficiencies in the early components of the classic pathway (C2 and C4) are associated with autoimmune diseases (e.g., systemic lupus erythematosus or glomerulonephritis)

- Of these, **C2 deficiency,** is the most commonly identified complement deficiency.

- **C3 deficiency** is associated with frequent, serious pyogenic bacterial infections that may be fatal.

- Patients with deficiencies in the terminal components of the complement pathway (C5, C6, C7, C8, or C9) have an increased susceptibility to infections by *Neisseria* species.

Hereditary angioedema is an autosomal dominant deficiency in **C1 inhibitor**, leading to edema in the skin and mucosa. Steroids may be helpful in increasing C1 inhibitor concentrations.

Paroxysmal nocturnal hemoglobinuria is a rare disease that causes hemoglobinuria (brownish urine), particularly upon awakening. It is caused by a defect in the ability to attach decay-accelerating factor (DAF) and CD59 to cell membranes. DAF and CD59 are molecules that protect host cells (including RBCs) from activating the alternative complement pathway. Their absence leads to complement-mediated intravascular red blood cell lysis.

Acquired Immunodeficiency

Acquired immunodeficiency is a decrease in the immune response that may occur as a result of another disease process, such as neoplasia, malnutrition, infection, or as a complication of treatment, such as chemotherapy.

Drug-induced immunosuppression is used to treat inflammatory diseases, autoimmune diseases, and to prevent allograft rejection.

- **Corticosteroids** cause selective lysis of T-cells and lymphoid precursor cells, leading to decreased antibody responsiveness, reduction in phagocytosis by macrophages, and decreased cytokine production.

- **Cyclosporin A** selectively affects CD4 helper T-cells and acts to block the IL-2–dependent growth and differentiation of T-cells.

- Other immunosuppressive drugs include metabolic toxins, such as **azathioprine** and **cyclophosphamide.** Likewise, chemotherapeutic drugs and radiation therapies administered to cancer patients are usually cytotoxic to both mature and developing leukocytes.

- Newer medications include **FK506,** which resembles cyclosporin A in its mode of action and **kanamycin,** which blocks T-cell growth in response to IL-2.

Acquired Immunodeficiency Syndrome

Acquired immunodeficiency syndrome (AIDS) is caused by the **human immunodeficiency virus (HIV).** HIV infects CD4-expressing cells, which are primarily T-helper cells, but also include macrophages, monocytes, and follicular dendritic cells in lymph nodes. CD4 cells are destroyed by the virus, which leads to loss of cell-mediated immunity and B-cell abnormalities. Patients have increased susceptibility to opportunistic infections, such as *Pneumocystis jirovecii* pneumonia, and certain tumors, such as Kaposi's sarcoma and lymphoma. Severe neurologic problems, such as dementia or neuropathy, can also arise due to HIV infection of brain monocytes and macrophages or as the result of overwhelming opportunistic infection.

The HIV genome contains the three typical retroviral genes—*gag, env,* and *pol*—that encode the core structural proteins, envelope glycoproteins, and enzymes required for viral replication, respectively. HIV enters cells via fusion of the viral envelope with the cell membrane after binding of the virion gp120 envelope protein to the CD4 protein on the target cell surface. The virus integrates into the host genome and may enter a stage of latency that can last for months or years (Figure 17). Initiation of HIV gene transcription and HIV replication appears to be stimulated by the same mechanisms, such as antigen or cytokine stimulation, that promote growth of the host T-cell. The virions assemble in the cytoplasm and are released from the cell by budding.

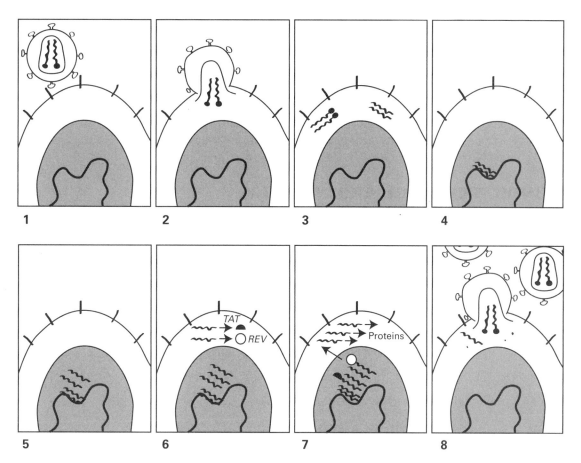

Figure 17 The life cycle of human immunodeficiency virus in CD4+ T-cells.
(**1**) Adherence of viral particle to CD4 molecule on T-cell. (**2**) Fusion of viral envelope with cell membrane; entrance of viral genome. (**3**) Copying of viral RNA in to double-stranded cDNA by reverse transcriptase. (**4**) Integration of viral cDNA into host DNA; quiescent until T-cell activation. (**5**) T-cell activation; induction of provirus transcription at a low level. (**6**) Multiple splicing of RNA transcripts; translation of early genes (TAT and REV). (**7**) Amplification of viral RNA transcription by TAT; transport of viral RNA to cytoplasm by REV. (**8**) Translation of late proteins (GAG, POL, ENV) and assemblyinto virus particles; budding from cell.

The clinical picture of HIV infection can be divided into three stages:

- The **early, acute stage** usually begins 2–4 weeks after infection and is characterized by a mononucleosis-like picture of fever, lethargy, sore throat, rashes, and generalized lymphadenopathy

- A **middle, latent stage** of several years usually follows, during which patients may be asymptomatic or may develop clinical features known as **AIDS-related complex.** The most frequent manifestations of this complex are persistent fevers, night sweats, weight loss, chronic diarrhea, and generalized lymphadenopathy.

- The **late stage** of HIV infection is AIDS, manifested by a decline in the number of CD4 cells in the peripheral blood, from a normal amount of about $1,000/ml^3$ to fewer than $400/ml^3$, and an increase in the frequency and severity of opportunistic infections.

Transmission of HIV occurs primarily by sexual contact and by transfer of infected blood. Perinatal transmission from infected mother to neonate also occurs, either at birth or, less frequently, via breast milk. Preliminary diagnosis of HIV infection is made by the detection of antibodies by enzyme-linked immunosorbent assay (ELISA) and is confirmed by Western blot analysis. Antibodies to HIV typically appear 2–3 months after infection, but polymerase chain reaction (PCR) can be used to directly detect viral presence before this time. **Protease inhibitors**, such as saquinavir and indinavir, when combined with **nucleoside analogues** (e.g., AZT) that inhibit reverse transcriptase activity, are effective in inhibiting viral replication and increasing CD4 cell counts. No human vaccine is widely available at this time.

IMMUNOLOGICALLY MEDIATED DISORDERS

Hypersensitivity

Hypersensitivity reactions result from uncontrolled immune reactions that occur after foreign antigens interact with antibodies or sensitized cells. The individual is sensitized after the first antigen contact. Subsequent contacts elicit the hypersensitivity reaction or allergic response. Hypersensitivity reactions are divided into four types:

- Types I, II, and III are antibody mediated

  - Type I reactions are mediated by IgE

  - Types II and III are mediated by IgM and IgG

- Type IV is cell mediated (T-cells and macrophages)

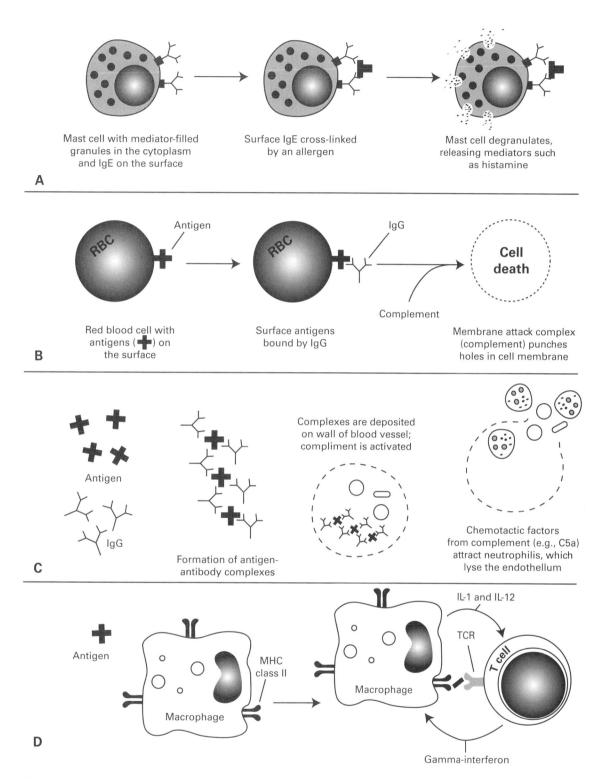

Figure 18 The four types of hypersensitivity reactions. (**A**) Type I, immediate/anaphylactic hypersensitivity. (**B**) Type II, antibody/complement-mediated cytotoxic hypersensitivity. (**C**) Type III, immune complex-mediated hypersensitivity. (**D**) Type IV, delayed hypersensitivity.

Type I: Immediate Hypersensitivity

Type I is an **immediate hypersensitivity,** or anaphylactic, reaction, which occurs within minutes after re-exposure to an antigen. Cross-linking of **antigen-bound IgE** on the surface of sensitized mast cells or basophils leads to cellular degranulation and release of pharmacologic mediators, such as histamine, prostaglandins, thromboxanes, and leukotrienes. Symptoms of anaphylaxis include erythema, urticaria (hives), asthma, rhinitis, conjunctivitis, and eczema. Injection of protein antigens, such as antitoxins or drugs (particularly antimicrobial agents, such as penicillin), can cause systemic anaphylaxis leading to severe bronchoconstriction and hypotension.

Type II: Antibody-Mediated Hypersensitivity

Antibodies against acetylcholine receptors in **myasthenia gravis** and against thyroid-stimulating hormone receptors in **Graves disease** are also examples of type II hypersensitivity reactions.

Type II hypersensitivity is induced by IgM or IgG. Antibodies bind to antigens of the cell membrane, activating complement, and leading to target-cell lysis. Notable examples include the anti–glomerular basement membrane antibody that develops in Goodpasture's syndrome and antibodies that develop during Rh incompatibility. Type II hypersensitivity can also be characterized by the following:

- NK cells, which kill target cells by antibody-dependent-cellular cytotoxicity.

- Phagocytosis of antibody-coated target-cells.

- Antibodies that cause pathologic effects by binding to functionally important cell surface molecules.

Type III: Immune Complex–Mediated Hypersensitivity

Type III hypersensitivity reactions are caused by persisting antigen-antibody immune complexes. The simultaneous presence of excess antigen and antibody (or IgG) leads to the formation of soluble immune complexes. The Arthus reaction and serum sickness are type III hypersensitivity reactions. In the tissues, the complexes deposit mainly in arteries, renal glomeruli, and the synovia of the joints, leading to complement fixation and neutrophil activation. Subsequent vasculitis, nephritis, and arthritis associate immune complexes with clinical disorders, such as glomerulonephritis, rheumatoid arthritis, and systemic lupus erythematosus.

Type IV: Delayed Hypersensitivity

Type IV is a form of hypersensitivity resulting from antigen contact with specifically sensitized T-cells and macrophages. Contact sensitivity is a type IV reaction that occurs after sensitization with simple chemicals, such as plant materials (e.g., poison ivy, poison oak), metals and topically applied drugs. The tuberculin skin test (PPD) for prior exposure to mycobacterium tuberculosis is another example of a delayed, type IV reaction. In both instances, the response is delayed and may take 24–48 hours to appear.

Summary of Hypersensitivity Reactions

Mechanism	Chronology	Signs/Symptoms	Examples	Treatment
Type I				
Cross-linking of IgE antibodies on mast cells/basophils releases histamine and other anaphylactic factors	Immediate	Erythema, hives, respiratory distress	Bee stings, food allergies, Penicillin allergy	Epinephrine, antihistamines, corticosteroids
Type II				
IgG or IgM directed toward cellular antigens. May be cytotoxic (through activation of complement/NK cells) or noncytotoxic.	Variable	Cytotoxic: loss of tissue function.	Goodpasture's syndrome, Pernicious anemia, Pemphigus vulgaris.	Corticosteroids
		Noncytotoxic: may mimic the effects of that given tissue	Graves disease	
Type III				
IgM forms complexes with soluble antigen and fall out of solution and deposit on tissues. Deposition initiates local inflammatory response.	5–12 hours	Presentation is dependent largely on the primary site of immune complex deposition Vasculitis Glomerulonephritis Arthritis.	Arthus reaction (from tetanus vaccine), Serum sickness	Corticosteroids
Type IV				
T-cells become sensitized on primary exposure to antigen. On secondary exposure, cell-mediated damage takes place.	24–48 hours	Localized rash (contact dermatitis). Loss of tissue function.	Diabetes mellitus type 1, Multiple sclerosis, PPD test, contact dermatitis (ex. poison ivy)	Corticosteroids

Table 7 Summary of hypersensitivity reactions

Transplantation

Transplantable organs include kidney, liver, heart, lung, pancreas (including pancreatic islets), intestine, and skin. Bone marrow, bone matrix, cardiac valves, and corneas are also transplanted. In most situations, donors and recipients must be matched for blood group ABO compatibility and HLA antigens to avoid graft rejection. HLA-A, -B, and -DR are the most important HLA antigens to match in transplantation.

Tissue typing by sequence analysis of the HLA genes, or serologic reactions between HLA antigens and specific antibodies, are used to select donors with compatible HLA types. A test called the **mixed leukocyte reaction (MLR)**, which measures the proliferation of recipient lymphocytes in response to donor lymphocytes, can be used to determine if individuals are well matched. There are different categories of transplants, and each has a different success rate. An **autograft** is the transfer of an individual's own tissue (skin, blood), which is always accepted. A **syngeneic graft** is the transfer of tissue between genetically identical individuals (monozygotic twins) and has a low risk of rejection. An **allograft** is the transfer of tissue between genetically different individuals of the same species, which is the most common type of human transplant. Allografts have a high risk of rejection and require long-term immunosuppression of the recipient. **Xenografts** are transplants between different species (human, primates, pigs) and are only experimental in humans.

Transplant Rejection

Transplant rejection is an immune response to an allograft, which occurs when the recipient cells recognize the donor cells as foreign. The immune response to alloantigens may lead to graft failure, necessitating its removal. The severity and rapidity of rejection varies, depending on the degree of HLA differences between the donor and the recipient, the immunocompetence of the recipient, and the type of tissue being transplanted. In cell-mediated rejection, CD8 T-cells are activated by recognition of foreign class I alloantigens expressed by cells in the graft, and CD4 T-cells are activated by class II alloantigens. Humoral responses against foreign HLA antigens can generate antibodies that target the graft vasculature, causing immune complex deposition and associated tissue injury.

Type of rejection	Onset	Histology	Gross
Hyperacute	Minutes to hours	Vascular occlusion neutrophils, antibodies	Engorged cyanotic
Acute	Days to weeks	Molecular cell infiltration necrotizing vasculis	—
Chronic	Months to years	Fibrous, mononuclear infiltration	Fibrosis, shrinkage

Table 8 Graft rejection chart

Graft rejection is usually classified as hyperacute, acute, or chronic rejection (Table 8). **Hyperacute (white graft) rejection** is mediated by pre-existing antibodies (e.g., anti-ABO antibodies) that bind to endothelium and activate complement. It is characterized by rapid thrombotic occlusion that begins within minutes after vascular anastomosis is complete. **Acute rejection** occurs within days to weeks of transplantation and is characterized by extensive lymphocyte and macrophage infiltration and tissue necrosis. **Chronic rejection** can occur months or years after transplantation and is characterized by fibrosis and loss of normal organ structure. A T-cell–mediated reaction is the main cause of rejection of many types of grafts, but antibodies contribute to the rejection of certain transplants, especially bone marrow.

Transplant recipients may also display **graft-versus-host (GVH)** reactions if grafted immunocompetent T-cells attack host cells. The GVH reaction can be either acute or chronic and is particularly common after bone marrow transplantation. Target organs include the skin, liver, and GI tract. Patients develop skin rash, jaundice, and diarrhea. GVH disease can be minimized by pre-transplantation or T-cell depletion of donor tissue with drugs or radiation.

Tumor Immunology

Many tumor cells develop new antigens on their surface, which can be recognized by T-cells or antibodies. These **tumor-associated antigens** and **tumor-specific antigens** may be unique antigens found only on tumor cells, or they may be antigens found on both tumor and normal cells.

Tissue-specific antigens include **S-100** protein expressed by melanoma, common acute lymphoblastic leukemia antigen (CALLA) expressed in B-cell leukemia/lymphoma, and **CA-125** and **CA-19-9** glycoproteins expressed by ovarian and pancreatic cancer cells, respectively. **Carcinoembryonic antigen (CEA)** and **a-fetoprotein (AFP)** are proteins that occur normally in fetal tissue but are expressed abnormally in tumor cells of hepatocellular carcinoma and carcinoma of the colon, pancreas, breast, ovary, lung, and stomach.

Macrophages and NK cells respond to tumor cells by releasing TNF-a and lysing cells, respectively. T- and B-cells may also participate in a more specific immune response. To escape immunosurveillance by cytotoxic T-cells, MHC class I expression may be down-regulated in some tumor and virally infected cells.

Tumor immunotherapy is still somewhat experimental. One method is to stimulate the immune system by local injection of killed or irradiated tumor cells together with nonspecific adjuvants (e.g., bacillus Calmette-Guérin mycobacterium) or high-dose administration of cytokines, such as IL-2, TNF-a, IFN-a, and IFN-g. Passive immunity can also be induced by administering "magic bullets," or monoclonal anti-bodies against tumor-specific antigens, which are linked to toxic molecules, radioisotopes, or drugs to selectively kill tumor cells (a kind of immunologic "Trojan horse"). A modification of this approach is to use hybrid monoclonal antibodies, with one component specific for tumor antigen and the other for the TCR. These heteroconjugates allow activated T-cells to confront tumor cells, potentially leading to tumor regression.

Lymphatic Drainage

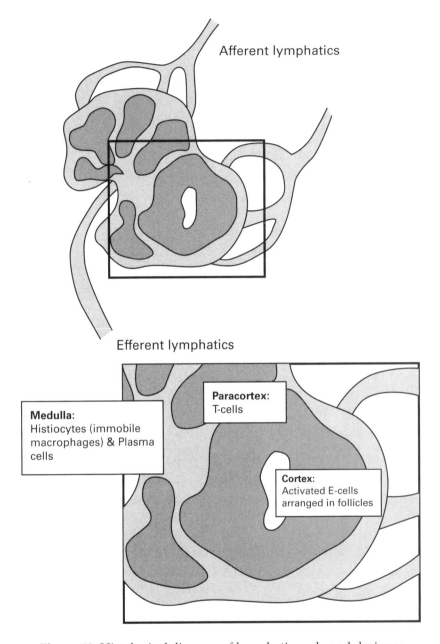

Figure 19 Histological diagram of lymphatic node and drainage

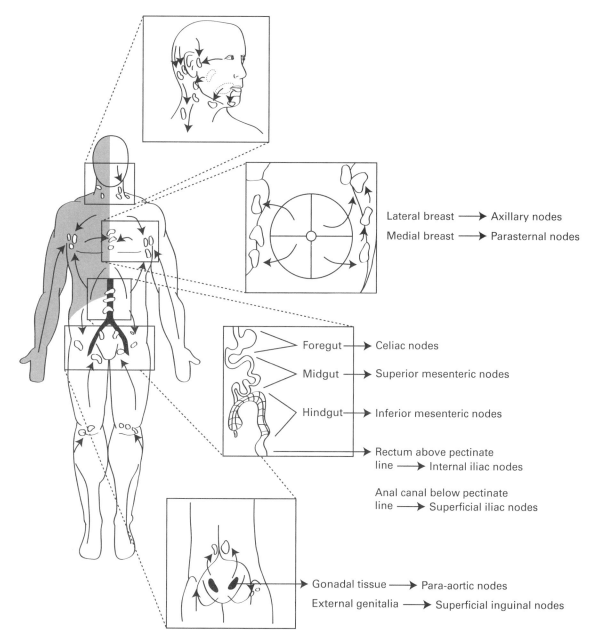

Lateral breast ⟶ Axillary nodes

Medial breast ⟶ Parasternal nodes

Foregut ⟶ Celiac nodes

Midgut ⟶ Superior mesenteric nodes

Hindgut ⟶ Inferior mesenteric nodes

Rectum above pectinate line ⟶ Internal iliac nodes

Anal canal below pectinate line ⟶ Superficial iliac nodes

Gonadal tissue ⟶ Para-aortic nodes

External genitalia ⟶ Superficial inguinal nodes

Figure 20 Important anatomic considerations of lymphatic drainage

Vaccines provide prophylactic immunization against infectious diseases. Vaccination can induce active or passive immunity, or a combination of both. **Active immunity** is acquired through vaccination with killed or attenuated microorganisms or their products. Purified antigen vaccines contain a suspension of structural components, such as capsular polysaccharides or inactivated toxins (toxoids). In general, live, attenuated vaccines (which contain live micro-organisms that are unable to cause disease but retain their antigenicity) induce longer-lasting immunity and produce a more effective cell-mediated response than killed vaccines. Killed vaccines—containing a suspension of inactivated, intact microorganisms—induce a predominantly humoral response. A successful active vaccine should lead to the production of memory T- and B-cells. **Passive immunity** is provided by the administration of preformed antitoxin or antiviral antibodies in preparations called immune globulins.

Combined immunization is widely used—for example, the diphtheria-tetanus-pertussis vaccine (purified bacterial antigen vaccine) or the measles-mumps-rubella vaccine (live attenuated viral vaccine). Snake and spider antivenins are equine (horse) immunoglobulins that provide passive immunity.

Diagnostic Tests

Antigen-antibody reactions reflect physical characteristics of the antigen or antibody. **Affinity** refers to the strength of the attraction between a single antigenic epitope and the antibody-binding site. **Avidity** refers to the strength of the interaction between multivalent antigens and complementary antibodies. Diagnostic tests determine the presence of unknown antigen or antibody in patient serum by complementarity with specific standard antigens or antibodies.

Test	Description	Representative Example
Agglutination	Particulate antigen (e.g., bacteria) combines with specific antibody and forms and aggregate	Widal test to diagnose enteric *Salmonella* infection
Hemagglutination inhibition	Antiviral antibody-inhibition of red blood cell agglutination	Diagnosis of viral infections
Precipitation	Soluble antigen combines with specific antibody and forms and aggregate	Serum test for antibody to diphtheria toxoid
Double diffusion (Ouchterlony technique)	Precipitation reaction in agar, leading to viable lines of precipitate	Diagnosis of hypersensitivity pneumonitis (e.g., pigeon breeder's lung)
Immunoelectrophoresis	Precipitation in agar with an electric field identifies antigens by charge, size, and specificity	Diagnosis of selective globulin immunodeficiencies
Antiglobulin	Visible aggregation due to bridging of anti-body-coated cells by anti-y globulin	Coombs' test for erythroblastosis fetalis
Radioimmunoassay (RIA)	Antigen bound to specific antibody is quantitated by comparison to radio-labeled antigen standards competitively bound to the same antibody	Detection of antibodies to hepatitis B surface antigen
Enzyme-linked immunosorbent assay (ELISA)	Similar to RIA but antigen-antibody binding is quantitated by colorimetric detection of an enzyme substrate	Human immunodeficiency virus antibody screening
Immunoflourescence	Microscopic detection of fluorescently labeled antigen or antibodies in histologic tissue sections	Identification of antinuclear antibodies in systemic lupus erythematosus

Western blot	Antigenic proteins separated by electrophoresis are blotted to a membrane and detected by reaction with labeled antibodies	Confirmatory test for HIV
Complement fixation	Complement is added to identify either partner in an antigen-antibody complex if the other is known; hermolysis constitutes a negative reaction	Wasswerman test for syphilis
Mixed lymphocyte culture	Responder T-cells proliferate and/or lyse irradiated target cells in response to foreign human leukocyte antigens	Test of transplant donor and recipient compatibility
Fluorescence-activated cell sorting (FACS)	Blood cell enumeration by laser detection of fluorescently labeled monoclonal antibodies directed against cell surface markers	CD4+ T-cell counts in HIV patients

Table 9 Antigen-antibody diagnostic tests

CHAPTER 11

MICROBIOLOGY

INTRODUCTION

Bacterial Structure and Function

The average bacterial size is 0.2–5.0 µm in diameter. Bacteria can be classified according to their structure. **Cocci** are spheres that are often found in pairs, rows, or clusters. **Bacilli** are rod shaped. **Spirochetes** are curved or spiral shaped. These structural distinctions are identifiable through microscopy, allowing one to narrow the possible type of bacteria that is in question.

The bacterial genome is a single, circular piece of double stranded DNA (dsDNA) with approximately 2,000 genes. Prokaryotes have no true nucleus, so the circular DNA floats in the cytoplasm of the cell. Some cells may contain one or more **plasmids**, which are extra-chromosomal pieces of circular dsDNA that replicate independent of genomic DNA. Plasmids can confer resistance to antibiotics, heavy metals and UV light; and can encode exotoxins and nitrogen fixation enzymes. **Transmissible plasmids** are large, containing genes for the synthesis and use of sex pilus. **Non-transmissible plasmids** are small and contain fewer genes, having many copies per cell.

The prokaryotic ribosome is 70S (composed of 50S and 30S subunits). They are unique from the eukaryotic ribosome, which is 80S (composed of 60S and 40S subunits). This distinction permits some antibiotics to harm bacterial ribosomes without affecting host ribosomes.

Protein synthesis occurs on **polyribosomes** (i.e. many ribosome molecules per RNA strand), resulting in parallel production of multiple copies of a given protein.

Bacteria are surrounded by a cytoplasmic membrane, composed of a phospholipid bilayer (similar to eukaryotic membrane, but does not contain sterols).

Invaginations of the cytoplasmic membrane, **mesosomes**, contain enzymes necessary for chemical fixation.

Peptidoglycan makes the cell wall of bacteria. It is composed of a sugar backbone with cross-linked peptide side chains. The main function is to provide structure and support that protects it from osmotic pressure. This layer is much thicker in Gram-positive bacteria. Bacteria with unusual cell membranes/walls include: **mycoplasma**, containing sterols and have no cell wall; and **mycobacteria**, which contain mycolic acid and have high lipid content.

Between the cell wall and the cytoplasmic membrane is the **periplasmic space**, which may contain enzymes called β-lactamase that are important in bacterial resistance to penicillins. The periplasmic space is only found in Gram-negative bacteria.

Think of encapsulated organisms having a capsular "swelling" reaction

Some bacteria are surrounded by **capsules** composed of a gelatinous, polysaccharide layer outside of the cell wall. These capsules are frequently used to determine serologic type within a species. They can act as virulence factors and are often immunogenic allowing them to be used as vaccines. They can also be involved in adhesion to human tissues. A **Quellung reaction** is the swelling of a capsule due to antibody binding.

Flagella are long, whip-like protrusions made of many subunits of flagellin protein used for motility.

Pili, or fimbriae, are short, hair-like projections composed of subunits of pilin protein. Pili are found mainly on gram-negative bacteria. They mediate the attachment of bacteria to human tissue.

Sex pilus is used for conjugation between bacteria (bacteria sex).

Glycocalyx is a secreted slime layer, made up of polysaccharides that allow adhesion to certain tissues and materials, such as catheters.

Spores made by genus *Bacillus* and genus *Clostridium* are metabolically inactive forms of bacteria. They are highly resistant to heat and chemicals due to a thick, keratin-like coat containing **dipicolinic acid** (a calcium chelator), which is responsible for resistance to adverse conditions.

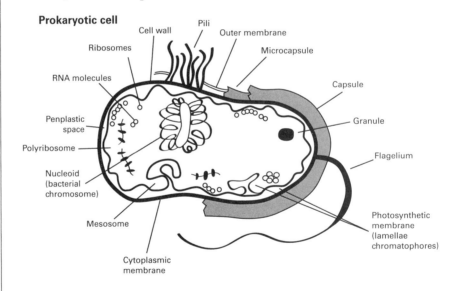

Figure 1 Prokaryotic Cell

Bacterial Cell Wall and Gram Staining

Gram staining is frequently used to identify organisms. First, crystal violet and iodine are used to stain all the cells blue. Then the cells are washed with ethanol or acetone. Finally, they are stained with a red counter-stain, such as safranin. Bacteria stain different colors due to differences in the composition of their cell wall.

- **Gram-positive** organisms are blue/purple on Gram stain due to their thick, multilayered peptidoglycan layer that absorbs the crystal violet stain well and resists staining by organic solvents. Some gram-positive organisms have techoic acid for an outer membrane.

- **Gram-negative** organisms are red on Gram stain. These organisms have a thin peptido-glycan layer and a complex outer membrane containing **lipopolysaccharide (LPS),** which absorbs the crystal violet stain poorly and is easily stained by organic solvent. **LPS** is also known as **endotoxin,** and can cause fever and shock. LPS is composed of lipid A (the cause of toxic effects), a core polysaccharide, and an outer polysaccharide (O antigen).

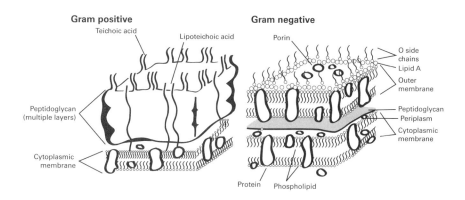

Figure 2 Gram Positive & Gram Negative

- **Acid-fast bacteria**, such as Mycobacteria, do not change color on Gram stain but rather stain with carbolfuchsin (**Ziehl-Neelsen stain**). Their cell walls have a high lipid content (**mycolic acid**).

Bacterial Oxygen Requirement Classification

Obligate aerobes require oxygen for growth. Examples include *Nocardia, Pseudomonas aeruginosa, Mycobacterium tuberculosis,* and *Bacillus.* **Facultative anaerobes** can use oxygen if available but otherwise can survive on fermentation. **Obligate anaerobes** can't grow in the presence of oxygen because they do not have the enzymes **catalase** or **superoxide dismutase,** which are important in neutralizing toxic reactive oxygen metabolites. Examples include *Clostridium, Bacteroides,* and *Actinomyces.*

Cellular Respiration

In aerobic respiration, the final electron acceptor is oxygen, whereas in anaerobic respiration, the final electron acceptor is an inorganic molecule. Both are used by facultative anaerobes. Other electron acceptors include nitrate, fumarate, sulfate and carbonate.

Fermentation

Fermentation describes the combustion of substrate in the absence of oxygen. It uses an incomplete oxidation pathway and results in the accumulation of an end product made to regenerate nicotinamide adenine dinucleotide (NAD). This end product may be useful in the identification of bacteria. *Clostridium* species can use amino acids for fermentation.

Bacterial Reproduction and Growth Cycle

Bacteria reproduce via **binary fission**. The **doubling time** can range from 20 minutes (e.g., *Escherichia coli* in ideal conditions) to longer than 24 hours (*Mycobacterium tuberculosis*).

Bacterial growth has four phases:

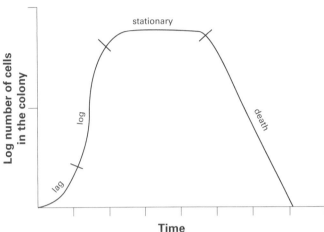

The four phases of a bacterial growth curve

Figure 3 Four phases of bacterial growth

- **Lag phase**—little division, but lots of internal metabolic activity as the cells prepare copies of everything for duplication.

- **Log phase**—period of optimal cell division.

- **Stationary phase**—occurs when there is nutritional depletion and the number of new cells made equals the number of old cells dying, growth curve plateaus.

- **Death phase**—occurs when there is a decrease in the viable cell number due to buildup of toxins and lack of nutrients.

GENETICS

Bacteria are haploid—that is, they have only one copy of their genome. As a result, mutations caused by radiation, chemicals, viruses, or transposons are more likely to affect the genome and alter function.

Bacterial DNA Transfer

1. **Conjugation**—the "mating" of two cells, controlled by the **F (fertility) plasmid**.

The F plasmid contains information for a sex pilus, which acts as the conjugation tube. During conjugation, the pilus on an F+ bacterium binds to a receptor on the F- bacterium. The cells are then in close contact and linked by a conjugation tube. A single strand of the F plasmid DNA is cleaved, and goes through the conjugation tube to the F- cell. Complementary strands are then made in both cells, to produce complete plasmids, identical to each other. The resulting cells will both be F+ (see Figure 4).

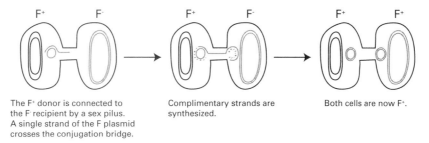

The F⁺ donor is connected to the F⁻ recipient by a sex pilus. A single strand of the F plasmid crosses the conjugation bridge.

Complimentary strands are synthesized.

Both cells are now F⁺.

Figure 4 Bacterial

The F plasmid can also be integrated into the host genome so that "mating" can transfer pieces of genomic DNA from one bacterium to another. This is called **high-frequency recombination** (Hfr). The mating complex is unstable, usually only a portion of the genome is transferred. The transferred segment can recombine with the recipient's genomic DNA (see Figure 5 below).

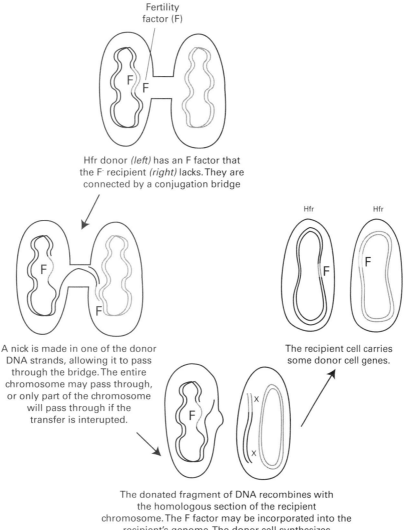

Fertility factor (F)

Hfr donor *(left)* has an F factor that the F⁻ recipient *(right)* lacks. They are connected by a conjugation bridge

A nick is made in one of the donor DNA strands, allowing it to pass through the bridge. The entire chromosome may pass through, or only part of the chromosome will pass through if the transfer is interrupted.

The donated fragment of DNA recombines with the homologous section of the recipient chromosome. The F factor may be incorporated into the recipient's genome. The donor cell synthesizes DNA to replace the single-standed fragment.

The recipient cell carries some donor cell genes.

Figure 5 Bacterial Conjugation with High Frequency Recombination

2. **Transduction**—occurs via a **bacteriophage**, a virus that infects bacteria.

The bacteriophage then can enter either the lytic or lysogenic cycle.

In the **lytic cycle**, the virus replicates in the bacterium and is released with lysis of the bacterium.

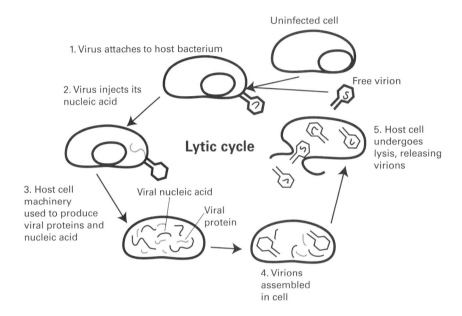

Figure 6 Lytic Cycle

In the **lysogenic cycle**, the virus is integrated into the host genomic DNA (now called a **prophage**) and is dormant for some time before entering the lytic cycle.

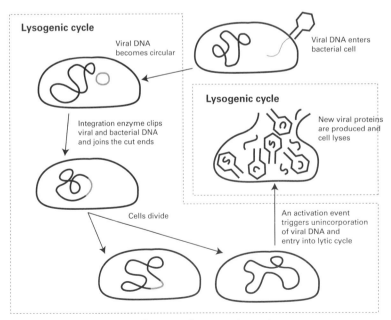

Figure 7 Lysogenic cycle

- *Generalized* transduction occurs from a packaging error when a **lytic phage** carries with it a random piece of bacterial DNA that is then transferred to other bacterium. This can lead to antibiotic resistance.

- *Specialized* transduction occurs with **lysogenic phages** when the integrated virus genome takes along an adjacent piece of bacterial DNA when it enters the lytic cycle. This can lead to DNA recombination.

3. **Transformation**—the direct uptake of naked DNA. Bacterial lysis may release their DNA, which can then be taken by other bacteria. Although not an important process in disease, this is often used as a laboratory technique with purified DNA.

Sterilization and Culture Technique

Disinfection is the elimination of *pathogenic* microorganisms. **Sterilization** occurs when *all* microorganisms die, including spores (often the hardest organisms to kill!). With sterilization, metabolic activity may still exist, but reproduction is impossible. Sterilization may be achieved through the following methods:

- **Autoclaving** is the most effective method of sterilization. Moist heat (steam) for 15 minutes at 121 C, under pressure of 15 psi. Alternatively, dry heat (180 C for 2 hours) can be used.

- **Radiation** can also be used for sterilization. Ionizing radiation (e.g., X-ray, gamma ray) has good penetration but requires high energy. UV light uses less energy than does ionizing radiation but is less penetrating; it is effective in sterilizing surfaces.

- **Filtration**, using a 0.22-μm cellulose ester filter, is performed to sterilize heat-labile substances, such as drug solutions.

Boiling and the use of chemicals are less reliable methods, which may leave behind the hardy spores. **Chemical agents** show a wide variability in effectiveness. They are compared using the phenol coefficient (i.e., the ratio of concentration of the agent to concentration of phenol needed for the same amount of killing). They have three types of effects:

Mechanism	Examples
Disruption of cell membranes	Alcohols (e.g., 70% Ethanol)
	Detergents (e.g., benzalkonium chloride)
	Phenols
Modification of important proteins	Chlorine, iodine, hydrogen peroxide (oxidizing agents)
	Heavy metals (block enzymatic activity)
	Glutaraldehyde and ethylene oxide (alkylating agents)
	Acids and alkalis
	Alcohols and phenols can also denature proteins
Modification of DNA	Crystal dyes and malachite green
	Glutaraldehyde and ethylene oxide

Table 1 Effects of chemical agents

Virulence Factors

Virulence factors are the characteristics of the microorganism that determine its pathogenic potential, both in terms of efficiency (how few or many organisms are required to cause disease) and symptoms. Examples of virulence factors are as follows:

1. **Adherence**—occurs via pili; if pili are lost, bacteria are usually non-pathogenic.

2. **Invasiveness**—mediated by enzymes secreted by the bacteria that lead to tissue destruction and disease.

   - **Collagenase** and **hyaluronidase** allow spread through subcutaneous tissue. They are important in cellulitis, especially in *Streptococcus pyogenes* infection.

   - **IgA protease** allows adherence to mucous membranes
     - *Neisseria gonorrhoeae, Haemophilus influenzae,* and *Streptococcus pneumoniae*

   - **Leukocidins** that are toxic to neutrophils and macrophages

3. **Anti-phagocytic** traits may allow bacteria to resist destruction.

   - **Capsules** make phagocytosis difficult. However, there are vaccines with capsular antigens to promote anticapsule-antibody formation, which allow opsonization and subsequent phagocytosis.
     - *Neisseria meningitides, S. pneumoniae, Klebsiella pneumoniae, Salmonella,* and *Haemophilus influenzae.*

   - **Cell wall proteins** are found in some gram-positive cocci, such as *S. aureus* (**protein A**) and *S. pyogenes* (**M protein**).

   - **Coagulase,** secreted by *Staphylococcus aureus,* enhances clot formation and may protect bacteria from phagocytosis by formation of a fibrin coat.

   - **Invasins** are seen in intracellular organisms. Invasins bind the integrin-family protein on reticuloendothelial cells, allowing the organism to enter the cell. Once inside, other factors protect the bacteria from digestion.

4. **Toxins** present in bacteria may affect pathogenicity:

Endotoxins (LPS)	Exotoxins
Found in cell wall of gram-negative bacteria	Found in certain species of both gram-posiive and gram-negative bacteria
A component of the outer cell membrane of Gram negative bacteria that is released with cell lysis	Protein is secreted and is usually extremely toxic
Polypeptide	Gene is usually encoded on plasmid or phage DNA
Encoded in the bacteria genome	High toxicity
Low toxicity	High immunogenicity
Low immunogenicity	Used in vaccines
Not used in vaccines	Mostly the **A-B type** (the B subunit is for **binding** and entry into the target cell; the A subunit does the damage).
Lipid A is the active component	
Causes fever via macrophage release of:	Purified, inactivated toxins, known as toxoids, are also immunogenic and are used in vaccines
• Interleukin 1 (IL-1)	
• Tumor Necrosis Factor (TNF) (antibodies to TNF can block endotoxin symptoms)	Examples:
	• Neurotoxins
Cause hypotension, septic shock by bradykinin (and nitric oxide) mediated vasodilation	• Enterotoxins
	• Pyrogenic toxins
Disseminated intravascular coagulation (DIC), after activation of factor XII, results in thrombosis and ischemia	• Tissue invasive toxins
	(Examples described below)
Activates the alternate complement pathway, resulting in inflammation	
Activates macrophages and B cells	
These manifestations are seen in meningitis (by gram-negative cocci) and sepsis (by gram-negative rods)	
Endotoxin-like effects are seen with some cases of gram-positive sepsis (*S. aureus, S. pyogenes*) due to some other component of the cell wall that may activate IL-1, TNF and other factors	

Table 2 Endotoxins & Exotoxins

B-binding
A-action/activity

Examples of Exotoxins

Neurotoxins

- **Tetanus toxin** is made by *Clostridium tetani.* This toxin is encoded by a plasmid and inhibits the release of glycine, an inhibitory neurotransmitter. This results in tetanus, consisting of muscle spasm and lockjaw (trismus). The toxin travels from a wound to the anterior horn of the spinal cord in the blood or by retrograde axonal transport.

- **Botulinum toxin** is made by *Clostridium botulinum*. It is encoded by a bacteriophage and blocks the release of acetylcholine at the neuromuscular synapse, resulting in paralysis. Ingestion of honey in babies an cause **floppy baby syndrome**. It is very toxic; 1 μg is lethal.

Enterotoxins

- **Heat-labile enterotoxin** is made by *E. coli* and encoded on plasmid DNA. In the small intestine, this toxin causes ADP-ribosylation of a G_s protein, resulting in constitutive activation of **adenylate cyclase** → Cyclic adenosine monophosphate (cAMP) increases → increased Cl⁻ excretion and decreased Na⁺ absorption. The increased Na⁺ in the lumen pulls water into the lumen leading to increased water and electrolyte loss, resulting in diarrhea. Toxins from *Vibrio cholerae, Campylobacter jejuni,* and *Bacillus cereus* act in a similar manner to cause diarrhea.

- **Heat-stable toxin**, produced by *E. coli*, results in the activation of **guanylate cyclase**, which leads to an increase in cyclic guanosine monophosphate and decreased Na⁺ absorption, ultimately resulting in diarrhea. *Yersinia enterocolitica* makes a similar toxin.

- **Verotoxin** (Shiga-like toxin) is made by the 0157:H7 *E. coli* serotype. It acts by removing adenosine from 28S ribosomal RNA (rRNA) from the 60S subunit of the ribosome, thus stopping protein synthesis. It is found in undercooked contaminated meat and causes outbreaks of bloody diarrhea. **Shiga toxin**, produced by *Shigella dysenteriae*, also acts by blocking protein synthesis.

- **Heat-stable toxin** produced by *Staphylococcus aureus*, results in diarrhea and vomiting that lasts less than one day. *Bacillus cereus* also produces a heat-stable toxin that results in vomiting that lasts for one day, and limited diarrhea when ingested.

Pyrogenic toxins

- **Erythrogenic toxin**, made by *S. pyogenes,* is encoded by a lysogenized phage. This toxin causes scarlet fever by an unknown mechanism.

- **Toxic shock syndrome toxin** (TSST) is made by some strains of *S. aureus*. It is known as a *superantigen* (SAg). TSST binds major histocompatibility complex class II (MHC II) and stimulates large populations of T cells. These activated T cells release inflammatory cytokines and interleukins, resulting in toxic shock.

Tissue Invasive toxins

- **Diphtheria toxin** is made by *Corynebacterium diphtheriae*. This toxin, encoded by the *TOX* gene of the lysogenized phage, causes adenosine diphosphate (ADP)-ribosylation of elongation factor 2 (EF-2), which inhibits protein synthesis and results in cell death. The diphtheria toxin exhibits specificity for eukaryotic EF-2 by its unique amino acid diphthamide (a modified histidine) and does not inhibit prokaryotic EF-2. EF-2 is found in all cells, and thus there is no toxin-tissue specificity. This toxin is extremely potent: One molecule can kill a cell within hours. *Pseudomonas aeruginosa* **exotoxin A**, acts with a similar mechanism to cause liver damage.

- **Pertussis toxin** is made by *Bordetella pertussis*. It activates adenylate cyclase by ADP-ribosylation.

- *Clostridium perfringens toxin*, called the **alpha toxin** (lecithinase), is a phospholipase that hydrolyzes lecithin in the cell membrane, resulting in cell death and causing gas gangrene.

- *Clostridium difficile* produces **toxin A** and **toxin B**, which act in concert to produce pseudomembranous enterocolitis, characterized by colonic inflammation, fever, abdominal pain, and bloody diarrhea. Commonly occurs following antibiotic therapy (most commonly, *clindamycin* or *ampicillin*)

- **Anthrax toxin**, produced by *Bacillus anthracis*, has three components. **Edema factor** is the A subunit, which increases cAMP levels in phagocytes to inhibit phagocytosis. **Protective antigen** is the B subunit, which allows entry into target cells. **Lethal factor** kills macrophages.

- *Staphylococcus aureus* and *Streptococcus pyogenes* make a number of toxins, including streptokinase, DNases, hyaluronidase, lipases, etc., that result in tissue destruction in the form of abscesses, skin infections and systemic infections. **Exfolatin** from *S. aureus*, for example, produces scalded skin syndrome in infants.

Principles of Laboratory Diagnosis

- **Blood cultures** are used in the diagnosis of sepsis, endocarditis, meningitis, pneumonia, and osteomyelitis. The most commonly grown organisms in blood cultures are gram-positive cocci (*S. aureus* or *S. pneumoniae*) or gram-negative rods (*E. coli, Klebsiella pneumoniae, Pseudomonas aeruginosa*). Skin flora, such as *Staphylococcus epidermidis*, may grow as a contaminant resulting from the blood draw itself.

- **Throat cultures** are performed in cases of suspected *S. pyogenes* and in cases of thrush (*Candida*), diphtheria, and gonococcal pharyngitis. A swab of the posterior pharyngeal exudate is spread onto a blood agar plate, which is subsequently checked for beta-hemolysis and bacitracin sensitivity.

- **Sputum cultures** are used in the diagnosis of pneumonia, tuberculosis (TB), or lung abscesses. Commonly isolated organisms include *S. pneumoniae* (community-acquired) or *K. pneumoniae* (nosocomial).

- **Spinal fluid culture** is done for suspected meningitis. Common organisms include *N. meningitides, S. pneumoniae,* and *H. influenzae.*

- **Stool cultures** are performed in cases of enterocolitis. Usual organisms are *Shigella, Salmonella,* and *Campylobacter*. Common stool cultures include MacConkey eosin-methylene blue (EMB), triple sugar iron (TSI) and Skirrow's agar.

- **Urine culture** is performed for suspected urethritis, cystitis, or pyelonephritis. By far the most common organism in urine cultures is *E. coli*, followed by *Enterobacter, Proteus,* and *Streptococcus faecalis. Staphylococcus saprophyticus* is seen in urinary tract infections (UTIs) in sexually active women. Midstream specimens are used for analysis to avoid contamination with normal flora.

- **Genital tract cultures** are used in the detection of sexually transmitted infections (STIs). Urethral discharge can be gram stained directly and inspected for *N. gonorrhoeae* infection. *Chlamydia trachomatis* is an intracellular organism that must grow in human cells and therefore requires a special transport medium. *Treponema pallidum*, which causes syphilis, cannot be grown in culture and diagnosed by dark-field microscopy (visualizing motile spirochetes) and serology.

- Both aerobic and anaerobic cultures must be performed because wounds and abscesses may be caused by aerobic organisms, anaerobic organisms, or a mixture of the two (depending on the site of the infection).

Immunologic Methods to Identify Known Antigens

The **Quellung reaction** consists of capsular swelling in the presence of homologous antiserum.

A **slide agglutination test** is performed when an antibody to O antigen on *Salmonella* and *Shigella* causes clumping of the organism. A **latex agglutination test** is similarly performed, except the antibodies used are latex coated.

Counter immunoelectrophoresis tests are used to detect the presence of capsular antigens in spinal fluid. The antigen and antibody move toward each other in a gel. Subsequent binding causes precipitation.

Immunologic Methods to Identify Serum Antibodies

A slide or tube agglutination test requires serial dilutions of patient serum with bacterial suspensions to determine the organism and antibody titer. A fourfold rise in serum titer is needed for diagnosis.

Serological methods used to diagnose Syphilis (*T. pallidum* infection):

- **VDRL** (venereal disease research laboratory) and **rapid plasma regain (RPR)** tests use beef antigen (cardiolipin) to detect cross-reactive antibody to *T. pallidum*. These tests are not specific, but they are relatively inexpensive.

- Laboratory tests using treponemal antigens include fluorescent treponemal antibody-absorbed (**FTA-ABS)** and microhemagglutination-*T. pallidum* (**MHA-TP**).

The **cold agglutinin test** is performed in suspected cases of *Mycoplasma* infection. *M. pneumoniae* infection induces autoantibodies that agglutinate red blood cells (RBCs) at 4 C, but this test is not specific to *M. pneumoniae.*

IMMUNIZATION

Vaccinations provide active immunity with bacterial antigens to stimulate a protective immune response. They are divided into three types:

1. **Capsular polysaccharide vaccines** are composed of the outer capsules of organisms.

   - *S. pneumoniae* **vaccine**—contains polysaccharide antigens from the 23 most prevalent serotypes. It is given to people older than age 60 and those at high risk of developing pneumonia. (Known as Pneumovax 23)

   - *N. meningitides* **vaccine**—composed of antigens from four strains. It is given to high-risk individuals and during periods of meningitis outbreaks. It is given to close-contacts of an individual with a confirmed diagnosis with N. meningitides.

   - *H. influenzae* **vaccine**—usually given in combination with diphtheria-pertussis-tetanus (DPT) triple vaccine to infants. The *b* polysaccharide is poorly immunogenic, therefore, it is coupled with diphtheria toxoid to increase its immunogenicity.

2. **Toxoid vaccines** are composed of inactivated toxin.

   - Commonly used toxoid vaccines include *C. diphtheriae* and *C. tetani*.

3. Whole bacteria or protein vaccines are used for a variety of organisms, including *B. pertussis, Salmonella typhi, Vibrio cholerae*, and *Yersinia pestis.*

- *Bacillus anthracis* **vaccine** is a purified "protective antigen" vaccine given to populations at risk. The **bacillus Calmette-Guérin (BCG)** vaccine, used outside the United States, consists of live attenuated *Mycobacterium bovis*. It is used for TB vaccination, although its efficacy has not been proved, and those who get the vaccine will later have a positive PPD test.

- Vaccines that provide passive immunity consist of preformed antiserum to provide immediate defense against a pathogen.

- **Tetanus antitoxin antibody**—given to wound and injury patients who have not been adequately immunized with tetanus toxoid.

- **Botulinum antitoxin antibody**—derived from horse antisera, is effective against the A, B, and E types of toxin.

- **Diphtheria antitoxin antibody**—also synthesized in horses. The botulinum or diphtheria antisera may elicit a hypersensitivity reaction to horse serum.

GRAM-POSITIVE COCCI

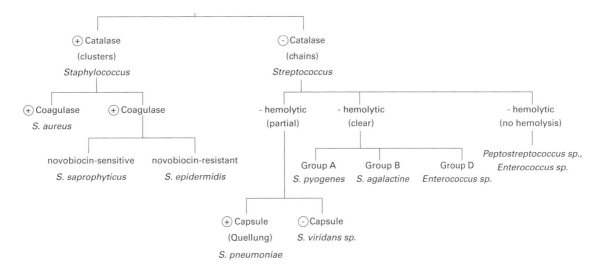

Figure 8 Gram-positive cocci

Staphylococcus Aureus

Fast Facts	**Protein A** in the cell wall binds immunoglobulin G (IgG) Fc, thereby preventing complement activation. **Teichoic acid** is present for cell adherence. **Enterotoxin**, classified as types A–F, stimulates the release of IL-1 and IL-2. **Toxic shock syndrome toxin (TSST)** is enterotoxin F and acts as a super antigen **Alpha toxin** causes skin necrosis and hemolysis *S. aureus* is part of normal human flora and is found in the nose and on skin. Transmission occurs via hands and fomites.
Signs and Symptoms	Inflammatory Pathway <ul><li>Skin infections—impetigo, cellulitis, folliculitis, furuncles, carbuncles</li><li>Abscesses—skin and organs</li><li>Acute endocarditis (especially in IV drug users, causing right-sided heart disease)</li><li>Osteomyelitis and septic arthritis</li><li>Meningitis</li><li>Pneumonia</li><li>Empyema</li></ul>Toxin-mediated Pathway <ul><li>Food poisoning (heat-stabile toxin)—short course vomiting and watery diarrhea</li><li>Toxic shock syndrome (TSST-1)—fever, rash, desquamation of palms and soles, and hypotension</li><li>Scalded skin syndrome (exfoliation toxin)—epidermis layer of skin sloughs off</li></ul>
Diagnosis	Gram-positive cocci in clusters Catalase positive; coagulase positive Cultures reveal yellow colonies ("aureus" means golden)
Treatment	Most strains are penicillin-resistant because they carry a plasmid-mediated β-lactamase Drugs of choice include third-generation penicillins, such as nafcillin, methicillin, and dicloxacillin; some cephalosporins; and vancomycin An increasingly worrisome strain of *S. aureus*, known as **methicillin-resistant S. aureus (MRSA)**, has altered penicillin-binding proteins that make it resistant even to third generation penicillins; vancomycin is given for MRSA

Staphylococcus Epidermidis and Staphylococcus Saprophyticus

Fast Facts	*S. epidermdis* is part of normal human skin flora; produces biofilm via glycocalyx
Signs and Symptoms	*S. epidermidis* • Catheter infections • Endocarditis, especially in patients with prosthetic heart valves. *S. saprophyticus* • UTIs, especially in young, sexually active women
Diagnosis	Blood or urine culture Coagulase negative Only *S. saprophyticus* is sensitive to novobiocin
Treatment	*S. epidermidis* is resistant to many antibiotics. If specific sensitivities are not available, treat with vancomycin. *S. saprophyticus* is treated with a quinolone or trimethoprim-sulfamethoxazole (TMP/SMX).

Streptococcus Pyogenes: Group A

Fast Facts	Found on skin and in the throat Transmitted by respiratory droplets Hemolytic exotoxins **streptolysin O** and **S** causes complete RBC lysis (β hemolytic) leaving a halo around a blood agar colony **M protein** within cell wall **Streptokinase**, activates plasminogen to plasmin, causing subsequent clot lysis **Hyaluronidase** helps bacteria move through connective tissue **Erythrogenic toxin** if it contains a lysogenic phage. Causes scarlet fever **Streptolysin O** is a an oxygen-labile hemolysin that causes beta-hemolysis in colonies growing under a blood agar surface • It is immunogenic (antibodies against it are antistreptolysin O [ASO]) • Responsible for the "sandpaper" rash of scarlet fever **Pyrogenic exotoxin A** acts similarly to TSST **Exotoxin B** destroys tissue causing necrotizing fasciitis

Signs and Symptoms	**Pharyngitis** (Strep Throat)
	- If left untreated, it may develop into otitis, sinusitis, meningitis, rheumatic fever, and glomerulonephritis
	Skin infections—Cellulitis, Impetigo
	Necrotizing fasciitis—a severe superficial infection
	Rheumatic fever may develop 2 weeks or more after infection
	- Fever, polyarthritis, carditis (especially damaging the mitral and aortic valves), subcutaneous nodules, chorea.
	- Manifestations occur due to cross-reactivity between bacterial and self-antigens, causing an auto-immune reaction
	- Rheumatic sequelae may be prevented by treating the acute infection with antibiotics
	Acute glomerulonephritis occurs approximately 2–3 weeks after skin infection in children
	- Results from deposition of immune complexes in the glomeruli
	- Patients develop hypertension, edema of ankles and face, and dark urine
Diagnosis	Gram-positive cocci found in pairs or chains
	Catalase-negative
	Bacitracin sensitive
	Beta-hemolytic
	Smears are performed for wound and skin infections
	For suspected pharyngitis, a culture swab is plated on blood agar and colonies are tested for beta-hemolysis and bacitracin sensitivity
	ASO antibody titers help diagnose a recent *Streptococcus* infection
Treatment	Penicillin
	Antibiotics are not helpful in the treatment of autoimmune sequelae

Streptococcus Agalactiae: Group B

Fast Facts	Commonly found as normal flora of the vagina Transmitted during birth. Most common cause of meningitis in newborns
Signs and Symptoms	**Neonatal sepsis** **Meningitis**—especially in premature babies **Neonatal Pneumonia**
Diagnosis	Genital tract culture in mother. Gram stain of CSF, urine, or blood in neonates Gram-positive cocci in chains Catalase-negative, Beta-hemolytic, Bacitracin resistant
Treatment	Penicillin G, with the possible addition of an aminoglycoside

Group "B" Strep, causes sepsis in "Babies"

Streptococcus Faecalis: Group D

Fast Facts	Also known as enterococci Found in the colon and occasionally in the genitourinary (GU) tract (Think 'D' for doo-doo.) Common cause of nosocomial infections in U.S. No known virulence factors
Signs and Symptoms	**UTIs**—especially in patients with urinary catheters **Subacute Endocarditis**—especially on previously abnormal valves after bacteremia caused by gastrointestinal (GI) or urinary tract surgery
Diagnosis	Gram stain and culture of urine or blood Catalase-negative Grows in hypertonic NaCl (6.5%) Makes a black pigment on bile-esculin agar
Treatment	Penicillin—with the possible addition of an aminoglycoside Patients with damaged prosthetic heart valves should be given ampicillin and gentamicin before GI or GU surgery

Viridans Streptococci

Fast Facts	*S. viridans* species, such as *S. mutans* and *S. sanguis*, are found in the oropharynx
	Use **dextrans** for adherence on teeth
Signs and Symptoms	Infective endocarditis *(S. sanguis)*
	• Fever, anemia and a heart murmur
	• Especially likely in patients with damaged or prosthetic heart vales who experience bacteremia during a dental procedure
	Dental caries *(S. mutans)*
	• Ferments sugars in teeth to lactic acid which demineralizes tooth enamel
Diagnosis	Multiple blood cultures are often necessary to detect the organism
	Cocci in chains, Alpha-hemolytic, Catalase-negative
	Optochin resistant
Treatment	Penicillin G
	Prophylactic amoxicillin treatment should be given to high-risk patients before **dental procedures**

Streptococcus Pneumoniae

Fast Facts	Also known as pneumococci
	Spread via respiratory droplets
	Up to 50% of people carry this in their oropharynx
	Have capsular polysaccharides, which can determine serotype
	IgA protease—promotes adhesion to mucous membranes.
Signs and Symptoms	Pneumococcal pneumonia
	• Sudden chill, fever, and **rusty sputum**
	• Predisposing factors include alcohol intoxication (suppresses the cough reflex and can lead to aspiration) and respiratory tract injury from irritants or viral infection
	Other infections such as bronchitis, otitis media and meningitis
	• *S. pneumoniae* is the most common cause of otitis media in young children
	Immunocompromised patients, whose who have undergone splenectomy and sickle-cell patients (self-splenectomized), are at increased risk of infection with encapsulated organisms, especially *Pneumococcus*
Diagnosis	Alpha-hemolytic oval diplococci
	Gram stain and **Quellung reaction** of sputum sample bile-soluble or sensitive
	Optochin sensitive (scared to go "up to chin" from lungs!)
Treatment	Penicillin is the treatment of choice
	Resistance may be developing
	Erythromycin is also used

GRAM-NEGATIVE COCCI

Neisseria Meningitidis

Fast Facts	Also known as meningococci
	Kidney bean-shaped diplococci
	Capsule; 13 serotypes based on capsular polysaccharides
	Found in the flora of the upper respiratory tract
	Transmitted by airborne droplets
	Antibodies against the capsule are protective, but group specific
	Complement activation in host defense is important • Deficiency in this places patient at higher risk for infection IgA protease
	Meningococcus is the second most common cause of sporadic meningitis in children ages 6 months to 6 years and is the most common cause of epidemic meningitis
Signs and Symptoms	Meningitis • Fever, headache, stiff neck Severe cases result in meningococcemia known as **Waterhouse-Friedrichsen syndrome** • Characterized by fever, shock, purpura, disseminated intravascular coagulation (DIC), and adrenal insufficiency
Diagnosis	Oxidase-positive
	Gram stain and latex agglutination tests are performed on Cerebrospinal fluid (CSF)
	Blood or CSF culture is plated on chocolate agar • To differentiate from *N. gonorrhoeae*, remember that meningococci ferments maltose in addition to glucose
Treatment	Penicillin G
	Rifampin prophylaxis is used for close contacts of patients, and patients with suspected meningitis should be in respiratory isolation until *Meningococcemia* is ruled out
	Prevention of outbreaks is performed with a vaccine made from capsular antigens

Neisseria Gonorrhoeae

Fast Facts	Also known as gonococci
	No polysaccharide capsule, pili, contains lipo-oligosaccharide (LOS)
	Organism is serotyped by pilus type (> 100 serotypes)
	Transmission occurs sexually or to newborns during birth
	It is found in the genital tract, anorectal area, and pharynx
	IgA protease
	IgA, IgG, complement (C5-C8), and neutrophils are important in host defense
Signs and Symptoms	**Gonorrhea**—most common reportable bacterial disease in the United States
	• Men: Urethritis with dysuria and purulent discharge
	• Women: asymptomatic or cervicitis that results in purulent vaginal discharge and bleeding
	Ascending infection can cause salpingitis, **pelvic inflammatory disease (PID)**, with risk of infertility, ectopic pregnancies, and may also spread and infect the liver capsule (Fitz-Hugh–Curtis syndrome)
	Disseminated infection includes **septic arthritis** and **pustules**
	Neonatal conjunctivitis can occur when organism is acquired by the newborn during delivery. Risk for blindness!
	Other infections include proctitis and pharyngitis
Diagnosis	Culture and Gram stain of the discharge is performed
	Oxidase-positive diplococci
	In men: gram-negative diplococci within neutrophils in the discharge is diagnostic
	Culture is performed on **Thayer-Martin medium**, which has antibiotics to inhibit normal flora
	Enzyme-linked immunosorbent assay (ELISA), searching for gonococcal antigens and PCR tests for bacterial ribosomal genes are also performed
Treatment	Ceftriaxone is the treatment of choice, with spectinomycin and ciprofloxacin used if the patient is penicillin allergic
	Penicillinase-producing strains have been isolated
	If concurrent *C. trachomatis* infection is suspected (and it usually is), tetracycline is given as well
	Neonatal conjunctivitis is preventable with prophylactic erythromycin eye ointment at birth

Moraxella Catarrhalis

Fast Facts	Gram-negative diplococcus
	Member of the normal flora of the upper respiratory tract
	Common cause of **otitis media** (after *S. pneumoniae* and non-typable *H. influenzae*)
Signs and Symptoms	Otitis media, sinusitis, pneumonia and bronchial infections
	• In children and immunocompromised patients
Diagnosis	Gram stain of sputum or culture
Treatment	TMP/SMX
	Many strains are penicillin resistant

GRAM-POSITIVE RODS

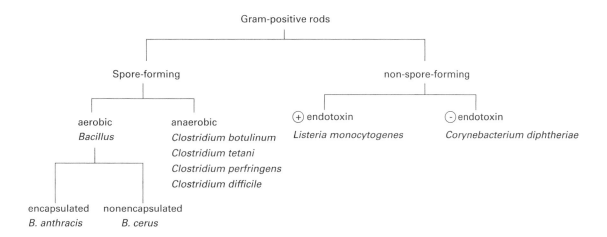

Figure 9 Gram Positive Rods

Bacillus Anthracis

Fast Facts	Non-motile, spore-forming organism
	Spores are present in soil; human infection occurs from spores on animals or animal products
	Entry occurs through the skin, mucous membranes, or respiratory tract
	Unique capsule made of **D-glutamate**; inhibits phagocytosis
	Produces toxin composed of three parts: <ul><li>Edema factor (Adenylate cyclase)</li><li>Lethal factor—cell death</li><li>Protective factor—facilitates the entry of the other two toxin parts into host cells</li></ul>
Signs and Symptoms	**Anthrax**—seen mostly in animals, but sometimes in humans
	Skin abrasions—Symptoms include edema and a black, necrotic painless ulcer known as a malignant pustule.
	Untreated cases result in bacteremia and death
	Inhalation of the spores can cause fatal pneumonia, known as **Woolsorters' disease**
Diagnosis	Gram stain shows bacteria in chains with a protein capsule
Treatment	Penicillin
	Disease transmission can be prevented by proper disposal of dead animals and sterilization of animal products
	Workers at risk should wear masks and protective clothing and can receive vaccination (anti-PA vaccine) against the disease

Bacillus Cereus

Fast Facts	Spore-forming, motile organism
	Resides on grains and is ingested
	Classic test question asks you to associate *B. cereus* with food poisoning after eating reheated fried rice
Signs and Symptoms	Food poisoning of one of two types <ul><li>Heat-stable enterotoxin- Short incubation—develops within 4 hours, characterized by nausea and **vomiting**</li><li>Heath-labile enterotoxin- Long incubation—develops within 18 hours, with associated **diarrhea**</li></ul>
Diagnosis	History
Treatment	Symptomatic treatment of fluid loss and diarrhea

Contains two enterotoxins, which act by unknown mechanisms

Clostridium Tetani

Associate Clostridium "tetani" with a "Tennis" racket

Fast Facts	Anaerobic, spore-forming organism present in the soil
	Microscopically, it resembles a tennis racket, with a terminal spore
	Enters through broken skin and is often seen in IV drug users
	Grows well in necrotic tissue (which has poor blood supply)
	Disease is caused by tetanus toxin, which is made at the wound site and carried by retrograde axonal transport to the CNS
	Toxin blocks the release of inhibitory neurotransmitters, glycine and y-aminobutyric acid (GABA) at spinal synapses of Renshaw cells, causing unopposed hyperexcitability or spastic paralysis.
Signs and Symptoms	**Tetanus** characterized by violent muscle spasms and lockjaw (mouth cannot be opened)
	Patients have exaggerated reflexes and are at severe risk of respiratory failure
Diagnosis	History of injury
	All motor vehicle injuries are presumed to be infected and are treated accordingly
Treatment	Immediate treatment with immune globulin against the toxin is necessary
	Bacteria can be treated with penicillin
	Benzodiazepines are used to prevent spasms
	Prevention, using vaccines with tetanus toxoid booster shots, should be performed every 10 years in adults after they have received the initial series of injections in childhood

Clostridium Botulinum

Fast Facts	Anaerobic, spore-forming organism found in soil
	These spores can contaminate foods, especially beans, raw honey, mushrooms, and smoked fish, that are improperly sterilized and canned
	Bacteria grow in anaerobic conditions and produce preformed toxin, which is then ingested and absorbed into the blood
	Toxin travels to synapses in the peripheral nervous system and blocks acetylcholine release
Signs and Symptoms	**Botulism** is characterized by weakness and flaccid paralysis, including diplopia, dysphagia, and respiratory failure
	Infant botulism, which results in a **Floppy Baby Syndrome** (constipation and flaccid paralysis), may develop from ingestion of raw honey, after which the bacteria grows in the gut and secrete toxin
Diagnosis	Mouse protection assay, in which a mouse is given a serum sample from the patient and dies if toxin is present
Treatment	Immediate antitoxin administration
	Respiratory support
	The toxin is heat-labile, so foods should be heated thoroughly before they are eaten

Clostridium Perfringens

Fast Facts	Anaerobic, spore-forming, non-motile bacteria found in soil and on food
	Part of normal flora of the colon and vagina
	Alpha toxin (lecithinase), which is made by bacteria growing in an infected wound—causes muscle cell necrosis
	Gas is produced by other enzymes in the tissue, resulting in **gas gangrene**
	Enterotoxin is made in the GI tract during sporulation, resulting in **food poisoning**
Signs and Symptoms	**Gas gangrene** occurs in contaminated wounds
	• Cellulitis, pain, edema, hemolysis and skin crackling upon pressure (crepitus) due to gas production of the bacteria
	• Black fluid exudate from skin
	• Associated with high mortality rate
	Food poisoning occurs by bacterial growth in reheated foods, and causes watery diarrhea 8-16 hours after ingestion, which resolves within 24 hours

Diagnosis	Organism can be seen on smear of an exudate
	Anaerobic cultures and tests for sugar fermentation should be done
Treatment	Gas gangrene is treated with penicillin or clindamycin and wound debridement
	Food poisoning requires only supportive care

Clostridium Difficile

Fast Facts	Anaerobic, spore-forming, motile organism
	Part of the normal GI flora in up to 30% of hospitalized patients
	Transmission route is fecal-oral exotoxin A—causes watery diarrhea exotoxin B—causes mucosal damage, resulting in pseudomembrane formation
	• Exotoxin B functions by ADP-ribosylation of protein r, a G protein that regulates actin
	Antibiotic therapy can alter normal flora and allow *C. difficile* overgrowth, resulting in exotoxin formation. A major cause of hospital-acquired diarrhea
Signs and Symptoms	**Pseudomembranous colitis** can develop after broad-spectrum antibiotic therapy especially with clindamycin or aminoglycosides
	Patients experience watery, non-bloody diarrhea
Diagnosis	Exotoxin B can be isolated from stool
	ELISA tests for both exotoxins are available
	Colonoscopy shows pseudomembranes
	Because the toxin is difficult to detect, a minimum of three separate stool samples should be analyzed before ruling out *C. difficile* infection
Treatment	Withdraw causative antibiotic treatment
	Treat with metronidazole or vancomycin

Corynebacterium Diphtheriae

Fast Facts	Non-motile, non-spore-forming, club-shaped rods
	Present in upper respiratory tract
	Transmission occurs by airborne droplets
	Diphtheria toxin causes ADP-ribosylation of EF-2, which results in inactivation and cell death
	• The toxin is produced from a lysogenized bacteriophage-β prophage (Bacteria that do not have the integrated phage are not pathogenic)
	• The host can make antibody to fragment B of the exotoxin (this fragment is necessary for entry into the cell)
Signs and Symptoms	**Diphtheria** results in fibrinous, adherent, gray pseudomembrane over the tonsils and throat
	Patients also experience fever and cervical adenopathy
Diagnosis	Methylene blue stain on smear from a throat swab shows metachromatic granules
	Throat swab cultured on Löffler's coagulated serum, a tellurite plate (which turns from gray black if organism is present), and blood agar
	Toxin production is verified from cultured plates
Treatment	The antitoxin antibodies neutralize unbound toxin
	• The antiserum is made in horses and may cause hypersensitivity problems in sensitized individuals
	Penicillin or erythromycin is used to slow growth of bacteria
	Widespread vaccination with inactivated toxoid (DTaP) has resulted in very low incidence of disease
	Warning: do not try to scrape the pseudomembrane because bleeding and toxin spread can occur!

Listeria Monocytogenes

Fast Facts	Non-spore-forming rod in V or L shapes; tumbling motility via several flagella
	Beta-hemolytic; facultative intracellular
	The only Gram + with **endotoxin**
	Can colonize the GI and female GU tract
	Transmission is via contact with animals or feces, contaminated vegetables, and unpasteurized milk, soft cheeses (the classic test question scenario) and lunch meats
	Transmission can occur to newborns *in utero* or at delivery
	Listeriolysin O—makes holes in membranes
	Suppressed cell-mediated immunity predisposes affected patients to infection
Signs and Symptoms	**Meningitis** and sepsis can develop in newborns and immunocompromised patients
	• Third most common cause of meningitis in newborns (after Group B Streptococcus and *E. coli*)
	Infected mothers are usually asymptomatic
	Can cause spontaneous abortion in pregnancy
Diagnosis	Gram stain and culture
	Culture shows small gray colonies on blood agar as well as beta-hemolysis and tumbling motile organisms
Treatment	Amipicillin and gentamicin
	TMP-SMX

GRAM-NEGATIVE

Escherichia Coli

Fast Facts	Facultative anaerobe, fast lactose fermenter, pili, capsule
	Found in the GI tract, although vaginal colonization may occur
	Transmission route is fecal-oral and can occur during birth
	O (cell wall), H (flagellar) and K (capsule) antigens
	More than 1000 serotypes are possible based on variations in these antigens
	Enterotoxin-producing strains cause watery diarrhea by releasing one or both of the two enterotoxins
	• **Heat-labile enterotoxin**—stimulates adenylate cyclase via ADP-ribosylation of a stimulatory G protein, causing increased cAMP and protein kinase activity, resulting in excretion of electrolytes and fluids (watery diarrhea)
	• **Heat-stable enterotoxin**—stimulates guanylate cyclase, increasing cGMP and decreasing reabsorption of NaCl, water remains in lumen causing watery diarrhea
	Verotoxin (Shiga-like toxin)—made by the 0157:H7 strain
	• Found in undercooked hamburger meat and can cause life-threatening DIC or **hemolytic-uremic syndrome (HUS)**
	Like all gram-negative organisms, contains LPS endotoxin, which causes fever, shock and DIC
Signs and Symptoms	Most common cause of **UTI**—especially in women due to the short female urethra
	Cystitis and pyelonephritis may result from an ascending infection
	Neonatal meningitis may develop from exposure during birth because approximately 25% of women have vaginal colonization (Second most common cause of neonatal meningitis)
	Traveler's Diarrhea—caused by enterotoxigenic *E. coli* (ETEC)—causes self-limited, water, non-bloody diarrhea
	EIEC: Invades intestinal mucosal layer and secretes Shiga-like toxin; causes fever, inflammation, and dysentery.
	Bloody diarrhea, with associated abdominal cramping and fever is caused by enteropathogenic *E. coli*

Associate the "T" in ETEC with Traveler's Diarrhea

Remember the "I" in EIEC indicates it is "Invasive"

Diagnosis	Cultures are performed on blood agar, EMB, and MacConkey agar
	E. coli produces lactose-fermenting pink colonies that are green metallic sheen on EMB agar
Treatment	UTI- TMP/SMX or quinolones
	Sepsis—parenteral cephalosporin's
	Neonatal meningitis—ampicillin and cefotaxime
	Diarrhea treated symptomatically
	Travelers can be given prophylactic doxycycline
	Water supplies are routinely tested for the presence of *E. coli* to avoid fecal contamination

Salmonella Typhi

Fast Facts	Facultative anaerobe found in the GI tract; motile via flagella
	Has O (cell wall; type A-1), H (flagellar; phase 1 and 2) and Vi (virulence) polysaccharide capsule antigens
	Transmission route is fecal-oral from contaminated sources (e.g. food contaminated by animal feces, pet turtles)
	Gastric acidity is an important defense mechanism Enters in the small intestine, multiples in phagocytes of Peyer's patches and travels within phagocytes to the liver, spleen and gallbladder
	3% of infected persons are carriers (like Typhoid Mary!), with asymptomatic colonization in the bladder (esp. in gallstones)
Signs and Symptoms	**Typhoid Fever**—slow onset of fever, malaise, diffuse abdominal pain, and constipation
	1 week after exposure—high fever, delirium, abdominal pain that is either diffuse or mimic appendicitis. May progress to intestinal hemorrhage and perforation causing bloody diarrhea
	Spleen enlargement
	"Rose spots" are rare; consist of red macules on the abdomen
	Osteomyelitis in sickle cell children

Diagnosis	Gram stain and culture from blood are performed on EMB and MacConkey agar
	Colorless, non-lactose-fermenting colonies oxidase negative; produces H_2S
	Agglutination tests with anti-sera for O, H, Vi antigens
Treatment	Ceftriaxone is used, as are ciprofloxacin, ampicillin and TMP/SMX
	Can develop resistance to chloramphenicol and ampicillin by plasmid-encoded genes
	Cholecystectomy can be performed to treat the carrier
	Vaccines are available but give limited protection

Salmonella Enteritidis

Fast Facts	Similar to *S. typhi*
	Facultative anaerobe in the GI tract; motile via flagella
	Has O, H, and Vi antigens
	Transmission is fecal-oral from contaminated sources such as poultry and eggs; pet turtles
	Ingestion of at least 100,000 organisms is needed for disease
	Gastric acidity is an important defense mechanism
	Disease-causing strains invade the mucosa to the lamina propria; resulting in inflammation and diarrhea
Signs and Symptoms	Enterocolitis
	Incubation is 6–48 hours, during which the patient develops nausea, vomiting, abdominal pain, diarrhea
	Usually self-limiting
	Sepsis with metastatic abscesses can occur, although rare
	Osteomyelitis—seen in sickle cell patients
Diagnosis	Gram's stain and culture from stool samples on EMB and
	MacConkey agar show colorless, non-lactose-fermenting colonies
	oxidase negative, Produce H_2S
	Agglutination tests can be performed for known antigens
Treatment	Enterocolitis can be treated conservatively
	Severe infection requires ceftriaxone

Shigella Dysenteriae and Shigella Sonnei

Fast Facts	Non-motile, facultative anaerobe
	Found in the GI tract (always pathogenic- not part of normal flora)
	Transmission route is fecal-oral by the four F's:
	• Fingers, flies, food, feces
	Very virulent—ingestion of only 10–100 organisms is needed for disease
	Cell wall O antigen divides the genus into four groups:
	• A, B, C, D
	Shiga toxin—inactivates 60S ribosomes; can cause HUS like EHEC
	Invades the mucosa of the distal ileum and colon which results in inflammation and ulceration
Signs and Symptoms	**Enterocolitis** develops with a 1–4 day incubation
	• Fever, abdominal cramps, bloody diarrhea
	• Young children and elderly get more severe disease
	S. sonnei causes milder disease
Diagnosis	Gram stain and culture from stool sample on EMB and MacConkey agar show colorless, non-lactose-fermenting colonies
	Oxidase negative; does not produce H_2S
	Methylene blue stain of the stool sample reveals neutrophils in invasive disease
Treatment	Ciprofloxacin and TMP/SMX may be used
	Resistance to multiple antibiotics is common
	Antibiotics may prolong shedding
	Otherwise, conservative therapy is used

Vibrio Cholerae

Fast Facts	Comma-shaped, gram-negative rod; motile via a single flagella
	Both human and marine reservoirs
	Transmitted via fecal-oral route by contaminated food, water, or undercooked shellfish
	An asymptomatic carrier state exists
	Adherence to the small intestine is dependent on a mucinase enzyme—dissolves glycoprotein in intestinal cells
	Organisms then multiples and make two subunit toxin known as *choleragen* (AB_5 toxin) • A subunit: ADP-ribosylates G protein causing chronic activation of adenylate cyclase and increased cAMP, chloride ion, and water secretion • B subunit: binds a receptor on the enterocyte
Signs and Symptoms	Watery diarrhea ("rice water stools") with no associated blood or abdominal pain
	Death occurs from dehydration and electrolyte imbalance if left untreated
Diagnosis	Colorless colonies are seen on MacConkey agar
	Oxidase-positive, glucose fermenter
	Comma-shaped Gram stain—rods with a single flagella in stool culture
	Flat yellow/orange colonies on TCBS agar
	Agglutination tests with antiserum to O antigen are performed
Treatment	Fluid and electrolyte replacement is critical
	Tetracycline may shorten the duration of illness or eliminate the carrier state
	Currently available vaccine is not very effective

Vibrio Parahaemolyticus

Fast Facts	Marine organism transmitted through improperly cooked seafood
	Makes enterotoxin similar to choleragen from *V. cholera* and is a major cause of diarrhea in Japan due to raw seafood consumption
Signs and Symptoms	Patients develop explosive watery diarrhea, nausea, vomiting and abdominal cramps. Sometimes fever also develops.
	Symptoms are self-limited and typically last 3 days
Diagnosis	Distinguished from *V. cholera* by its ability to grow in 8% NaCl
Treatment	Symptomatic only

Campylobacter Jejuni

Fast Facts	Microaerophilic, motile, comma-shaped or S-shaped rods, polar flagellum
	Domestic animals and humans are the reservoirs
	Transmission is fecal-oral or ingestion of unpasteurized milk; Carried by poultry, cattle, domestic animals
	Pathogenesis is unclear, but some strains make an entero-toxin similar to choleragen and cytotoxin
	Tissue invasion occurs, results in bloody diarrhea
Signs and Symptoms	Ill-smelling, watery diarrhea, nausea, vomiting, and abdominal cramps. May be followed by bloody diarrhea
	May be associated with Guillian-Barré Syndrome
	Systemic infection, seen in neonates and adults in poor health is caused by *C. intestinalis*
Diagnosis	Stool sample is cultured on a blood agar plate with antibiotics (Skirrow's agar) to inhibit normal flora
	Urease negative
Treatment	Symptomatic therapy
	Erythromycin or ciprofloxacin

Incubation is done at 42°C "Camp fires are HOT!"

Helicobacter Pylori

Fast Facts	Curved, gram-negative rods; motile via polar flagellum
	Resemble *Campylobacter* in many ways
	Natural habitat is the stomach; transmission is likely oral
	Attaches to gastric mucosa, causing inflammation
	Contains **urease** enzyme, which makes ammonia from urea, resulting in increased pH (i.e. less acidity) to protect itself from gastric acid
	Inflammation and ammonia cause mucosal damage

Signs and Symptoms	**Gastritis** (esp. antral gastritis in U.S.) • Watery diarrhea, nausea, vomiting, and abdominal cramps Peptic ulcers: **duodenal > gastric** Chronic gastritis can lead to gastric adenocarcinoma and MALT. Systemic infection, seen in neonates and adults in poor health is caused by *C. intestinalis*
Diagnosis	Gram stain and culture of a biopsy specimen Urease-positive (unlike *C. jejuni*, which is urease-negative) Radiolabeled urea breath test can be performed, in which labeled CO_2 is expelled if bacteria are present
Treatment	Triple therapy is needed for eradication: • Amoxicillin • Metronidazole • Bismuth subsalicylate (Pepto-Bismol)

Klebsiella Pneumoniae

Fast Facts	Encapsulated, gram-negative rod, non-motile Found in upper respiratory and GI tracts Transmission to lungs occurs by aspiration or inhalation Transmission to the GU tract can occur by ascending infection from fecal flora Large capsule has a **mucoid appearance** and inhibits phagocytosis Endotoxin is also present in the cell wall
Signs and Symptoms	Pneumonia • Especially right upper lobe due to aspiration in **alcoholics**. • Also seen in patients with weakened immune systems (i.e. diabetics) Both community-acquired and hospital acquired pneumonia can occur • Product of thick and bloody "**currant-jelly**" sputum due to necrotizing lung tissue (abscesses) Less common: UTIs, meningitis, sepsis
Diagnosis	Colored, lactose-fermenting, mucoid-like colonies grow on EMB or MacConkey agar Urease +, indole -
Treatment	Antibiotic resistance is common Empiric treatment with gentamicin and cefotaxime is given until cultures are tested for specific sensitivities

Proteus Mirabilis and Proteus Vulgaris

Fast Facts	Motile via many flagella
	Its motility gives a "swarming" effect on agar and may aid in the spread of infection
	Organisms are found in soil, water, and the human colon
	UTI develops by ascending spread of fecal flora
	Presence of urease results in ammonia production, which causes increased urinary pH; alkaline urine favors stone production ("struvites"), resulting in epithelial damage
Signs and Symptoms	Both community- and hospital-acquired **UTIs** may develop
	Vaginal colonization and urinary catheters predispose to infection
	Less common infections: wound infection, pneumonia, sepsis
Diagnosis	Colorless, non-lactose-fermenting colonies from on EMB agar
	Cultures on blood agar containing phenylethyl-alcohol inhibit swarming
	Indole-negative, phenylalanine deaminase-positive, urease-positive, produces H_2S
	Some O antigens cross-react with antigens from Rickettsiae in what is called the **Weil-Felix reaction**—used in laboratory screening for antirickettsial antibody
Treatment	Ampicillin

Pseudomonas Aeruginosa

Fast Facts	Strict aerobe that flourish in moist environments, has a capsule, pili, motile via flagella
	Very resistant to disinfectants
	Found in soil and water; 10% of people carry it in the colon, oropharynx, or on the skin
	Transmission occurs via respiratory droplets, contact with burned skin, fecal contamination or aspiration
	Nosocomial infections: contaminate hospital equipment and fluids easily (i.e. respiratory equipment, endoscopes)
	Synthesizes exotoxin A—inhibits protein synthesis via ADP-ribosylation of EF-2 (like C. diphtheriae).
	Endotoxin → shock and fever
	Makes pigments **pyocyanin** (which turns pus blue) and **pyoverdin** (fluorescent under UV light)
	Makes a slime layer called **glycocalyx**—adherence to mucosa

Signs and Symptoms	Opportunistic pathogen
	Commonly: nosocomial UTIs, pneumonia in cystic fibrosis, infection in wound and burn infections, the immunocompromised and patients with indwelling catheters
	Sepsis can develop from any of these causes and carries a 50% mortality rate. May see black lesions on the skin
	Other infections: Endocarditis (esp. IVDUs), Osteomyelitis (diabetics), external otitis media, folliculitis, osteochondritis of the foot, resulting from puncture wounds through shoes and corneal infections in contact lens wearers
Diagnosis	Colorless, non-lactose-fermenting colonies form on EMB and MacConkey agar
	Oxidase-positive and forms a metallic sheen on TSI agar
	Noted for its blue-green pigment and fruity aroma
Treatment	Ticarcillin + gentamicin
	Resistance is common and can arise during therapy

Bacteroides Fragilis

Fast Facts	Strict anaerobe, non spore forming, has large capsule
	Predominant organism in the colon 60% of women have vaginal colonization
	Transmission is endogenous from a break in the GI mucosal surface and requires a predisposing factor for disease such as surgery or trauma
Signs and Symptoms	**Peritonitis** or localized abdominal **abscesses** are the most common infections
	Others include pelvic or lung abscesses or bacteremia
Diagnosis	Growth occurs under anaerobic conditions on blood agar plates with kanamycin and vancomycin
Treatment	Resistance to multiple antibiotics is common
	Metronidazole or third generation cephalosporins are typically used
	Aminoglycosides are given to treat mixed infections
	Abscesses require drainage
	Cefoxitin is often given as prophylaxis before GI surgery

Haemophilus Influenzae

Fast Facts	Encapsulated coccobacillus with several serotypes
	Serotype b is the most pathogenic, causing meningitis in young children
	Transmission is by airborne droplets
	IgA protease
	Causes upper respiratory tract illnesses such as pneumonia, otitis media and sinusitis
	Asplenic patients (e.g., those with sickle-cell disease) are susceptible
	In chronic smokers—may cause exacerbations of chronic bronchitis
	In young children—may cause epiglottitis leading to fatal airway obstruction
Signs and Symptoms	Meningitis: • Leading cause of meningitis in children 6 mos-6 yrs (after S. pneumoniae and N. meningitides). Decreased in recent years due to childhood vaccination
	Pneumonia or other respiratory tract infections
	Epiglottitis presents with dysphagia, inspiratory stridor and excessive drooling. "Thumbprint" sign on X-ray
	Otitis media
	Other systemic infections: septic arthritis and cellulitis
Diagnosis	Culture and Gram stain of sputum or CSF is performed; otherwise, it is treated empirically
	Growth occurs on chocolate agar supplemented with **factors V** (NAD) and **X** (heme)
	Quellung reaction is used to ascertain encapsulation, and serotypes are determined by fluorescent antibody and agglutination tests
Treatment	Common upper respiratory tract infections are treated with ampicillin or TMP/SMX
	Meningitis must be treated promptly with third generation cephalosporin
	If left untreated, fatality rate exceeds 90%
	Current recommendations suggest that all infants less than 1 year of age should receive vaccination with type b antigen coupled with diphtheria toxoid
	Epiglottitis is a medical emergency and requires intubation to preserve the airway plus IV cephalosporin's
	Give rifampin to close contacts as prophylaxis

Legionella Pneumophila

Fast Facts	Gram-negative rods with pili
	Facultative intracellular organism
	Once phagocytized by alveolar macrophages, it proliferates and prevents phagolysosome fusion.
	Transmission occurs through airborne droplets
	Habitat is environmental water sources such as air conditioners and cooling towers (person to person spread does not occur)
	Typical host is usually predisposed by being immunocompromised or having a chronic illness
	Elderly men who smoke and drink are also at risk
Signs and Symptoms	**Legionnaire's disease** is an atypical pneumonia; can present with unusual symptoms such as diarrhea, confusion and proteinuria. Nonproductive cough has many neutrophils
	Pontiac fever is a milder flu-like illness that lasts 2–5 days
Diagnosis	Sputum shows neutrophils and few bacteria
	Visualized by silver stain
	Charcoal yeast extract culture growth with iron and cysteine added
	Diagnosis is made by an increase in antibody titer in convalescing patients or by detection of antigens in urine
Treatment	Erythromycin

Bordetella Pertussis

Fast Facts	Small, aerobic coccibacillus with filamentous hemagglutinin (FHA)—facilitates adherence to ciliated epithelium
	• Once anchored to the cilia, tracheal cytotoxin is released causing the cilia to stop beating → whooping cough
	Transmitted by respiratory air droplets
	Other toxins
	• Pertussis toxin—ADP-ribosylation of G_i protein, blocking inactivation of adenylate cyclase, resulting in increased cAMP → lymphocytosis
	• Bacterial adenylate cyclase—taken up by phagocytes and inhibits their activity
	Pertussis infection is largely prevented by vaccination as part of the DPT vaccine during childhood
	Both a killed bacteria and acellular toxoid vaccine are available
Signs and Symptoms	**Whooping cough**—primarily in children
	• Onset is usually mild symptoms, but most contagious (first 1–2 weeks), which progress to paroxysmal cough and the production of large amounts of mucus
	Symptoms may last for several weeks to months and can progress to pneumonia, which can be fatal
Diagnosis	Culture from a nasopharyngeal swab is placed on a Bordet-Gengou agar plate (consisting of 20–30% blood agar)
	Agglutination and fluorescent antibody test are also performed
Treatment	Prophylaxis with DTaP vaccine in children
	Erythromycin decreases the incidence of secondary complications but does not alter disease course because respiratory mucosa is already damaged
	Oxygen therapy and frequent suctioning are used as supportive care

Zoonotic Bacteria

Brucella Species

Fast Facts	Specifically *B. melitensis*, *B. abortus*, and *B. suis*, are aerobic, facultative intracellular gram-negative rods that can cause undulant fever Found in domestic livestock • *B. melitensis* in goats and sheep • *B. abortus* in cattle • *B. suis* in pigs Transmission occurs by ingestion of contaminated milk products or through the skin Classic patient is an animal handler or a traveler who has consumed unpasteurized milk or cheese products Infection can be prevented by pasteurization of milk and cheese products and livestock vaccination
Signs and Symptoms	**Undulant fever** (or brucellosis) is caused by infection of the reticuloendothelial system, including lymph nodes, spleen, liver, and bone marrow • Fever, diaphoresis, weakness, fatigue, lymphadenopathy, and splenomegaly • Fever undulates daily with a slow rise in temperature through the day, a temperature peak at night, and a return to normal temperature by morning • Symptoms last from months to years • Complications include osteomyelitis, endocarditis and caseating granulomas and abscess formation
Diagnosis	**Brucella** is cultured in enriched medium and 10% CO_2 Slide agglutination and serum antibody tests are used for diagnosis
Treatment	Tetracycline and gentamicin

Francisella Tularensis

Fast Facts	Pleomorphic, facultative intracellular, gram-negative rod
	Found in animals such as rabbits, deer, and rodents in most areas of the U.S.
	Transmission occurs between animals by lice, mites, and ticks, especially *Dermacentor* ticks (like R. rickettsii)
	Transmission to humans occurs from a bite by a vector or contact with the hide of an infected animal
	Skin entry leads to lymph node infection; potentially causing abscesses or ulceration
	Inhalation can cause pneumonia, and ingestion of infected mean can cause GI disease
Signs and Symptoms	**Tularemia** can be sudden and flu-like or prolonged
	May be an ulcer with a black base at the entry site and swollen, painful regional lymph nodes
	Other manifestations include conjunctiva, pulmonary, and GI
Diagnosis	Cultures are not usually done due to the high risk of laboratory worker inhalation
	Agglutination test with serum samples and a skin test similar to PPD are performed
Treatment	Streptomycin
	Live attenuated vaccine for the high risk

Yersinia Pestis

Fast Facts	Small, encapsulated (F-1 antigen), bipolar-staining organism with a clear central area
	Bubonic Plague—Endemic in wild rodents in Europe and Asia and in prairie dogs in the United States
	Transmission occurs with passage between wild rodents and fleas
	The rodents are generally asymptomatic carriers from which the fleas obtain the organism after a blood meal; bacteria then multiple in the flea and are regurgitated during the next meal
	Humans are accidental hosts
	Transmission via respiratory droplets may occur if the organism has invaded the bloodstream and causes abscess formation in the lung
	Infection can be prevented by avoiding dead rodents
	People in high risk occupations may be vaccinated with a killed bacteria vaccine
Signs and Symptoms	**Bubonic plague**—high fever, myalgias, painful swollen lymph nodes known as buboes
	Septic shock and death develop in more than half of untreated cases
	Pneumonic plague—characterized by lung abscesses that can develop from inhalation or bacteremia. Chest pain, difficulty breathing, blood-tinged cough
Diagnosis	Gram stain and cultures from blood or a bubo are done
	Giemsa or Wayson stain is best for demonstrating bipolar staining (looks like safety pin)
	Serology and immunofluorescence are also done
Treatment	Streptomycin

Pasteurella Multocida

Fast Facts	Short, coccobacilli, pleomorphic, bipolar-staining organism that is part of the normal oral flora of cats and dogs
	Humans are infected by animal bites, which cause localized **cellulitis** or even **osteomyelitis** if the bone is injured during the bite
Signs and Symptoms	Cellulitis Osteomyelitis Sutures may act as a nidus of infection and cause worsened cellulitis
Diagnosis	Wound culture Oxidase +; catalase +
Treatment	Penicillin G Clean and drain wound site. Animal bites should not be sutured

Also *Borrelia burgdorferi* (under spirochetes section)

OBLIGATE INTRACELLULAR

Chlamydia Trachomatis

Fast Facts	Obligate intracellular Gram-negative. Steals ATP from host cell for survival. No peptidoglycan or muramic acid Life cycle has two forms: • **Elementary body (EB)**—non-replicating, round infectious particles inside cytoplasmic inclusion bodies. Once cell bursts, and EB infects another host cell. Prevents phago-lysosomal fusion. • **Reticulate body**—forms once an EB enters the cell via endocytosis. The EB germinate to become a reticulate body and replicates by binary fusion. These are larger particles that require ATP, and then form into EB particles once again. Several serotypes: • A,B & C- trachoma • D-K: urethritis, PID, neonatal pneumonia, neonatal conjunctivitis • L1,L2, and L3: lymphogranuloma venereum Most frequent cause of bacterial STI in the U.S. Most common cause of blindness worldwide
Signs and Symptoms	**Trachoma**—chronic conjunctivitis that can lead to corneal vascularization and scarring. Inversion of eyelashes worsens scarring leading to blindness. (esp. in Africa.) **Urethritis** • Females: ascend to fallopian tubes and cause **PID**—increases risk of ectopic pregnancy. Spread to peritoneal cavity may cause **Fitz-Hugh—Curtis** • Males: can also develop prostatitis and epididymitis • Other complications: Reiter's syndrome (conjunctivits urethritis, and arthritis) **Neonatal conjunctivitis**—acquired through birth canal. Purulent yellow discharge and swollen eyelids comes 5–14 days postpartum. **Neonatal pneumonia**—acquired through birth canal. Symptoms develop 4–11 weeks postpartum. **Lymphogranuloma venereum (LGV)**—Sexually transmitted causing painless ulcer at site of infection that heals but bacteria spreads to local lymph nodes → buboes form and drain pus.

Diagnosis	Nucleic acid amplification tests (NAAT)
	Intracellular growth cultures have largely been replaced by NAATs
	Frei test for LGV
Treatment	Doxycycline (contraindicated in pregnant women)
	Erythromycin in neonates and pregnant women. Also used prophylactically as eye drops in neonates.
	Azithromycin

Chlamydia Psittaci

Fast Facts	Life cycle similar to *C. trachomatis*
	Reservoir birds (i.e. parrots)
	Bird feces shed bacteria and spread via aerosol → enters upper respiratory tract, causing atypical pneumonia
Signs and Symptoms	**Atypical pneumonia**- fever, dry cough
Diagnosis	Serology (immunofluorescence tests)
Treatment	Doxycycline

Rickettsia Rickettsii

Fast Facts	Obligate intracellular
	Reservoir in dogs and rodents- transmission via wood tick (Dermacentor) → infects endothelial cells of small blood vessels
	Rocky Mountain spotted fever
Signs and Symptoms	**Rocky Mountain spotted fever**—fever, conjunctivitis, severe headache, maculo-papular rash on palms & soles that spread toward the trunk.
Diagnosis	Direct immunofluorescent test on skin biopsy
	Positive Weil-Felix test
Treatment	Doxycycline
	Chloramphenicol

Other Rickettsia Species

Fast Facts	*R. prowazekii*—carried on flying squirrels and humans; transmitted by human body louse. Causes **epidemic typhus** *R. typhi*—carried on rats and transmitted by rat fleas. Causes **endemic typhus** *R. tsutsugamushi*—from rodents to humans via mite larvae (chiggers). Causes **Scrub typhus** *Coxiella burnetii*—from cattle, sheep, and goats that shed endospores from cow hide or dried placenta. Can also acquire from consumption of contaminated un-pasteurized milk. Causes **Q fever** *Ehrlichia*—From deer, dogs and coyotes transmitted to humans via ticks (Ixodes). Causes human **Erlichiosis**
Signs and Symptoms	**Epidemic typhus** (R. prowazekii)—rash that spares palms, soles and face; abrupt fever and headache. Can lead to vascular necrosis, which can also cause CNS changes (delirium/stupor) and gangrene **Endemic typhus** (R. typhi)—fever, headache and rash (starts and trunk then to extremities but spares palms and soles **Scrub typhus** (R. tsutsugamushi)—fever, headache, eschar at bite site then rash **Q fever** (Coxiella burnetii)—Fever, headache and atypical pneumonia. NO RASH **Erlichiosis**—Similar to rocky mountain spotted fever, but rarely get rash
Diagnosis	Weil-Felix reaction positive: R. prowazekii, R. typhi, R. tsutsugamushi PCR for Coxiella burnetii and Ehrlichia Ehrlichial inclusion bodies in leukocytes in blood smears
Treatment	Doxycycline

CELL WALL VARIABLES

Mycobacterium Tuberculosis

Fast Facts	**Mycolic acid cell wall**; non-motile; no pili; aerobic
	Acid-fast staining
	Facultative intracellular growth
	Virulence factors: Cord factor, sulfatides, wax D, iron siderophore
	Transmission through aerosol droplets
	Ghon complex—granulomas called Ghon focus (lower lobes) with calcified hilar nodes. Seen in primary infections
	Primary TB—Lower lobes; Ghon complexes; lives and proliferates in macrophages; caseous granulomas → calcified scars. Can spread via lymphatics and blood to other organs. PPD positive test
	Secondary TB—reactivation of dormant TB; apex of the lungs (more O_2); caseous granulomas that cause lung cavitations. Dissemination can cause military TB
Signs and Symptoms	**Primary TB**—asymptomatic or symptomatic
	• Asymptomatic—bacteria are walled off inside caseous granulomas and eventually heal with fibrosis and calcification (Ghon focus). Ghon complexes
	• Symptomatic—more common in children and immunocompromised Atypical pneumonia
	Secondary TB—Chronic low-grade fever, night sweats, weight loss, and productive cough (may contain blood). Can disseminate to CNS, pericarditis, vertebral bodies (Pott's disease), lymph nodes kidneys, skeletal, joints. Also, can cause military TB
Diagnosis	Acid-fast stain of sputum
	PPD test
	Ghon complexes on X-ray
Treatment	Isoniazid (INH)
	Rifampin
	Pyrazinamide
	Ethambutol
	Streptomycin

Mycobacterium Leprae

Fast Facts	Mycolic acid cell wall; non-motile; no pili; obligate aerobe; facultative intracellular
	Acid-fast staining; grows in low temperatures; phenolase +
	Causes leprosy (tuberculoid or lepromatous leprosy)
	Can spread via respiratory secretions or contact with skin lesions → infects skin (cooler areas like tip of nose and superficial nerves, testes). Pathogenesis depends on host immune system
Signs and Symptoms	**Tuberculoid leprosy**—Occurs in people with intact cell- mediated immunity. May develop one to two skin lesions that are hypopigmented and hairless. En-larged nerves near the lesions may be palpable
	Lepromatous leprosy—Occurs in the immunocompromised. More severe symptoms. Thickened skin nodules all over body, leonine facies (face looks like a lion), destruction of nasal cartilage, involved testes can lead to infertility, blindness, sensory loss in the face and extremities
Diagnosis	Skin and nerve biopsy: acid-fast bacilli (lepromatous) or granulomas (tuberculoid)
	Cultures in mouse footpad or armadillo
	Lepromin skin test (+ in tuberculoid –in lepromatous)
Treatment	Combination: dapsone, rifampin, and clofazamine

Mycoplasma Pneumoniae

Fast Facts	**No cell wall**; pleomorphic; motile; facultative anaerobe
	Contains **cholesterol** in the membrane
	CXR looks worse than symptoms. Also known as "walking pneumonia"
	Transmission through respiratory droplets
	Protein P1: causes adherence to epithelial cells of the respiratory tract and destroys the mucosa by inhibiting cilia motion
	IgM cold agglutinin
	Common in military bases and prison
Signs and Symptoms	**Atypical pneumonia** (walking pneumonia)—Mostly seen in younger people. Fever, dry cough, and headache **Tracheobronchitis**
Diagnosis	Cold agglutinins (4 C)
	Growth on Eaton's agar—fried egg appearance
Treatment	Erythromycin or tetracycline

SPIROCHETES

Borrelia Burgdorferi

Fast Facts	Gram-negative spirochete; motile
	Reservoir include white-footed mouse and deer; Vector is tick Ixodes
	Causes **Lyme disease** (most common vector-borne disease)
Signs and Symptoms	Lyme disease
	Three stages:
	1. Stage 1—erythema chronicum migrans, flu-like symptoms
	2. Stage 2—Neurologic (Bell's palsy, peripheral neuropathy), Cardio (carditis, AV nodal block), and joint pain (esp. knee)
	3. Stage 3—Chronic arthritis, encephalopathy, skin atrophy
Diagnosis	Skin biopsy → dark field microscopy
	ELISA
Treatment	Doxycycline or amoxicillin
	Ceftriaxone if involves CNS

Treponema Pallidum

Fast Facts	Gram-negative spirochete; motile (endoflagellum)
	Causes **syphilis**
	Infects humans only; sexually transmitted disease and a **TORCH** infection
Signs and Symptoms	Syphilis
	• 1 (6 weeks after exposure)—painless chancre
	• 2 (6 weeks after healing)—dissemination causing macular red lesions throughout body, including palms and soles. Lesions may form condyloma lata in moist areas (i.e. vulva and scrotum). Other organ involvement and lymphadenopathy
	• 3 (years later)—Gummas, aortitis, tabes dorsalis (neurosyphilis), meningitis, Argyll Robertson pupil
	Congenital syphilis—CN VIII deafness, saber shins, saddle nose, Hutchinson's teeth, mulberry molars, "snuffles" which are blood tinged nasal secretions, stillbirth
Diagnosis	Dark field microscopy
	VDRL—detects antibodies to beef cardiolipin. Nonspecific and can give false positives.
	FTA-ABS—more specific since it detects anti-treponemal antibodies
Treatment	Penicillin G

GRAM-VARIABLE

Gardnerella Vaginalis (Bacterial Vaginosis)

Fast Facts	Gram-variable; pleomophic; facultative anaerobic
	Causes **vaginitis**. Can be due to a disruption of normal vaginal flora
	Likes to grow in a more alkaline environment. The vagina is normally acidic so when there is a disruption in the vaginal flora causing a more alkaline environment, it becomes favorable for *G. vaginalis*
	Not considered an STI
	Clue cells—vaginal epithelial cells surrounded by the bacteria
Signs and Symptoms	**Vaginitis**—vaginal discharge (grayish) with a "fishy" odor and pruritis
Diagnosis	Clue cells
	Clinical history
Treatment	Metronidazole

BRANCHING BACTERIA

Nocardia

Fast Facts	Gram-positive rods that are branching; beaded filaments
	Weak acid-fast staining; obligate aerobe
	Found in soil and transmitted by inhalation
	Immunocompromised are susceptible
Signs and Symptoms	Nocardiosis:
	pneumonia, brain abscess, CNS (headache, lethargy, confusion, seizures), cellulitis
Diagnosis	Gram +, aerobic, beaded filaments
	Weakly acid-fast
Treatment	TMP-SMX

Actinomyces Israelii

Fast Facts	Gram +; beaded filaments
	NOT acid-fast; anaerobe; sulfur granules
	Normal oral flora, GI and vagina
	Known as the most misdiagnosed disease because it can resemble tumors
Signs and Symptoms	Actinomycosis • Formation of abscesses and empyema, tissue fibrosis, and formation of drainage sinuses. Most commonly involves the mouth and face, but can also involve the thorax, abdominopelvic and CNS. • Can spread hematogenously
Diagnosis	Gram +, anaerobic
	Beaded filaments with yellow sulfur granules
Treatment	Penicillin G

yellow sand granules of Israelli

VIROLOGY

Introduction

Viruses are obligate intracellular parasites that require host cells to replicate. They consist of nucleic acids surrounded by a protein capsid. The genome can be either DNA or RNA and can be single or double-stranded. Viruses are usually haploid (one copy of each gene), with the exception of retroviruses, which are diploid. The majority of viruses have either an icosahedral (20 equilateral triangular sides) or helical capsid. Viral RNA is either a positive-sense/plus-strand or negative-sense/minus-strand. Positive sense RNA can be directly translated into protein, as if it is viral mRNA whereas negative-sense RNA requires an extra step and needs to be made into positive sense via RNA polymerase before it can be translated. The genome and capsid may be surrounded by a lipoprotein envelope.

Viral lytic and lysogenic cycles are described below. Lysogenic viruses are able to integrate their DNA into the host cell for a period of time and remain latent. When they excise, they can convert back to the lytic cycle. Viruses also produce a cytopathic effect (CPE) on cells, which causes them to deform in a specific way. Light microscopy can reveal inclusion bodies (areas of high virus concentration) and giant cells (cell fusion caused by the virus). Specific tests for viral antigens or antibodies are used for diagnosis.

Virus	Type of vaccine
Adenovirus	Live attenuated
Hepatitis A	Killed
Hepatitis B	Recombinant protein
Influenza	Killed
Measles	Live attenuated
Mumps	Live attenuated
Polio	Live (OPV) and killed (IPV)
Rabies	Killed
Rubella	Live attenuated
Smallpox	Live attenuated
Varicella-zoster	Live attenuated
Yellow fever	Live attenuated

OPV = live oral poliovirus vaccine; IPV = inactivated poliovirus vaccine
Table 3 Vaccines and viruses

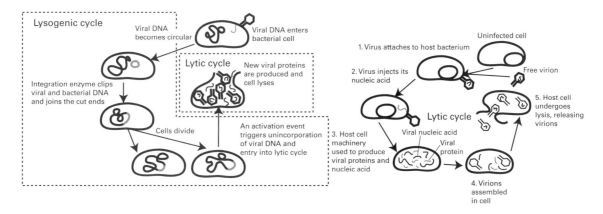

Figure 10 Lysogenic and Lytic Life Cycles

Vaccinations for viral diseases can be made from live, attenuated virus, killed virus, or recombinant viral protein. Live virus vaccinations result in a stronger immune response and longer-lasting memory. The virus can regain virulence within the host, however, causing disease, especially in immunocompromised individuals. Thus, live vaccines should be avoided in certain vulnerable populations, such as pregnant women and HIV patients. A killed virus vaccine induces a weaker immune response but cannot revert to virulence. Finally, passive immunity may be provided by immune globulin and is given to exposed persons at high risk for developing disease.

Virus Classification

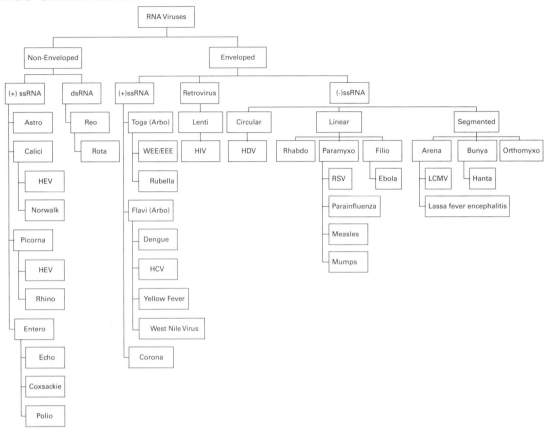

Figure 11 RNA Viruses

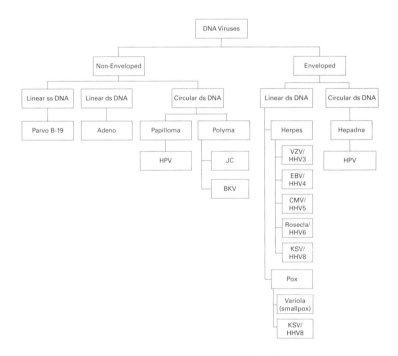

Figure 12 DNA Viruses Classification

HERPES VIRUSES

Herpes-Simplex Virus 1

Herpes simplex virus 1 (HSV-1) is a double-stranded DNA virus commonly seen in children. Patients who are infected develop recurrent lesions that can be triggered by sunlight, stress, and other infections. Transmission occurs by contact with the infected vesicle. The virus has the ability to reside in a latent state located in the sensory ganglia.

Signs & Symptoms	Diagnosis	Treatment
HSV-1 causes herpes labialis (cold sores), gingivostomatitis & keratoconjuctivitis. Complications include blindness & encephalitis. Most common cause of viral encephalitis in US!	Cell cultures shows CPE & multinucleated giant cells. Tzanck smear is positive in all herpesvirus infections. Serology & immunofluorescence can be used for diagnosis of primary infections.	Acyclovir

Herpes-Simplex Virus 2

HSV-2 is a double-stranded DNA virus that is sexually transmitted and causes genital, anal, or oral infection, which is dependent on the mode of transmission. Like HSV-1, recurrences are common, and the virus resides in the sensory ganglia in a latent state.

Signs & Symptoms	Diagnosis	Treatment
HSV-2 causes genital herpes, with painful vesicular genital, anal, or oral lesions. Neonatal herpes can develop in the newborns of mothers with active lesions. Neonatal encephalitis and congenital defects. A ToRCHeS infection.	As with HSV-1, cell culture shows CPE, multinucleated giant cells, and a positive Tzanck smear. Serology and fluorescent antibodies are used for viral detection.	Acyclovir shortens duration of recurrence and reduces viral shedding.

Varicella Zoster Virus

Varicella-zoster virus (VZV) is a double-stranded DNA virus that causes chickenpox in children and shingles in adults. It is transmitted by respiratory droplets and causes disease, which is generally more severe in older patients. As with other herpes viruses, the virus can remain latent in the sensory ganglia and reactivate later in life, resulting in **shingles**. Exposure to VZV in pregnant women can result in severe congenital birth defects and may cause fetal death. A live, attenuated VZV immunization is now available and is recommended for all children.

Signs & Symptoms	Diagnosis	Treatment
Three weeks after primary exposure, chickenpox develops with fever and malaise, followed by a pruritic vesicular rash that spreads from the trunk to the extremities and face. Rash looks like dew drops on a rose petal. Severe infections can progress to encephalitis and pneumonia. Shingles manifests by the development of vesicles along a sensory nerve dermatome, usually on the trunk or face. The lesions may last for several weeks to months and are very painful.	Clinical inspection. Tzanck smear shows multinucleated giant cells. Serology and immunofluorescent antibodies may also be used.	Conservative management, although aspirin should not be given to children because of the possibility of Reye's syndrome (potentially lethal with encephalopathy and liver failure). Severe cases of VZV are treated with acyclovir. Pregnant women who are exposed should receive varicella immune globulin.

Cytomegalovirus

Cytomegalovirus (CMV) is a common double-stranded DNA virus that usually causes asymptomatic infection. However, it can be lethal in immunosuppressed populations, such as transplant recipients, newborns, and acquired immunodeficiency syndrome (AIDS) patients. It is transmissible in all bodily fluids and is present in infected donor organs.

Signs & Symptoms	Diagnosis	Treatment
In fetuses and infants, CMV causes cytomegalic inclusion disease. Newborns with the disease have a "blueberry muffin" rash, with jaundice, petechiae, and growth retardation. Mental retardation, blindness, and hearing loss are common sequelae. In adults, CMV causes heterophil-negative mononucleosis, characterized by fever, lethargy, and abnormal lymphocytes. Can also cause pneumonia, hepatitis, and diarrhea. Common cause of retinitis in AIDS patients.	Cell culture shows a characteristic CPE. Inclusion bodies have an "owl's-eye" appearance. Fluorescent antibodies and serology are performed, although many people are CMV IgG–positive due to past exposure. **Figure 13** CMV Cytopathic Effects (CPE)	Gancyclovir or foscarnet. Immunosuppressed persons should receive CMV-negative blood transfusions.

Epstein-Barr Virus

Epstein-Barr virus (EBV) is a double-stranded DNA virus that is transmitted by saliva and responsible for mononucleosis. EBV is associated with the development of Burkitt's lymphoma in African populations. It has also been associated with nasopharyngeal carcinoma and thymic carcinoma, although the mechanism is not well understood.

Signs & Symptoms	Diagnosis	Treatment
EBV causes infectious mononucleosis, characterized by fever, sore throat, cervical lymphadenopathy, and splenomegaly. It usually resolves within a few weeks but can progress to hepatitis and encephalitis, especially in immunocompromised patients.	Diagnosis is made with the heterophil antibody test (Monospot test). This test takes advantage of the fact that antibodies against EBV cross-react and agglutinate with sheep RBCs. On blood smear, atypical lymphocytes with a large, lobulated nucleus and basophilic cytoplasm are present.	Avoid contact sports due to risk of splenic rupture.

Human Herpesvirus 6

Human herpesvirus 6 (HHV-6) causes **roseola infantum (sixth disease)**, which is one of the most common causes of infantile febrile seizures. The virus tends to infect infants six months to three years of age.

Signs & Symptoms	Diagnosis	Treatment
After a 10-day incubation period, infants develop an extremely high fever that lasts from three to five days, during which time they are at risk of experiencing a febrile seizure. As the fever subsides, a transient rash develops on the trunk.	The history of the disease progression is diagnostic. **Figure 14** Roseola skin lesions	—

Human Herpesvirus 8

Human herpesvirus 8 is putatively linked to **Kaposi's sarcoma**, an AIDS-associated malignancy found predominantly in homosexual men and rarely in elderly white men.

Signs & Symptoms	Diagnosis	Treatment
Kaposi's sarcoma appears as several violet plaques or nodules on the mucous membranes and skin all over the body. It can spread to the GI tract and lungs. Pulmonary Kaposi's sarcoma can be life-threatening.	Symptomatic **Figure 15** Kaposi's sarcoma skin lesion	The underlying immunosuppression (HIV, immunosuppressive medication) is addressed first. Cryotherapy, intralesional chemotherapy, radiation therapy, or laser surgery can be used to treat individual lesions. Intravenous chemotherapy is used for progressive disease.

POX VIRUSES

Variola Virus

The variola virus is a double-stranded DNA virus that causes **smallpox**. It was eradicated in 1977. It had a single stable serotype, which was the key to its eradication because people were vaccinated with a live, attenuated vaccine. Transmission occurred from respiratory droplets or contact with a skin lesion.

Signs & Symptoms	Diagnosis	Treatment
Smallpox was characterized by a sudden fever and rash that began as maculopapular but eventually became vesicular and crusted.	Cell culture (CPE) or immunofluorescence of fluid from the vesicles.	None available

Molluscum Contagiosum Virus

Molluscum contagiosum virus causes a papular lesion that is transmitted by direct skin contact or sexual contact. It can be an early manifestation of an opportunistic infection in HIV.

Signs & Symptoms	Diagnosis	Treatment
The translucent, umbilicated papules can be found on the face and trunk of children. When sexually transmitted, the papules can be found on genitalia.	Diagnosis is usually made by the characteristic appearance of the lesions.	The lesions usually resolve spontaneously in a few years and do not require treatment. Surgery or liquid nitrogen can be used to remove papules.

HEPATITIS VIRUSES

Introduction

The viruses that cause hepatitis come from different families of virus. All are RNA viruses except for the hepatitis B virus. All five viruses can cause **acute viral hepatitis**; HBV, HCV, and HDV are also responsible for **chronic viral hepatitis.**

Hepatitis A Virus

Hepatitis A is a single-stranded RNA virus of the picornavirus family that causes a form of hepatitis commonly seen in children. Transmission is fecal-oral, and patients usually recover without serious sequelae. There is no chronic carrier state. A killed vaccine is currently available to prevent infection in persons traveling to developing countries.

Signs & Symptoms	Diagnosis	Treatment
Most patients are asymptomatic or develop mild hepatitis symptoms, such as jaundice, nausea, and vomiting, which resolves spontaneously after a few weeks. In less than one percent of cases, fulminant hepatitis develops.	Clinical history and IgM and IgG serum antibody tests are used for diagnosis.	None. Immune serum globulin can be administered within two weeks of exposure to close contacts and travelers to endemic regions. A heat-killed vaccine is also available.

Hepatitis B Virus

Hepatitis B virus (HBV) is a double-stranded DNA virus (member of the hepa**dna**virus family) that has three important antigens. The s antigen (**HBsAg**) is a **S**urface antigen on the viral envelope that is used in diagnosis. The c antigen (**HBcAg**) is a nucleocapsid **C**ore antigen that is also used in diagnosis. The e antigen (**HBeAg**), also a nucleocapsid core antigen, is used as an indicator of transmissibility; high levels indicate that the patient is highly inf**E**ctious. The presence of anti-HBsAg antibody is a marker of immunity to the virus, and the presence of anti-HBeAg antibody is an indication of low transmissibility of the virus.

HBV is transmitted via sexual contact, blood or perinatally. There is a high incidence of HBV infection in Asia, and HBV has been associated with the development of **hepatocellular carcinoma.** Approximately 10% of infected persons become chronic carriers. Healthcare workers and persons at increased risk of exposure should receive the recombinant vaccine. Transfusions are routinely screened for HBV.

Signs & Symptoms	Diagnosis	Treatment
Infection with HBV can be asymptomatic but is usually accompanied by jaundice, fever, anorexia, nausea, and vomiting. Incubation period is approximately 12 weeks. Patients may develop arthritis, vasculitis, and glomerulonephritis due to immune complex deposition	Different antigens and antibodies are present at varying times after infection (See figure below). Serum alanine aminotransferase (ALT) and aspartate aminotransferase (AST) are elevated.	Acute hepatitis requires supportive care. Interferon-alpha is given in chronic infections and may decrease hepatocellular damage. Hepatitis B immune globulin can be administered soon after exposure to HBV to greatly reduce chances of acquiring symptomatic disease.

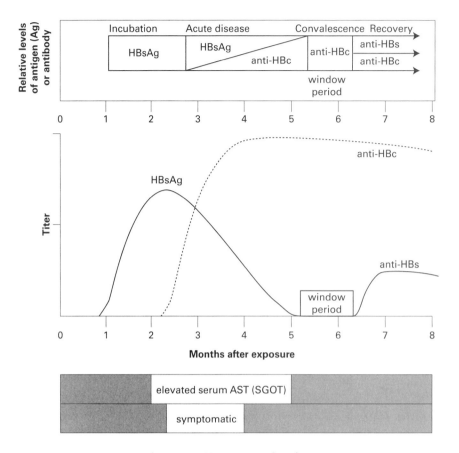

Figure 16 Hepatitis B Serologies

Note: The only serologic marker present during the window period of an acute infection is the IgM anti-Hepatitis B core antigen. IgG anti-Hepatitis B core antigen is elevated in the initial infection and is present for years after the infection.

Hepatitis C Virus

Hepatitis C virus (HCV) is a single-stranded RNA virus that is transmitted via blood and sexual contact. It is also associated with an increased incidence of **hepatocellular carcinoma**. Approximately one-half of infected patients become chronic carriers. Transfusions are routinely screened for possible HCV infection. A new agent, known as **hepatitis G**, has been linked to HCV infection and may be transmitted similarly.

Signs & Symptoms	Diagnosis	Treatment
As with other hepatitis viruses, patients experience jaundice, nausea, vomiting, and anorexia. Symptoms are usually less severe than with HBV infection, but a higher percentage (> 50%) develop chronic infection.	ELISA testing is used to detect IgM and IgG antibodies to HCV.	Supportive care. Interferon-alpha may decrease hepato-cellular damage in chronic carriers. There is no vaccine for Hepatitis C.

Hepatitis D Virus

Hepatitis D virus (HDV, **delta** agent) is a defective virus that requires co-infection with HBV for HDV viral production. It is a single-stranded RNA virus that is transmitted sexually, perinatally, or in blood products.

Signs & Symptoms	Diagnosis	Treatment
Co-infection with HDV causes symptoms more severe than does HBV alone. In addition to jaundice, nausea, and vomiting, patients may progress to fulminant hepatic failure.	Detection of serum delta antigen or anti-delta antigen IgM.	As in hepatitis B, supportive care is used. Co-infected carriers may receive interferon-alpha to prevent hepatic damage.

Hepatitis E Virus

Hepatitis E virus is a single-stranded RNA virus (calicivirus family) that causes disease primarily in developing countries. It has fecal-oral transmission, and outbreaks are common. Pregnant women are at increased risk of both fetal and maternal mortality if infected. There is no carrier state.

Signs & Symptoms	Diagnosis	Treatment
Asymptomatic cases are common. Patients who develop the disease experience anorexia, nausea and vomiting, and jaundice after a six-week incubation period. The illness is clinically indistinguishable from HAV infection. In 80% of pregnant women, fulminant hepatitis develops; otherwise, fulminant hepatitis is rare.	Exclusion of other causes of hepatitis, and serology.	—

SINGLE-STRANDED DNA VIRUSES

Parvovirus B-19

Parvovirus B-19 is responsible for **erythema infectiosum**, or **fifth disease**, a common infection among young children. It is spread via respiratory droplets or blood and infects and lyses RBC progenitor cells. This mechanism makes it dangerous to sickle cell patients, who run the risk of an aplastic crisis when infected. Infection of pregnant women can lead to **hydrops fetalis**. Immunocompromised patients may suffer from chronic anemia.

Signs & Symptoms	Diagnosis	Treatment
Erythema infectiosum is characterized by a "slapped cheek" red rash on the face followed by a lacy reticular rash on the extremities and trunk. Arthralgia may accompany the infection.	Presence of IgM B19 antibody in serology assays.	—

DOUBLE-STRAND DNA VIRUSES

Adenovirus

Adenovirus is a double-stranded DNA virus that causes both respiratory and enteric infections. Transmission is fecal-oral or by aerosol droplet. Outbreaks commonly occur in groups living closely together, such as the military, and a live vaccine is available to be given to these groups.

Signs & Symptoms	Diagnosis	Treatment
Some adenoviruses cause respiratory disease with fever, malaise, and pharyngitis. Lower respiratory infection can result in pneumonia. Infantile gastroenteritis with non-bloody diarrhea may also occur. Less common strains can cause conjunctivitis and hemorrhagic cystitis.	Diagnosis is usually made clinically, but cell cultures show CPE. Serology can be performed for definitive diagnosis.	—

Human Papillomavirus

Human papillomavirus (HPV) is a double-stranded DNA virus with more than 60 known serotypes. It is transmitted by direct contact and infects squamous epithelium. **Skin warts** are caused by HPV types 1 through 4, whereas **genital warts** are caused by HPV types 6 and 11.

Infection with HPV-16, -18, and -31 is associated with the development of cervical and penile carcinoma (note that these are not the subtypes that cause genital warts). Two genes, known as **E6 and E7**, may inhibit activity of p53 and the retinoblastoma gene, respectively.

Gardisil, the current vaccine against HPV serotypes 6, 11, 16 & 18, is recommended for girls ages 13–26.

Papeeeeelomavirus has two genes to note, E6 &E7. Just break down the name Papill(6) o (&) mavirus(7)

Signs & Symptoms	Diagnosis	Treatment
Depending on the subtype, infection can be asymptomatic or can manifest as warts, which are circumscribed, firm, grayish growths on the extremities or genitals. Laryngeal polyposis is an uncommon manifestation.	Microscopically, infected cells contain koilocytes, cytoplasmic vacuoles that are the hallmark of HPV infection. Koilocytes may be seen in skin biopsies or cervical Papanicolaou smears. **Figure 17** KoilocytesDiagnosis may be made by clinical inspection. DNA hybridization may be used as well.	Warts are removed with keratolytics such as liquid nitrogen or podophyllin. However, HPV infection is usually life-long. Genital transmission can be prevented with condoms.

JC Virus

This virus is seen only in immunosuppressed individuals, such as HIV or leukemia patients and transplant recipients. It is responsible for the **progressive multifocal leukoencephalopathy (PML)**, a demyelinating disease that is fatal within six months.

Signs & Symptoms	Diagnosis	Treatment
Depending on the site of demyelination, neurological disturbances can include speech impairment, dementia, cognitive dysfunction, motor impairment, loss of vision, and coma.	JC virus DNA in CSF or brain biopsy.	—

SINGLE-STRANDED RNA VIRUSES

Influenza Virus

Influenza virus is a single-stranded RNA virus that can undergo rapid **antigenic drifts** due to mutations of its genome; these cause slight changes in the antigenic natures of its surface glycoproteins. Antigenic drift allows the same individual to be reinfected with influenza virus after developing antibodies to the older strain, but the second illness tends to be milder.

Infections occur more commonly in winter and are transmitted by respiratory droplets. **Pandemics** occur when antigenic shifts produce new, previously unseen viral types. Types A, B and C are classified by internal capsid proteins. **Type A** infects **both** humans and animals. It is responsible for **antigenic shifts** by swapping RNA segments with animal strains of virus, thus producing influenza strains with antigens very different from those previously seen by the human immune system. Killed vaccines are available for types A and B, but protection is temporary and lasts only a few months. Nonetheless, elderly persons, persons with chronic respiratory disease, and health care workers should receive annual influenza vaccination.

Signs & Symptoms	Diagnosis	Treatment
Influenza A and B cause influenza outbreaks, whereas influenza C causes a mild upper respiratory tract infection. Influenza is characterized by sudden fever, myalgias, and cough that resolves within days or may progress to pneumonia.	Diagnosis is made clinically. Antibody titers may be used.	Supportive care. Children with possible influenza infections should not receive aspirin because they are at risk of developing Reye's syndrome, resulting in encephalopathic and liver failure. Amantadine or rimantadine are used to treat infection and to prevent influenza A outbreaks (e.g., nursing homes).

Measles Virus

Measles virus is a single-stranded RNA virus that is transmitted by respiratory droplets. It is very infectious and can cause severe disease in malnourished children and immunocompromised patients. In the United States, all children should receive a live, attenuated vaccine given in conjunction with mumps and rubella vaccine (MMR) at age 15 months. A rare late complication of measles infection is **subacute sclerosing panencephalitis** (SSPE), which can develop years after the primary infection and result in dementia and death.

Signs & Symptoms	Diagnosis	Treatment
Measles (rubeola) develops within 2 weeks of exposure. It begins with fever, photophobia, cough, and Koplik spots on the buccal mucosa, followed by a maculopapular rash, which starts on the face and neck and progresses downward. The lesions are red with a central white dot and frequently appear on the buccal mucosa. Severe infections can progress to pneumonia or encephalitis.	Diagnosis is made clinically, but serology may be used to assess immunity. **Figure 18** Koplik lesions on buccal mucosa	None. Persons born before 1980 may require an additional booster vaccination for adequate protection.

Mumps Virus

Mumps is a single-stranded RNA virus that is transmitted by respiratory droplets. A live, attenuated vaccine is given in conjunction with measles and rubella vaccine (MMR) in all children aged 15 months.

Signs & Symptoms	Diagnosis	Treatment
Mumps causes a flulike prodrome for about 3 weeks, followed by the development of tender, swollen parotid glands. Infection can spread to the ovaries, testes, and pancreas. Mumps orchitis can result in sterility.	Diagnosis is made clinically. Urine or saliva may be cultured. Serology indicates recent infection.	—

Respiratory Syncytial Virus

Respiratory syncytial virus (RSV) is a single-stranded RNA virus that is transmitted by respiratory droplets or hand to nose and mouth. It is often responsible for hospital outbreaks of pneumonia. It is prevalent in the winter and spring.

Signs & Symptoms	Diagnosis	Treatment
In older children and adults, RSV causes a mild upper respiratory infection. In infants and young children, RSV causes bronchiolitis, which is a severe lower respiratory tract infection that can progress to pneumonia. Children with bronchiolitis exhibit circumoral cyanosis and a hacking cough.	Immunofluorescent detection of the virus can be performed from a respiratory epithelium sample. Cultures show multinucleated giant cells. Serology is usually used for diagnosis. **Figure 19** Multinucleated giant cells in RSV	Ribavirin is used in hospitalized patients with severe infection.

Parainfluenza Virus

Parainfluenza virus is a single-stranded RNA virus that is transmitted by respiratory droplets. It is responsible for **bronchiolitis** in infants, **croup** in children, and is one of many viruses that can cause the common cold in adults.

Signs & Symptoms	Diagnosis	Treatment
Bronchiolitis is characterized by a hacking cough, hoarseness, and circumoral cyanosis. Croup, or laryngotracheitis, has a barking cough that may be accompanied by inspiratory stridor and wheezes. In adults, patients experience cough, rhinorrhea, and malaise. Severe cases can progress to pneumonia.	Clinical diagnosis and serology. Cell cultures show multinucleated giant cells.	Respiratory support is given if needed. Inhaled racemic epinephrine may help in severe cases.

Rubella Virus

Rubella is a single-stranded RNA virus that is transmitted by respiratory droplets. Congenital rubella infection, especially in the first trimester, is associated with multiple birth defects, including congenital cataracts, hearing loss, cardiac defects, and mental retardation. Rubella can be prevented with a live, attenuated vaccine, combined with measles and mumps (MMR), which is given at 15 months of age. It should also be given to all unimmunized young women before pregnancy. Although no documented cases of birth defects caused by immunization exist, the vaccine should not be given to pregnant women.

Signs & Symptoms	Diagnosis	Treatment
About 3 weeks after exposure, patients display a maculopapular rash that starts on the face and spreads downward (**German measles**). The characteristic physical finding is **posterior auricular lymphadenopathy**.	Diagnosis is performed with serology or ELISA. Antirubella IgM in pregnant women suggests recent infection, and amniocentesis may be done to see if the fetus is infected.	—

Rabies Virus

Rabies virus is a single-stranded RNA virus with a **bullet-shaped capsid** that can infect many mammals. Transmission occurs from the bite of a rabid animal, such as a bat, rodent, or dog, although most domestic animals are immunized against rabies. The bite causes infection of sensory neurons, which spreads to the CNS by retrograde axonal transport. Proliferation occurs in the CNS, and the virus travels down the peripheral nerve to the salivary glands, where it can be transmitted by bite. CNS infection causes encephalitis, which can be fatal. Workers at high risk of exposure (e.g., foresters) should receive a killed vaccine for prevention.

Signs & Symptoms	Diagnosis	Treatment
Time between exposure and manifestation of rabies can range from a few weeks to several months. Rabies progresses over several weeks, with patients developing fever, anorexia, confusion, and lethargy. Increased salivation occurs, and patients develop hydrophobia (fear of water) because the throat muscles go into painful spasms when trying to swallow. Symptoms eventually progress to seizures, paralysis, and coma. Death occurs due to vocal cord paralysis and respiratory distress.	The suspected animal is sacrificed, and brain sections are studied for **Negri bodies** (cell inclusions) or with anti rabies fluorescent antibodies. Infected patients are diagnosed with serology. **Figure 20** Negri body	No treatment is available. Exposed individuals receive a series of rabies immune globulin injections.

Human Immunodeficiency Virus

Human immunodeficiency virus (HIV) is a retrovirus containing single-stranded RNA. It carries reverse transcriptase, an RNA-dependent DNA polymerase, and integrase in its core. The *env* gene encodes **gp160**, which is cleaved to make the envelope proteins gp120 and gp41. gp120 binds the **CD4** receptor, providing its selectivity for **T helper cells**, and gp41 is involved in fusion with the host cell membrane. The *pol* gene encodes reverse transcriptase, integrase, and protease. The *gag* gene encodes core proteins, of which p24 is the most important and is used in diagnostic tests. The *tat* gene encodes proteins that activate the transcription proteins.

HIV causes AIDS, which is associated with an extremely high mortality rate. Transmission occurs by sexual contact, blood, or perinatally. Groups who have been at increased risk of contracting HIV in the United States include homosexual men, IV drug abusers, and hemophiliacs. Around the world, however, HIV infection is seen most commonly in heterosexuals. HIV infection results in the loss of cell-mediated immunity, which predisposes patients to opportunistic infections, TB, lymphomas, and Kaposi's sarcoma. HIV infections can be prevented through condom use and by not sharing needles. HIV-positive mothers should take zidovudine (AZT) during pregnancy to avoid passing the virus to the fetus. Vaccines are currently being developed but are difficult to produce due to antigenic shifts in the virus.

Signs & Symptoms	Diagnosis	Treatment
The acute phase of HIV infection is associated with fever, lethargy, and lymphadenopathy. Patients are then typically asymptomatic, with normal CD4 counts, although viremia persists. Some patients develop fever, lymphadenopathy, and weight loss with no obvious cause. The late phase of HIV infection (AIDS) is characterized by CD4 counts below 400/mm3, and patients develop opportunistic infections with agents such as *Pneumocystis jirovecii* (formerly known as *P. carinii*), MAC, and *Candida*.	Presumptive diagnosis is made by ELISA for antibodies to HIV and HIV proteins. Definitive diagnosis is made by Western blot.	HIV-infected individuals are usually given combination therapy with two nucleoside analogues (such as AZT, d4T, and 3TC) and one protease inhibitor (e.g., saquinavir).

Poliovirus

Poliovirus is a single-stranded RNA virus that is transmitted by the fecal-oral route. The virus replicates in the motor neurons of anterior horns in the spinal cord, resulting in motor neuron damage and muscle paralysis. Widespread vaccination has eradicated poliovirus from the Western hemisphere, although exposure is still common in developing countries. Two vaccines are available. The Sabin vaccine, or oral polio vaccine (OPV), is a live, attenuated vaccine that is given orally. It is used commonly in the United States and provides a long-lasting immunity to recipients and contacts through viral shedding. However, this vaccine carries the possibility of viral reversion to wild type, which then causes polio in the recipient. As such, it should not be given to immunocompromised individuals. The Salk vaccine, or inactivated polio vaccine (IPV), is a killed vaccine that is injectable.

Signs & Symptoms	Diagnosis	Treatment
The vast majority of infected persons are asymptomatic or develop mild symptoms, such as fever, nausea, and vomiting. Less than 1% go on to develop nonparalytic poliomyelitis, resulting in meningitis, or paralytic poliomyelitis, which leads to muscle paralysis. "Bulbar" poliomyelitis can cause brain stem infection and lead to respiratory paralysis. Exposure as an adult is more likely to lead to symptomatic infection.	Diagnosis is made with cultures of throat, stool, or CSF. Serology is also useful.	No antiviral treatment is available. Physical therapy after infection may limit the extent of disability.

Coxsackievirus

Coxsackievirus is a single-stranded RNA virus that is transmitted by the fecal-oral route and respiratory droplets. Infections are more common in the summer and fall. As with poliovirus, it infects the GI tract and travels to the anterior horn motor neurons. Two different types, **group A and B**, cause different disease entities.

Signs & Symptoms	Diagnosis	Treatment
Group A: virus primarily infects skin and mucous membranes, causing fever, sore throat, and tender vesicles in the oropharynx. Children also develop a vesicular rash on the hands and feet (hence the name, Hand, foot, and mouth disease) Group B: virus infections can cause myocarditis and may be implicated in the development of diabetes mellitus. Both groups can cause mild upper respiratory tract infections.	Diagnosis is by culture or serology.	—

Echoviruses

ECHO stands for enteric cytopathic human orphan virus. It is a single-stranded RNA virus that is transmitted by the fecal-oral route. The term orphan originally signified that they were not associated with any disease, but it is now thought that echoviruses are the most common cause of **viral meningitis.**

Signs & Symptoms	Diagnosis	Treatment
Echoviruses cause aseptic viral meningitis, upper respiratory tract infections, and diarrhea in infants.	Cell Culture.	—

Rhinoviruses

Rhinoviruses are single-stranded RNA viruses that are transmitted by respiratory droplet or from hand contact with the eyes, nose, or mouth. Because they prefer low temperatures, they can infect the nose but are unable to infect the lower respiratory tract. Rhinoviruses cause the common cold, along with adenoviruses, coronaviruses, influenza C virus, and coxsackievirus.

Signs & Symptoms	Diagnosis	Treatment
Symptoms include nasal discharge, fever, sore throat, and headache.	Clinical diagnosis. Cell cultures from nasal secretions are rare.	—

Yellow Fever Virus

Yellow fever virus is a single-stranded RNA virus seen in Africa and South America. There are two types of yellow fever: jungle yellow fever and urban yellow fever. **Jungle yellow fever** is seen in the tropical areas. The reservoir is monkeys, and the vector is the *Haemagogus* mosquito. **Urban yellow fever** has a human reservoir and has the *Aedes aegypti* mosquito as the reservoir. A live, attenuated vaccine is suggested for visitors to endemic areas.

Signs & Symptoms	Diagnosis	Treatment
Yellow fever causes jaundice and fever, accompanied by headache and photophobia. Progression can lead to GI hemorrhage (black vomitus) as well as cardiac and renal sequelae.	Serology or Viral Culture.	—

Think: "Black and Yellow, Black and Yellow" for black vomitus and yellow jaundice

Dengue Fever

Dengue virus is a single-stranded RNA virus seen in tropical areas, including the Caribbean. The reservoir appears to be humans and other primates, and the vector is the *A. aegypti* mosquito.

Signs & Symptoms	Diagnosis	Treatment
Dengue fever, also known as **breakbone** fever, is characterized by sudden flu-like symptoms accompanied by severe muscle and joint pains. This usually resolves without sequelae. **Dengue hemorrhagic fever**, seen more commonly in South Asia, has the symptoms of breakbone fever, but progresses to GI and skin hemorrhage and shock.	Serology or Viral Culture.	—

Hantavirus

Hantavirus is a single-stranded RNA virus harbored by rodents and transmitted to humans through inhalation of rodent urine and feces. In Europe and Asia, it has been associated with hemorrhagic fever with renal failure. In the southwestern states, it is linked to hantavirus pulmonary syndrome.

Signs & Symptoms	Diagnosis	Treatment
Hantavirus pulmonary syndrome is characterized by high fever, myalgias, cough, nausea, vomiting, and pulmonary edema. Even with respiratory support, 80% of patients die of the illness.	Serology or Viral Culture. **Figure 21** Hantavirus	Ribavirin is currently under investigation as a possible treatment.

DOUBLE-STRANDED RNA VIRUSES

Rotavirus

Rotavirus is a double-stranded RNA virus that is transmitted via the fecal-oral route. The virus is resistant to stomach acid and is able to infect the small intestine, causing gastroenteritis. Most people are infected in their childhood.

Signs & Symptoms	Diagnosis	Treatment
Patients are usually young children who develop non-bloody diarrhea. If fluids are not replaced, this can lead to serious dehydration.	Diagnosis is made with ELISA or radioimmunoassay of stool sample, or serology.	Oral rehydration therapy.

Arboviruses

Arboviruses describe a variety of viruses transmitted by an arthropod vector (ArBo = arthropod-borne). Infection in animals or in the arthropod usually does not result in disease; however humans, as accidental hosts, may develop disease. Arboviruses can be classified regionally.

- **Eastern equine encephalitis virus** (EEE) occurs in the Atlantic Coast and Gulf Coast states during summertime. The reservoir is wild birds, and the vector is the *Aedes mosquito*. Humans and horses are accidental hosts that develop severe encephalitis with a high mortality rate. This disease is rare, with less than 10 human cases per year.

- **Western equine encephalitis virus** (WEE) occurs west of the Mississippi. The reservoir is wild birds, and the vector is the *Culex* mosquito. Humans and horses develop a mild encephalitis that is rarely fatal.

- **St. Louis encephalitis virus** is seen in the southern and western United States. The reservoir is wild birds, and the vector is the *Culex* mosquito. The virus can be asymptomatic or cause encephalitis in humans.

- **California encephalitis virus** is seen in the north central states (not California, where it was discovered). The reservoir is small mammals, such as rodents, and the vector is the *Aedes* mosquito. The virus causes a range of symptoms, including (of course) encephalitis, but it is rarely fatal.

- **Colorado tick fever virus** is seen in the Rocky Mountains. The reservoir is wild rodents, and the vector is the American dog tick. Infection in humans causes symptoms such as headache, muscle pain and fever. This disease is seen in hikers and campers and can be prevented by wearing long sleeves and inspecting skin for tick bites.

Oncogenic Viruses

A number of viruses have been implicated in the development of human cancers. The most commonly associated ones are described here:

- **Human T-cell leukemia virus** (HTLV-I and II) preferentially infects CD4 T cells, as HIV does. It causes **cutaneous T-cell lymphoma** and **tropical spastic paraparesis**, an autoimmune disease.

- **HPV** infect squamous epithelium and cause warts. Not all HPV subtypes are associated with cancer development, but HPV-16, -18, and -31 are associated with **cervical** and **penile cancer**.

- **EBV** infects B-cells and has been associated with **Burkitt's lymphoma** in Africa, although cases of Burkitt's lymphoma in the United States have not been associated. **Nasopharyngeal carcinoma** in China and **thymic carcinoma** in the United States have also been associated.

- **HSV-2** is seen more commonly in women with **cervical cancer**, but because both HSV and cervical cancer are associated with increased sexual activity, it is unclear whether HSV plays a causative role. In vitro, HSV has shown the ability to transform cells in culture.

- **HBV and HCV** are associated with the development of **hepatocellular carcinoma**. Both viruses can cause chronic hepatitis, which may play a role in cancer progression.

- **Human herpesvirus 8** has been detected in **Kaposi's sarcoma** lesions in HIV-infected patients.

PRION DISEASES

General Information

Prions are infectious agents composed only of protein with no nucleic acids. They are highly resistant to heat and chemicals. Prions have been implicated in **Creutzfeldt -Jakob disease** (CJD) and **kuru** in humans as well as **bovine spongiform encephalitis**, or "mad cow" disease, in cattle.

CJD is characterized by a spongiform (Swiss-cheese) appearance of brain; patients develop dementia and ataxia, which progress to coma and death. CJD has been transmitted iatrogenically (e.g., during brain surgery or corneal transplant).

Kuru has been transmitted through the ingestion of the brains of infected people, performed mostly in New Guinea. Kuru patients develop ataxia and tremors but do not develop dementia.

Gerstmann-Sträussler-Scheinker syndrome (GSS) and **Fatal Familial Insomnia** (FFI) are thought to be familial forms of prion diseases. GSS has a long course of illness and is characterized by cerebellar ataxia. FFI does not demonstrate spongiform lesions, but instead is characterized by thalamic atrophy resulting in untreatable insomnia and dysautonomia.

FUNGI AND FUNGAL INFECTIONS

General Information

Fungi are eukaryotic organisms that have cell walls containing **chitin**, a polymer of N-acetylglucosamine. The fungal cell membrane contains **ergosterol** and **zymosterol**, in contrast to animal cells, which contain cholesterol. Fungi can exist as yeasts or molds, but some fungi are **dimorphic**, having the ability to grow as a yeast or mold, depending on environmental conditions.

Yeasts grow as single cells, which reproduce by budding. Some produce **pseudohyphae**, which are buds that do not detach. Molds grow as filaments known as **hyphae** and form mats known as mycelia. Septate hyphae form transverse walls and nonseptate hyphae have multinucleate cells. Fungi are typically aerobic. Some fungi reproduce sexually, but most medically important fungi reproduce asexually, forming spores called **conidia**.

The typical host response to fungal infection is a cell-mediated immune response, resulting in granuloma formation. Fungal skin tests are delayed-type hypersensitivity reactions (type IV), but allergies to fungi are mediated by IgE and are type I hypersensitivity reactions

Laboratory diagnosis is done through microscopy by the identification of characteristic spores and hyphae. Fungal cultures are usually grown on **Sabouraud dextrose agar**, which inhibits bacterial growth. Serology and fungal antigens are also used in diagnosis.

Dermatophytoses

Dermatophytoses are caused by a variety of species, including *Epidermophyton*, *Trichophyton*, and *Microsporum*. These fungi are spread by direct contact and infect superficial structures, such as skin, nails, and hair. **Tinea pedis** (athlete's foot), **tinea cruris** (jock itch), and **tinea corporis** (ringworm) are examples of dermatophytoses.

Signs & Symptoms	Diagnosis	Treatment
Patients develop pruritic papules and vesicles as well as broken hair and thickened nails. Lesions occurring from an allergic response to the infection are known as dermatophytid ("id") reactions. These patients develop vesicles on their fingers, although the primary infection is elsewhere.	Microscopy shows hyphae and conidia. Affected areas fluoresce under UV light.	Topical antifungals, such as miconazole, are used. Griseofulvin can be used for severe infections.

Tinea Versicolor

Tinea versicolor is a superficial skin infection caused by *Malassezia furfur* (also known as *Pityrosporum orbiculare*), which occurs frequently in humid climates.

Signs & Symptoms	Diagnosis	Treatment
Patients develop areas of hypopigmentation and scaling on the neck, arms, and upper trunk.	Microscopy examination of a skin scraping shows hyphae and budding yeast. **Figure 22** Skin scraping associated with Tinea Versicolor	Topical miconazole.

Sporothrix Schenckii

Sporothrix schenckii causes sporotrichosis. The organism grows on vegetation and is transmitted through a thorn prick. It is commonly known as "rose-gardener's disease." (classic test question scenario) or other injury.

Signs & Symptoms	Diagnosis	Treatment
Infection causes a localized pustule and lymphadenopathy	Microscopy shows cigar-shaped, unequal budding yeasts **Figure 23** Classic pattern of unequal budding yeast	Potassium iodide or itraconazole.

Coccidioides Immitis

Coccidioides immitis is a dimorphic fungus that takes the form of a mold in soil but forms spherules within the body. It is present in the soil of the southwestern United States and Latin America. Infection occurs from inhalation of arthrospores, which spread by direct extension or through the circulation to the bone and CNS, where they form granulomatous lesions. People in endemic areas usually have positive skin tests.

Signs & Symptoms	Diagnosis	Treatment
Coccidioidomycosis is a lung infection that is usually symptomatic but can manifest flulike symptoms, known as valley fever. Some people develop arthralgias, and meningitis can develop in immunosuppressed patients. The development of erythema nodosum—red, tender nodules on the extensor surfaces of extremities—is due to a delayed-type hypersensitivity response to fungal infection.	Microscopy of tissue sample shows spherules. Serology is used for detecting past infection and recovery. **Figure 24** Coccidioides spherules	Ketoconazole is given for respiratory symptoms, and amphotericin B is used for disseminated disease.

Histoplasma Capsulatum

Histoplasma capsulatum is a dimorphic fungus that forms mold in the soil and yeast in tissue. It is found in the soil in the Ohio and Mississippi River valleys. Infection occurs from inhalation of the spores, which are ingested by macrophages and become yeast. They form granulomas in tissue.

Signs & Symptoms	Diagnosis	Treatment
Histoplasma infection is usually asymptomatic but can also cause pneumonia and produces disseminated disease in infants or the immunocompromised.	Microscopy shows oval, budding yeast in macrophages. Cultures and RNA probes are also used. **Figure 25** Histoplasma capsultam in a macrophage	Ketoconazole is given in lung disease and amphotericin B for disseminated disease.

Blastomyces Dermatitidis

Blastomyces dermatitidis is a dimorphic fungus that forms mold in the soil and yeast in tissue. It is found in moist soil in both North and South America. Infection occurs from inhalation of the spores.

Signs & Symptoms	Diagnosis	Treatment
Blastomycosis is usually asymptomatic but can form lung granulomas. Disseminated disease causes ulcerated granulomas of the skin and bone.	Microscopy shows thick-walled yeast with a **broad-based bud.** Cultures grow hyphae with conidia. Serology is not performed. **Figure 26** Blastomyces broad based budding	Ketoconazole.

Paracoccidioides Brasiliensis

Paracoccidioides brasiliensis is a dimorphic fungus that forms mold in the soil and yeast in tissue. It is found in the soil in South America. Infection occurs from inhalation of the spores.

Signs & Symptoms	Diagnosis	Treatment
Paracoccidioidomycosis is usually asymptomatic but may cause oral lesions, lymphadenopathy, and widespread dissemination.	Microscopy shows a thick-walled yeast with multiple buds. Serology is also useful. **Figure 27** Multiple buds of yeast	Itraconazole or Ketoconazole.

OPPORTUNISTIC MYCOSES

Candida Albicans

Candida albicans is part of the normal flora of the upper respiratory tract, GI tract, and female genital tract. Candidal overgrowth can occur normally, but diabetics and persons taking antibiotics are predisposed to overgrowth. Candidiasis also occurs commonly in immunosuppressed patients.

Signs & Symptoms	Diagnosis	Treatment
Thrush occurs in the mouth, forming white patches that cannot be easily scraped off. Candidal overgrowth can also cause vaginitis, diaper rash, and intertrigo in skin folds. Immunosuppressed patients can develop esophageal or disseminated candidiasis, and IV drug users can develop endocarditis.	Microscopy shows budding yeasts and pseudohyphae. **Figure 28** Budding yeasts and pseudohyphae	Mucous membrane infection is treated with fluconazole or ketoconazole. Skin infections are treated with topical antifungal agents.

Cryptococcus Neoformans

Cryptococcus neoformans is an encapsulated, oval, budding yeast that grows in soil contaminated with **pigeon droppings**. Infection occurs from inhalation of the yeast cells.

Signs & Symptoms	Diagnosis	Treatment
Cryptococcosis is usually asymptomatic but can cause pneumonia or meningitis. Immunocompromised persons develop disseminated disease.	Microscopy; India ink stain reveals yeast with wide unstained area caused by the capsule CSF cultures and serology are also performed. **Figure 29** India ink stain reveals capsules	Amphotericin B and flucytosine are used to treat meningitis. Fluconazole is given to AIDS patients for long-term meningitis prophylaxis.

Aspergillus Fumigatus

Aspergillus fumigatus is a mold that grows on decaying vegetation. Infection occurs by inhalation or contact with airborne spores.

Signs & Symptoms	Diagnosis	Treatment
A. fumigatus can infect wounds and burns, especially in immunocompromised patients. It can infect the lungs and form a fungal ball known as an **aspergilloma,** which causes hemoptysis. Patients can also develop **allergic bronchopulmonary aspergillosis**, which causes asthmatic symptoms.	Microscopic examination shows septate, branching hyphae. **Figure 30** Aspergillus branching hyphae	Amphotericin B and surgical debridement.

Mucor and Rhizopus

Mucor and Rhizopus are molds that are found widely in soil. Infection occurs from inhalation of spores

Signs & Symptoms	Diagnosis	Treatment
These fungi cause invasive infection in immunocompromised patients, especially persons with **diabetic ketoacidosis** and burns. Proliferation in the endothelium of sinuses and lungs causes severe tissue necrosis.	Microscopy shows nonseptate hyphae with wide-angle branches.	Amphotericin B and surgical debridement.

PARASITES

Entamoeba Histolytica

Entamoeba histolytica exists in two forms. The **trophozoite** form is motile and exists in lesions and diarrheal stool. **Nonmotile cysts** are found in nondiarrheal stool. Transmission is fecal-oral. Ingestion of the cysts causes colonization of the colon, which can invade through the gut wall and enter the portal circulation, resulting in liver abscesses.

Signs & Symptoms	Diagnosis	Treatment
The vast majority of infected persons are asymptomatic, although the cysts are still shed in the feces. Some develop amebic dysentery with bloody, mucus-containing diarrhea. Liver abscesses cause right upper quadrant pain, weight loss, and fever.	Stool samples show trophozoites or cysts with four nuclei **Figure 31** Entamoeba histolytica trophozoite with one ingested blood cell and one nucleus.	Metronidazole and iodoquinol.

Giardia Lamblia

Giardia lamblia exists in two forms. The trophozoite has a suction disk for attachment to the intestinal wall. Nonmotile cysts are found in stool. This is found in wild mammals and humans, and transmission is fecal-oral. The classic case of Giardia is a hiker who drinks stream water that is contaminated with infected animal feces.

Signs & Symptoms	Diagnosis	Treatment
Giardiasis causes a foul-smelling, greasy, nonbloody diarrhea. Symptoms can last for several weeks.	Pear-shaped, flagellated trophozoites and cysts are found in stool. The "string" test is performed by having the patient swallow a string and removing it, with the trophozoites adhering to the string.	Metronidazole.

Trichomonas Vaginalis

Trichomonas vaginalis resides in the human vagina and prostate and is transmitted by sexual contact. Condom use can prevent transmission.

Signs & Symptoms	Diagnosis	Treatment
In women, trichomoniasis causes a thin, malodorous (fishy-smelling), frothy discharge with pruritus. Men may be asymptomatic or can develop urethritis.	Wet mount of discharge shows motile, pear-shaped, flagellated trophozoites. **Figure 32** Trichomonas with apparent flagella	Metronidazole—both partners must be treated to prevent reinfection.

Cryptosporidium Parvum

Cryptosporidium parvum is transmitted by the fecal-oral route and is a concern in immunocompromised patients because water supplies can become contaminated despite chlorination. The **oocytes** attach themselves to the small intestine and release **trophozoites**, which then become **schizonts** and **merozoites**. The latter make **microgametes** and **macrogametes**, which unite to make an oocyte.

Signs & Symptoms	Diagnosis	Treatment
Cryptosporidiosis causes a copious, watery diarrhea, which is more persistent in immunocompromised patients.	Acid-fast stain of stool sample reveals oocytes.	—

Plasmodium Species

Plasmodium species that cause infection in humans are *P. vivax*, *P. ovale*, *P. malariae*, and *P. falciparum*. They have a complicated life cycle, with a sexual stage in the *Anopheles* mosquito as vectors and an asexual stage in humans. Briefly, **sporozoites** are introduced into the human bloodstream by mosquito bite and are quickly taken into the hepatocytes, where they infect RBCs and differentiate into **gametocytes**. These are then ingested by the mosquito in a blood meal and reproduce sexually within the mosquito, forming sporozoites. Symptoms occur as the RBCs rupture, which occurs every 72 hours with *P. malariae* and every 48 hours with the other Plasmodium species.

Malaria is a global public health problem, causing more than a million deaths per year in developing countries. **Chloroquine resistance** is widespread in Southeast Asia, South America, and East Africa. Mefloquine prophylaxis is recommended for people traveling to endemic areas, but reports of neurologic and psychiatric symptoms in mefloquine users have kept some people from taking the drug.

Signs & Symptoms	Diagnosis	Treatment
Malaria causes abrupt fever, chills, and headaches a few weeks after infection, with a spiking fever pattern. Patients develop splenomegaly, hepatomegaly, and anemia. *P. falciparum* causes the most severe disease and can be life-threatening due to brain and kidney damage. Malaria from other Plasmodium species is self-limited but can still cause relapses after several years.	Microscopy of blood smear shows crescent-shaped or spherical gametes within the blood cells. **Figure 33** **A.** Plasmodium vivax signet-ring trophozoite within a red blood cell. **B.** P. vivax amoeboid trophozoite within a red blood cell, with Schüffner's dots.	If sensitive, chloroquine is used. Otherwise, mefloquine or quinine plus pyrimethamine-sulfadoxine is used. Primaquine is used to rid the liver of hypnozoites from *P. vivax* and *P. ovale*.

Falciparum can be Fatal

Toxoplasma Gondii

Toxoplasma gondii results from eating infected meat or exposure to **cat feces** that carry *Toxoplasma gondii* cysts. Persistent asymptomatic infection can occur in the cells of brain, muscle, and liver, which can cause disease again when the host is immunocompromised. Transplacental transmission can occur if primary infection occurs during pregnancy (TORCHES infection). Disease can be prevented by properly cooking meat and avoiding cat litter boxes if pregnant or immunocompromised.

Signs & Symptoms	Diagnosis	Treatment
Toxoplasmosis is usually asymptomatic or causes flulike symptoms. In immunosuppressed patients, the disease can disseminate and cause brain abscesses or encephalitis. Congenital infection can cause intrauterine growth restriction (IUGR), hydrocephalus, cerebral calcifications, and chorioretinitis.	Serology is used to determine previous or current exposure. Otherwise, biopsy of the affected tissue shows cysts within the cells. **Figure 34** MR image reveals multiple "ring-enhancing" lesions.	Sulfadiazine and pyrimethamine.

Trypanosoma Cruzi

Trypanosoma cruzi has two life cycles. The first cycle is within the **reduviid bug**, also known as a kissing bug, in which the insect ingests **trypomastigotes** from a blood meal, which undergo multiplication within the bug and are shed in its feces. If the feces are shed on a host, the trypomastigotes can enter the host's bloodstream by being scratched into the site of a bite or rubbed into a mucous membrane, especially the eyes. They then transform into **amastigotes** and reside in cardiac tissue, glial tissue, and esophageal tissue. Further conversion to trypomastigotes in the bloodstream allows the organism to be spread by the next bug bite. The disease is typically found in Central and South America but is occasionally found in the southern United States.

Signs & Symptoms	Diagnosis	Treatment
T. cruzi causes **Chagas disease** (American trypanosomiasis). During acute infection, patients develop an edematous **chagoma** at the site of the bite. This progresses to lymphadenopathy, fever, and hepatosplenomegaly. If the feces are rubbed into the eyes, edema of the eyes ensues (called **Romaña's** sign). Chronic disease is rare and leads to myocarditis and neuronal injury resulting in loss of muscle tone in the colon and esophagus, causing megacolon and mega-esophagus, respectively. Death usually occurs from cardiac complications.	Blood smear, bone marrow, or muscle biopsy reveals the organism. Serology is also performed. **Figure 35** **A.** *Trypanosoma cruzi* trypomastitgote in human blood. **B.** *T. cruzi* amastigotes found in cardiac muscle.	Nifurtimox.

Trypanosoma Brucei Gambiense and Trypanosoma Brucei Rhodesiense

Trypanosoma brucei gambiense and *T. brucei rhodesiense* have two life cycles. The first cycle occurs in the **tsetse** fly, in which the insect ingests **trypomastigotes** from a blood meal. These multiply in the tsetse fly and infect the host through the insect's saliva at the time of a bite. The organism then infects locally, in the bloodstream, and in the CNS. The organism evades the host immune system by repeatedly varying its surface antigens through **variant surface glycoproteins** (VSGs). The disease is found in Africa.

Signs & Symptoms	Diagnosis	Treatment
African trypanosomiasis causes **sleeping sickness**. Disease from *T. brucei gambiense* is low grade and chronic, but disease from *T. brucei rhodesiense* is rapidly progressive. Patients develop a chancre at the site of the bite, followed by headache and somnolence, which leads to coma and death. **Winterbottom's sign**, or posterior cervical lymphadenopathy, is a common finding.	Blood and CSF examination shows the organism. Serology is useful in acute infection.	Suramin and melarsoprol.

Leishmania Donovani

Leishmania donovani has two life cycles. The first cycle in the **sandfly** occurs during ingestion from a blood meal. The organism undergoes multiplication within the bug and is shed in its saliva during a bite. The organism infects the macrophages and reticuloendothelial system, including the spleen, liver, and bone marrow. The disease is found in Asia and Africa.

Signs & Symptoms	Diagnosis	Treatment
Visceral leishmaniasis, or **kala azar**, causes periodic fevers, weakness, pancytopenia, weight loss, and hepatosplenomegaly. Months later, hyperpigmentation of the extremities and a warty, ulcerative facial rash can develop. The disease tends to be chronic and, if untreated, leads to death by secondary infection.	Microscopy of the lymph nodes, bone marrow, or spleen tissue shows amastigotes. Cultures and serology are also done. **Figure 36** Leishmania donovani amastigotes within splenic macrophages.	Sodium stibogluconate.

Leishmania Braziliensis, L. Mexicana, and L. Tropica

The life cycle of these organisms is similar to that of *Leishmania donovani*, and the vector is the **sandfly**. However, the infection is limited to the skin and mucous membranes. *L. braziliensis* and *L. mexicana* are found in South America, whereas *L. tropica* is seen in Asia and Africa.

Signs & Symptoms	Diagnosis	Treatment
L. braziliensis causes **espundia**, a mucocutaneous disease that forms ulcers at the bite site and spreads to the nose and mouth, where it can cause total destruction of the nasal cartilage. *L. mexicana* and *L. tropica* cause a localized ulcer and rash at the site of the bite.	Microscopy of the skin lesion shows amastigotes.	Sodium stibogluconate.

Pneumocystis

Although *Pneumocystis carinii* is genetically a fungus, it is considered a parasite because it does not grow on fungal media and is not treated with antifungals. *P. carinii* cysts are ubiquitous in the environment, and transmission occurs by cyst inhalation. Most people are infected during childhood but are asymptomatic and carry the cysts in their lungs until they trigger infection when patients are in an immunocompromised state. HIV-infected patients are placed on TMP/SMX as prophylaxis against *Pneumocystis* infection

Signs & Symptoms	Diagnosis	Treatment
P. carinii pneumonia (PCP) is common in immunocompromised patients. It is characterized by sudden fever, cough, and dyspnea with bilateral rales and rhonchi.	Chest X-ray shows a diffuse interstitial infiltrate. Sputum sample from bronchial lavage shows cysts with sporozoites (which appear boat-shaped).	TMP/SMX. Pentamidine is used in sulfa-allergic patients.

CESTODES

Taenia Solium

Taenia solium is a species of tapeworm that causes disease through the ingestion of undercooked pork. The pig ingests food that has been fecally contaminated with *T. solium* eggs. These form **cysticerci**, larvae that invade muscle tissue (meat), CNS, and the gut. Once in the gut, the cysticerci form worms that release the segmented body parts (proglottids) full of eggs.

Signs & Symptoms	Diagnosis	Treatment
Taeniasis or intestinal tapeworm, can be asymptomatic or cause diarrhea and anorexia. It results from eating undercooked pork that contain cysticerci. Disseminated disease is called **cysticercosis** and causes space-occupying lesions in the brain and eyes. It is due to ingestion of eggs (fecal-oral).	Stool sample shows gravid proglottids with five to ten uterine branches. Cysticerci may be seen on CT scan or X-ray, if calcified.	Niclosamide is used for intestinal infection. Cysticercosis is treated with praziquantel or albendazole.

Taenia Saginata

Taenia saginata is similar to *T. solium*, except transmission occurs by ingestion of undercooked beef. *T. saginata* does not cause disseminated disease to the CNS.

Signs & Symptoms	Diagnosis	Treatment
T. saginata is asymptomatic or causes postprandial nausea.	Stool sample shows gravid proglottids with 15–25 uterine branches.	Niclosamide.

Diphyllobothrium Latum

Diphyllobothrium latum is ingested in raw fish. Patients who harbor *D. latum* can develop vitamin B$_{12}$ **deficiency** because the worm preferentially absorbs it, causing megaloblastic anemia. The fish ingest the larvae or other fish (who have already ingested the larvae). The host ingests these and the tapeworm resides in the small intestine, shedding eggs in proglottids, which eventually contaminate the water and form larvae. *D. latum* can be killed if the infected fish is cooked adequately.

Signs & Symptoms	Diagnosis	Treatment
Diphyllobothriasis is usually symptomatic but may cause diarrhea.	Stool sample reveals oval eggs with operculae (small "lids").	Niclosamide.

Echinococcus Granulosus

Echinococcus granulosus is a parasite of dogs, and humans are a dead-end host. Infected dogs shed the eggs in their feces and humans ingest them through fecal contamination. The larvae hatch in the small intestine and produce cysts in the liver, lung, and brain. *E. granulosus* is endemic to the Mediterranean, Middle East, and western United States.

Signs & Symptoms	Diagnosis	Treatment
Hydatid cysts form in the liver, lung, and CNS. Hypersensitivity can develop due to continual exposure, which can cause anaphylaxis if the cyst ruptures.	Microscopy of affected tissue and serology.	Careful surgical removal of the cyst and treatment with albendazole. The organisms are killed before removal to prevent possible rupture.

TREMATODES

Schistosoma Mansoni and Schistosoma Japonicum

Schistosomes are blood flukes transmitted by swimming in infected water. Free-swimming **cercaria** penetrate the skin and enter the portal circulation to the liver, where they mature into adults. These then travel through the mesenteric veins into the gut lumen and shed eggs into the feces. The eggs then have a cycle in snails before producing cercaria into the water. *Schistosoma mansoni* is seen in Central and South America, and *S. japonicum* is seen in southeast Asia and Japan. Infection can be prevented by proper waste disposal and avoiding swimming in endemic areas.

Signs & Symptoms	Diagnosis	Treatment
Schistosomiasis is usually asymptomatic or causes pruritus and rash soon after infection. Fever, chills and diarrhea follow this. Patients develop a granulomatous response to the eggs, causing hepatosplenomegaly, portal hypertension, and GI hemorrhage through varices.	Stool sample reveals eggs with large or small lateral spine. **Figure 37** Schistosoma mansoni ovum with lateral spine.	Praziquantel.

Schistosoma Haematobium

The life cycle of *Schistosoma haematobium* is similar to that of the other schistosomes, but the adult organism resides in the venous plexus of the bladder and is excreted in the urine. It is endemic to Africa and the Middle East. It is associated with the development of **squamous cell bladder carcinoma**.

Signs & Symptoms	Diagnosis	Treatment
Patients may experience **hematuria** and develop obstructive symptoms if there are too many eggs in the urethra.	Urine sample shows eggs with a large terminal spine X-rays may show calcification of the bladder. Schistosoma haematobium ovum with terminal spine.	Praziquantel.

Clonorchis Sinensis

Clonorchis sinensis, the Oriental liver fluke, is contracted by ingesting raw fish. The larvae hatch into the small intestine and mature in the bile duct. Eggs are passed into the feces, where they contaminate the water in which the fish live. Snails act as intermediate hosts before the organism encysts onto fish scales and enters the fish muscle. *C. sinensis* is endemic to Japan, China, and southeast Asia. *Clonorchis* infection has been associated with the development of **cholangiocarcinoma**.

Signs & Symptoms	Diagnosis	Treatment
Clonorchiasis is usually symptomatic but can cause abdominal pain and hepatomegaly.	Stool sample shows eggs with opercula.	Praziquantel.

Paragonimus Westermani

Paragonimus westermani, the lung fluke, is ingested in undercooked crabmeat. The worms hatch in the small intestine and travel to the lung. Eggs are present in sputum and are coughed up or swallowed and shed in feces, where they contaminate water. Snails act as intermediate hosts before the organism encysts onto crabs and enters the meat.

Signs & Symptoms	Diagnosis	Treatment
Paragonimiasis causes a **chronic cough** with bloody sputum, which is similar to tuberculosis.	Microscopy shows operculated eggs in the sputum or feces.	Praziquantel.

NEMATODES (ROUNDWORMS)

Enterobius Vermicularis

Enterobius vermicularis causes pinworm infection, which usually affects children. The eggs are picked up on the hands and ingested. The eggs mature into worms in the colon and migrate to the perianal area, where they lay eggs that are picked up by direct contact.

Signs & Symptoms	Diagnosis	Treatment
Pinworm causes perianal pruritus.	Cellophane tape on the perianal region collects eggs, which can be examined microscopically. Worms can be found in the stool.	Mebendazole. Reinfection is common.

Trichuris Trichiura

Trichuris trichiura, or whipworm, is transmitted via the fecal-oral route. Eggs are ingested from contaminated food or soil, and they hatch and mature in the small intestine. Eggs are then passed in the feces. The disease occurs in tropical areas and in the southern United States

Signs & Symptoms	Diagnosis	Treatment
Whipworm infection is usually asymptomatic but it can cause diarrhea and **prolapsed rectum**.	Stool sample shows barrel-shaped eggs with plugged ends.	Mebendazole.

Think of the "i" from the end switching locations, or prolapsing... this bug causes rectal prolapse!

Ascaris Lumbricoides

Ascaris lumbricoides is ingested in contaminated food and travels through the gut wall into the bloodstream to the lungs and heart. In the lungs, the organism is coughed up and swallowed and eventually settles in the small intestine. Eggs are then shed in the feces. The disease occurs in tropical areas and in the southern United States.

Signs & Symptoms	Diagnosis	Treatment
Ascariasis is usually asymptomatic, but a heavy worm burden can cause malnutrition. Lung infection causes fever and cough.	Stool sample reveals oval eggs and occasionally worms.	Mebendazole or pyrantel pamoate.

Think "Lumb" in the Lung!

Ancylostoma Duodenale and Necator Americanus

Ancylostoma duodenale and *Necator americanus* are hookworms. Contaminated soil carries larvae that enter through the skin and migrate to the lungs, where they are coughed up and swallowed. Maturation occurs in the small intestine and eggs are shed in the feces, where they hatch in moist soil. **A. duodenale** is seen in Africa and Asia, whereas N. americanus is seen in tropical areas of South America and the southern United States. Infection can be prevented by wearing shoes.

Signs & Symptoms	Diagnosis	Treatment
Hookworm causes a pruritic papule at the site of infection. Lung infection can cause pneumonia. While the hookworm is in the small intestine, it secretes an anticoagulation factor that causes blood loss and subsequent **anemia**.	Stool sample shows eggs and blood cells.	Mebendazole or pyrantel pamoate.

Strongyloides Stercoralis

Strongyloides stercoralis has two life cycles. It has a free-living cycle in the soil, during which **filariform larvae** can penetrate the skin. It travels into the bloodstream to the lungs, where it is coughed up and swallowed. **Rhabditiform** larvae then develop in the small intestines and are shed in the feces. Disease occurs mainly in the tropics and in the southeastern United States. Autoinfection may occur, when larvae penetrate the gut wall and enter the bloodstream to travel to the lungs. Wearing shoes can prevent infection.

Signs & Symptoms	Diagnosis	Treatment
Strongyloidiasis is usually asymptomatic but causes a pruritic papule at the entry site. Lung infection can cause pneumonia, and gut irritation may cause watery diarrhea. Autoinfection can lead to sepsis from the simultaneous entry of enteric bacteria and is especially dangerous in immunocompromised patients.	Laboratory tests show **eosinophilia**. Stool sample shows larvae.	Thiabendazole.

Trichinella Spiralis

Trichinella spiralis is ingested in undercooked pork. The calcified larvae are present in pig muscle, which is ingested, and then they live in the small intestine. **Larvae** are hatched and then migrate to the heart, CNS, and striated muscle. Humans are a dead-end host. The disease can be prevented by not feeding pigs undercooked infected meat.

Signs & Symptoms	Diagnosis	Treatment
Trichinosis causes gastroenteritis followed by fever, muscle pain, and periorbital edema. Cardiac and CNS infection can result in **granuloma formation**.	Laboratory tests show eosinophilia. Serology is also useful.	Thiabendazole or mebendazole.

Wuchereria Bancrofti and Brugia Malayi

Wuchereria bancrofti and *Brugia malayi* are transmitted by the *Anopheles* and *Culex* mosquitoes. The mosquito deposits larvae during a bite, which then enter the lymphatic system. The larvae mature in the lymph nodes and produce **microfilariae**, which enter the bloodstream and are ingested by a biting mosquito. **W. bancrofti** infection occurs in Africa, South America, and southeast Asia while *B. malayi* is found in Malaysia.

Signs & Symptoms	Diagnosis	Treatment
Filariasis causes inflammation of the lymphatic system, leading to obstruction and edema. Persistent and severe infection causes massive lymphatic obstruction, resulting in **elephantiasis**, usually of the lower extremity and scrotum.	Blood smears taken at night show microfilariae.	Diethylcarbamazine kills microfilariae.

Onchocerca Volvulus

Onchocerca volvulus is transmitted by the **black fly**, which leaves the organism in subcutaneous tissue after a bite. The organisms develop into nodules and spread throughout the subcutaneous tissue, where they are taken up by other biting black flies. These organisms do not enter the bloodstream, although lesions close to the eye may cause infection and blindness. Most disease is found along rivers in Africa and Central America.

Signs & Symptoms	Diagnosis	Treatment
Onchocerciasis causes a pruritic papule and subsequent nodule development. "**River blindness**" occurs when microfilariae concentrate in retina, cornea, and conjunctiva.	Skin biopsy reveals microfilariae.	Ivermectin. Suramin is used in ocular lesions.

Loa Loa

Loa loa is transmitted by the deer fly *(Chrysops),* which deposits larvae into the subcutaneous tissues during a bite. The organism spreads to the eyes and the bloodstream during the daytime, when it is ingested by a biting deerfly. It is seen in Africa.

Signs & Symptoms	Diagnosis	Treatment
Loiasis causes transient, nonerythematous swellings on the extremities called **Calabar swellings**. Adult worms may be seen crawling across the conjunctiva.	Blood smear shows microfilariae.	Diethylcarbamazine.

Dracunculus Mmedinensis

Dracunculus medinensis infection is transmitted by **copepods**, tiny crustaceans that can be found in contaminated drinking water. Once ingested, the larvae penetrate the small intestine and enter the subcutaneous tissue, where they travel to the lower extremities and mature. The adults live in the skin but create ulcers for the larvae to pop out of the skin and into the water, where they are ingested by copepods. Disease occurs in Africa, the Middle East, and India, and can be prevented by boiling drinking water.

Signs & Symptoms	Diagnosis	Treatment
Dracunculiasis causes skin ulceration and pruritus at the exit site.	The head of the adult worm can be visualized in the ulcer.	The worm is slowly wound out on a stick over several days. Niridazole or metronidazole may make this easier.

Toxocara Canis

Toxocara canis infection occurs in dogs. Eggs are present in infected dog feces, which are ingested by humans. These eggs hatch and the larvae enter the small intestine and travel to the liver, CNS, eyes, and other organs. Humans are dead-end hosts. Infection control is performed by treatment of infected dogs.

Signs & Symptoms	Diagnosis	Treatment
T. canis produces **visceral larva migrans**, a creeping eruption caused by granulomatous hypersensitivity to the larvae. It can also cause blindness and encephalitis.	Serology or tissue microscopy to visualize larvae.	Thiabenzadole and steroids.

ANTIMICROBIAL AGENTS

Antibiotics

Antibiotics can be difficult to study for the Step 1 examination. We recommend that you know the classic side effects, mechanisms of action, and coverage of each class of antibiotics, without spending too much time on the fine details. You are not expected to know dosages.

Drugs

SULFONAMIDES, TRIMETHOPRIM AND RELATED COMPOUNDS

Action: Prevent nucleotide synthesis inhibit DNA synthesis

- Block Folic Acid Synthesis

- **Sulfonamides** are bacteriostatic competitive analogues of para-aminobenzoic acid (PABA) that bind to the enzyme *dihydropteroate synthetase*, which is needed to make dihydropteroic acid in the folic acid synthesis pathway.

- **Trimethoprim** and related compounds (**pyrimethamine and methotrexate**) inhibit the reduction of dihydrofolic acid to tetrahydrofolate, by blocking *dihydrofolic reductase*.

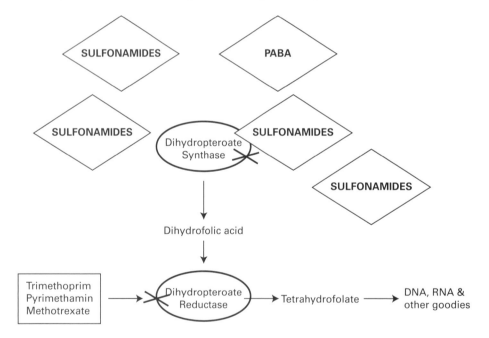

Figure 38 Mechanisms of action for TMP-SMX

Clinical Use:

- **Note**: **Trimethoprim** are often used with sulfonamides (TMP-SMX) because of their synergism: They attack two separate steps in the synthesis of folic acid.

Activity	Uses	Adverse reactions
Klebsiella sp.	Uncomplicated	Hemolytic anemia (especially in G6PD* deficiency)
Escherichia coli	UTI	
Enterobacter sp.	Cystitis	Nephrotoxicity—Crystalline aggregates in kidney (must increase fluid intake)
Pneumocytis carinii	P. carinii	
Shigellla sp.	Prophylaxis	Photosensitivity
Salmonella sp. "KEEPSS"	Diarrhea	Kernicterus (infants)
		Stevens-Johnson syndrome
		Allergic reactions, drug fever, skin reaction (common)

G6PD = glucose-6-phosphate dehydrogenase

Resistance:

- Develops by reduced drug uptake, increased intracellular PABA, lowered affinity in the dihydropteroate synthase enzyme.

PENICILLINS
(PENICILLIN G, PENICILLIN V, PROTOTYPE β-LACTAM ANTIBIOTICS)

Action: Inhibit peptidoglycan cross-linking → block bacterial cell wall synthesis

- Penicillins are bactericidal only to growing bacteria since they block cell wall synthesis, resulting in bacterial cell lysis. Penicillin binds penicillin-binding proteins in the bacterial cell wall, which inhibits peptidoglycan cross-linking.

PenciLLins block ceLL waLLs and are good for T. paLLidum (syphilis)

Clinical Use:

Aminopenicillins
Aim farther

Agents	Activity	Uses	Adverse reactions
Limited Spectrum Penicillin G (IM/IV) Penicillin V (oral)	Streptococcus Pyogenes Neisseria menigitidis Clostridium sp. (except C. difficile) Treponema pallidum	Pharyngitis Meningitis (some cases) Syphilis	Allergic reaction Hemolytic anemia
(Aminopenicillins) Ampicillin Amoxicillin	Broader spectrum than penicillin G HEELP*	Otitis Media Pharyngitis Sinusitis Pneumonia	Diarrhea *Ampicillin* can cause rash in parts with viral infections, including mononucleosis
Fourth Generation (Anti-Pseudomonal ureidopenicillins) Ticarcillin Mezlocillin Piperacillin	As Above and better Pseudommonas sp. Klebsiella pneumoniae	Pseudomonal infections Resistant gram-negative infections	Neutropenia Anemia
Beta-Lactamase Resistant Penicillin Methicillin Nafcillin Oxacillin Dicloxacillin	Resistant staph. infections (except MRSA)		Nephropathy

HEELP: **_Haemophilus influenza_**, **_Escherichia coli_**, Enterics (Shingella, Salmonella), Listeria, Proteus

Resistance:

- Resistance is usually caused by the presence of *beta-lactamases*, which break the beta-lactam ring found in penicillin. In gram-negative organisms, plasmids usually account for resistance and allow the accumulation of beta-lactamases in the periplasmic space. Gram-positive resistance can be either chromosomal or plasmid derived. **Clavulanic acid** (also sulbactam and tazobactam) inhibit beta-lactamases. Given with penicillins, clavulanic acid can broaden the spectrum and increase drug activity. An example is Amoxicillin given with clavulanic acid. Beta-lactamase–resistant penicillins, such as **methicillin**, are also used, but resistance to these drugs has already developed.

CEPHALOSPORINS

Action: Beta-lactam drugs similar to penicillins → inhibit cell wall synthesis

Clinical Use:

- **Note**: There are four generations of cephalosporins. The newer generations are more effective against Gram-negative bacteria, but less effective against Gram-positive organisms. Third-generation cephalosporin, Ceftriaxone crosses the blood-brain barrier therefore useful against meningitis.

Agents	Activity	Uses	Adverse reactions
First Generation Cefazolin Cephalexin	Gram-positive cocci (S. aureus & Streptococcus sp.) Some *E. coli* Klebsiella sp. Proteus sp.	Back-up penicillin for strep and staph Used for prophylaxis before surgery	Cephalosporin allergy seen in 10% pen-allergic patients GI upset (pseudomembranous enterocolitis via C. difficile) Anemia Nephrotoxicity
Second Generation Cefoxitin Cefaclor Cefuroxime Cefamandole Cefmetazole Cefotetan	Gram-positive Mild Gram-negative infections Cefoxitin, Cefmetazole, Cefotetan have some anaerobic coverage	Pharyngitis Otitis media Sinusitis Skin infections	Same as above Cefamandole, Cefmetazole, Cefotetan have a methyle-thio-tetrazole side chain that interferes with the synthesis of Vitamin K dependent clotting factors (poor coagulation)

Third Generation Ceftriaxone Cefotaxime Ceftazidime Moxalactam	Severe gram-negative Infections Ceftazidime has antipseudomonal activity	Gonorrhea Lyme disease Gonorrhea	Same as above
Fourth Generation Cefepime	Pseudomonas Gram-positives	Same as above	Same as above

AMINOGLYCOSIDES
(GENTAMICIN, NEOMYCIN, AMIKACIN, TOBRAMYCIN, STREPTOMYCIN)

Action: Bacteriostatic drugs that block **30S** ribosomal subunit → inhibit protein synthesis

Clinical Use:

- Note: They are synergistic with beta-lactam antibiotics, which allow for increased uptake of aminoglycosides.

Activity	Uses	Adverse reactions
Aerobic gram-negative *Escherichia coli* Klebsiella sp. Pseudomonas sp.	Severe gram-negative infec-tions Tularemia Plague	Ototoxicity due to loss of co-chlear hair cells, irreversible **Nephrotoxicity** (reversible) Teratogen

Resistance:

- Resistance develops due to altered ribosomal structure or the development of enzymatic deactivation (by group transferases) of the antibiotic by the bacteria. Aminoglycosides have little activity against strict anaerobes because they rely on oxygen-dependent transport to enter bacteria.

TETRACYCLINES

Action: Bind to **30S** subunit → decreased protein synthesis

Clinical Use:

Agent	Activity	Uses	Adverse reactions
Tetracycline	Rickettsia sp. Mycoplasma sp. Chlamydia sp.	Atypical pneumonia Chronic bronchitis Acne Lyme disease	GI irritation Hepatotoxicity Renal Toxicity **Discoloration of teeth** in children ("Tet and teeth")
Doxycycline Minocycline Demeclocycline (ADH antagonist)	Enteric Bugs Diarrhea	Lyme disease—Meningococcal carrier state	Less Renal Toxicity

Resistance:

- Resistance can develop through decreased uptake by energy-dependent transporters or through the development of a protein "**pump**" that actively excretes the drug.

MACROLIDE ANTIBIOTICS
(ERYTHROMYCIN, AZITHROMYCIN, CLARITHROMYCIN, TELITHROMYCIN)

Action: Bind to **50S** ribosome → inhibit protein synthesis

- **Note**: **Erythromycin** also acts as an analogue to motilin, an endogenous hormone that causes increased GI motility, so its ability to cause diarrhea is no surprise.

Big Mac binds to the Big ribosome and inhibits translocation

Clinical Use:

Agent	Activity	Uses	Adverse reactions
Erythromycin	Community-acquired pneumonia & atypicals Mycoplasma sp Legionella sp. Chlamydia sp. Corynebacteria	Alternative to penicillin if allergic Pneumonia	GI Irritation Pneumonia
Azithromycin	Same as above	same as above	Fewer GI problems than erythromycin
Clarithromycin	Same as above	Mycobacterium avium complex	Fewer GI problems than erythromycin

Resistance: Demethylation on the 23s rRNA leads to macrolide antibiotic resistance

LINCOSAMIDES
(CLINDAMYCIN, LINCOMYCIN)

Action: Bind to **50S** subunit of ribosome → inhibit protein synthesis

- **Note**: The classic **toxicity** associated with clindamycin use is **pseudomembranous colitis**, in which overgrowth of *Clostridium difficile* causes an invasive colitis. Although this can develop in anyone on long-term antibiotics, clindamycin is the classic drug, and therefore a common test question. It works well against anaerobic bacteria.

Clinical Use:

Activities	Uses	Adverse reactions
Same as erythromycin Anaerobic bacteria Bacteroides sp. Clostridium sp.	Mixed **anaerobic** infections Lung infections Intra-abdominal infections	Diarrhea Pseudomembranous colitis

Resistance: Similar to Macrolides: methylation on the 23s portion of the 50S bacterial ribosome

FLUOROQUINOLONES AND QUINOLONES
(FLUOROQUINOLNES: CIPROFLOXACIN, NORFLOXACIN, OFLOXACIN;
QUINOLONES: NALIDIXIC ACID)

Action: Bacteriocidal drugs that inhibit **DNA gyrase** and **DNA IV topoisomerase** → prevents future DNA replication

Clinical Use:

- **Note**: Children and pregnant women should not use these drugs because they cause cartilage erosion. A classic case associated with fluoroquinolone use is the rupture of a tendon (e.g., the Achilles tendon) following the course of antibiotics.

Agents	Activity	Uses	Adverse reactions
Ciprofloxacin Ofloxacin Norfloxacin	All gram-negative rods Pseudomonas sp. Mycoplasma sp. Neisseria	UTIs STIs Otitis Sinusitis Bronchitis Osteomyelitis	GI discomfort **Tendonitis** photosensitive rash
Nalidixic Acid	Gram negative rods ex. Pseudomonas sp	UTIs	GI discomfort Photosensitive rash Growth plate toxicity in children

Resistance: Mutations may significantly limit the effectiveness of these medications. Resistance develops from overuse of a single agent.

ANTI-TUBERCULAR AGENTS

Clinical Use:

- **Note**: Because mycobacteria are slow-growing, treatments are usually very long term. As a result, problems of resistance and patient compliance have emerged. Granulomatous lesions also pose a problem since they are often difficult to penetrate with drugs due to their avascular nature. Antimycobacterial drugs are used in combinations (e.g., simultaneous administration of isoniazid, rifampin, and pyrazinamide, with possible addition of ethambutol) in an effort to combat drug resistance.

Agent	Mechanism	Uses	Adverse reactions
Isoniazid (INH)	Inhibits synthesis of mycolic acids*	TB (with other drugs for active disease; alone for prophylaxis)	Peripheral neuritis and neurotoxicity from pyridoxine deficiency Rash Hepatotoxicity Inactivated by N-acetylation; eliminated in urine Genetic difference in acetylation: "fast" and "slow" Fast type gives poorer responses, slow type gives toxicity
Rifampin	Binds beta subunit of RNA Pol → inhibits translation	TB, pox virus Prophylaxis for meningitis in close contacts	Tears, urine turns orange Induces cytochrome P-450 enzymes Hepatotoxicity Hypersensitivity Mutation (RNA pol that does not bind to rifampin) No cross-resistance Reduces efficacy of oral contraceptives.
Ethambutol	Inhibits mycolic acid transfer to cell wall	TB	Optic neuritis (dose-dependent; reversible; red & green color blindness) Peripheral neuropathy Hyperuricemia
Pyrazinamide	Unknown	TB	Irreversible hepatic injury Hyperuricemia

Mycolic acids make up mycobacterial cell walls

Miscellaneous Antibiotic Agents

Agent	Mechanism	Activity	Uses	Adverse reactions
Bacitracin	Inhibits dephosphorylation of lipid pyrophosphate	Gram + cocci	Topical skin infections Eye Infections	Nephrotoxic
Vancomycin	Inhibits transfer of disaccharides during cell wall synthesis	**MRSA** Clostridium difficile	A "**Big Gun**": Use only needed serious multi-drug resistant infections S. aureus called VRSA is resistant (Resistance: D-ala/D-**ala** → D-ala/D-**lac**) Only good for Gram +	"Red man" syndrome or "red neck" syndrome Histamine release with rapid IV infusion
Telavancin	New analog of Vancomycin: Disrupts bacterial cell wall synthesis	Same	—	Renal damage Fetal damage
Aztreonam (monobactam)	Inhibits cell wall cross-linking by binding to PBP3. β-lactamase resistant	Gram—rods Pseudomonas sp.	A really big gun!	Very minimal
Imipenem	Inhibits cell wall cross-linking. Usually given with cilastatin, which prevents renal drug inactivation	Everything except MRSA & mycoplasma	The Last Resort!	Same as penicillin Seizures (can use meropenem instead)
Chloramphenicol	Inhibits peptidyltransferase of bacterial ribosome to stop protein synthesis	Gram—except: Pseudomonas sp.	Not used much due to toxicity Used mostly in developing countries	Reversible, dose related bone marrow supression Irreversible aplastic anemia "Grey baby syndrome"

ANTI-VIRAL AGENTS

Miscellaneous Anti-Viral Agents

Agent	Mechanism	Uses	Adverse reactions
Acyclovir	Viral **thymidine kinase** (tk) converts drug to triphosphate nucleoside analogue, which inhibits DNA synthesis and causes chain termination	Oral and genital HSV and herpes zoster	Skin irritation Renal crystal formation if given too rapidly
Ganciclovir	Similar to acyclovir	CMV retinitis and severe CMV infections	Granulocytopenia Thrombocytopenia
Vidarabine	Nucleoside analogue Activated drug inhibits viral DNA pol	HSV encephalitis	Flulike symptoms Anorexia Hepatotoxicity Encephalopathy
Iododeoxyuridine	Viral DNA strand breakage; not selective to viral polymerase so only used topically	HSV keratitis	Photophobia Conjunctivitis
Foscarnet	Pyrophosphate analogue: inhibits viral DNA polymerase and reverse transcriptase	CMV retinitis and severe CMV infections	Renal toxicity Hypocalcemia Anemia Diarrhea Deposits in bone and teeth
Amantadine & Rimatodine	Binds influenza matrix protein and inhibits viral uncoating	Influenza A prophylaxis Parkinsonism	Depression Congestive heart failure Urinary retention Use rimatidine in patients with renal failure
Ribavirin	Competitively inhibits IMP dehydrogenase resulting in decreased synthesis of guanine nucleotides	Severe respiratory syncytial virus infection Chronic hepatitis C Influenzas, viral hemorrhagic fevers	Decreased pulmonary function Severe teratogen Hemolytic anemia

Note: HSV = Herpes Simplex Virus; CMV = cytomegalovirus; HBV = Hepatitis B virus

HIV DRUGS

Human immunodeficiency virus (HIV) is a retrovirus that utilizes the enzyme *reverse transcriptase* to convert its RNA genome into DNA. Nucleoside analogues are converted to nucleotides in the cell and inhibit reverse transcriptase, resulting in DNA chain termination. Protease inhibitors are the latest addition to the drugs used for HIV treatment. The protease in HIV is encoded on the pol gene and is used to cleave precursor proteins during viral synthesis. Protease inhibitors therefore block viral production. As with tuberculosis, multiple drugs are used simultaneously in HIV to decrease viral load and prevent development of resistance.

HAART: Highly Active Antiretroviral Therapy-This is aggressive treatment, which suppresses HIV replication. Treatment usually consists of 3 anti-HIV agents. Combinations include: 2 nucleoside reverse transcriptase inhibitors (NRTIs) + 1 protease inhibitor (PI); 2 NRTI + 1 Non-Nucleoside Reverse Transcriptase Inhibitor (NNRTIs)

Nucleoside Analogs (NRTIs)

Agents	Additional Comments and Toxicity
Zidovudine (AZT or ZDV)	Thymidine analogue Headaches, nausea, myalgias, anemia, and neutropenia
Dideoxyinosine (ddl)	Converted to ddATP Peripheral neuropathy, pancreatitis, diarrhea, headache
Dideoxycytosine (ddC)	Converted to ddCTP Peripheral neuropathy, pancreatitis, bone marrow suppression
Lamivudine (3TC)	Headache, malaise, nausea, pancreatitis
Stavudine (d4T)	Converted to stavudine triphosphate Peripheral neuropathy, liver enzyme elevations

Notes: ddATP = dideoxy adenosine triphosphate; ddCTP = dideoxy cytosine triphosphate

Protease Inhibitors (PI)

Agents	Additional Comments and Toxicity
Indinavir	Kidney stones, hyperbilirubinemia, neutropenia, GI effects
Nelfinavir	Diarrhea and other GI effects
Ritonavir	GI effects; many drug interactions
Saquinavir	GI effects

Non-Nucleoside Reverse Transcriptase Inhibitors (NNRTIs): Nevirapine, Efavirenz, Delavirdine

Fusion Inhibitors: Enfuvirtide

ANTI-FUNGAL AGENTS

Ampho-toxic (Amphotericin B is extremely toxic and should be avoided if possible)

Agent	Activity	Uses	Toxicities
Amphotericin B	Binds ergosterol in fungal membrane, blocking synthesis	Systemic fungal infections, fungal meningitis	Very toxic—fevers, chills, headache, nausea; renal toxicity, hypokalemia; basal metabolism suppression; anemia; thrombophlebitis
Griseofulvin	Interferes with microtubule function, arresting mitotic activity	System drug for Tinea infections	Teratogenic, carcinogenic, GI effects, headache, allergic reactions
Nystatin	Destroys fungal membrane	Topical drug for Candida sp. and mixed fungi Rinse & swallow for thrush	Few side effects
Miconazole	Inhibits ergosterol synthesis	Topical drug for Candida sp. and mixed fungi	Topical irritation
Ketoconazole	Blocks demethylation of lanosterol to ergosterol and blocks cholesterol synthesis	Candida sp., Coccidioides sp., Histoplasma sp., Paracoccidiodes sp.	Nausea, vomiting, hepatitis, testosterone suppression; poor CSF penetration
Itraconazole	Inhibitor of fungal P-450, causing membrane damage	Aspergillus, Histoplasma, Blastomyces sp., Coccidiodes sp., Cryptococcus sp., Candida sp., cryptococcal meningitis prophylaxis	Nausea, vomiting, hepatitis; poor CSF penetration
Fluconazole	Similar to itraconazole	Similar to itraconazole	CSF penetration; GI distress

Terbinafine	Inhibits sterol metabolism	Systemic drug for tinea corporis and onychomycosis	Diarrhea, skin irritation
5-Fluorouracil & flucytosine	Incorporated into DNA and inhibits thymidylate synthesis	Second-line drug for Cryptococcus sp., Aspergillus sp., and Candida sp.	Teratogenic; renal toxicity; hepatotoxicity, myelosuppression, GI effects
Potassium Iodide	Unknown	Sporothrix sp.	Rash, drug fever, parotitis

ANTI-PARASITIC AGENTS

Agent	Mechanism	Uses	Toxcities
Quinine	Similar to chloroquine	Malaria (Plasmodium falciparum) that is resistant to Chloroquine	Cinchonism; headache, tinnitus, nausea; bitter taste; uterine contractions; cardiovascular depressant
Chloroquine	Allows buildup of heme product, which is toxic to the plasmodium	Malaria prophylaxis and treatment in nonresistant areas (P. falciparum)	Same as above, strange & vivid dreams
Mefloquine	Unknown	Malaria prophylaxis and treatment in chloroquine-resistant areas	Weird neuropsychiatric disturbances have been reported
Primaquine	Affects glutathione levels and protein synthesis	Malaria treatment for strains resistant to other medicines, esp. P. vivax and P. ovale	Hemolytic anemia in people with G6PD deficiency; GI effects, CNS effects
Fansidar (sulfadoxine and pyrimethamine)	Affects parasite's reductase enzyme	Resistant P. falciparum, toxoplasmosis	Anemia
Metronidazole	Metabolized to a toxic radical, which targets DNA	Giardia sp., Trichomonas sp., amebiasis Also, bacterial anaerobes	Metallic taste, nausea, vertigo, leukopenia; must avoid alcohol

Quinine Fun Fact:
Quinine is a component of tonic water. British soldiers in India were more willing to consume quinine when its bitter taste was mitigated with gin. Hence, the popular *Gin and Tonic* cocktail was born.

Iodoquinol	Unknown	Amebiasis in GI tract	Mild GI effects
Pyrantel pamoate	Nerve depolarization and paralysis of organism	Ascaris sp., hookworm, Enterobius sp.	GI effects, somnolence
Thiabendazole	Inhibits fumarate reductase in parasitic mitochondria	Strongyloides sp., other roundworms	Malaise, hepatitis, dizziness
Mebendazole	Inhibits glucose uptake and microtubule formation	Trichuria sp., other roundworms	Diarrhea, rash, neutropenia, hepatitis
Suramin	Unknown	Roundworms	Vomiting, peripheral neuropathy, proteinuria
Ivermectin	Causes GABA release resulting in toxic paralysis	Strongyloides sp., Onchocerca sp.	Rash, edema, visual loss; can be used during pregnancy
Niclosamide	Inhibits glucose uptake, allows worm to be digested	Diphyllobothrium latum, Hymenolepis nana, and Taenia saginata	Nausea/vomiting, abdominal pain, itching
Praziquantel	Stimulates motility and impairs suckers	D. latum, H. nana, T. solium, and T. saginata	Cannot operate machinery because over 30% of patients get dizziness and headache

CHAPTER 12

MUSCULOSKELETAL SYSTEM

MUSCULOSKELETAL ANATOMY

The Upper Extremity

The Shoulder

The shoulder joint (i.e. glenohumeral joint) is the convergence of three bones and a ring of four muscles, which are all enclosed in a capsule and cushioned by several bursae. The shoulder girdle is composed of the **scapula, clavicle**, and **humerus**. The scapula is situated on the posterior aspect of the thorax, between the 2nd and 7th rib. Extending from the upper sternum medially is the clavicle, which acts as a brace to keep the shoulder joint laterally to allow arm movements. The four rotator cuff muscles, **supraspinatus, infraspinatus, teres minor,** and **subscapularis muscles**, all attach onto the humerus, allowing the shoulder joint to have a wide range of motion.

BURSITIS

Bursae are fluid-filled sacs that cushion the rotator cuff muscles. Bursitis occurs where these sacs become inflamed from muscle overuse.

ROTATOR CUFF TEAR

This is a common injury for the elderly where the rotator cuff is strained or torn with overuse. A torn supraspinatus tendon results in limited arm abduction with a characteristic shrug during attempted abduction.

CLAVICULAR FRACTURES

The most frequently fractured bone in the body is the clavicle. Clavicular fractures usually result from falling on the shoulder or on an outstretched hand. The point of fracture usually occurs at the junction of the outer and middle third of the clavicle. Due to the weight of the arm, the lateral fragment will be depressed and pulled medially and anteriorly by the pectoralis major muscle. Meanwhile, the medial fragment is tilted upward by the sternocleidomastoid muscle. Fracture of the clavicle resulting from a sharp anterior blow may jeopardize the underlying subclavian vessels. However, the brachial plexus is protected from clavicle injuries by the subclavius muscle.

Anatomy Mnemonics for the Rotator Cuff Muscles
SITS:
S—supraspinatus
I—infraspinatus
T—teres minor
S—subscapularis

SHOULDER DISLOCATIONS

Shoulder dislocations are either glenohumeral or acromioclavicular injuries caused by a fall or direct blow to the shoulder. Glenohumeral dislocations can be anterior or posterior; possible axillary nerve damage should be assessed in anterior dislocations. Posterior dislocations are high energy and associated with seizures and electrical shocks. Patients younger than 25 with shoulder dislocations will most likely have recurrent instabilities or dislocations after initial injury. Additionally, patients younger than 40 will have labral tears and patients older than 40 have associated rotator cuff tears. Patients have tenderness and swelling over the joint with fullness of the affected shoulder or elevation of the outer portion of the clavicle. It is important to test the axillary and radial nerve function after all shoulder dislocations.

The Brachial Plexus

The brachial plexus is a complex network of nerves that innervate the shoulder and upper extremity. It derives from the ventral rami from C5 to T1.

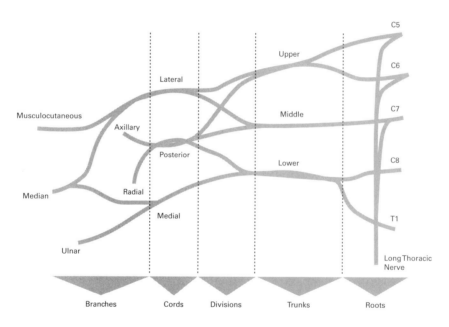

Figure 1 The Brachial Plexus

The **radial nerve** (C5-T1)—travels in the spiral groove on the back of the humerus and stays in the posterior arm and posterior forearm region. The radial nerve's functions include shoulder extension, forearm extension, wrist extension, metacarpophalangeal joint extension, forearm supination, and thumb abduction and extension.

The **musculocutaneous nerve** (C5-C6)—supplies the arm flexors (biceps, brachialis) and cutaneous innervations to the lateral forearm. Located in the anterior portion of the arm, musculocutaneous nerve's functions include shoulder flexion, forearm flexion, and supination.

The **axilliary nerve** (C5-C6)—wraps around the humerus at the surgical neck and supplies sensory to lateral proximal arm. It supplies motor function to the deltoid and teres minor.

The **median nerve** (C5-T1)—travels through the anterior forearm and passes under the flexor retinaculum, a fibrous wristband, to supply the thenar muscles as well as the flexors of the forearm.

Its innervations lead to wrist flexion, metacarpophalangeal joint flexion, and thenar eminence abduction, flexion, and opposition to thumb.

The **ulnar nerve** (C8-T1)—supplies the intrinisic muscles of the hand, the distal interphalangeal joints, and the proximal interphalangeal joints to allow joint extensions. The ulnar nerve innervates abductor digiti minimi, flexor digiti minimi brevis, and opponens digiti minimi. It also innervates the adductor pollicis to allow thumb adduction.

The **long thoracic nerve** (C5-7)—runs along with the lateral thoracic artery on the anterior surface of the serratus anterior muscle. It only supplies the motor function of the serratus anterior muscle.

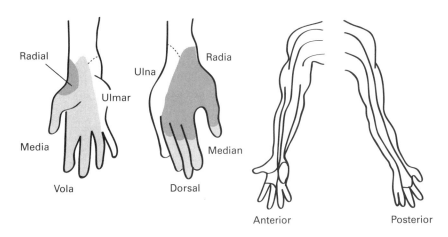

Figure 2 Cutaneous distribution of the nerves and spinal roots

Nerve	Common Injury	Motor Deficit	Sensory Deficit
Radial nerve	Midshaft humerus fracture	Wrist drop—flaccid hand flexion, difficulty with hand extension	Decreased sensation on posterior and lateral arm, posterior forearm, and dorsum of hand
Musculocutaneous nerve	—	Difficulty flexing elbow	Decreased sensation on lateral forearm via lateral cutaneous nerve of forearm
Axilliary nerve	Shoulder dislocation	Difficulty abducting the arm greater than 90°	Numbness over the dome of the shoulder
Median nerve	Carpal tunnel syndrome, wrist fracture, or supracondylar humerus fracture	Decreased thumb function, can't abduct or oppose thumb, unopposed radial nerve, lack of flexion for index and middle finger	Numbness or decrease sensation over the palmar aspect of the thumb, index, middle, and medial half of the ring finger

Ulnar nerve	Fractures of the medial epicondyle of the humerus, wrist fracture	Clawhand sign—inability to adduct thumb, plus the inability to abduct or adduct fingers	Numbness and decreased sensation over both palmar and dorsal aspect of the lateral half of the ring finger and pinky
Long thoracic nerve	Mastectomies with axillary node dissection, thoracic nerve impingement	Winged scapula—medial border of scapulae protrude like wings due to reduced contraction of the serratus anterior muscles on the anterior-medial aspect of the scapula	—
C5-C6 root	Traction or tear of the upper trunk, blow to shoulder, trauma from delivery	Erb-Duchenne palsy/waiter's tip: paralysis of the abductors, lateral rotators, and loss of biceps. Arm will be medially rotated, with forearm pronated and hanging by the side	—
Inferior trunk: C8, T1	Thoracic outlet syndrome—subclavian artery and inferior trunk are compressed	Atrophy of the interosseous muscle, thenar eminence, and hypothenar eminence	Decreased sensation over the medial aspect of the hand and forearm

Table 1 Common nerve injuries

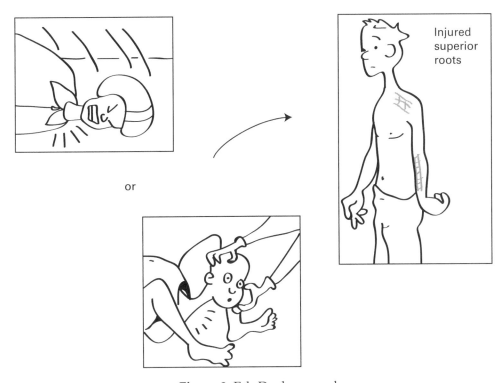

Figure 3 Erb-Duchenne palsy

Arm, Elbow, and Forearm

The arm is divided into the extensor and flexor compartments, which are separated by intermuscular septae. The flexor muscles of the arm are **biceps**, **brachii**, **brachialis**, and **coracobrachialis**. All three muscles in this flexor compartment are innervated by the musculocutaneous nerve. The extensor muscles consist of **triceps brachii** and the **anconeus**; both are supplied by the radial nerve.

The elbow joint is where the humerus forms a hinge joint with the **radius** and **ulna**. The head of the radius is strapped to the ulna by the annular ligament. In a subluxated or "pulled" elbow, the ligament is damaged, and the radius is pulled out of position ("Nursemaid's elbow").

The skeletons of the forearm consist of ulna and the radius. The interosseous membrane is a strong connective tissue that extends between the radius and the ulna. As the weight-bearing bone, the radius is more susceptible to fractures. The most common fracture of the radius is Colles' fracture, which often results from falling on an outstretched hand. This is a complete transverse fracture within the distal portion of the radius. The distal fragment is usually displaced dorsally, leading to a typical "silver-fork deformity".

ELBOW DISLOCATION

Posterior dislocations of the elbow occur due to a fall on an outstretched hand. Avulsion fractures of the medial epicondyle and distal radial (Colles') fractures are associated. The median nerve, the ulnar nerve, and the brachial artery are at risk during these dislocations. Another common form of elbow dislocation is the **subluxation of the head of the radius** and tearing of the annular ligament when a parent forcefully pulls or yanks on the arm of a child. Pronation and supination are markedly restricted in this case.

The forearm can also be divided into the flexor and extensor compartments. The flexor muscles are located on the anterior and the medial aspect of the forearm, while the extensor compartment is situated on the posterior and lateral surfaces.

Flexor Muscles of the forearm	Extensor muscles of the forearm
Superficial layer	*Superficial layer*
Pronator teres	Brachioradialis
Flexor carpi radialis	Extensor carpi radialis longus
Palmaris longus	Extensor carpi radialis brevis
Flexor carpi ulnaris	Extensor digitorum
—	Extensor carpi ulnaris
Intermediate layer	—
Flexor digitorum superficialis	—
Deep layer	*Deep layer*
Flexor digitorum profundus	Supinator
Flexor pollicis longus	Abductor pollicis longus
Pronator quadratus	Extensor pollicis longus
—	Extensor pollicis brevis
—	Extensor indicis

Table 2 Muscles of the forearm

The extensor carpi radialis brevis originates from the lateral epicondyle. Lateral epicondylitis, or tennis elbow, is often seen in middle-aged athletes who overexert their elbow, causing an inflammation to the extensor tendon.

WRIST AND HAND

There are eight carpal bones in the wrist, and they roughly line up in two rows. The proximal row consists of **pisiform** and three carpal bones that articulate with the radius: **scaphoid**, **lunate**, and **triquetrum**. The ulna does not articulate with any carpal bones. The distal row consists of **trapezium**, **trapezoid**, **capitates**, and **hamate**.

The scaphoid fracture is the most commonly fractured carpal bone, usually resulting from falling on an outstretched hand. It is located in the "anatomic snuffbox" on the lateral side of the hand at the base of the thumb. The anatomic snuffbox is enclosed posteriorly by the extensor pollicis longus and anteriorly by the extensor pollicis brevis and abductor pollicis longus. Due to its poor blood supply, a fractured scaphoid may undergo avascular necrosis. Lunate dislocation also may occur from falling on an outstretched dorsiflexed hand.

The flexor retinaculum, or transverse carpal ligament, bridges the concavity of the carpal arch and forms a carpal tunnel with the bones. The flexor tendons and median nerve pass through this tunnel to enter the hand.

Carpal tunnel syndrome occurs when the median nerve is compressed as it passes through the tunnel, resulting in loss of sensation or paresthesia in the lateral 3½ digits. Additionally, loss of coordination and strength in the thumb may also occur since the median nerve sends fibers to the abductor pollicis brevis, flexor pollicis brevis, and opponeus pollicis. Compression of the median nerve may be due to edema, infection, hypothyroidism, pregnancy, or arthritic changes in the carpal bones. Hypothyroidism, pregnancy, and acromegaly are associated with bilateral carpal tunnel syndrome. The Phalen's test (reproducible pain when dorsal surfaces of the hands are pressed together with wrist flexion) and Tinel's sign (pain with tapping of the median nerve at the wrist) may be used to diagnose carpal tunnel syndrome. Treatments include activity modification, night splints, NSAIDS, corticosteroid injections, and in severe cases, surgical release of the carpal tunnel.

Both the radial and ulnar arteries traverse the wrist and supply the hand. They arc around the hand and loop in a circle. The Allen's test may be performed to test the blood supply to the hand. To perform the Allen's test, the patient needs to make a fist for 15–30 seconds while both the radial and ulnar arteries are compressed. After the patient opens his or her hand, the ulnar artery is released. Color and warmth should return within 7–10 seconds for a normal test. This is a subjective way to guarantee adequate blood flow to the hand if the radial artery is used to draw ABG, or for catheterization or bypass surgery.

The fascial spaces of the hand are areas of loose connective tissues within the central compartment of the hand, which is located between the long flexor tendons and the adductor pollicis and interossei.

The thickening of the palmar fascia may result in Dupuytren's contracture, where the digits are flexed. Dupuytren's contracture occurs more commonly in the 4th and 5th fingers of the hand. It may also occur in other fingers as well as in the feet. Additionally, infection of the fascial spaces may results in painful swelling and lead to tenosynovitis.

BLOOD SUPPLY TO THE UPPER LIMB

The blood supply to the arm begins with the subclavian artery, which branches off the brachiocephalic trunk on the right side and directly off the aorta on the left side. The subclavian artery becomes the axillary artery after crossing the first rib. As it travels past the posterior edge of the teres major muscle, it becomes the brachial artery, which splits into the radial and ulnar arteries after crossing the elbow joint.

Collateral circulations exist throughout the upper limb in the shoulder, elbow, and hand. In the shoulder, collateral circulation occurs between the subscapular and suprascapular arteries. The subscapular artery stems from the axillary artery, while the suprascapular artery originates from the thyrocervical trunk via an early branch of the subclavian artery. Collateral circulation also occurs around the elbow: anastomoses occur between the profunda brachii artery and the radial recurrent artery laterally and the ulnar collateral arteries and ulnar recurrent arteries medially. In the hand, the superficial palmar arch from the ulnar artery and the deep palmar arch from the radial artery form collateral circulation.

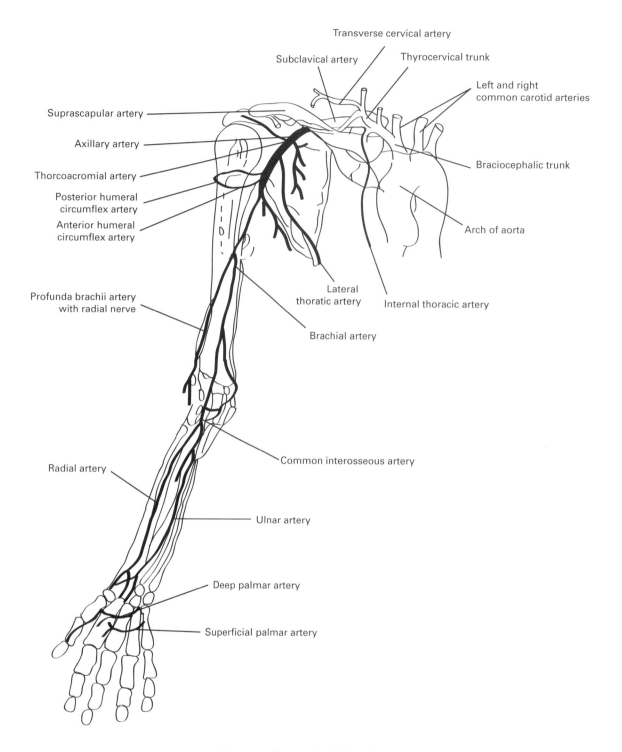

Figure 4 Upper limb blood supply

The Back and Lower Extremity

The Spine

The human vertebral column is composed of 33 vertebrae and 31 pairs of spinal nerves. The vertebrae of the cervical, thoracic, and lumbar region make up approximately 75% of the total length of the presacral column. The sacrum vertebrae fuse to form a single bony plate while the coccyx vertebrae also unite to form a single bone.

Region	Vertebrae
Cervical	7
Thoracic	12
Lumbar	5
Sacral	5
Coccyx	4 (3–5)

Table 3 Vertebral column

The spinal cord ends around L1 or L2, and the remaining nerves dangle down as the cauda equina. Hence, lumbar punctures are done at the L4-L5 or L5-S1 level to prevent laceration of the spinal cord.

The vertebral column in a normal adult is characterized by four anteroposterior curves. The primary curves which persist from birth to adulthood are the thoracic and sacral curves. Both of these curves concave anteriorly. The secondary curves are the cervical and lumbar curves. The cervical curve develops to allow the ability to hold the head erect. The dorsolumbar curve develops throughout childhood as one learns to stand erect and walk. Both secondary curves have concavity facing posteriorly.

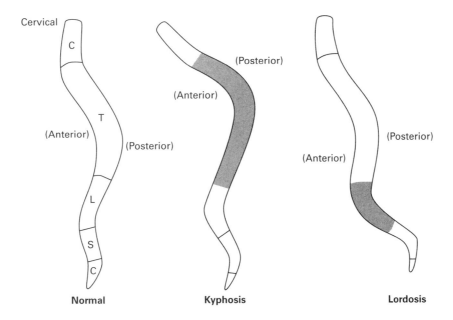

Figure 5 Curves of the spinal column

Abnormal curvatures of the spine may be due to congenital factors, trauma, compensation, or muscle imbalance. Excessive curvature with concavity facing anteriorly is called kyphosis. Kyphosis usually occurs in the thoracic region. Excessive curvature with concavity facing posteriorly is called lordosis. As a rule, lordosis is always a compensatory curve.

Scoliosis occurs when the spine curves laterally. As the most complex abnormal curvature, scoliosis curvatures frequently originate in the thoracic region and have associated rotational components. Scoliotic curves may be functional from compensatory effect of the afflicted part of the column. They may also be structural, resulting from abnormal development such as hemi-vertebra. For severe cases of scoliosis, surgical corrections may be necessary to reduce pain and prevent development of restrictive lung disease.

Muscles of the back may be roughly grouped into five groups. They are all supplied by the dorsal rami of the spinal nerves.

Groups/Location	Function	Muscles
Spinotransversales group		
Extends from spine to transverse process	Rotates head and vertebral column Extends head and neck	Splenius capitis Splenius cervicis
Sacrospinalis group		
Extends from sacrum and iliac crest to neck and skull	Extends the vertebral column	Iliocostalis Longissimus Spinalis
Transversospinalis group		
Extends from transverse process inferiorly to spinous process of the vertebrae located superiorly or to the skull	Rotates the vertebral column Allows lateral flexion of the column	Semispinalis Multifida Rotators
Segmental muscle		
Extends between adjacent vertebrae	Extensors of the column Lateral flexion of the column	Interspinalis Intertransversarii
Suboccipial muscles		
Located in cervical region	Rotation of the head Extension of the head and upper cervical region	Rectus capitis posterior major Rectus capitis posterior minor Obliquus capitis inferior Obliquus capitis superior

Table 4 Muscles of the back

Lumbosacral Plexus

The lumbosacral plexus is a complicated network of nerves. The lumbar part consists of nerves branching from T12 to L4 while the sacral portion involves L5-S4. Together, they innervate the pelvis and the legs. The sacral nerves (S2-S4) also supply some parasympathetic fibers. A few high-yield nerves have been selected and are presented below with their motor innervations.

The **femoral nerve** and the **lateral femoral cutaneous nerve** may be compressed by prolonged sitting in tight jeans. Pelvic fractures often compromise the femoral nerve, leading to leg extension and thigh flexion deficits, as well as decrease in sensation over the anterior thigh and medial leg. The **iliohypogastric** and **ilioinguinal nerves** swing around the flank and down into the pubic region. The **obturator nerve** supplies the thigh adductors. In anterior hip dislocation, the obturator is damaged, leading to difficulty with thigh adduction as well as decreased sensation over the medial aspect of the thigh.

Region	Action	Nerve
Gluteal region	Thigh extension	Interior gluteal nerve
Gluteus maxius	Thigh abduction	Superior gluteal nerve
Gluteus medius and minimus		
Posterior thigh (Hamstrings)	Hip extension Knee flexion	Sciatic nerve (tibial division)
Anterior thigh (Quadriceps)	Hip flexion Knee extensions	Femoral nerve
Posterior leg	Foot plantar flexion and inversion Toe flexion	Tibial nerve
Anterior leg	Foot dorisflexion and inversion Toe flexion	Deep peroneal nerve (Branch of common peroneal nerve)
Lateral leg	Foot eversion	Superficial peroneal nerve (Branch of common peroneal nerve)

Table 5 Lower extremity motor innervations

The **sciatic nerve** (L4-S3) is the largest offshoot of the sacral plexus. It runs down the back of the leg and gives off the **common peroneal** and **tibial nerves**. To avoid the sciatic nerve during gluteal intramuscular injections, the shots should be given in the upper outer buttocks. The common peroneal wraps around near the top of the fibula. It is susceptible to injuries such as trauma to the lateral aspect of the leg or fracture of the fibula neck. Damages to the common peroneal nerve result in difficulty with toe extension and dorsiflexion of the foot (foot drop). Trauma to the peroneal nerve also presents with sensory deficit over the anteriolateral leg and the dorsal aspect of the foot.

The tibial nerve supplies the posterior leg muscles and the sole of the foot. Knee trauma often results in tibial nerve damage, which leads to difficulty with foot inversion or plantarflexion. Additionally, toe flexion and sensation of the sole of the foot are also compromised.

Other nerves of the sacral plexus include the **superior gluteal nerve**, which innervates muscles of thigh abduction (gluteus medius and minimus), and the **inferior gluteal nerve**, which innervates the gluteus maximus (hip extension). Posterior hip dislocation may also compromise the superior and inferior gluteal nerves. As a result, patients have difficulties with thigh abduction and extension and may be positive for Trendelenburg sign.

Pelvis, Hip, and Thigh

The pelvis is composed of three bones: two coxal bones (**ilium** and **ischium)**, and the **symphysis pubis,** which articulate posteriorly with the **sacrum**. The **acetabulum** is the cup-shaped depression where the head of the **femur** sits in the pelvis. The lunate surface is smooth and covered with hyaline cartilage. A fibrocartilaginous ring called the acetabular labrum deepens the hip joint. The hip joint is held together by the iliofemora ligament, ischiofemoral ligament, and pubofemoral ligament. The femur is also attached to the pelvis by the ligament of the head of the femur, which extends from the acetabular fossa to the fovea of the head.

The head of the femur may be dislocated from the acetabulum either congenitally or by injury. Femoral head fracture in the trochanteric area usually results from direct trauma and most commonly occurs in children or middle-aged patients. These patients have good blood supply and avascular necrosis seldom occurs. However, intracapsular fracture of the femoral neck often occurs in the elderly, leading to avascular necrosis of the femoral head. These patients are commonly treated with hip replacement to prevent recurrent fracture or further development of degenerative joint disease.

There are several sources of blood supply to the hip joint. The major sources are the medial and lateral femoral circumflex arteries, the first perforating branch of teh profunda femoris, and the obturator artery.

HIP DISLOCATIONS

Hip dislocations are usually posterior and often occur during an automobile accident, as the body flies forward and the hip joint hits the steering wheel or dashboard. Fracture of the acetabulum often accompanies this injury. Patients hold their legs in flexion, adduction, and internal rotation. The affected leg appears shorter than the non-affected leg. Avascular necrosis of the femoral head is a common complication that can be prevented if reduction of the dislocation occurs within 6 hours. Possible damage to the sciatic nerve should be assessed. Patients with hip dislocations may demonstrate a positive Trendelenburg sign, a downward tipping of the pelvis on the opposite side from the stepping leg, due to faulty hip abduction on the side of the stepping leg. This is also seen in superior gluteal nerve injury and fracture of the neck of the femur.

Anatomy Mnemonics for the Femoral Structures

In the groin area, the NAVEL structures may be palpated:

N—femoral **n**erve
A—femoral **a**rtery
V—fem Biopsy oral **v**ein
E—**e**mpty space
L—**l**ymphatics

In brief, there are three muscle groups in the thigh. The anterior group is supplied by the femoral nerve and extends the leg along with the flexors of the thigh. The anteromedial group primarily adducts the thigh and is innervated by the obturator nerve. Lastly, the posterior group flexes the leg along with thigh extension. Leg flexion is supplied by the sciatic nerve, while thigh extension is supplied by the inferior gluteal nerve, which innervates the gluteus maximus.

The Knee

The knee joint consists of the **femur** at the distal end, the **tibia** at the proximal end, and the **patella**. The fibrous capsule over the joint is made of strong connective tissues that are reinforced by ligaments and tendons. Anteriorly, the capsule is supplied by tendon of the quadriceps and patellar ligament. Posteriorly, it is strengthened by oblique and arcuate popliteal ligaments.

There are two collateral ligaments. The fibular (lateral) collateral ligament extends from the lateral epicondyle of the femur to the head of the fibula. The tibial (medial) collateral ligament extends from the medial epicondyle to the medial aspect of the proximal tibia.

With forceful abduction of the tibia, the medial collateral ligament may be torn at its attachment sites. To test for the integrity of the collateral ligaments, the leg can be forced into abduction (valgus stress) or adduction (varus stress). Exaggerated medial opening with valgus stress may represent injury to the medial collateral ligament, while exaggerated lateral opening with varus stress may represent injury to the lateral collateral ligament. To ensure proper assessment, always compare the exam with the contralateral knee.

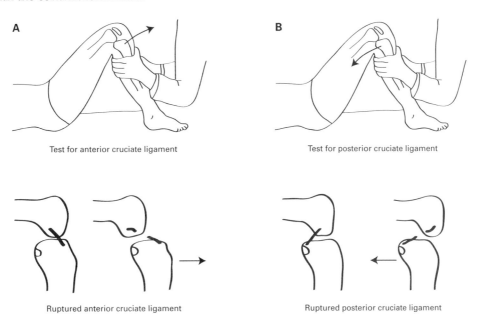

Figure 6 The drawer
(Adapted from *High-Yield Gross Anatomy*)

The cruciate ligaments are strong bands extending between the femur and tibia and are identified by its tibial attachment. The anterior cruciate ligament (ACL) arises from the anterior inter-condylar area of the tibia and attaches to the medial surface of the lateral condyle of the femur. The ACL limits hyperextension of the knee and are often damaged from sports injuries. The "drawer test" shown above tests the integrity of the ACL by pulling the tibia forward with respect to the femur. The posterior cruciate ligament (PCL) arises from the posterior intercondylar area of the tibia and attaches to the lateral surface of the medial condyle of the femur. Similarly, the PCL may be tested with the posterior drawer's test. A classic triad of knee injury from a blow to the lateral side of the knee results in damage of the medial collateral ligament, medial meniscus, and ACL.

The Leg and Ankle

Tibia and **fibula** are united by an interosseous membrane which lends support to the fibula and provides additional surface for the origin of leg muscles. The distal end of the tibia is expanded, forming prominent medial malleolus and laterally the fibular notch for articulation with the fibula. Both the tibia and the fibula articulate with the **talus**. Shin splints are commonly used to refer to stress fractures of the tibia. Another common leg injury is malleolar fracture, which results from severe twisting of the ankle.

There are three muscle groups in the leg: anterior, lateral, and posterior. The anterior group is innervated by the **deep peroneal nerve** while the lateral group arise largely from the fibula and is innervated by the **superficial peroneal nerve**. The posterior group is innervated by the **tibial nerve**.

At the ankle, the flexor retinaculum and the tendon sheaths of the deeper layer of the muscles of the calf holds the tibialis posterior, flexor digitorium longus, and flexor hallucis longus.

The tarsus is made of seven bones: **talus**, **calcaneus**, **navicular**, three **cuneiform** bones, and the **cuboid** bone. The metatarsal and phalanges make up the rest of the foot along with the tarsus. Ankle sprain is very common and may result in either partial or complete rupture of the collateral ligaments.

Inversion sprain is the most common type of sprain, resulting from forceful foot inversion. The lateral collateral ligaments are called upon to bear a higher load, resulting in ligament damage. Inversion sprains may cause an avulsion of the lateral malleolus and the proximal end of the fifth metatarsal. Lateral ankle sprains are more common due to limited ligament support. The most common ligament injury from ankle sprains is the anterior talofibular ligament.

Eversion sprains are less common and mostly involve the medial collateral ligament. Avulsion of the medial malleolus, or Pott's fracture, may result from eversion sprain.

Blood Supply to Lower Limb

The aorta splits into two **common iliac arteries** which further divide in the pelvis to form the **external iliac artery**, the main blood supplier to the leg, and the **internal iliac artery**. The interal iliac artery gives off the **obturator artery** which supplies the adductor muscles and the head of the femur and the **inferior gluteal artery**, which supplies the gluteal

Anatomy Mnemonics for **O**rder of the **T**endons at the **M**edial **M**alleolus

Order of the tendons from proximal to distal of the mallelolus:

Tom, Dick, and Harry

T—**T**ibialis posterior
D—Flexor **d**igitorum longus
H—Flexor **h**allucis longus

muscles. The external iliac artery becomes the **femoral artery** and travels under the inguinal ligament midway through the anterior superior iliac spine and the symphysis pubis. The femoral artery is readily palpable and may be an accessible as a source of emergency blood draws. The femoral artery travels through the adductor hiatus and becomes the **popliteal artery**. The popliteal artery gives off **genicular arteries** (blood supply for the knee), and the **anterior** and **posterior tibial arteries**.

Compromise to the femoral artery from trauma such as a car accident may end in severe loss of function. The collateral blood supply provided by the obturator and inferior gluteal arteries are inadequate to maintain leg perfusion.

Muscle pain and fatigue from exercise due to reduced blood supply is known as claudication. Atherosclerosis of the follow vessels may lead to claudication.

Artery	Area of pain
External iliac artery	Gluteal, thigh, and leg
Femoral artery proximal to profundal femoris artery	Thigh and leg
Femoral artery distal to profunda femoris artery	Leg
Popliteal artery	Leg
Anterior and posterior tibial arteries	No pain!

Table 6 Sources of claudication and presentation

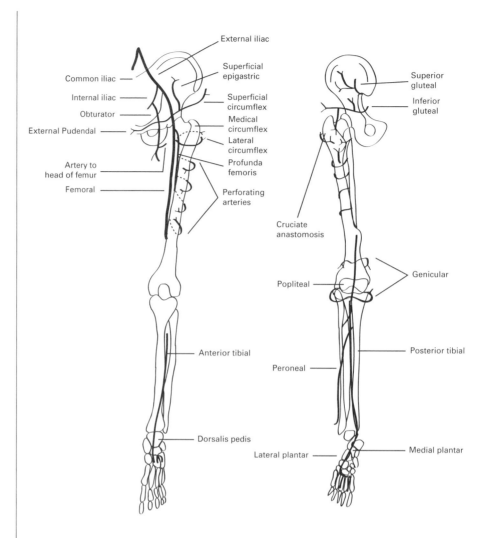

Figure 7 Lower extremity arterial supply
(Adapted from *High-Yield Gross Anatomy*)

EMBRYOLOGY AND GROWTH

Muscle

Muscle tissue derives from the **mesoderm** ([*meso-* means middle], the middle embryologic tissue layer in between the endoderm and ectoderm), which gives rise to **mesenchyme** tissue, which will differentiate into muscle, bone, connective tissue, and blood.

There are 3 types of muscle: **skeletal** muscle, **smooth** muscle, and **cardiac** muscle.

Mesodermal defects are associated with a syndrome of birth defects known as **VACTERL Association**: **V**ertebral defects, **A**nal atresia, **C**ardiac defects, **T**racheo-**E**sophageal fistula, **R**enal defects, **L**imb defects (bone + muscle).

	Skeletal	Smooth (e.g. abdominal organs)	Cardiac
Embryological Growth Pattern	Derived from **somites** (blocks of mesoderm organized next to the notochord; **Figure 8**)	Derived from **mesenchyme** surrounding the endoderm of the primitive gut	Derived from **splanchnic** (visceral) **mesoderm** surrounding the primordial heart tube
Additional Information	Most skeletal muscle forms by 1 year old Develops via fusion of many cells (in contrast to the cardiac muscle) Size increases via **hypertrophy**, not hyperplasia (i.e. an increase in the size of muscle cells as opposed to formation of new cells)	—	Develops from single cells (in contrast to the skeletal muscle) Some cardiac muscle cells differentiate into highly specialized conducting fibers, e.g., Purkinje cells

Table 7 The Three Different Types of Muscle

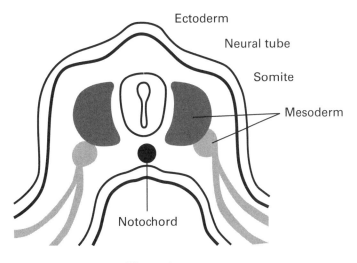

Figure 8

Bone and Cartilage

Like muscle, bone and cartilage develop from mesoderm and its resulting mesenchyme. Mesenchyme develops into bone in two ways: 1) **Intramembranous ossification**, and 2) **Endochondral ossification**.

	Intramembranous Ossification	Endochondral Ossification
Growth Pattern	Flat bone growth Bone forms spontaneously in the mesenchyme without cartilage Begins as woven bone then remodeled to lamellar bone	Long bone growth Formation of cartilaginous model by chondrocytes, which are subsequently converted into bone by osteoclasts and osteoblasts (Figure 9)
Examples	Flat bones (skull, face, axial skeleton)	Limbs, ribs, and other long bones

Table 8 The Two Types of Ossification

Endochondral ossification occurs in the following manner (**Figure 9**):

1. **Hyaline cartilage** model forms via condensation of mesenchyme around blood vessels. The **epiphyseal plate** (EP) forms at the end of the bone as a factory for elongation.

   - Within the EP, chondrocytes (cartilage cells) grow in the **zone of proliferation**, which allows for bone lengthening.

   - Adjacent to the zone of proliferation is the **zone of hypertrophy**, where chondrocytes swell and die in response to calcification of the distal future metaphysis by osteoblasts, leaving a marrow cavity.

   - In the future metaphysis, **osteoblasts** derived from the mesenchyme produce a hard matrix of calcium and phosphate called **hydroxyapatite**, which cuts off nutrient supply to the chondrocytes. This causes them to swell and die, forming the zone of hypertrophy.

2. Cartilage continues to grow in the zone of proliferation, while the **bone collar** of hydroxyapatite in the metaphysis follows close behind until puberty. After puberty, the EP fuses and only **appositional growth** or thickening of bone is possible.

3. Eventually, all cartilage will be replaced by bone, except for the **articular cartilage**, which remains at the end of the bone and facilitates smooth joint movement.

This is why excess growth hormone causes **gigantism** (long bones) in youth and **acromegaly** (thick bones) after puberty.

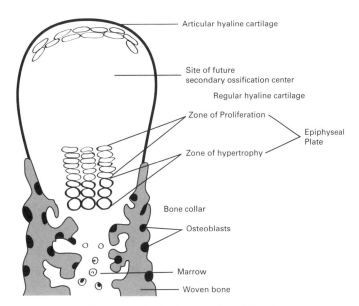

Figure 9 Endochondral ossification

Intramembranous ossification occurs in the following manner:

1. When bone is first made, the collagen is laid down somewhat randomly, and the bone is called **woven bone** (primary bone).

2. Eventually, this haphazardly arranged collagen is remodeled into **lamellar bone** (secondary bone), in which the collagen is neatly organized into layers or **lamellae**.

Limbs develop in the growing embryo by **tissue induction** by overlying ectoderm, causing budding to occur.

HISTOLOGY

Skeletal Muscle

Skeletal muscle histology is confusing because there is a lot of confusing terminology. Fortunately, these names are not particularly high-yield for Step 1, but they are worth being familiar with. One way to think of it is that a **muscle** is a large bundle of **fasciculi**, which in turn are a bundle of **fibers**, which are a bundle of **myofibrils**, which are finally bundles of **myofilaments**, which are contractile proteins (actin and myosin). In other words, a bunch of bundles. This is visually described below (Figure 10):

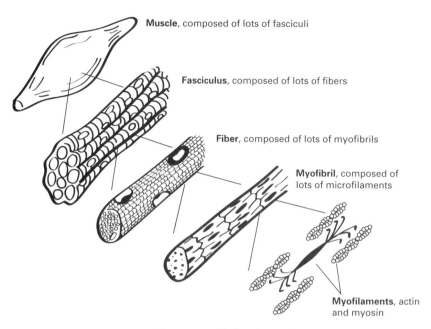

Muscle, composed of lots of fasciculi

Fasciculus, composed of lots of fibers

Fiber, composed of lots of myofibrils

Myofibril, composed of lots of microfilaments

Myofilaments, actin and myosin

Figure 10 Skeletal muscle

Each *fasciculus* is multiple muscle *fibers* covered by a membrane called the **perimysium.** Furthermore, a bundle of fasiculi is surrounded by **epimysium**, which is the tough fibrous coat you may remember cutting through in Gross Anatomy.

Even the cellular structures in muscle cells have special names: **sarcoplasm** is the cytoplasm, **sarcolemma** is the plasma membrane, and **sarcoplasmic reticulum** is the smooth endoplasmic reticulum. Again, not very high-yield, but it is good to be familiar with these terms, as they are referred to in muscle physiology.

Each muscle fiber (or cell) is comprised of multiple mesenchymal cells fused together to form a long, cylindrical **syncytium** with many nuclei. Each cells has numerous myofibrils, which are long, contractile threads composed of subunits called sarcomeres.

The **sarcomere** is the fundamental unit of muscle contraction. Take a look at the structure of the sarcomere (**Figure 11**). Notice the different bands, lines, and the arrangement of actin and myosin. Don't worry about the details of how they work yet. These will be discussed in the Physiology section of the chapter. For now, note that on microscopy, one will see "dark" lines wherever there is *any* myosin, even when overlapping with actin (i.e. the A-Band) and "light" lines where there is *only* actin (i.e., the I-band); see **Figure 12.** Also, note that **M**yosin is anchored to the **M**-line, while **A**ctin is anchored to the **Z**-line (think "A to Z").

A-band = d**A**rk band.
I-band = L**I**ght band.

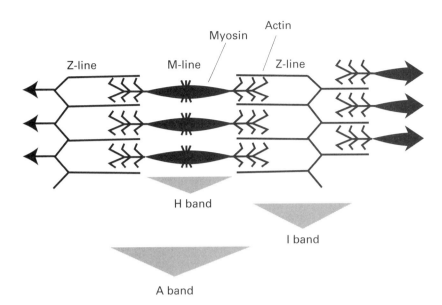

Figure 11 Sarcomere

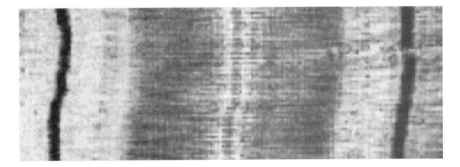

Figure 12 The I-band

Smooth Muscle

Smooth muscle is found in the walls of hollow organs (e.g., gut, uterus, bladder, bronchioles) and blood vessels. Smooth muscle gets its name from its lack of striations, which are visible in skeletal and cardiac muscle as linearly arranged myofibrils. Smooth muscle does have actin and myosin, but they are not arranged in sarcomeres. Rather, they are anchored into **dense bodies** (see Figure 13), which are the equivalent of Z-lines (further discussed in the Physiology section).

Unlike syncytial, multi-nuclear skeletal muscle, smooth muscle cells have only one nucleus, and they are connected electrically by **gap junctions** (Figure 13).

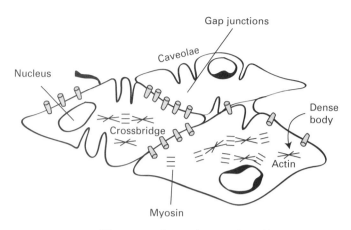

Figure 13 Smooth muscle cell

Smooth muscle is under autonomic control. There are three basic types: 1) **Multi-unit** smooth muscle, **2) Unitary** smooth muscle, and **3) Vascular** smooth muscle (**Table 9**).

	Multi-unit	Unitary	Vascular
Structure	Electrically uncoupled cells (i.e., few or no gap junctions), all supplied by nerves Thus, each cell contracts independently, allowing for fine muscle control	Electrically coupled cells (many gap junctions) that act autonomously with only minor modulation by neurotransmitters The cells contract as one unit, allowing for strong force production (e.g., propelling food, liquid, or babies)	Combination of multi-unit and unitary smooth muscle, having coordinated contractions, as well as substantial neural control
Examples	Iris, ciliary muscle of the lens, vas deferens	GI tract, bladder, uterus, and ureter	Blood vessels

Table 9 The Three Types of Smooth Muscle

Cardiac Muscle

Cardiac muscle combines features of skeletal and smooth muscle. Like skeletal muscle, it contains sarcomeres and is striated. Each cell has one or two nuclei, and the cells may be branched. Like smooth muscle, the cells are electrically connected via **intercalated discs**, which have gap junctions for coordinated contraction. Additionally, cardiac muscle is under involuntary, autonomic control.

Connective Tissue

Like bone and muscle, connective tissue is derived from mesenchyme; in fact, bone is a special type of connective tissue! Connective tissue is composed of cells and matrix. **Fibroblast** cells secrete the **matrix**, which is composed of fibers (**collagen** and **elastin**) and ground substance (**proteoglycans**, which are sugar chains on a protein backbone) that fills in the gaps between cells.

Elastin helps structures that get stretched by returning them to their original shape (e.g. lung, face, arteries, bladder… think elastic recoil).

Collagen is an extremely versatile and ubiquitous protein (the most common in the human body), made from bundles of **tropocollagen** triple helices. Collagen molecules assemble into fibrils by **cross linking via lysyl oxidase** which requires **copper. Menkes disease** (**kinky hair syndrome**) is a **functional copper deficiency** where cross linking is affected, leading to coarse, "kinky" hair and impaired physical and nervous system growth and development.

There are four principal types of collagen:

Type of Collagen	Found In	Associated Diseases (when abnormal)
I	Skin, bone, tendon, wound repair	Osteogenesis imperfecta
II	Cartilage, vitreous body, nucleus pulposus	
III	Reticulin (skin, blood vessels, lymph node)	Ehlers-Danlos syndrome
IV	Basement membrane, basal lamina.	Alport syndrome

Table 10 Collagen Type

Collagen fibers are cross-linked by vitamin C. A deficiency causes unstable collagen, leading to scurvy (capillary rupture and poor wound and fracture healing).

"Don't drop your **BCR** ["VCR"] on the **Floor**." (Type I = Bone, Type II = Cartilage, Type III = Reticulin, Type IV = "floor" i.e. basement membrane [also rhymes with "four"]).

Cartilage

Cartilage is a specialized connective tissue that is comprised of **chondrocytes** (cells that secrete matrix), collagen, and ground substance. There are three types of cartilage:

	Hyaline ("glassy cartilage")	Elastic (contains elastin fibers)	Fibrocartilage (contains type I collagen)
Found In	Developing skeleton (endochondral ossification) Articular surfaces Trachea Larynx	Epiglottis Pinna of the ear	**Annulus fibrosus** of the intervertebral disks Tendon insertion site on bones

Table 11 Types of Cartilage

Bone

Bone plays two roles: 1) structural rigidity and strength secondary to its composition of inorganic matter (**hydroxyapatite** crystals of calcium and phosphate), and 2) calcium level regulation by acting as a reservoir of calcium in the body.

Bone is covered by a connective tissue sheet called the **periosteum**, where tendons insert; note that the periosteum is highly sensitive (think about how badly it hurts to get kicked in the shin!). Lining the inner surfaces of the bone is a connective tissue sheet called the **endosteum**. The cells that are responsible for bone remodeling (osteoblasts and osteoclasts) are found in both the periosteum and endosteum (**Figure 14**).

There are two major cells involved in bone remodeling: **osteoblasts** and **osteoclasts**, which have opposing roles and unique characteristics (**Table 12**).

	Osteoblasts	Osteoclasts
Derived from:	Osteoprogenitor cells	Fusion of cells from the monocyte-macrophage lineage → multi-nucleate Tip: Osteoclasts are multi-nucleate, so they are hungry, i.e., they break bone down
Function	Synthesize **osteoid** from type I collagen and proteoglycans, which is the organic part of the bone matrix that quickly becomes calcified Essentially, osteoblasts **build the bone up** and **store calcium** Eventually, they secrete so much bone matrix that they become encased in osteoid, at which point they are called **osteocytes**, the major mature cell in bone **Osteocytes** have cytoplasmic "telephone lines" that extend through bone **canaliculi** to allow chemical communication with other osteocytes via gap junctions	Resorb calcium in the bone by dissolving it with acids, thereby allowing it to enter the blood Essentially, osteoclasts **break the bone down** and **release calcium**

Table 12 Osteoblasts vs. Osteoclasts

The two types of lamellar bone (remember: this type of bone is formed via intramembranous ossification) are **compact** (dense) **bone** and **cancellous** (spongy) **bone** (**Figure 14**). Compact bone is made of concentric, cylindrical lamellae arranged around a central canal that contains blood vessels.

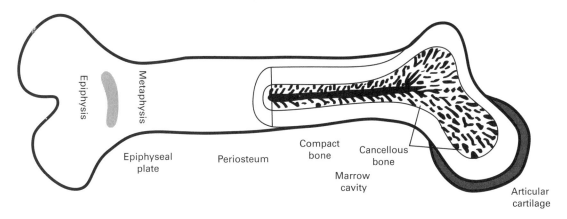

Figure 14 Lamellar bone

The whole apparatus is called a **Haversian system**, or an **osteon**. These long columns of mineral along the bone axis are very strong. Cancellous bone consists of networking spicules of lamellar bone with lots of space in between for bone marrow (**Figure 15**).

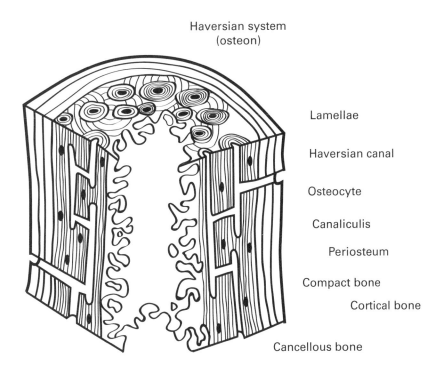

Figure 15 Compact bone and cancellous bone

Other Musculoskeletal Tissues

There are several other musculoskeletal tissues, which you should be familiar with.

- **Ligaments** are fibrous collagen bands that connect bone to bone and provide joint stability.

- **Tendons** are extremely strong collagen bands between muscle and bone.

- **Joints** are collections of tissue found where bones articulate.

If a joint has to move a lot, it has a **synovium**, which is a layer of cells on the inner surface of the joint that secretes lubricating **synovial fluid**. Joints that do not move much (e.g., the sutures in your skull or the pubic symphysis) do not have a synovium.

The **intervertebral joint** is a special joint in which the spine bodies are connected by a disk and the arches articulate via synovial joints. The disk has a gelatinous, central **nucleus pulposus** (derived from the notochord) and a cartilaginous, outer **annulus fibrosus** ring. If this fibrous ring is weakened by age or injury, the nucleus pulposus can herniate out and impinge on a spinal nerve (**disk herniation** or "slipped disk") (Figure 16).

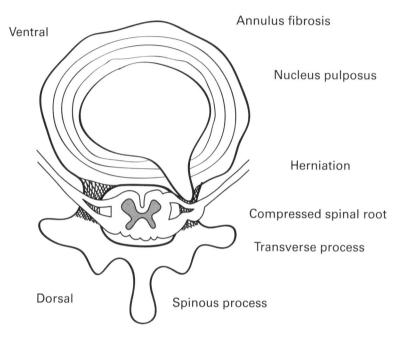

Figure 16 Intervertebral

PHYSIOLOGY

Muscle Excitation-Contraction Coupling (Skeletal muscle and Cardiac muscle)

Muscles are innervated by nerves, which command the muscle to contract via the action potential. The area at which a nerve interacts with a muscle is called the **neuromuscular junction** (**Figure 17**). The following describes how skeletal and cardiac muscle contract.

1. When the action potential depolarizes the nerve terminus, voltage-gated calcium channels open, causing acetylcholine release into the neuromuscular junction.

2. Acetylcholine then binds to ion channels on the **sarcolemma** (muscle cell membrane), causing sodium to enter the muscle cells, and a new action potential to start.

3. This new action potential travels along the sarcolemma until it reaches the **T-tubule**, a cell membrane invagination, which allows the signal to dive further down toward the interior of the muscle fiber.

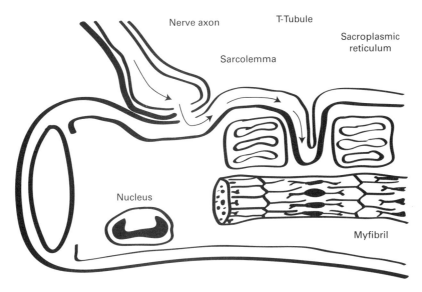

Figure 17 Path action potential

4. The T-tubule (short for **transverse tubule** because it is perpendicular to the sarcolemma) abuts the **sarcoplasmic reticulum** (smooth endoplasmic reticulum of muscle), which contains a lot of calcium ions.

5. As the action potential travels down the T-tubule, the calcium stored in the sarcoplasmic reticulum is released.

This calcium release occurs in *skeletal* muscle via depolarization of the **dihydropyridine receptors** in the T-tubule membrane, which then cause a **conformational change** in the **ryanodine receptors** ("foot processes" are pulled away from the ryanodine receptors). In this manner, dihydropyridine receptors act as depolarization "sensors" for the ryanodine receptors. This conformational change causes calcium to be released into the muscle cells.

In *cardiac* muscle, the ryanodine receptor is not hooked up to the T-tubule. Instead, **extracellular calcium ions** diffuse into the T-tubule after a depolarization and cause the ryanodine receptor to undergo conformational change and release calcium (**Figure 18**). Because of this, **the heart depends on a good supply of extracellular calcium.**

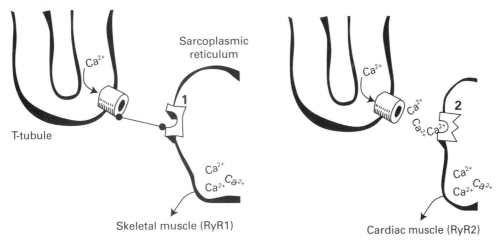

Figure 18 The ryanodine receptor

1. The calcium ions released from the sarcoplasmic reticulum then bind to **troponin C** (C for calcium). Troponin C is one of the proteins on the actin filament, along with **tropomyosin,** and **troponins T** and **I.** Actin is a double-stranded chain of protein that has binding sites for another chain-like protein, myosin. When calcium binds to troponin C, a conformational change occurs in which tropomyosin shifts out of the way and allows myosin to bind to actin (**Figure 19**).

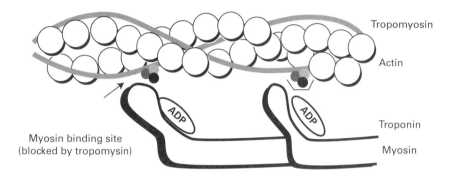

Figure 19 Actin, troponin, and tropomyosin

2. The actin microfilaments are anchored to the Z-lines at the end of the sarcomere (think **A**ctin = **A**nchored). The sarcomere shortens (and the muscle contracts) when myosin pulls an actin ("power stroke") and brings the Z- lines close together, shrinking the width of the H band and I band (Figure 20). The A band width always remains unchanged.

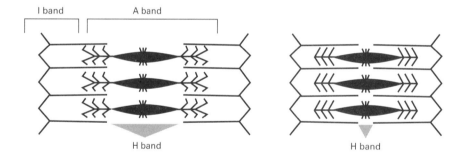

Figure 20 Contraction of a sarcomere. Notice: The H-band and I-band shorten while the A-band does not change.

3. The myosin microfilaments lie in the center of the sarcomere (think **M**yosin = **M**iddle). The myosin has a light-chain tail and a mobile **heavy-chain** head, which carries a molecule of **ADP**. When the head binds to the actin (as described earlier), the ADP falls off and the head swings down. This causes the actin to move relative to the myosin (Figure 21).

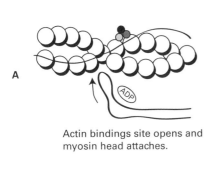

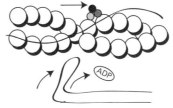

Actin bindings site opens and myosin head attaches.

When ADP is kicked off, myosin head moves and actin shifts (contraction).

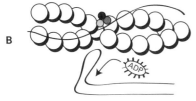

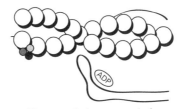

ATP binds to myosin, knocking it off the actin and recocking the head.

The myosin is now ready for another round of contraction.

Figure 21 A. Action of myosin. **B**. Release and recocking of myosin.

4. The Z-bands have now moved a little bit closer together. For another contraction to occur, however, the band of actin must be released, i.e., the muscle must relax. To release the actin, the myosin requires **ATP** to bind to it. The **hydrolysis of ATP to ADP** (which stays bound to the myosin heavy chain) causes the head to **recock (Figure 21B)**. Also during this relaxation, calcium is sequestered into the sarcoplasm via an ATP-powered calcium pump, i.e., ATP is involved in both actin release and calcium re-sequestration.

As you can see, calcium is a crucial component of normal muscle contraction. It is also implicated in abnormal muscle contractions: **Malignant hyperthermia** is a genetic disorder that results in **excessive calcium release** from the sarcoplasmic reticulum of skeletal muscles, causing uncontrolled contractions that raise the body temperature. **General anesthesia** often **triggers** it in these people. Treatment is IV **dantrolene** to inhibit calcium release from the sarcoplasmic reticulum.

Smooth Muscle Contraction

Many of the components of smooth muscle are the same as those for skeletal muscle, including actin, myosin, and tropomyosin. However, the actin is anchored to dense bodies rather than the Z-line. **Calmodulin** also plays an important role in muscle contraction, as described below:

Without ATP (e.g., in death), the muscles contract but are unable to release the myosin from the actin. This is what causes **rigor mortis**.

1. The action potential (either from a nerve or from a neighboring smooth muscle cell via gap junctions) opens up calcium channels on the cell membrane.

2. The calcium enters the cell, binds to the sarcoplasmic reticulum, and releases more calcium.

This calcium then binds to calmodulin, which activates a protein kinase called **myosin light-chain kinase** whose job is to **phosphorylate myosin**, allowing the myosin head to bind to actin and **contract**.

Dephosphorylation by another enzyme called **myosin light-chain phosphatase** lets the smooth muscle relax.

1. The myosin head stays attached to the actin much longer than it does in skeletal muscle. It still requires ATP to reset, but because it resets so infrequently, smooth muscle uses much less energy than its skeletal counterpart.

   - This is great because it allows smooth muscle to stay contracted all day (convenient for maintaining blood pressure), whereas skeletal muscles would tire in a fraction of the time

Skeletal Muscle Fiber Types

There are two types of skeletal muscle fibers that have specialized roles: 1. Slow Twitch (Type I), and 2. Fast Twitch (Type II) (Table 13):

	Type I: SLOW Twitch	Type II: FAST Twitch
Specialized for:	Prolonged, weak contractions, i.e., endurance For example: postural muscles.	Rapid, powerful contractions
How so?	Lots of mitochondria and blood vessels	Large fibers with many glycolytic enzymes and glycogen stores, but relatively few mitochondria → anaerobic metabolism (short bursts of energy)
Appearance	Red	White
Think of it like…	Cows = RED meat, i.e., they are slow and stay standing up in fields for long times (in contrast to chickens)	Chickens = WHITE meat, i.e., they are fast and move around a lot (in contrast to cows)

Table 13 Types of Skeletal Muscle Fiber

If you are a sprinter, you need a lot of fast-twitch fibers for quick, rapid forceful contractions which require anaerobic metabolism. On the other hand, if you run marathons, you need lots of mitochondria and vascularization in your muscles for aerobic metabolism via slow-twitch muscle fibers.

Muscle Metabolism

Muscle utilizes different energy sources depending on the duration of contraction:

- Muscle needs **ATP**, but it only has enough to sustain maximal contractions for **a second or two.**

- When ATP runs out, the first place muscle turns is **phosphocreatine**, which has high-energy phosphate bonds that can be converted to ATP. This lasts **7 or 8 seconds**.

- Next, muscle turns to **glycogen** for ATP, snipping off stored glucose residues and converting them to lactic acid and pyruvic acid. This provides **a minute** of contractions at the expense of a little lactic acidosis.

- If you want to go further, you need **oxidative metabolism**, which gets as much ATP as possible from carbohydrates, proteins, and fats through electron transport.

Growth Hormone

Growth hormone (GH, aka **somatotropin**) has many effects in the body, most visibly on the musculoskeletal system. Naturally, it promotes growth of both muscle and bone. GH has direct and indirect anabolic effects. It mainly acts on liver, muscle and adipose tissue. Through the liver it promotes synthesis of somatomedins (ie IGF-1) which act directly on bone promoting chondrogenesis in the growth plates of long bones.

GH is inhibited by **somatostatin**, which is the treatment for acromegaly.

Repair and Regeneration

While damaged muscle and bone cannot regenerate, they can be repaired. The mechanism of muscle repair is beyond the scope of Step 1, but bone repair is a good topic to be familiar with:

1. After you fracture a bone, the osteoblasts in the bone and periosteum leap into action, laying down new bone matrix.

2. The osteoprogenitor cells start churning out even more osteoblasts.

3. Pretty soon, a **callus** composed of cells and matrix forms at the fracture site.

4. Over **4–6 weeks**, osteocytes and osteoclasts get involved in **bone remodeling** so that it looks as good as new!

Kids with **GH deficiency** (or deficiencies in GH-releasing hormone, insulin-like growth factors, or GH receptors) have **dwarfism** (short stature, delayed puberty, and obesity).

An **excess of GH** causes **gigantism** (long bones) *before* **puberty** and **acromegaly** (thick bones) *after* **puberty**, i.e., after the epiphyses have fused.

CONGENITAL AND METABOLIC DISORDERS

Congenital Dislocation of the Hip

Congenital dislocation of the hip is seen more commonly in females and in infants with a family history of hip dislocation. The cause is unknown, but it may be related to ligamentous laxity or breech positioning in utero. Examination for hip dislocation is part of the **standard newborn examination**.

Signs and Symptoms

If dislocation is unilateral, the affected leg appears **shorter**.

On examination:

1. **Barlow maneuver:** hip flexion and posterior force dislocates the hip.

2. **Ortolani test:** abduction and anterior pressure reduces the femoral head into place. You may hear a "**clunk**" as the hip joint slips back into normal position.

Diagnosis

Ultrasound or X-rays may confirm the diagnosis.

Treatment

• Braces and splints during growth.

• Surgical correction in severe cases.

Osteogenesis Imperfecta

Osteogenesis imperfecta is a disease of **abnormal bone fragility** caused by a disorder of **type I collagen** formation. It is also known as "**Brittle Bone Disease**." The most serious type is osteogenesis imperfecta congenital (aka type II), which is often fatal in infancy due to trauma during delivery. It is an **autosomal dominant** disease.

Signs and Symptoms

Osteogenesis imperfect causes type I collagen deficiencies. Therefore, everything in the body that contains type I collagen, e.g., bones, will be weak! Here are the most common findings:

• **Multiple limb fractures** (→ abnormally short extremities, aka dwarfism)

• **Blue sclera**

• The **skull feels like a "bag of bones"** (i.e., **soft**) when palpated.

Note: A history of multiple fractures should also lead you to suspect child abuse.

• **Hearing loss** due to abnormal formation of the ossicles.

• **Dental defects**

Pathology

Microscopically, the bony tissue is osteopenic with abnormally thin cortices and trabeculae.

Diagnosis

Radiologic studies are diagnostic.

Treatment

No treatment currently exists.

Achondroplasia

Achondroplasia is secondary to **retarded endochondral bone formation** → abnormally short bones (Dwarfism). The majority of cases are spontaneous mutations, but a small percentage are hereditary (autosomal dominant, recessive, or X-linked). Type II collagen defects have been implicated in a small number of cases.

Signs and Symptoms

- **Bones** appear **short** but have **normal width**.

- The **spine and skull appear normal**.

- Fingers may appear **stubby**, and the patient generally looks **bow-legged**.

Diagnosis

History and radiographic findings

Treatment

Surgical hip replacement may be helpful.

Due to abnormal cervical spine formation, care must be taken during neck hyperextension (as during intubation) or spinal cord compression may result.

Muscular Dystrophy

Muscular dystrophy refers to a group of genetic disorders that result in **muscle wasting**. There are several different types of muscular dystrophy: those transmitted as autosomal or X-linked mutations.

The **most common** muscular dystrophy is **Duchenne muscular dystrophy**, an **X-linked recessive** disease that occurs during childhood, particularly in **males**. This disease has been linked to the absence of the gene for **dystrophin**, a protein that is usually found in the sarcolemma.

Another commonly tested muscular dystrophy is **Becker muscular dystrophy**, which like Duchenne's, is an X-linked mutation of the dystrophin gene. However, Becker's dystrophy is **less severe** and has **later onset** (adolescence or early adulthood as opposed to childhood).

Signs and Symptoms

- The typical patient is a **5-year-old boy** who experiences **frequent falls and difficulty climbing stairs**, due to proximal muscle weakness.

- **Gowers' sign**: the characteristic use of arms to compensate for hip extensor weakness when rising from a supine to standing position.

- **Pseudohypertrophy** of the calves is seen, and **cardiac involvement** is common.

Pathology

Cardiac and skeletal muscle biopsy show **necrosis and fatty replacement** of muscle tissue.

Diagnosis

- Serum **creatine kinase is markedly elevated**.

- Cardiac and skeletal muscle biopsy

Treatment

- None

- Patients are usually wheelchair-bound by age 12, and life expectancy is about 20 years; the most common cause of death is heart failure.

- Patients who have a family history of muscular dystrophy should receive **genetic** counseling before planning a pregnancy.

Rhabdomyolysis

Rhabdomyolysis is a skeletal muscle injury that causes muscle cell contents to enter the bloodstream. It can be caused by overexertion, seizures, and hypoxia, as well as **drugs,** such as *cocaine* and *statins*.

Myoglobin, the carrier of oxygen in muscle tissue, is released into the bloodstream during rhabdomyolsis. It is a nephrotoxin and can cause **renal failure**. The mechanism is unclear, but it may be due to intratubular precipitation of myoglobin, causing obstruction or concomitant release of proteases from the muscle cells.

Signs and Symptoms

- Patients with rhabdomyolysis have **myalgias** and **pain** in the affected muscles, with a **"doughy" feeling** of the muscle masses.

- Patients also develop **dark brown urine** (**myoglobinuria**) from excess myoglobin excretion.

Keep rhabdomyolysis high on the differential diagnosis for a patient taking **statins** (i.e. patient with history of hyperlipidemia) who presents with **muscle pain!**

- Note that urinalysis can be "heme" positive, but there are no RBC's . This is because the color dipsticks react with the iron-containing porphyrin ring present in both hemoglobin and myoglobin, even in the absence of red blood cells, as is the case in myoglobinuria.

Diagnosis

- **Creatine phosphokinase** and **aldolase** levels are elevated.

- **Myoglobinuria**

- Patients are **hyperkalemic** and **hyperphosphatemic** due to release of potassium and phosphate from injured muscle.

- **Calcium** may be **low** due to calcium deposition in the injured tissues.

Treatment

Aggressive hydration

Osteomalacia and Rickets

Osteomalacia in adults and **r**ickets in children produce defective mineralization of the bone. Both are caused by **vitamin D deficiency**, which may result from poor dietary intake (breast milk has little vitamin D, so **exclusively breastfed infants are at risk**!), malabsorption, lack of exposure to sunlight, or renal disease.

Note that **Vitamin D** is a fat-soluble vitamin. *Any* **fat malabsorption condition** (chronic pancreatitis, sclerosis cholangitis, Crohn's disease, short bowel syndrome) can put **patients at risk.**

Signs and Symptoms

- Children may have **bowed legs**, and infants with the disease may have reduced skull mineralization, known as **craniotabes**.

- Costochondral beading, known as rachitic rosary appearance, and kyphoscoliosis may be present, as well, in children.

- Adults may be asymptomatic or have soft bones.

Pathology

Microscopically, osteomalacia has **thickened trabeculae** but **deficient mineralization** of **cartilaginous** material. Contrast with osteoporosis (see the next section).

Diagnosis

Serum vitamin D levels are low.

Treatment

Vitamin D supplementation

McArdle's Disease

McArdle's disease is caused by a genetic deficiency of glycogen phosphorylase in skeletal muscle, resulting in an inability to break down glycogen.

Signs and Symptoms

- Cramping and skeletal muscle weakness after exercise

- Myoglobinuria

Diagnosis

- Muscle **biopsy** shows absence of glycogen phosphorylase with increased amount of glycogen.

- Exercise does not cause a rise in lactate level.

Treatment

Severe exertion should be limited.

Osteoporosis

Osteoporosis is **decreased bone mass** despite the presence of **normal bone and lab values**, resulting in an increased risk of bone fracture. It develops in **postmenopausal women** due to **lack of estrogen** needed to help replace bone. Patients on **chronic corticosteroid treatment** are also at risk. Asian and **Caucasian women** are at increased risk, whereas African-American women are at decreased risk. **Smoking** may also contribute to osteoporosis development.

Signs and Symptoms

- Patients may be asymptomatic or develop kyphosis.

- The classic fractures associated with osteoporosis are **hip** (femoral neck)**, vertebral crush,** and **Colles' fractures**.

Pathology

Bone tissue appears normal, although the number and size of trabeculae are reduced.

Diagnosis

- Bone density studies show decreased bone mass.

- Normal lab values

If the patient has a uterus, she also needs progestin therapy in conjunction with the estrogen to prevent the development of endometrial cancer.

Treatment

Several measures have been found to decrease bone loss and delay the development of osteoporosis:

1. Calcium supplementation in the diet

2. Exercise

3. Estrogen replacement therapy (including Selective-estrogen receptor modulators [SERM], which are estrogen agonists in bone and antagonists in breast tissue):

   • **Tamoxifen**: prevents breast cancer and osteoporosis, but **increases risk of endometrial cancer** secondary to partial estrogen agonist effects at the endometrium. (Think "That TAM [damn] Tamoxifen! Gives you endometrial cancer!").

   • **Raloxifene:** like tamoxifen, prevents breast cancer and osteoporosis with **no effect on endometrium** (not an agonist at the endometrium).

4. Bisphosphonates (e.g., alendronate) may also be used to preserve bone.

Gout and Pseudogout

Gout is a form of arthritis caused by the deposition of **uric acid** crystals in the joint. Patients may inadequately excrete uric acid due to renal disease or overproduce uric acid, as with **Lesch-Nyhan syndrome** (a nucleic acid metabolic deficiency).

Pseudogout is caused by **calcium pyrophosphate** deposition in the joints. The etiology is not clear, but **trauma** and **endocrine disorders**, e.g., diabetes mellitus, obesity, and hypothyroidism are commonly associated with the disease.

As a quick reminder of biochemistry, the specific pathology in **Lesch-Nyhan syndrome** is an X-**linked** recessive condition of **HGPRT deficiency**, resulting in elevated uric acid levels, **self-mutiliation**, mental retardation, and poor muscle control.

As the two diseases may present similarly (e.g. both are acute monoarthritides), it is important to able to distinguish between the two (Table 14):

	Gout	Pseudogout
Mechanism of Disease	Deposition of **monosodium urate** crystals into joints, most commonly due to **underexcretion** (90%) vs. overproduction (10%) Common causes are **Lesch-Nyan Syndrome** and use of **thiazide diuretics** Also occurs after alcohol use, as products of alcohol metabolism can block uric acid excretion from the body	Deposition of **calcium pyrophosphate** in the joints Associated with **trauma**
Epidemiology	**Men** are more commonly affected Most common in 20's and 30's	Men and women are affected **equally** Most common after age 50
Signs and Symptoms	Arthritis affecting the big toe (known as **podagra**) is classic Affected joint is red, hot, swollen, and tender Patients may also develop **tophi** (uric acid deposition in the tissues), especially on the **ear**	Rather than the big toe, arthritis of the **knee** is classic
Diagnosis	Joint aspiration shows <u>**negative**</u> **birefringent crystals** (yellow when polarized light is parallel, and blue when perpendicular, to crystals Uric acid levels may be normal during a gouty attack	Joint aspiration shows <u>**positive**</u> **birefringent crystals** (blue when polarized light is parallel, and yellow when perpendicular, to crystals
Treatment	**Acute** treatment is very different from **chronic** treatment. This is important; using the wrong treatment can worsen an acute attack! Nonsteroidal anti-inflammatory drugs (NSAIDs) and colchicine are used in **acute** attacks High-dose colchicine, allopurinol, and uricosuric agents (e.g., probenecid) should be started after the attack has resolved (i.e., **chronically**)	Very similar to Gout

Table 14 Gout and Pseudogout

INFLAMMATORY DISEASES

Rheumatoid Arthritis

Rheumatoid arthritis (RA) is an **autoimmune** arthritis (Type III Hypersensitivity) seen predominantly in women. It appears to have a genetic association with the **HLA-DR4** haplotype.

Signs and Symptoms

- RA usually affects the hand joints, especially the wrist, proximal interphalangeal (**PIP**), and metacarpophalangeal (**MCP**) joints, with **ulnar deviation** of the wrists.

- Joint involvement is usually **symmetric**.

- Patients develop **morning stiffness for at least 1 hour** after waking.

- The affected joints show **subluxations** (incomplete dislocations) and **limitation of movement.**

- Patients may develop subcutaneous **rheumatoid nodules** on bony prominences or extensor surfaces, such as the elbow.

Diagnosis

- Erythrocyte sedimentation rate (**ESR**) is elevated.

- Serum **rheumatoid factor** is positive.

- X-rays may show **erosion** of the joint space.

Treatment

- Pain relievers such as **NSAIDs** are used.

- **Corticosteroids** (both oral and local injection)

- Disease-modifying Antirheumatic Drugs **(DMARDs)**, such as methotrexate and hydroxychloroquine, may induce remission of symptoms.

For Step 1, it is important to distinguish RA from osteoarthritis. Classic signs of RA (as opposed to osteoarthritis) include **symmetric MCP involvement** (not affected in osteoarthritis, which is usually assymetric), **morning stiffness lasting longer than 60 minutes that improves as the day goes on** (not typical of osteoarthritis), and **systemic symptoms** (e.g., fever).

Septic Arthritis

Septic arthritis is caused by bacterial infection of the joint space. The likely infecting organism is based on history:

- **Staphylococcus aureus** is **the most common cause** of septic arthritis.

- **Young, sexually active** persons are more likely to develop **gonococcal arthritis**.

- **IV drug users** may have **gram-negative rod** infections.

- Persons with **prosthetic joints** are at high risk of developing septic arthritis from common **skin or oral flora**.

- Also, systemic diseases, such as **Lyme disease** (*Borrelia burgdorferi*) and **hepatitis B**, may cause septic arthritis.

- **Pott's disease** is a **tuberculosis** infection in the joint spaces of the spine.

Signs and Symptoms

- The ensuing arthritis usually affects only one or a few joints and is associated with **fever, swelling, and pain.**

- **Gonococcal** arthritis may be associated with a pustular **rash** or **genital** symptoms and classically presents as a **monoarticular**, "**migratory**" arthritis (i.e., arthritis that moves from one joint to another).

- **Lyme disease** is associated with "**target lesions**" at the bite site and is discussed in more detail in Chapter 19.

Diagnosis

- Drainage of the joint fluid shows many white blood cells (usually neutrophils).

- Gram stain may reveal an organism, but not always, e.g., in the case of gonococcal arthritis.

Treatment

- Appropriate antibiotic treatment

- Surgical drainage may be necessary

Spondyloarthropathies

The spondyloarthropathies share a number of common features.

- They are associated with **HLA-B27.**

- They frequently involve the **sacroiliac joint** in addition to **peripheral joints**.

- Unlike rheumatoid arthritis, they occur in the **absence of rheumatoid factor** (RF) [hence, they are also known as **seronegative spondyloarthropathies**], and the pathologic changes begin not in the synovium, but rather in the **ligamentous attachments to bone**.

There are four types of seronegative spondyloarthropathies:

1. **Ankylosing spondylitis** is the prototypical spondyloarthropathy highly associated with **HLA-B27**. It is a chronic arthritis that affects the spine and sacroiliac joints, ultimately leading to a rigid spine from bone fusion ("**bamboo spine**"). It is also associated with **uveitis** and **aortic regurgitation**.

2. **Reiter's syndrome** aka **reactive arthritis** features a classic triad of conjunctivitis, urethritis, and arthritis, often following **sexually transmitted** urethritis or diarrhea from a bacterial **GI infection**. The arthritis is **asymmetric** and commonly affects the **ankles, knees, and feet**.

3. **Psoriatic arthritis:** Affects approximately 10% of individuals with **psoriasis** and associated with dactylitis, commonly described as "**sausage fingers**," i.e., swollen, painful fingers. Classic findings on x-ray are "**pencil-in-cup**" deformity.

4. **Spondylitis with inflammatory bowel disease**: A complication of **Crohn's disease** and **ulcerative colitis**.

Osteomyelitis

Osteomyelitis, or bone infection, can result from direct trauma, localized infection, or hematogenous spread. **S. aureus** is a common infecting organism, especially in children. Patients with **sickle cell anemia** are at **increased risk** of the development of **Salmonella** osteomyelitis, although **S.aureus remains the most common infecting organism**, i.e., sickle cell patients most commonly have osteomyelitis secondary to S.aureus, BUT if a patient has Salmonella osteomyelitis, he or she is more likely to have sickle cell anemia.

Signs and Symptoms

Patients have **fever** and **localized pain** at the affected bone.

Pathology

- Microscopic examination shows **inflammation** followed by **necrosis** and **fibrotic replacement**.

- *Sequestrum* refers to an area of **necrotic bone without vascular supply**, and *involucrum* is **new periosteal bone formation** in response to the infection that surrounds the inflammatory area.

Diagnosis

- X-rays are **often normal** but may show "**mottling**."

- Nuclear bone scans show **increased white blood cell concentrations** in the affected areas.

- Elevated ESR and C-reactive protein (CRP)

Treatment

- Antibiotics are directed at the causative organism.

- Surgical drainage may be required in severe cases.

Polymyalgia Rheumatica

Polymyalgia rheumatica is a syndrome of joint pain affecting individuals **over age 50**. Etiology is unknown, and it may be a **diagnosis of exclusion** in some cases. It is considered an **autoimmune** disease but has not been definitively linked to any HLA types.

Signs and Symptoms

- Patients complain of pain and stiffness (but *no weakness*) in the neck, shoulders, upper arms, and hips that lasts **at least a month**.

- **Morning stiffness**, **symmetric** joint involvement, and systemic symptoms (e.g., fever, fatigue, weight loss) is common.

- Associated with **temporal** or **giant cell arteritis**

Diagnosis

ESR and CRP may be elevated, but other laboratory tests are normal.

Pathology

- Muscle biopsies are normal.

- Joint examination may reveal mild inflammation.

Treatment

- *Low-dose* **prednisone** is usually curative (vs. high-dose for temporal arteritis).

- If you suspect temporal arteritis, you **must** get temporal artery biopsy and NOT delay treatment if visual symptoms occur, lest the patient become blind.

Osteochondritis Dessicans

Osteochondritis dessicans occurs when a portion of subchondral bone undergoes **avascular necrosis**. The affected bone segment then **breaks off and floats** in the joint space. It commonly affects the knees (the lateral portion of the **medial femoral condyles** is most common site), hips, elbows, and ankles. The cause is **unknown**, and it is seen primarily in **young male adults**.

Signs and Symptoms

- Patients experience pain and stiffness that **worsen with activity**.

- The joint may **lock** if the fragment becomes completely detached.

Diagnosis

X-rays are diagnostic.

Treatment

- Weight is kept off joints with crutches for several months to promote healing.

- Surgery is often necessary.

Osgood-Schlatter Disease

Osgood-Schlatter disease is an inflammatory disorder that involves the **tibial tuberosity** at the insertion of the patellar tendon. It is characteristically seen in **physically active adolescents 10 to 17 years** old and is believed to be secondary to **repetitive stress and trauma,** e.g, constant **sports activity**.

Signs and Symptoms

Knee pain aggravated by vigorous exercise

Diagnosis

X-ray reveals irregularity of the tubercle contour, with possible haziness of the adjacent metaphyseal border.

Treatment

- **Rest and stretching** of the hamstrings and quadriceps.

- In severe cases, **casting or bracing** may help reduce pain by reducing strain on the tibial tubercle.

- **Surgical excision** is also used, but rarely.

DEGENERATIVE JOINT DISEASES

Osteoarthritis (OA)

Osteoarthritis, also known as degenerative joint disease, is very common in the aging and obese populations. It is a non-inflammatory arthritis caused by collagen breakdown and chondrocyte injury. The most commonly affected joints are knees and hips but OA can be seen in the distal interphalangeal joints (DIP), proximal interphalangeal joints (PIP), the thumb carpometacarpal joint, and the spine. The presentation is usually asymmetric. OA occurs either idiopathically or secondary to trauma, hip dysplasia, or even repetitive use.

Signs and Symptoms

Symptoms include gradual onset of joint pain, with little or no morning stiffness. DIP (Heberden's nodes) and PIP (Bouchard's nodes) bony protuberances are common. Patients have decreased ROM and crepitus. Medial aspect of knee is most commonly affected, leading to varus deformity. There are no systemic signs.

Diagnosis

X-rays show joint space narrowing, with flaking of cartilage. Areas of excessive smoothness, known as eburnation, may form at contact points. Osteophytes and subchondral cysts are seen on X-rays.

DIP involvement signifies osteoarthritis but not rheumatoid arthritis.

Treatment

NSAIDs, muscle strengthening, joint protection, and even surgery (arthoplasty or arthrodesis)

Osteitis Deformans

Also known as **Paget's disease**, osteitis deformans is caused by osteoclastic over-activity followed by abnormal bone deposition by osteoblasts. Patients usually develop the disease in the fifth decade, and it is usually diagnosed incidentally, when the patient receives X-rays for another medical problem. Patients with Paget's disease are at increased risk of developing osteosarcoma. It's believed that Beethoven may have had Paget's disease.

Signs and Symptoms

Patients are often asymptomatic but may develop gait abnormalities or abnormal bone swelling, especially of the skull leading to lionlike facies and increased head size. Back pain may develop from malformation of the articular facets, and hearing loss may occur from destruction of the ossicles. Patients are predisposed to pathological fractures.

Diagnosis

Serum alkaline phosphatase is elevated and is pathognomonic. Urine hydroxyproline levels are increased because the hydroxyproline and hydroxylysine from the destroyed bone is not used in the manufacture of new bone. X-rays show a characteristic mosaic appearance with lytic lesions.

Pathology

Lamellar bone is replaced by woven bone, and the trabeculae are thickened. A mosaic pattern is present microscopically as well.

Treatment

Calcitonin and etidronate may be used to retard activity of osteoclasts.

Slipped Capital Femoral Epiphysis

The typical presentation of slipped capital femoral epiphysis is a painful limp or knee pain in an overweight teenage boy. The cause is a growth disturbance of the proximal femoral growth plate that causes the femur to rotate externally under the capital epiphysis. This phenomenon is rarely seen in prepubescent children.

Signs and Symptoms

Limb shortening and limited internal rotation may also be present, along with decreased hip external rotation with flexion and antalgic gait.

Diagnosis

X-ray taken in the frog-leg and lateral positions.

Treatment

Pin fixation prevents further misalignment. Osteotomy is required in chronic cases.

Legg-Calvé-Perthes

Legg-Calvé-Perthes disease is characterized by avascular necrosis of the femoral epiphysis due to unknown causes. Like slipped capital femoral epiphysis, a limp is often the presenting complaint, although in this case the limp tends to be painless. It is seen more commonly in boys than girls and tends to occur in a younger age group (children 4–8) than does slipped capital femoral epiphysis. It can be bilateral.

Signs and Symptoms

Limp, usually without pain. Pain, if present, is referred to the knee. Range of motion is limited upon internal rotation, abduction, and flexion.

Diagnosis

The femoral head is flattened. The initial X-ray may be normal, with later studies revealing epiphyseal radiolucency.

Treatment

Young children with minimal involvement may be observed. Older children with more femoral head changes require orthotic bracing or surgery to protect the fragile femoral head and maintain normal range of motion. Prognosis depends on the amount of ischemic damage. Long-term disability results from abnormal or asymmetric growth.

	SCFE	Legg-Calvé-Perthes
Pathology	Displacement of femoral epiphysis	Idiopathic osteonecrosis of femoral head
Patient	Obese adolescent male 10–16 years old	Boys usually 4–8 years old
Presentation	Decreased internal rotation, painful limp, limb shortening	Painless limp. Pain can be referred to knee
Imaging	X-ray shows slipped epiphysis	Sclerosis and subchondral collapse
Treatment	Percutaneous *in situ* screw fixation	Young children: observation, reduced weight bearing Older patients: femoral or acetabular osteotomy

Table 15 SCFE and Legg-Calvé-Perthes

Fractures

Fracture healing occurs in the following three stages.

1. **Inflammatory phase**: a hematoma forms at the fracture site and supplies site with hematopoietic and osteoprogenitor cells. Neovascularization occurs, and the formation of a soft **procallus** begins with the presence of pluripotent stem cells that differentiate into osteoclasts and osteoblasts.

2. In the **intermediate phase**, the procallus becomes a fibrocartilaginous callus with the removal of necrotic tissue by the osteoclasts and the deposition of new osteoid by the osteoblasts.

3. The **remodeling phase** occurs when the fibrocartilaginous tissue is replaced by osseous tissue. This may continue for months after clinical improvement because woven bone is replaced by lamellar bone, which is more suitably oriented for weight bearing. Restoration of the medullary cavity also occurs during this phase.

Bones need a good blood supply to heal and also stability.

Smoking and NSAIDS can inhibit fracture healing

Stage	Primary Process
Inflammatory	Hematoma develops presence of hematopoetic/osteoprogenitor cells
Intermediate	Soft Callus: cartilage that bridges bone ends Hard Callus: replacement of soft callous into woven bone and endochondral ossification
Remodeling	Woven bone to lamellar bone

Table 16 Stages of fracture healing

Complications of fractures include the following

Six Ps:
pain,
pallor,
pulselessness,
paresthesia,
poikilothermia, and
paralysis.

- **Neurologic** and **vascular damage** can occur through laceration or excessive traction. These are surgical emergencies.

- **Compartment syndrome** occurs when bleeding or swelling occurs within a closed fascial space. The resulting pressure can compress the vascular supply, resulting in tissue necrosis. This occurs most commonly in the forearm or leg. Surgical fasciotomy relieves the pressure. Most sensitive test is extreme pain on passive extension. Three general causes for compartment syndrome are the following: constriction of a compartment (scarring or contracture), increased fluid in a compartment (hemorrhage or edema), and external compression (like a cast) of a compartment.

- **Disuse atrophy** and **joint contractures** are common. These can be prevented with early physical therapy, including range-of-motion, and exercises.

- **Deep venous thrombosis** may occur due to prolonged immobilization combined with previous trauma. Breakage of the clot may cause a fatal pulmonary embolus. Hence, all patients should be on deep venous thrombosis prophylaxis, with pneumatic compression boots or subcutaneous heparin injections daily.

Fractures are a common cause of morbidity in elderly patients, and about 20% of cases lead to death from prolonged immobility. Elderly women with osteoporosis are predisposed to developing fractures after falling. The most common fractures in the elderly population are hip, spine, and distal forearm (Colles') fractures. Vertebral fractures may occur gradually and may be asymptomatic or cause varying degrees of back pain.

The following are characteristically found in certain fractures:

- **Rib**: Fractures result in local pain and tenderness, which can be distinguished from soft-tissue injury by increased pain at the fracture site by compressing the chest anteroposteriorly (simultaneously pressing on the sternum and thoracic spine); this maneuver should not elicit increased pain in the tender site in soft tissue injury. Sometimes a step off can be felt. Lower rib fractures should lead to suspicion of possible kidney, liver, or spleen damage.

- **Femur**: A fracture at the neck of the femur results in shortening and lateral rotation of the leg (compared to hip dislocation, which produces shortening, **medial** rotation, and flexion of the leg). Fractures in other parts of the femur can pull the pieces in different directions, depending on the relative locations of the fracture site and the muscles attached to the femur.

Sprains

Sprains are injuries to a joint ligament or joint capsule. Common sites are the wrist and the ankle. Ankle sprains are usually caused by hyperinversion or eversion of the foot with foot plantar flexion. The anterior talofibular, calcaneofibular, and the deltoid ligaments are often involved.

Signs and Symptoms

Patients give a history of injury with pain and swelling at the affected site.

Diagnosis

Routine X-rays are usually performed to rule out "hidden" fractures, such as navicular, hook of hamate, or avulsion fractures. A common avulsion fracture is the proximal end of the fifth metatarsal by the peroneus brevis tendon during an inversion sprain of the foot.

Treatment

The mnemonic is "RICE"—rest, ice or heat application, compression (as with an Ace bandage), and elevation. Serious ligamentous injuries may require surgical correction.

Neoplasm	Location	Benign vs Malignant
Giant Cell Tumor	Epiphysis	Benign
Osteosarcoma	Metaphysis	Malignant
Osteochondroma	Metaphysis	Benign
Ewing's Tumor	Diaphysis	Malignant
Chondrosarcoma	Diaphysis	Malignant

Table 17 Neoplasms

	Blastic Lesions	Lytic Lesions
Characteristic	—	—
Associated Cancers	Breast and Prostate	Kidney, lung, colon, melanoma, and thyroid

Table 18 Bone Neoplasms

Osteosarcoma

Osteosarcomas (osteogenic sarcomas) are the most common primary malignant bone tumors. Malignant cells arise directly from the osteoid. Cases occur in teens and the elderly. Osteosarcoma is associated

Codman's triangle on X-ray is indicative of osteosarcoma.

with the familial retinoblastoma gene, Paget's disease, *p53* mutations, and history of irradiation. These lesions frequently metastasize by hematogenous spread to the lungs, liver, and brain.

Signs and Symptoms

Most cases occur in the metaphysis of long bones, particularly the proximal tibia and distal femur, and have associated pain and swelling. Patients may complain of unrelenting knee pain after minor trauma.

Pathology

Lesions may be lytic or blastic, depending on the cells involved. Histology typically shows highly pleomorphic cells and malignant osteoid with neoplastic cells between the osteoid deposits. Malignant osteoid is typically characterized by a "lace-like" pattern of deposits.

Diagnosis

Codman's triangle on x-ray is indicative of osteosarcoma.

X-rays show periosteal elevation (**Codman triangle**). A characteristic "sunburst" appearance due to periosteal inflammation may also be seen on X-ray. Serum alkaline phosphatase is elevated two- to threefold. Biopsy is diagnostic. A CT of the chest should be performed to detect pulmonary metastases.

Treatment

Combination surgery, radiation, and chemotherapy lead to 5-year survival rates of about 60%.

Ewing's Sarcoma

Unlike osteosarcoma which occurs more commonly in teenage years, **Ewing's sarcoma** is a malignant tumor that tends to occur in boys under 15 years of age. In addition to pain and localized swelling, it presents with the systemic symptoms of fever, weight loss, and fatigue. All of these symptoms are rarely seen in osteosarcoma. It is a primitive round cell tumor believed to be of neurogenic origin.

Signs and Symptoms

Common symptoms of Ewing's sarcoma include pain and swelling locally, along with fever, weight loss, and fatigue. The tumor tends to occur in the diaphyseal regions of long bones and in flat bones. Common sites include the diaphysis of long bones: femur, tibia, and pelvis.

Diagnosis

Seen in 11;22 translocation. Onion Skinning Appearance = Ewing's Sarcoma

Biopsy is diagnostic. Radiographs reveal a lytic bone lesion with "onion-skin" periosteal elevation (due to calcifications). Biopsy shows sheets of primitive cells with scant cytoplasm aka "round blue cells". Histology will also occasionally reveal Homer-Wright rosettes.

Treatment

Chemotherapy

Osteochondroma

Osteochondroma, the most common benign tumor of the bone, occurs most frequently in males under 25 years of age. It consists of a bony growth covered by a cap of cartilage that projects from the surface of a bone. The growth tends to emerge from the metaphysis, near the growth plate of long bones. Its progression is slow, and growth tends to stop when normal skeletal growth is complete, which lends credence to the belief that it is a malformation rather than a neoplasm. Malignant transformation to chondrosarcoma is incredibly rare. Usually an osteochondroma is asymptomatic, and the main concern is cosmetic deformity. Pain can result if the growth impinges on a nerve or if its stalk is fractured. Histological cross section will show trabecular or cortical bone with a cartilaginous cap composed of mature chondrocytes.

Giant Cell Tumors

Giant cell tumors, or **osteoclastomas**, are the second-most common benign tumor of the bone. They have the distinction of occurring more often in females than in males, and usually between the ages of 20 and 40.

Signs and Symptoms

Presentation is usually localized pain that can be mistaken for arthritis because the tumors tend to occur at the epiphyseal ends of long bones, such as the proximal tibia, distal femur, proximal humerus, or distal radius.

Diagnosis

Biopsy is diagnostic. X-ray reveals a characteristic "soap bubble" appearance. Histological examination shows poorly defined cytoplasmic borders and nuclei that resemble multiple giant cells that resemble osteoclasts.

Treatment

Currettage. Local recurrences are common. Malignant transformation is rare.

Metastatic Bone Disease

Most metastatic bone lesions come from primary tumors in the prostate, breast, kidney, and lung. Most lesions are lytic, and don't forget that multiple myeloma can cause similar bone lesions.

Signs and Symptoms

Bone pain may be the presenting symptom of the primary cancer, particularly in prostate cancer. Another indication for metastatic disease is a pathological fracture.

Diagnosis

X-rays and nuclear bone scans are useful.

Treatment

Because these lesions represent distant metastasis, prognosis is poor. Local irradiation of the lesion may provide palliative relief.

Soft Tissue Tumors

Lipoma

As the most common soft tissue tumor, **lipoma** is a benign, solitary, sporadic growth that can appear anywhere on the body, usually in the subcutaneous tissue of adults. It tends to be well-circumscribed. Excision is the cure.

Malignant Fibrous Histiocytoma

As the most common soft tissue sarcoma of adults, **malignant fibrous histiocytoma** tends to occur in the deep muscular tissues of the extremities or retroperitoneally. It is usually found in adults between 50 and 70 years of age. It appears as a gray-white, encapsulated mass, but is highly infiltrative and very aggressive, with frequent local recurrence. Metastases occur in half of patients.

Rhabdomyosarcoma

Rhabdomyosarcoma is a tumor of childhood, usually occurring in the first decade of life. It is the most common soft tissue sarcoma of childhood. The presentation is variable, ranging from the grape-like **sarcoma botryoides** that arise near mucosal surfaces of the genitourinary tract and in the head and neck, to a less well-defined, infiltrating mass. This tumor is differentiated from other small round cell tumors of childhood by the presence of sarcomeres in electron microscopic examination or the presence of muscle-associated antigens in immunocytochemical preparations. Dactinomycin is effective in treating rhabdomyosarcomas.

PHARMACOLOGY

Drug	Mechanism	Use	Toxicity
Asprin	Irreversibly inhibits cyclooxygenase, leading to decreased synthesis of prostaglandins and thromboxane	Low dose (< 300 mg/day): reduces platelet aggregation Intermediate dose (300–2,400 mg/day):antipyretic and anal gesic effects High dose (2,400–4,000 mg/day): anti-inflammatory	Adverse effects include gastrointestinal disturbances and increased risk of bleeding Causes increased bleeding time for coagulations (no change in PT or PTT) Bronchospasm Higher doses cause tinnitus, vertigo, hyperventilation, respiratory alkalosis, metabolic acidosis Reye's Syndome (Hepatic fatty degeneration and encephalopathy) occurs when aspirin is given to children with viral infections
Ibuprofen, Indomethacin, Naproxen,	Reversibly inhibit cyclooxygenase Ibuprofen has low potency, duration of action of 4–8 hours, and half life of 2 hours Naproxen has longer action Indomethacin has high potency action	Dysmenorrhea, inflammation (rheumatoid arthritis, gout), patent ductus arteriosus in premature infants	Indomethacin has increased toxicity Aplastic anemia Renal toxicity especially in the elderly GI distress, ulcers Cox 2 inhibitors have increased thrombotic risk
Slow-acting antirheumatic drugs (methotrexate, gold compounds, hydroxychloroquine, penicillamine)	Unknown	Benefits may require several months to manifest Used for patients with rheumatoid or other immune complexes in their serum Controversial	**Methotrexate**: bone marrow depression, hepatotoxicity, teratogenic fetal damage, or abortion **Gold**: dermatitis, bone marrow depression, gastrointestinal disturbances **Hydroxychloroquine**: mastitis, bone marrow depression, retinal degeneration **Penicillamine**: renal damage, aplastic anemia

Corticoste-roids	Enter cell, bind to receptors in cytosol and translocate to nucleus Alter gene expression Decrease lymphocytes, eosinophils, basophils, and monocytes Inhibit migration of leukocytes Suppress production of prostaglandins and leukotrienes due to inhibition of phospholipase	Autoimmune Disorders	Cushing's Syndrome Fat deposition, protein catabolism, skin wasting, osteoporosis, growth inhibition (in children) Immunosuppresive Large doses for long periods may cause behavioral disturbances; may increase risk of ulcer formation
Acetamino-phen	Inhibitor of prostaglandin synthesis mainly in the CNS, but exact mechanism unknown	Minor musculoskeletal pain	Rash Overdose can cause fulminant hepatic failure Metabolites deplete glutathione; N-acetylcystine is antidote and regenerates glutathione

Table 19 Anti-Inflammatory Agents

TNF-α Inibitors

These drugs are disease modifying agents that directly inhibit the actions of the cytokine TNF-α by either acting as a decoy receptor such as etanercept or by acting as anti-TNF antibodies such as infliximab and adalimumab.

Drug	Mechanism	Use	Toxicity
Etanercept	TNF receptor that binds to TNF to prevent it from binding to the actual receptor	Seronegative arthropaties and rheumatoid arthritis specifically psoriatic arthritis and ankylosing spondylitis Infliximab can also be used to treat inflammatory bowel disease	Predisposes to infection if patient has latent TB Always do a PPD prior to intiating treatment with TNF alpha inhibitors
Infliximab	Anti-TNF antibody		
Adalimumab			

Table 20 TNF-α Inibitors

Muscle Relaxants

Skeletal muscle relaxants are discussed in chapter 14. These include drugs such as curare derivatives and succinylcholine that block nicotinic receptors at the motor end plate; they are used for muscle relaxation during surgery. The drugs listed in Table 19 are used for less complete muscle relaxation.

Drug	Mechanism	Use	Toxicity
Baclofen	Acts on GABA receptors in the CNS Decreases pain in	Decreases pain in spastic patients	Somnolence, increased seizure activity
Dantrolene	Blocks calcium release from the sarcoplasmic reticulum	Muscle spasticity and malignant hyperthermia	Generalized weakness, sedation, hepatitis
Valium and Other Benzodiazepines	Bind to GABA receptors to cause increased-firing frequency	Mild muscle spasm, patients with spinal cord injury	Sedation, ataxia, addictive potential, withdrawal can be fatal

Table 21 Muscle Relaxants

Drug	Mechanism	Use	Toxicity
Colchicine	Inhibits microtubule assembly decreasing WBC actions	Acute gouty arthritis	Gastrointestinal effects; liver and kidney damage
Allopurinol	Inhibition of xanthine oxidase, an enzyme in uric acid synthesis	Recurrent renal stones; chronic gout	Not to be given in acute gout attack; gastrointestinal upset; peripheral neuropathy
Uricosuric acid (probencid, sulfapyrazine)	Inhibits uric acid absorption in the proximal convoluted tubule kidney	Chronic gout	May worsen acute attacks, can also block renal secretion of penicillin
Phenylbutazone	Prostaglandin inhibitor	Pain relief in acute gout	Aplastic anemia

Table 22 Gout Medications

Acute gout medications = NSAIDS, colchicine, phenylbutazone

Chronic gout medications= allopurinol, probenecid, febuxostat

Febuxostat inhibits xanthine oxidase

Allopurinol can be used in cancer patients recieveing cytotoxic therapy to prevent tumor lysis syndrome

Bone Homeostasis

Drug	Mechanism	Use	Toxicity
Bisphosphonates (etidronate, pamidronate, alendronate)	Binds hydroxyapatite crystal and prevents bone resorption and formation	Postmenopausal osteoporosis, Paget's disease, bony metastases, malignant associated hypercalcemia	Hypocalcemia leukemia, lymphopenia
Calcitonin (salmon)	Decreases bone resorption and serum calcium and phosphate by osteoclasts inhibition	Acute treatment of Paget's disease and hypercalcemia	Flushing, GI distress
Estrogen	Prevents or delays loss in postmenopausal women, possibly by inhibiting PTH-induced bone resorption by osteoclasts	Postmenopausal osteoporosis prophylaxis	Breast tenderness, discomfort, and headaches Possible cardiovascular thrombotic risk Increased risk of breast and endometrial carcinoma Should not be given in the long term

Table 23 Drugs that effect bone homeostasis

CHAPTER 13

NEUROLOGY & NEUROANATOMY

EMBRYOLOGICAL ORIGINS

The majority of the nervous system stems from **ectoderm**. During the third week of development, the **neural plate** forms from a thickened area of ectoderm near notochord. The neural plate invaginates and forms the **neural tube**. Eventually, parts of the ectoderm are pinched off and joined to form the **neural crest** that overlies the tube.

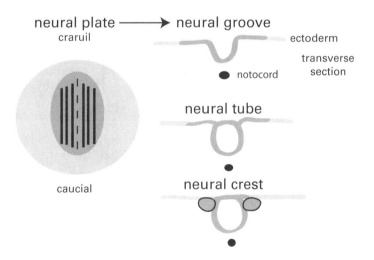

Figure 1 Formation of Neural Tube by Neurulation

Ectoderm—Majority of the CNS neurons and supporting glial cells, such as astrocytes, oligodendrocytes and ependymal cells are derived from the ectoderm.

Neural Crest—Schwann cells, PNS and enteric neurons arise from the neural crest, along with melanocytes and craniofacial bones.

Mesoderm—Microglia is derived from mesoderm.

In the fourth week, three bulges, or **primary vesicles** develop in the nervous system. From top to bottom, these primary vesicles are the **prosencephalon** (forebrain), the **mesencephalon** (midbrain), and the **rhombencephalon** (hindbrain).

During the fifth week, the primary vesicles divide into **secondary vesicles**, which further develop into various brain and brain stem structures. Each secondary vesicle retains a cavity that becomes part of the ventricular system (Table 1).

Primary vesicle	Secondary vesicle	Neural tube derivatives	Cavity
Prosencephalon	Telencephalon	Cerebral hemispheres	Lateral ventricles
	Diencephalon	Thalamus, hypothalamus	Third ventricle
Mesencephalon	Mesencephalon	Midbrain	Cerebral aqueduct
Rhombencephalon	Metencephalon	Pons and cerebellum	Fourth ventricle
	Myelencephalon	Medulla	Fourth ventricle and central canal

Table 1 Neural tube derivatives

In Guillain-Barré syndrome, antibodies cause an inflammatory response in the endoneurium.

Reconnection of perineurium is important in microsurgery.

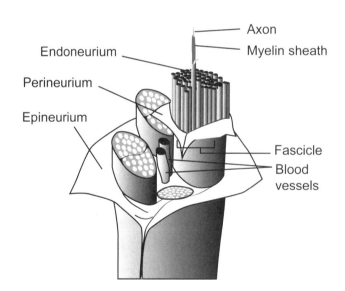

Figure 2 Microanatomy of a nerve fiber

Anatomy of a Peripheral Nerve

1. Inner: **Endoneurium** encases single layer of nerve fibers.

2. Middle: **Perineurium** is the permeable layer in the middle that encases multiple nerve fibers.

3. Outer: **Epineurium** encases the blood vessels and nerve fascicles.

CELL TYPES

1. **Neurons**: Neurons are the cells that serve as the foundation of the nervous system. Neurons are permanent cells stuck in G0 phase and do not undergo mitosis. Hence, no brain tumors arise in adults from neurons. Histology of neurons shows large cells with big nucleoli with cell body that can be stained with Nissl substance.

2. **Glial Cells**: Glial cells are the support cells of the neurons in the nervous system that make up the majority of cells.

Type of Glial Cell	Description
Astrocytes	• Physical Support—Astrocytes are the janitors of the synapse and clean up excess neurotransmitters and prepare for the next round of "neural firing." Also function in repair synapse during injury. • Reactive gliosis—Astrocytes respond to acute brain injury, especially during stroke. • Blood Brain Barrier—Astrocytes maintain and support the cells that make up the BBB. • **GFAP**—Marked by the GFAP stain, stands for glial fibrillary acidic protein which is an intermediate filament protein expressed in most astrocytes. • Cleans up excess potassium—Depolarization of neurons release potassium. Astrocytes are very permeable to potassium and suck up extra potassium around neurons. This function is critical to avoid interference in neuron depolarization.
Ependymal Cells	Ependymal cells form the inner lining of the ventricles and secrete CSF into the ventricles.
Microglia	• Phagocytosis—Microglia cells are the phagocytes of the CNS. • Giant Cell Formation—In response to infection from viruses, microglial cells can form huge multinucleated giant cells.

Astrocytes are the most abundant cell in the human brain.

Oligoden-droglia	• Oligodendroglia myelinate axons in the CNS. Note that one oligodendrocyte myelinates multiple CNS axons, in contrast to Schwann cells that envelops a single axon in the PNS. Oligodendroglial cells make up the majority of the white matter. • H&E stain—"Fried egg appearance"

Table 2 Cell types

3. **Schwann Cells**—Schwann cells myelinate PNS axons. PNS neurons are myelinated individually by one Schwann cell. Schwann cell precursors are neural crest cells.

Remember *PNS* neurons are myelinated by *Schwann cells* individually and *CNS* neurons are myelinated by *oligodendroctyes* in bundles.

Sensory Receptors

Location	Receptor	Sensation
Hair follicles	Merkel's Disks	Position sense. Slow adapters
Hairless skin (like the palms of your hands)	Meissner's corpuscles—large fibers	Position sense, dynamic fine touch
Skin	Free nerve endings • C fibers—these are SLOW unmyelinated fibers. • Delta fibers—fast and myelinated.	Pain and temperature

Table 3 Sensory Receptors

Neuro-transmitter	Role in pathology	Location	Drugs
NE (norepi-nephrine)	Lower in depression Higher in anxiety	Locus ceruleus	TCA's, ma-protiline and mirtazapine are NE reuptake inhibitors
Dopamine	Increased in schizophrenia, decreased in Parkinson's and depression	Ventral tegmen-tum and substantia nigra pars compacta (SNc)	Levodopa and carbidopa increase level of dopamine while selegiline pre-vents dopamine breakdown
Serotonin (5-HT)	Decreased in anxiety and depression	Raphe Nucleus	SSRI's
Ach	Reduced in Alzheimer's, Huntington's, REM sleep	Neuro-muscular junction, Basal nucleus of Meynert	Organophos-phates and nerve agents in-hibit breakdown of Ach
GABA	Reduced in anxi-ety, Huntington's	Nucleus accumbens	Benzodiaze-pines are GABA agonists and reduce anxiety

Table 4 Neurotransmitters

Memnonic to remember the drugs that are used to treat Parkinson's:

BALSA
Bromocriptine/
Benztropine
Amantadine
Levodopa
Selegilene
Antimuscarinics

ACh Receptor Agonists are used to treat myasthenia gravis and Alzheimer's disease.

PITUITARY

The pituitary is divided into anterior and posterior portions.

1. Posterior pituitary (neurohypophysis)—The posterior pituitary does not make its own hormones. Instead, it releases two hormones them from the axonal projections of the hypothalamus.

   - **Oxytocin**—From paraventricular axonal projections of the hypo-thalamus. Oxytocin regulates uterine contractions and milk let down during breastfeeding.

   - **ADH**—From supraoptic axonal projections of the hypothalamus. Also known as **vasopressin**; and regulates water reabsorption from the collecting duct.

2. Anterior Pituitary—Produces and secretes its own **FLAG TOP** hormones.

3. Pathology

- **Sheehan's Syndrome**—infarction of pituitary during childbirth due to mismatch of increased demand and perfusion due to blood loss

- Adenomas—pituitary can grow tumors divided into two classes: functioning and non-functioning. Functioning adenomas grow and secrete excess amount of hormones like **prolactinomas**. Prolactino mas are the most common type of adenomas

DIENCEPHALON

The diencephalon is composed of the thalamus and the hypothalamus.

Thalamus

The thalamus is the relay station for all senses going to the cerebral cortex, with the exception of smell. The thalamus relays senses to three main areas of the brain: cerebral cortex, basal ganglia and hypothalamus. Part of the thalamus is divided up by the internal medullary lamina.

- **Ventral posterolateral nuclei (VPL)**—Body and limb sensory tracts from the dorsal column and spinothalamic tract (PTPTV) is sent to primary somatosensory cortex.

- **Ventral posteromedial nuclei (VPM)**—Sensation from the face and taste via CN V is also sent to primary somatosensory cortex.

- **Ventral Anterior Nuclei (VAN)**—Receives afferent connections from basal ganglia and cerebellum.

- **Lateral geniculate nuclei**—Vision via CN II is sent to through the optic radiations to occipital cortex and calcarine sulcus.

- **Medial geniculate nuclei**—Hearing sensation from the inferior colliculus is sent to the auditory cortex in the temporal lobe.

- **Dorsal Medial Nucleus (DMN)**—Plays an important role in memory formation.

- **Anterior Thalamus**—Input is the limbic system and output is the mamillary bodies.

Hypothalamus

1. Lies on the floor of the third ventricle.

2. Functions of the hypothalamus can be summarized by **TAN HAT**

Damage to ventromedial area leads to hyperphagia.

Damage to lateral area leads to anorexia.

Medial for **M**usic

DMN is damaged with alcohol in Wernicke Korsakoff syndrome.

- Thirst

- Adenohypophysis control (control of the anterior pituitary)

- Neurohypophysis control (control of the posterior pituitary)

- Regulates hunger

  ○ Satiety is regulated by ventromedial area and activated by leptin.

  ○ Hunger is regulated by lateral area and inhibited by leptin.

- Autonomic regulation

- Temperature control

  ○ Anterior hypothalamus regulates cooling.

  ○ Posterior hypothalamus regulates heating.

- Suprachiasmatic nucleus: circadian rhythm

3. Major inputs

- OVLT—area around third ventricle that lacks a BBB and detects increases in blood osmolality and releases ADH.

- Area postrema—area on floor of fourth ventricle that acts as the vomit center and responds to emetics.

CEREBELLUM

The cerebellum regulates **m**uscle tone, coordinates **v**oluntary motor movements and governs **p**osture. However, cerebellum is NOT responsible for starting and stopping voluntary movements.

1. Anatomy: Composed of cerebellar hemisphere and cerebellar vermis.

2. Composed of two main layers: cerebellar cortex and deep nuclei.

   - Cortex is further divided into three layers: molecular, purkinje and granular. Purkinje layers dive deep into the deep nuclei.

   - Deep nuclei are the main exits out of the cerebellum. From lateral to medial, **Dentate, Emboliform, Globose, Fastigal**. The lateral side controls voluntary movements of the hands and feet while the medial side controls balance via truncal coordination.

3. Input: Receives contralateral cortical information from the middle cerebellar peduncle and ipsilateral proprioceptive information from the **i**nferior cerebellar peduncle. Inputs are carried via climbing and mossy fibers.

Cerebellum is the **MVP** of the brain.

Muscle tone
Voluntary movement
Posture

Deep Nuclei
Don't Eat
Greasy Foods!

Dentate **E**mboliform
Globus
Fastigial

4. Output: Purkinje fiber (contain GABA, inhibitory) → deep nuclei of cerebellum → superior cerebellar peduncle → contralateral ventral thalamic nuclei → cortex.

Pathology

A lesion in one hemisphere will result in ipsilateral intention tremor, nystagmus and falling to ipsilateral side when eyes are closed due to hypotonia of ipsilateral limbs. This is primarily regulated via the medial nuclei because they control truncal coordination. A lesion in the cerebellar vermis will result in truncal ataxia and dysarthria. It will also lead to "drunken sailor stance" where the patient presents with a wide set gait and has trouble turning.

Limbic system

The limbic system consists of hippocampus, fornix, cingulate gyrus, mammillary bodies, and septal nucleus.

- Plays an important role in evolutionarily important emotions and motivations, particularly those that are related to survival.

- 5 F's: Feeding, Fleeing, Fighting, Feeling, and Sex

Cerebral cortex

The cerebral cortex is the thin strip of gray matter overlying the deeper white matter of the brain. It is responsible for many functions and forms higher cognitive processes, such as abstract thinking and complex organization skills.

Cerebellar signs

PINARD'S
Past pointing
Intention tremor
Nystagmus
Ataxia
Rebound
Dysdiadokinesia
Slurred speech

Ipsilateral proprioception
from **I**nferior peduncle

**Stand up on your legs
and stick your tongue
out to side!**
Leg is medial and the
tongue is lateral
Anterior cerebral artery
will most likely affect the
contralateral leg
Middle cerebral artery
will most likely affect the
speech

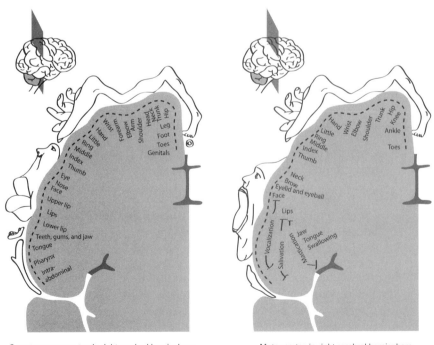

Somatosensory cortex in right cerebral hemisphere   Motor cortex in right cerebral hemisphere

Figure 3 Right and left motor and sensory homonculus

Homunculus

The homunculus shows a "map" of critical sensory and motor areas in the brain and the associated areas of the body.

It is important to know the relative locations of sensory and motor areas for its role during brain lesions and strokes.

Basal Ganglia

Basal ganglia receive cortical input and provide a unique negative feedback system to control voluntary movement and posture. Striatum consists of putamen and caudate. Putamen is motor while **C**audate is **C**ognition. Lentiform consists of putamen and globus pallidus.

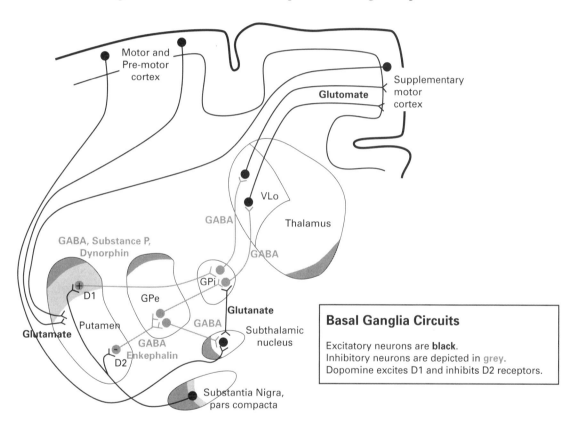

Figure 4 Basal Ganglia Circuits

- **Excitatory pathway**: Cortical input stimulates striatum causing it to release Ach.

  ○ Ach disinhibits the thalamus globus pallidus internus

  ○ Disinhibition of thalamus increases movement!

  ○ **Inhibitory Pathway**: Cortical inputs stimulate striatum and activates globus pallidus externus (Gpe)

    ■ GPe disinhibits subthalamic nucleus, which in turn inhibits thalamus

- ■ Inhibition of the thalamus decreases movement!

   ○ Dopamine: facilitates movement

   - ■ **D1** receptor: **D1**rectly activates excitatory pathway

   - ■ D2 receptor : Indirectly inhibit inhibitory pathway

Remember Parkinson's disease result from the death of dopamine generating cells in the substantia nigra!

Location	Function	Function
Frontal Lobe	Responsible for "executive functions." Controls voluntary motor movements	Key effect of an overall lesion in this area is **disinhibition**, lack of social judgment, proper planning, and improper mood.
Parietal Lobe	Responsible for integrating sensory information, spatial sense and navigation. Responsible for sensation throughout the body.	Lesions here will cause **hemispatial** neglect-agnosia of the contralateral side to the lesion. Contralateral apraxia may also result.
Frontal Eye Fields	Located in the prefrontal cortex. It is responsible for contralateral pursuit eye movements.	Left frontal eye field lesion will cause the eyes to slowly drift left, to the side of the lesion.
Broca's Area	Broca's area is responsible for language production	Lesion in the **inferior frontal gyrus** will cause broca's aphasia. Presents as nonfluent speech with intact comprehension.
Wernicke's Area	Wernicke's area is responsible for forming coherent speech and understanding language.	Lesion in the **superior temporal gyrus** will cause Wernicke's aphasia. Presents as fluent nonsensical speech.
Arcuate Fasciculus	Connects Broca's and Wernicke's area	Causes **conduction aphasia**— can't repeat phrases but can speak.

Think Phineas Gage!

Frontal = "motor strip"

Parietal ="sensory strip"

Broken Boca
Boca is Spanish
for mouth

Wernicke is Wordy but
doesn't make any sense!
What? mouth!

Broca's area Wernicke's area Arcuate fasciculus		Global Aphasia
Amygdala	Located deep within the medial temporal lobes and responsible for emotion and memory	**Kluver-Bucy syndrome**: hypersexuality, disinhibited behavior
Mammilary bodies	Anterior arches of the fornix	**Wernicke-Korsakoff syndrome**
Cerebellar Vermis	In cerebellum	**Truncal ataxia**
Hippocampus	In limbic system— role in memory	**Anterograde amnesia**
Paramedian pontine reticular formation	PPRF in center of pons	**Eyes look away from lesion**

Table 5 Critical areas of the cerebral cortex can be correlated with lesions.

Common middle cerebral artery infarcts results in global aphasias.

In frontal eye field lesion, eyes look towards lesion.

BRAIN TUMORS

Brain tumors may be primary or metastatic, or from non-CNS source.

Primary brain tumors arise from glia, neurons, or meninges and almost never spread to other areas of the body. In the brain, even benign tumor can be fatal due to mass effect and involvement of critical brain structures.

Brain tumors are usually **infratentorial** in children and **supratentorial** in adults.

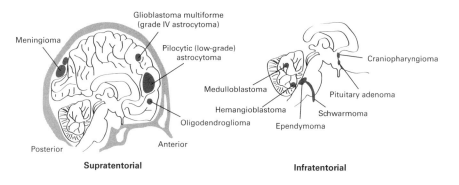

Figure 5 Distribution of brain tumors

Glioblastoma multiforme is the **most common primary brain tumor**.

Tumor	Origin/ Frequency/ Location	Clinical signs
Glioblastoma multiforme **(grade IV astrocytoma)**	Origin: Glial Cells Location: Usually grows at cerebral hemispheres. Supratentorial	Poor prognosis. Symptoms depend on location of tumor and result secondary to mass effect of tumor on cerebrum. CT scan will show a heterogeneously enhancing and branching lesion, the lack of smooth borders is highly suspicious of malignancy. Histology: Cells around areas of brain necrosis and are pleomorphic in shape Treatment: chemotherapy, radiation therapy, resection
Metastatic brain tumor	Origin: these tumors come from remote sites, separate from the brain and are called secondary brain tumors. The likely origin of the tumor is the following from most likely to least: Lung > breast > melanoma > kidney > gastrointestinal > lymphoma	Symptoms are variable and tend to evolve slowly over time. These include seizures, headache, nausea and vomiting, drowsiness, focal deficits, and mental impairment. CT scan will show m etastasis at junction of grey and white matter
Pituitary Adenoma	Origin: Due to excessive growth of pituitary gland. Location: This is an **infratentorial tumor** adult brain tumor. Note embryologyically the anterior pituitary is derived from **Rathke's pouch**. Frequency: rare	Signs and Symptoms: Hyper or hypo pituitarism. Most common tumor is prolactinoma. Treatment: can be surgically resected

Due to pressure on the optic chiasm, **bitemporal hemianopia** can result from pituitary adenoma.

Schwannoma	Origin: Arise from Schwann cells Location: Cerebellopontine angle and **Infratentorial** Frequency: **3rd most common** brain tumor	Frequently around CN VIII and presents as an acoustic schwannoma. Treatment: Surgical resection
Meningioma	Origin: Arachnoid cells of the meninges Location: Parasagittal and falx regions or the convexities of the cerebrum Frequency: **2nd most common** type of tumor	Headache and problems with vision. Most symptoms present due to mass effect. Histology: concentric spindle cells with calcifications called **psammoma bodies**. Treatment: Surgical resection
Oligodendroglioma	Origin: oligodendrocytes of axons Location: Frontal lobes Frequency: rare	Histology: cells have clear cytoplasm with round nuclei—there are often calcifications

Vestibular schwannoma presents with ipsilateral sensorineural hearing loss and disturbed sense of balance

Table 6 Typical adult tumors

Tumor	Origin/Location/Frequency	Clinical Signs
Ependymoma	Origin: Ependymal cells Location: Most commonly in fourth ventricle, however it can take place in all ventricles	Hydrocephalus is a common symptom due to blocked drainage of CSF by tumor. Poor prognosis. Histology: Rod shaped **blepharoplasts** are seen near the nucleus

Pheochromocytoma,
Renal cell carcinoma

Craniopharyngioma is the
most common supraten-
torial tumor in children.

Medulloblastoma's symp-
toms are often mistaken
for GI upsets in children.

Hemangioblastoma	Origin: Stromal cells of small blood vessels in the central nervous system. Location: Most frequently in the cerebellum, brain stem, and spinal cord	This tumor is associated with Von Hippel-Lindau syndrome. Histology: highly vascularized tumors with **foam cells**
Craniopharyngioma	Origin: remnant of Rathke's pouch Location: area of Rathke's pouch, therefore sometimes confused with pituitary adenoma	Bitemporal hemianopia due to its proximity to the optic chiasm.
Medulloblastoma	Origin: Primitive neuroectodoerm Location: cerebellum, can compress the 4th ventricle	Symptoms are variable but are mainly due to blockage of 4th ventricle and increased ICP. Nausea, vomiting and headache. Histology: **Solid small blue clusters and rossettes** seen.
Pilocytic astrocytoma **Figure 6**	Origin: astrocytes Location: cerebellum near the brain stem Frequency: frequent in NF1 patients	Symptoms: headache, nausea, vomiting, failure to thrive, lack of coordination, nystagmus Histology: characteristic bipolar cells with long **pilocytic (hair-like) processes**.

Neuroblastoma	Origin: can arise from any neural crest element of the sympathetic nervous system	Symptoms are vague but most common are loss of appetite, fatigue, fever and joint pain.
Figure 7	Location: most common in adrenal glands but also in neck, chest, abdomen and pelvis	Histology: see **blue, solid rosette cells**.
	Frequency: most common extracranial childhood tumor	

Table 7 Typical Pediatric Tumors

DEMENTIA

Neurodegenerative diseases that cause dementia are often tested in the USMLE. However, reversible and treatable causes of dementia are also critical. Other causes of cortical decline and dementia include multi-infarct dementia, Wilson's disease, and vitamin B12 deficiency. Infections with HIV and syphilis can also cause early dementia.

The neurodegenerative diseases in the table are emphasized on STEP 1.

Remember DEMENTIA!
Drug toxicity
Emotional (depression, anxiety)
Metabolic (electrolytes, liver disease, kidney disease, COPD)
Eyes/ Ears (peripheral sensory restrictions)
Nutrition (vitamin 12, Wilson's, iron deficiencies, NPH)
Tumors/ Trauma (including chronic subdural hematoma)
Infection (meningitis, encephalitis, pneumonia, syphilis, HIV)
Arteriosclerosis and other vascular disease

Disease	Signs and Symptoms	Causes	Pathology
Alzheimer's Disease	This disease is the **most common cause of dementia**. Patients tend to have a progressive loss of cognitive function, which begins with recent memory, followed eventually by aphasia. Often associated with depression, agitation and apraxia. Death generally occurs in 5–10 years.	1. Sporadic with unknown cause 2. **Down's Syndrome** patients (trisomy 21) 3. Mutations in chromosomes 14 (presenilin gene) and 21 (APP gene) 4. Late onset Alzheimer's is caused by a mutation in chromosome 19 (ApoE4).	1. Beta amyloid plaques 2. Insoluble tau proteins seen intracellularly 3. **Reduced Ach in CNS** Treatment: Acetylcholinesterase inhibitors: Tacrine, Rivastigmine and Donepezil **Memantine Donezepil Galantamine Rivastigmine** NMDA receptor antagonist: Memantine
Creutzfeldt-Jakob Disease	Sudden onset dementia that progresses within weeks to a debilitating cognitive deficit. **Jerky movements**, myoclonus with seizures, speech impairment and rigid posture. Death occurs within 6 months.	Caused by abnormal buildup of prion protein plaques in the brain. Happens when the normal prions (PrPc) get transformed to abnormal **PrPsc prions**, which are prone to form protease resistant plaques.	Spongiform encephalopathy. Cortex has tiny holes where neurons have died, resembling a sponge.z
Pick's Disease	Seen with aphasia and dementia. **Personality changes** can help differentiate from Alzheimer's. Disinhibited behavior.	This is **fronto-temporal** dementia that spares the parietal lobe. There is no known genetic cause.	Build-up of tau proteins in neurons, accumulating into silver-staining, spherical aggregations known as **"Pick bodies."**
Lewy Body Dementia	This disease relates to Parkinson's and overlaps with Alzheimer's. Patient presents with both cognitive deficits of Alzheimer's and **motor deficits seen in Parkinson's**. Sudden onset of dementia with motor symptoms is highly suspicious of Lewy Body Dementia. **Hallucinations** may also be present.	Mostly sporadic and not hereditary.	Lewy body formation in the cortex. These **Lewy bodies** are formed from abnormal alpha-synuclein protein in the cytoplasm. This leads to destruction of dopaminergic (Parkinson symptoms) and cholinergic neurons (Alzheimer's symptoms).

Table 8 Neurodegenerative diseases

Neurocutaneous disorders—The following provides pathognomonic words to help memorize key symptoms and signs for high yield neurocutaneous disorders.

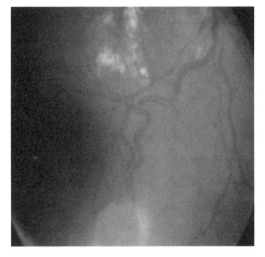

Figure 8 Retinal Hemagioblastoma seen in Von-Hippel-Lindau disease

Von Hippel-Lindau

- Angioma of the retina (blindness),

- Angioma of the brain (hemangioblastomas), cerebellum, brainstem.

- Pheochromocytoma, renal cell carcinoma, arteriovenous malformations

- Genetic disease: Chromosome 3 mutation

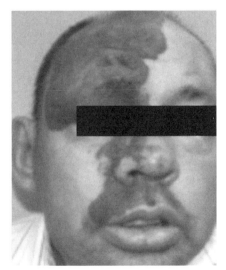

Figure 9 Port wine stain (nevus flammeus) in Surge-Weber Syndrome

Think **Bloody Tumors!**

Osler-Weber-Rendu is another disorder that has AVM but presents with systemic AVMs.

Sturge-Weber syndrome
- Typically occurs in the V1 area of trigeminal nerve
- Leptomeningeal angiomas
- Pheochromocytomas
- Also sporadically presents with: hemiparesis and mental retardation.

Neurofibromatosis Type I
- Skin—neurofibromas, café au lait spots
- Eyes—optic gliomas, Lisch nodules
- Adrenal glands—pheochromocytomas
- Autosomal dominant inheritance: mutation of the NF-1 gene on 17th chromosome

Think
CAFE SPOT!
Café-au-lait spots
Axillary, inguinal freckling
Fibroma
Eye: lisch nodules
Skeletal (bowing leg)
Pedigree/ family
Optic Tumor (glioma)

Tuberous Sclerosis
- CNS—seizures, hamartomas, mental retardation
- Integumentary—adenoma sebeceum, ash leaf spots, facial angiofibromas
- Cardiac—mitral regurgitation, cardiac rhabdomyoma
- Renal—angiomyolipoma on kidney
- Autosomal dominant inheritance of tumor suppressor genes

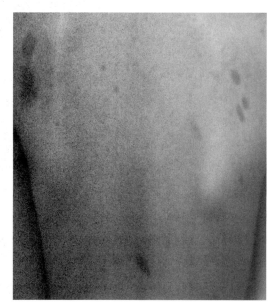

Figure 10 Cafe au-lait spots seen in NF-1

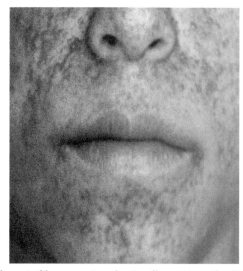

Figure 11 Facial angiofibromas in a butterfly pattern for Tuberous Sclerosis

Disease	Signs and Symptoms	Pathology and Treatment
Multiple Sclerosis *Miss or Ms. is for young female*	Most commonly affects young Caucasian women. Consists of autoimmune attack on CNS myelin cells. Symptoms include MLF syndrome, sensory and motor loss, loss of bowel and/or bladder control and sometimes, emotional changes. **Figure 12**	MRI with areas of demyelination. **Oligoclonal bands** of **IgG** in electrophoresis Periventricular plaques. Treatment: In a relapsing-remitting course, β-**interferon** is the most common treatment. Plasmapheresis can also be utilized.
Guillain–Barré	Autoimmune demyelinating disease that affects the peripheral motor nerves. **Ascending paralysis** with weakness beginning in the feet and hands and migrating towards the trunk.	Respiratory support is critical in these patients. Herpes and *campylobacter jejuni* have been known to trigger Guillain–Barré.
Progressive multifocal Leukoencephalopathy	Mainly seen in **AIDS** patients. Steady destruction of myelin sheaths due to infection by **JC virus**.	Demyelination symptoms vary but CNS lesions can result in severe neurological deficits. Fatal.
Acute disseminated encephalomyelitis	After **infection**, such as chicken pox, measles. Can also occur after small pox or rabies **vaccination**.	Multifocal periventricular inflammation and demyelination
Charcot-Marie-Tooth	**Hereditary motor and sensory neuropathy**	Defective protein production leading to **peripheral nerve** and myelin sheath dysfunction
Metachromatic leukodystrophy	Autosomal recessive lysosomal storage disease. **Arylsulfatase A deficiency**	Myelin production is impaired by buildup of sulfatase.

Table 9 Demyelinating Diseases

1. Spinal cord is composed of **31 spinal nerves** that give rise to multiple ascending and descending tracts.
2. C1-C7 all exit above corresponding vertebrae except for **C8**, which exits below.
3. Ventral rami of C5-C8+T1 form the **brachial plexus**.
4. There are 12 thoracic nerves, 5 lumbar nerves, 5 sacral nerves and 1 coccygeal nerve
5. Cell bodies of all sensory nerves are the **dorsal root ganglion** (DRG)
6. Spinal cord stops at L1-L2 vertebrae, anything below is **cauda equina**.
7. **Subarachnoid space** goes up to S2
8. **Lumbar puncture** is performed at L3-L4 or below.
9. **Disc herniations** usually take place between L5-S1 and occur when **nucleus pulposis** comes out of the **annulus fibrosis** and impinges on the nerve

C2: top of head
C3: Turtleneck
T4: Nipples
T7: Xyphoid process
T10: Belly but**TEN**
L1: Inguinal L1gament
L4: Down on alL 4 knees
S2,S3,S4: Erection and penile/anal sensations

SPINAL CORD

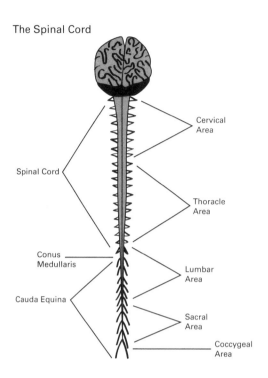

Figure 13 Areas of the spinal cord

Dermatomes

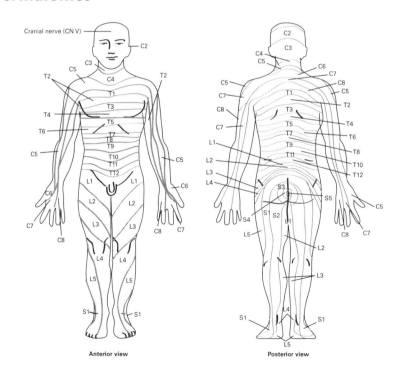

Figure 14 Sensory dermatomes

Reflexes

s1	Achilles reflex
l4	Patellar reflex
c5	Biceps
c7	Triceps
Primitive reflexes that disappear within 1 year of life	Moro reflex, Rooting, Sucking reflex, palmar reflex, Babinski reflex

Table 10 Reflexes

Spinal Cord Tract

Sensory Tracts	
Spinothalamic Tract 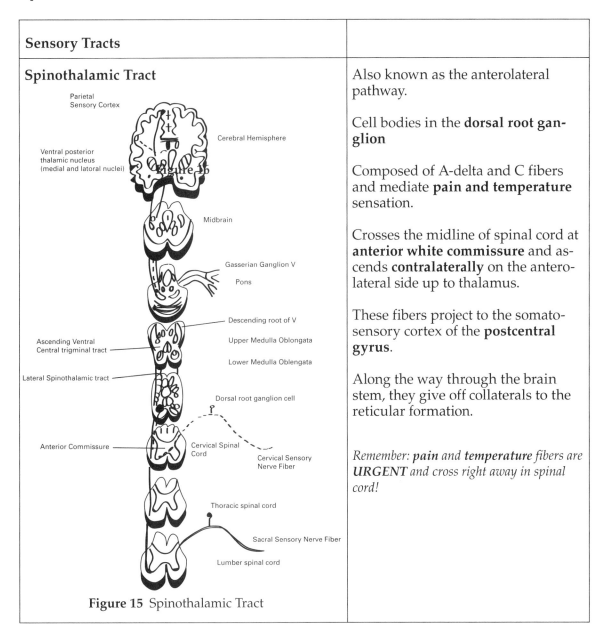 **Figure 15** Spinothalamic Tract	Also known as the anterolateral pathway. Cell bodies in the **dorsal root ganglion** Composed of A-delta and C fibers and mediate **pain and temperature** sensation. Crosses the midline of spinal cord at **anterior white commissure** and ascends **contralaterally** on the anterolateral side up to thalamus. These fibers project to the somatosensory cortex of the **postcentral gyrus**. Along the way through the brain stem, they give off collaterals to the reticular formation. *Remember:* **pain** *and* **temperature** *fibers are* **URGENT** *and cross right away in spinal cord!*

Dorsal column tract

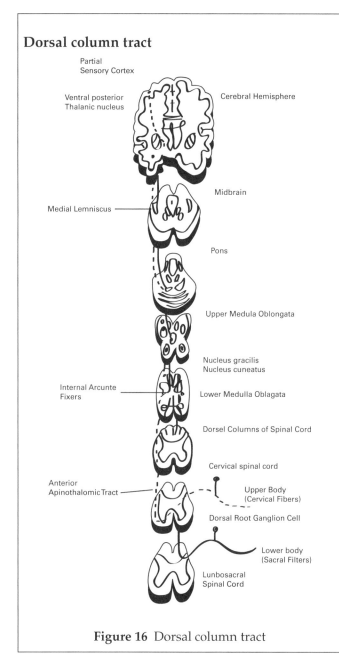

Partial
Sensory Cortex

Ventral posterior
Thalanic nucleus

Cerebral Hemisphere

Medial Lemniscus

Midbrain

Pons

Upper Medula Oblongata

Nucleus gracilis
Nucleus cuneatus

Internal Arcunte
Fixers

Lower Medulla Oblagata

Dorsel Columns of Spinal Cord

Cervical spinal cord

Anterior
Apinothalomic Tract

Upper Body
(Cervical Fibers)

Dorsal Root Ganglion Cell

Lower body
(Sacral Filters)

Lunbosacral
Spinal Cord

Figure 16 Dorsal column tract

Also known as medial lemniscus pathway

Detects **motion, vibration, pressure, and proprioception**.

These sensory fibers enter the **dorsal spinal cord** and synapse at specific dorsal nuclei that form the dorsal columns of the cord.

Nucleus gracilis carries sensations from the lower body; **nucleus cuneatus** does the upper body.

Fibers cross the midline to form the **medial lemniscus** and to form a synapse with the third-order neuron in the **ventroposterolateral nucleus of the thalamus**.

These fibers project to the somato-sensory cortex of the **postcentral gyrus.**

Motor Tract	
Lateral corticospinal tract **Figure 17** Lateral corticospinal tract	The corticospinal tract originates from the **precentral gyrus**, or primary motor cortex of the cerebral cortex The first-order neurons are **upper motor neurons** that arise in the motor cortex and descend in the brain stem to the medulla. Most (90%) undergo **pyramidal decussation** and give rise to the **lateral corticospinal tract.** These fibers descend through the **lateral funiculus** and synapse on the second-order neurons. The other 10% of the fibers that do not cross the midline descend in the anterior funiculus and form the **anterior corticospinal tract**. The **second-order neurons**, or lower motor neurons are the ventral horn motor neurons in the spinal cord They project through the ventral roots to synapse on **skeletal muscle fibers**. *Summary* *Motor cortex → internal capsule → cerebral peduncles at rostral pons → pyramid decussation → lateral corticospinal tract → synapse on gray matter of spinal cord at synapse on LMNs → impulse to skeletal muscle at NMJ*

Table 11 Spinal cord tract

Upper Motor Neurons vs. Lower Motor Neuron Lesions

- **Upper motor neuron damage** results in increased motor tone and increased resistance to passive movements with hyperactive reflexes. Positive Babinski sign, with fanning and dorsiflexion of the big toe when the sole of the foot is stroked firmly.

- **Lower motor neuron damage** results in decreased tone, absent or hypoactive reflexes with muscle atrophy.

Remember
STORM BABY!
In LMN lesion, everything decreases!

STORM BABY!	UMN	LMN
S: Strength	Lowers	Lowers
T: Tone	Increases (spastic)	Decreases (flaccid)
O: Others	Superficial reflexes absent Clonus	Fasciculation Fibrillation Reaction of degeneration
R: Reflexes	Increases	Decreases
M: Muscle mass	Only slight loss	Atrophy
B: Babinski sign	Positive	Negative

Table 12 Upper Motor Neurons vs. Lower Motor Neuron Lesions

Brown-Séquard Syndrome

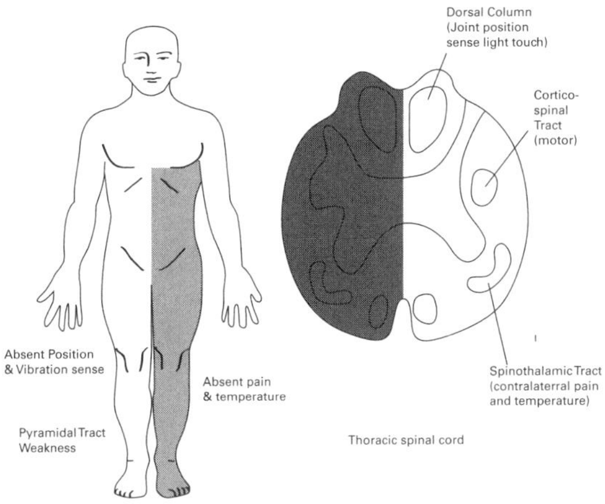

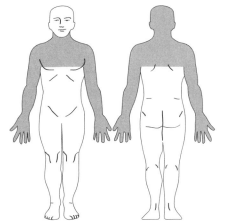

Figure 18

Hemisection of the spinal cord

Contralateral pain and temperature loss due to spinothalamic tract

Ipsilateral loss of vibration, motion and tactile sense due to dorsal column tract

UMN signs: hyper-reflexia below the lesion.

At the level of the lesion: ipsilateral loss of all sensation and LMN signs, such as paralysis.

Syringomyelia

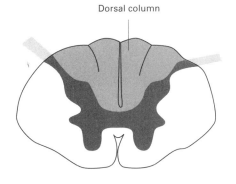

Figure 19

Damage of the **anterior white commissure** due to a syrinx, or cyst formation in the spinal cord.

Cape-like loss of pain and temperature along the C8-T1 area

Adversely affects the **spinothalamic tract** and causes bilateral loss of pain and temperature.

It does not affect the dorsal-medial lemniscus pathway because the spinothalamic tract crosses the midline and the anterior white commissure is on the midline!

Tabes dorsalis

Dorsal column

Figure 20

Destruction of dorsal roots and dorsal columns due to **tertiary syphilis**

Impaired motion, proprioception, vibration, and discriminative touch

- Caused by demyelination secondary to an untreated syphilis infection
- **"Tabetic gait"** is a characteristic where the patient's feet slap the ground as they strike the floor due to loss of proprioception."

Multiple Sclerosis	Destruction of the fatty myelin sheaths leading to demyelination and scarring of important spinal cord tracts.
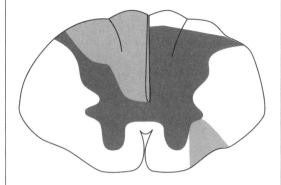 **Figure 21**	Presents in relapsing remitting format in young Caucasian females. *Remember DEMYELINATION!* • **D**iplopia/**D**ysmetria/**D**ysdiadochokinesis/**D**epression • **E**ye movement painful (Optic neuritis) **M**otor: Weakness; spasticity nystagmus • **E**levation in temperature (Uhthoff's phenomenon) • **L**hermitte's sign (electric sensation on back/limbs) • **I**ntention tremor • **N**europathic pain • **A**taxia • **T**alking is slurred; dysarthria • **I**mpotence • **O**veractive bladder (urinary urgency) • **N**umbness (sensory defect)
Amyotrophic lateral sclerosis (ALS)	Also known as **Lou Gehrig's Disease** Neurons contain proteinaceous inclusions within axons and cell bodies secondary to defect in **ubiquitin** protein. Combination of UMN and LMN defects Muscle weakness often starting at the limbs No sensory or cognitive defects. Congenitally acquired form is due to a defect in superoxide dismutase.
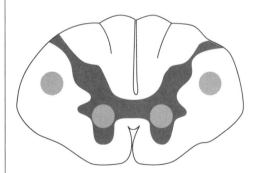 **Figure 22**	

Ventral Horn Diseases 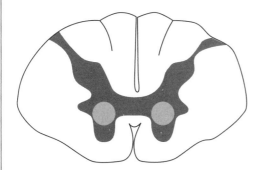 Figure 23	**Werdnig-Hoffman disease** Autosomal recessive mutation of a protein responsible for maintaining motor neurons. Results in destruction of ventral horns causing LMN lesion symptoms. Floppy baby, respiratory distress in newborns Tongue fasciculation, flaccid paralysis **Poliomyelitis** Poliovirus destroying ventral horns in the CNS. LMN lesion symptoms Fibrillation, hyporeflexia Headache
Subacute combined degeneration 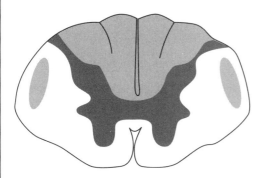 Figure 24	The word "combined" in SCD refers to demyelination of both the **dorsal columns** and **lateral corticospinal tracts**. Contrast this with tabes dorsalis, which has damage to only the dorsal columns. This condition is often caused by **vitamin B12** or **vitamin E** deficiency and is associated with pernicious anemia. Weakness in arms and legs with numbness that worsens Ataxic gait and motion, position and vibration sense negatively affected Positive Babinski sign and hyper-reflexia consistent with UMN lesions

High Yield Neurologic disorders	
Friedreich's Ataxia 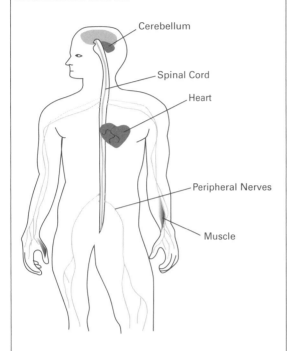 **Figure 25**	Similar presentation to SCD, however, it is an inherited recessive mutation in the gene that encodes frataxin. **Trinucleotide repeat mutation** (GAA repeats) The nerves degenerate and demyelinate in the spinal cord due to the mutation. **Hypertrophic cardiomyopathy** is frequently the cause of death. Ataxia with muscle weakness of arms and legs Scoliosis Hearing and vision impaired Presents between ages of 5 and 15 years old. *Remember neurological problems with cardiomyopathy should point to Friedreich's!*
Huntington's disease 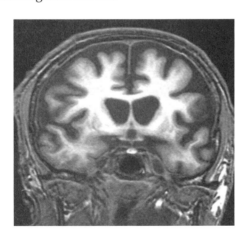 **Figure 26**	Autosomal dominant disorder characterized by strange movements, depression and aggression due to basal ganglia striatal nuclei damage. **Trinucleotide repeat mutation** CAG repeats = **C**audate – **A**ch & **G**ABA Chorea: Brief, sudden and jerky involuntary movements that are characteristic of Huntington's Athetosis: Slow, twisting and writhing movements Treatment: Reserpine, tetrabenazine, haloperidol *Remember **HUNT 4 DATE**:* ***HUNT**ington's on chromosome **4**, with cau**DATE** nucleus involvement!*

Table 13 Lesions of the spinal cord

Midbrain

Midbrain		Cranial nerve nuclei III & IV
Tectum (Dorsal)	Red nucleus Substantia nigra	Critical regions in the basal ganglia for **complex motor movements**
	Cerebral peduncles	Corticospinal and corticobulbar tracts run through
	Reticular activating system	Regulates **arousal and attention**
	Edinger-Westphal nucleus	Responsible for the **pupillary consensual reflex** When CN II receives light, its afferent fibers travel to the pretectal nucleus, which then activates bilateral Edinger-Westphal nuclei that cause the **constriction of both pupils** via CN III.
	Superior colliculus	The superior colliculus is responsible for visual processing and saccadic eye movements, smooth pursuit and **vertical eye movement.** Damage to SC leads to **Parinaud syndrome.** Vertical gaze paralysis Upward gaze nystagmus Lack of accommodation
	Inferior colliculus	The inferior colliculus is responsible for **auditory processing** and sends its output fibers to the medial geniculate nucleus of the thalamus.
Pons		Responsible for sleep paralysis Pneumotaxic center CN nuclei V-VIII

Locked-in syndrome can also result from basilar artery infarction

	Central pontine myelinolysis	Destruction of the white matter tracts Often due to rapid correction of hyponatremia Can result in locked in syndrome	
	Paramedian pontine formation	Responsible for horizontal gaze and saccadic eye movements Unilateral lesion will cause the eyes to deviate ipsilaterally towards the lesion with nystagmus. Bilateral lesion will cause horizontal gaze paralysis.	
Medulla Oblogata		Vomiting, vasomotor and respiratory centers CN nuclei IX-XII: Heart rate, breathing and autonomic control.	
	Medial medullary syndrome	Occlusion of the anterior spinal artery Ipsilateral flaccid tongue paralysis Contralateral hemiparesis Loss of motion, vibration, and proprioception of the trunk and extremities	

1. Midbrain
2. Pons
3. Medulla

Brain stem regulates consciousness, breathing, heart rate and sleep-wake cycles.

Locked-in syndrome can also result from basilar artery infarction.

A lesion in RAS can result in narcolepsy, ADD, Parkinson's.

Table 14 Midbrain

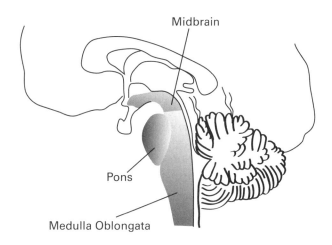

Figure 27

CRANIAL NERVES

There are 12 cranial nerves that can be memorized with the following mnemonic:
"Ooh, ooh ooh, to touch and feel very good vegetables, AH!"

In general, cranial nerves can be either sensory, motor or both.

"Some say marry money but my brother says big brains matter more."

CN	Description	Clinical Correlate
Olfactory (I) **"Ooh"** **Sensory** **"Some"**	Function: Sense of **smell**. Does not pass through thalamus and relays right to the brain. Course: Derives from the cerebral cortex, courses beneath the frontal lobe and exits through the **cribriform plate.**	Deficit presents as **anosmia**
Optic (II) **"Ooh"** **Sensory** **"Say"**	Function: **Sight** Course: Derived from the diencephalon, courses through the optic canal (along with ophthalmic artery and central retinal vein) and attaches to the retina. This nerve ends at the optic chiasm and called the optic tract. Some afferent fibers synapse on the pretectal nucleus to control consensual pupillary response.	**Marcus-Gunn pupil**: When light is shown in affected eye, there is a lack of pupillary constriction in both eyes. Indicates CN II is damaged and CN III is intact.

Oculomotor (III)	Function: **Most eye movement**, opening of eyelid (via levator palpebrae) and pupillary constriction.	**SO4 LR6 AR3** This nerve is composed of an inner and outer layer.
"Ooh" Motor "Marry"	Course: starts from oculomotor nuclei located in the superior colliculus, which goes through lateral wall of cavernous sinus and exits through the superior orbital fissure. Edinger-Westphal nucleus in the midbrain also provides parasympathetic input. Superior Rectus III — Inferior Oblique III — Superior Rectus III Lateral Rectus VI — Lateral Rectus VI R — L Inferior Rectus III — Superior Oblique VI — Inferior Rectus III **Figure 28**	The outer layer has parasympathetic fibers that **constrict the pupil**. Outer layer compression is the main cause of parasympathetic defect, such as tumor, uncal herniation, aneurysm, and hematoma causing a 'blown pupil.' The inner layer of CN III controls the eye muscles. Ischemia will affect this layer more than the outer layer; hence it is common to see a diabetic with palsy, but also with an intact pupillary response.
Trochlear (IV) "To" Motor "Money"	Function: controls **superior oblique** muscle of the eye. Course: nuclei in the midbrain, this is the **only cranial nerve that crosses the midline**. Goes through cavernous sinus. Exits through the superior orbital fissure.	Classic presentation with **CN IV palsy** is **"trouble walking down the stairs."** *Remember: a lesion in the trochlear nucleus will affect the contralateral eye!*

| Trigeminal (V) "Touch" Both (sensory and motor) "But" | Functions: main **sensation of the face** via three divisions

Motor—mastication muscles, tensor veli palatini, tensor tympani and myohyoid.

Course—Nuclei in the pons, the 3 divisions exit the skull through 3 different foramina:

Ophthalmic (V1)—**superior orbital fissure**

Maxillary (V2)—**foramen rotundum**

Mandibular (V3)—**foramen ovale**

Remember: Standing Room Only! | Lesion of this nerve presents **as jaw deviation to the side of the lesion** due to weak pterygoid muscle.
Trigeminal neuralgia- periods of intense pain on the face caused by CN V dysfunction.

Figure 29 The three branches of CN V |
| Abducens (VI) "And" Motor "My" | Function: controls the **lateral rectus muscle**.

Course: nuclei in the dorsal pons and courses through the corticospinal tracts in the ventral pons. It then runs through the cavernous sinus near the internal carotid artery and exits into the orbit via the **superior orbital fissure**. | Infarct in the **ventral pons** can cause **ipsilateral lateral rectus palsy** and **contralateral hemiparesis**. Infarct in the **dorsal pons** presents with **ipsilateral facial palsy** and **lateral rectus palsy**.

Lesion presents as diplopia due to unopposed medial rectus muscle. **Wernicke-Korsakoff** can cause nerve damage. **Internuclear ophthalmoplegia** can cause deficiency in lateral conjugate gaze. |

| Facial (VII) "Feel" Both (sensory and motor) "Brother" | Function: sensation—**taste** from anterior ⅔ of tongue.

Motor—controls muscles of facial expression and eye closing and the stapedius muscle in the ear.

Course: nucleus is in the pons and courses through the petrous temporal bone and then runs a torturous course in the facial canal before exiting through the **stylomastoid foramen** and running through the parotid gland. It divides into five branches and does not innervate the parotid gland.

• **Corda tympani**—part of the facial nerve but it splits off into the internal acoustic meatus, goes through the middle ear, and joins the lingual nerve (part of CN V). The corda tympani carries parasympathetic fibers that innervate the submandibular and sublingual salivary glands. | UMN Lesion: only lower contralateral face droops due to upper face having bilateral control from both facial nerves.
LMN Lesion (**Bell's palsy**): both upper and lower face droop.

Figure 30

Figure 31 |
| Vestibulocochlear (VIII) "Very" Sensory "Says" | Function: sensory nerve transmitting **sound** and **balance** information to the brain from the inner ear.

Course: Nuclei in the pons and courses through the internal **auditory meatus**. | Lesions in this nerve present as **vertigo, hearing loss**, nystagmus and tinnitus. |

Glossopharyngeal (IX) "Good" **Both (sensory and motor)** "Big"	Function—Sensory-*taste* from posterior ⅔ of tongue. Motor—**stylopharyngeus muscle**, swallowing muscles—critical muscle for swallowing. Also innervates the **parotid gland** through parasympathetic fibers from the otic ganglion. Nerve also contains carotid body chemoreceptors. Course: Nuclei in the anterior medulla. Sensory nucleus is **Nucleus solitarius**, which gets baroreceptor and taste input. Motor nucleus is **Nucleus ambiguous**, which aids in swallowing. Nerve exits through the **jugular foramen** and runs between the internal carotid and internal jugular vessels.	Lesion will produce a **taste defect** in the posterior ⅓ of the tongue along with **difficulty swallowing**.
Vagus (X) "Vegetables" **Both (sensory and motor)** "Brains"	Function: Motor—**swallowing**, **cough reflex**, **viscera** in thorax and abdomen, palatoglossus muscle. Sensory—**taste** in epiglottis, **baroreceptors** and **chemoreceptors** in the aortic arch. Course: Nuclei in the medulla. **Nucleus solitarius**—contains sensory information from the gut, **nucleus ambiguous**—motor innervation to the esophagus. **Dorsal nucleus** of the vagus nerve sends parasympathetic input to the abdominal viscera, heart and lungs. Nerve exits through the **jugular foramen** and enters the carotid sheath. There are many branches, but a unique one is the **recurrent laryngeal nerve**, which hooks under the aortic arch.	Due to so many vagal innervations lesion can present in many ways, one classic presentation can be seen with **uvula deviation** that is contralateral to the lesion. Normal Palsy of right palate **Figure 32** The vagus nerve also plays a key role in **vaso-vagal syncope** where some trigger stimulates the nucleus solitarius to withdraw sympathetic tone and increase parasympathetic tone. This sometimes causes people to pass out.

Accessory (XI) "AH" Motor "Matter"	Function: Motor—innervates the **SCM** and trapezius muscles, which function ipsilaterally in head turning and shoulder shrugging respectively. Course: The course is unique, this is the only cranial nerve to enter and exit the skull and it begins outside the skull. It forms in the **upper spinal cord** and enters the skull through the **foramen magnum** and then exits it through the **jugular foramen**. It then innervates the SCM and also pierces it while the going to innervate the trapezius.	In accessory nerve palsy classic presentation is **ipsilateral "shoulder droop"** and weakness turning head contralaterally. Advanced stages of the disease show atrophy of the SCM and trapezius muscle.
Hypoglossal (XII) "AH" Motor "More"	Function: Supplies motor innervation to **all muscles of the tongue except the palatoglossus muscle** (which is innervated by vagus). Course: Nuclei in the medulla, exits skull through **hypoglossal canal** and goes into the upper carotid sheath before innervating the muscles of the tongue.	Classical presentation of **LMN** lesion is tongue deviation to **ipsilateral** side of lesion due to unopposed genioglossus muscle. **UMN** lesions show **contralateral** deviation of the tongue.
CN reflexes	**Afferent**	**Efferent**
Corneal	V1 ophthalmic	VII temporal branch
Lacrimation	V1	VII
Jaw Jerk	V3 sensory	V3 motor
Pupillary	II **Marcus Gunn Pupil**: Afferent pupillary defect. When light is shone in affected eye, there is decreased bilateral constriction.	III *Remember!* *Miosis/Constriction: Pupillary sphincter muscle—Parasympathetic* *My**D**riasis/**D**ilation: Radial muscle-Sympathetic*

Table 15 Cranial nerves

BLOOD BRAIN BARRIER AND CEREBRAL PERFUSION

The brain is a protected space. The blood-brain barrier limits what molecules can enter the brain. The barrier is composed of astrocyte foot processes that wrap around CNS capillaries and form tight junctions. It is important to know which molecules can get through the blood brain barrier.

1. **Glucose**: specific carrier mediated transporters on endothelial cells of capillaries carries glucose into the brain. Glucose is the single largest source of energy for the brain.

2. **Amino Acids**: The brain needs these to make critical neurotransmitters, and often needs amino acids to do so.

Critical neurotransmitters and their links to amino acids

- Phenylalanine—Dopamine, NE

- Tryptophan—Gives rise to Serotonin and Melatonin via the serotonin pathway

- Glutamate—gives rise to GABA.

3. **Lipid soluble compounds** cross the BBB via diffusion into the brain.

- **Kernicterus** is a serious neurological condition that can affect severely jaundiced newborns. Indirect bilirubin builds up in the blood and crosses the BBB, piling up in the basal ganglia, cerebellum and brain stem causing permanent brain damage in newborns.

Exceptions to the BBB in the Brain

1. **Area postrema** is a highly vascular structure on the inferior-posterior side of the fourth ventricle. It lacks tight junctions and functions as the **"vomit center"** when it senses emetic substances in the blood, such as drugs in chemotherapy.

2. **OVLT** stands for the organum vasculosum of the lamina terminalis. This area is located in the anterior and ventral to the third ventricle. It has osmo-receptors that detect **osmotic pressure** in the blood and activate **vasopressin release** and thirst.

3. **Neurohypophysis** is the posterior pituitary. **ADH and oxytocin** are released in fenestrated capillaries that lack BBB tight junctions.

Fluorescent light therapy to help transform bilirubin into a form the body can more quickly eliminate.

CIRCLE OF WILLIS

- An area of huge anastomosis formed by the internal carotid and vertebral arteries.

- Remember the external carotid does NOT directly contribute to the circle of Willis.

- Blood can flow either way, which acts as collateral and help protect against ischemic damage as a result of occlusion.

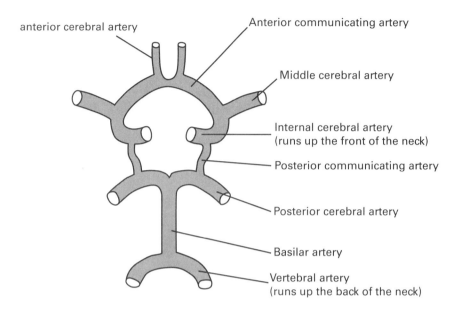

anterior cerebral artery

Anterior communicating artery

Middle cerebral artery

Internal cerebral artery
(runs up the front of the neck)

Posterior communicating artery

Posterior cerebral artery

Basilar artery

Vertebral artery
(runs up the back of the neck)

Figure 33 Regions of the Circle of Willis

Circle of Willis Component	Region Supplied	Symptoms if occulated	Clinical Correlate
Internal Carotid	This artery feeds into the circle of Willis. It also carries the sympathetic fibers of the **carotid plexus**, which innervates the pupillary dilator muscles.		
External Carotid	Branches are: superior thyroid, ascending pharyngeal, lingual, facial, occipital, posterior auricular, maxillary and superficial temporal arteries.	*Remember Mnemonic: Some Attendings Like Freaking Out Poor Medical Students*	
Middle Cerebral Artery	Anterior temporal lobe, insular cortex, lateral frontal and parietal lobes, motor cortex, sensory cortex, Wernicke's Area, Broca's Area *Remember: aphasia in these areas takes place only if lesion is on dominant side!*	**Contralateral paralysis** in the upper limbs and entire contralateral face. **Contralateral sensory loss** in the upper limb and entire contralateral side of face.	Right hand dominant patient shows **hemineglect** of left side.
Lateral Striate Artery or lenticulostriate arteries	Internal capsule and striatum, caudate nucleus, lentiform nucleus	Since posterior limb of internal capsule is damaged, contralateral motor defects but not sensory ones are affected. *Remember: most common cause of stroke in the basal ganglia/striatum is hypertension.*	A non-compliant hypertensive patient comes in with **hemiplegia** on his dominant side.
Basilar Artery	Feeds into the posterior part of the circle of Willis.	**"Locked-in Syndrome."** CN III not affected.	Patient is aware and awake but has complete paralysis of nearly all voluntary muscles in the body except for the eyes.

Anterior Cerebral Artery (ACA)	Medial surface of the frontal cortex, both sensory and motor cortex are supplied here.	Contralateral loss of sensation and paralysis in the lower limb.	Patient comes in with complaint of sensory and motor loss in the legs and feet. *Why not the hands? Because the medial side supplies the legs and feet!*
Anterior communicating artery	Serves as a connection between left and right anterior cerebral arteries.	**Paralysis and sensory loss in the lower limb** on only one side. Aneurysms arise here commonly can result in visual loss due to the proximity to the optic nerve.	Patient complains of right-sided leg weakness and sensory loss. He also reports vision problems.
Posterior communicating artery	Connection between the PCA and MCA	**CN III** palsy, due to its proximity, aneurysm can press on CN III.	Patient presents with slight weakness in upper limbs and an eye stuck. **"Down and out"**
Posterior Cerebral Artery	Mainly supplies the back of the brain, such as occipital cortex—main vision area and also inferior temporal lobe.	Contralateral hemianopia with macular sparing Figure 34	Patient presents with a "partial loss of vision" *Why are the centers of the visual fields spared? Macula also has blood supply from MCA!*
Anterior Spinal Artery	Lateral corticospinal tract, caudal medulla, medial lemniscus	**Contralateral hemiparesis** in the lower limbs and **ipsilateral tongue deviation** (hypoglossal nerve effected).	A 63-year old woman presents with right-sided leg weakness and upon examination she is found to have a left deviated tongue.

PICA	Supplies the lateral medulla and inferior cerebellar peduncle. Remember *SPAM* for Horner's syndrome! **S**: Sunken eye balls, **S**ympathetic cervical plexus affected **P**: Ptosis **A**: Anhydrosis **M**: Miosis	Occlusion at the lateral medulla causes **Wallenberg's syndrome** *Remember Wallenberg`s* **H**orny **ADVIC**e  • Ipsilateral Horner`s • Ataxia • Dyarthria, Dysphagia • Vertigo • Contralateral body sensory loss	Patient presents with pain and temperature loss of on the right side along with ataxia and lack of face pain on the left side. She also has a sense of vertigo and difficulty swallowing.
AICA	Lateral pons. Middle and inferior cerebellar peduncles.	**Lateral pontine syndrome** has similar presentation to Wallenberg, except for dysarthria and dysphagia.	Patient has ipsilateral facial paralysis, sudden onset vertigo, tinnitus and vomiting

Table 16 Circle of Willis

Watershed zones: MCA where it communicates with the ACA and PCA

Watershed Zones are special zones of the brain that receive dual blood supply from the distal branches of arteries. During an ischemic event, watershed areas have an advantage due to collateral blood supply. However, during times of hypoperfusion, these distal branches do not receive adequate blood supply. This creates focal deficits such as upper leg/arm weakness or lack of sensation in the face.

Berry aneurysms are outpouchings of blood vessels at arterial bifurcations with increasing risk of rupture over time. They are found most commonly in the anterior circle of Willis.

STROKE

It is important to differentiate between ischemic and hemorrhagic stroke, know the diagnosis, treatment, and the treatment contraindications. If the symptoms last more than 24 hours, it is most likely a stroke. If they last less the patient must be evaluated for a transient ischemic attack (TIA), which causes only brief episodes of neurologic defects. TIA patients are at high risk for stroke and must be further evaluated. Strokes are usually diagnosed with CT, but may also be diagnosed with MRI.

- **Ischemic Stroke** is due to blockage of a large vessel secondary to emboli from atrial fibrillation or carotid dissections. **tPA** is indicated within 3–5 hours of symptoms once hemorrhagic stroke has been ruled out by imaging.

- **Hemorrhagic stroke** is bleeding in the brain due to hypertension, aneurysm rupture, and abnormal vessels. It can also occur secondary to vasospasm and increased vessel fragility after ischemic strokes. The cause can also be iatrogenic with increased use of anticoagulants. tPA is contraindicated when the non-contrast CT scan shows bright areas of bleed. Hemorrhagic stroke can be classified depending on their location with respect to the dura.

Epidural Hematoma

Blood builds up between the skull and the dura mater.

Epidural hematoma occurs mostly due **to traumatic injury**. The **middle meningeal artery** will bleed and cause rapid expansion compressing brain tissue. Typical epidural hematoma case will present with lucid interval and CN III palsy, followed by unconsciousness.

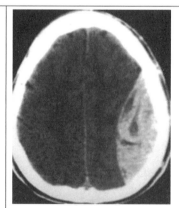

Figure 35

CT scan will show **E**pidural bleed that looks conv**Ex** and does not cross suture lines with midline shift.

Subdural Hematoma

Blood builds between the dura and the subdural space.

Subdural hematoma is due to rupture of **bridging VEINS** instead of an artery, hence there is slow bleeding spread throughout the space. Most often will present after **shaken baby syndrome**, **alcoholism** and **whiplash**, instead of outright trauma. Patient will present with a gradual confusion and loss of consciousness.

CT scan will show a con**C**ave shaped bleed that does cross suture lines and **C**rescent shaped.

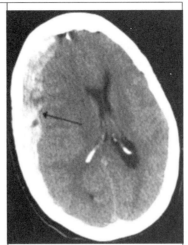

Figure 36

Subarachnoid Hemorrhage

Blood builds up between the sub-arachnoid space and the pia mater.

Most often due to aneurysm rupture, AV malformation or head trauma. Patient will present with the **"worst headache of my life"** or "thunderclap headache," seizure and loss of consciousness may also result.

CT scan will show the bleed, but an MRI may be more sensitive after several days. Angiography will show the origin of the bleed (aneurysm, AVM, etc). Lumbar puncture may show xanthochromia (yellow CSF due to blood breakdown in CNS).

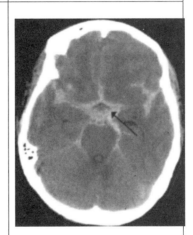

Figure 37

Table 17 Types of stroke

CSF AND VENTRICLES

Cerebrospinal fluid (CSF) is secreted by the **choroid plexus** into ventricles. The flow of CSF through the ventricle system is depicted below:

Two lateral ventricles
↓
Interventricular foramina
↓
Third ventricle
↓
Aqueduct of Sylvius
↓
Fourth ventricle
↓
Lateral foramen of Luschka
Medial foramen of Magendie
↓
Spinal cord

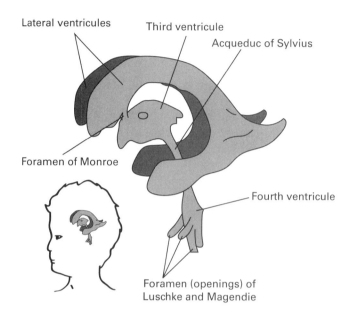

Figure 38 Ventricular System of the Brain

Under normal circumstances CSF is taken up by arachnoid villi and drained into the superior sagittal sinus, preventing a buildup of CSF in the central nervous system. **Hydrocephalus** results when there is a problem with CSF absorption or production.

1. **Normal-pressure hydrocephalus** (NPH) is known as a communicating hydrocephalus because the flow of CSF between ventricles is not obstructed. Rather, the increased fluid is likely due to impaired CSF absorption from arachnoid granulations.

   • NPH may be idiopathic or secondary to conditions that interfere with CSF absorption (e.g., meningitis, subarachnoid hemorrhage).

   • Key symptoms are urinary incontinence, dementia and ataxia.

2. Hydrocephalus in the presence of atrophy with normal intracranial pressure and the lack of "wet, wobbly and wacky" symptoms is called **Hydrocephalus ex-vacuo.**

"Wet, Wacky, Wobbly"

3. Noncommunicating or **obstructive hydrocephalus** is caused by blockade of CSF circulation in the ventricular system (e.g., by tumor, stenosis of aqueducts). It is associated with increased CSF pressure, headache, and papilledema.

HERNIATION SYNDROMES

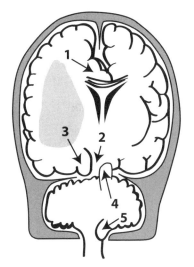

1. Subfalcine
2. Central
3. Uncal
4. Upward
5. Tonsillar

Figure 39 Cavernous Sinus Anatomy
(Adapted from *Toronto Notes*)

1. **Subfalcine** or cingulate herniation occurs under falx cerebri

2. **Central** herniation occurs downward

3. **Uncal** herniation

   - Ipsilateral ptosis due to stretching of CN III

   - Contralateral homonymous hemianopia due to compression of PCA

   - Ipsilateral paresis occurs due to compression of contralateral cruscerebri

   - Downward displacement of brain stem can lead to paramedian artery rupture and cause duret hemorrhages.

4. **Upward** herniation

5. **Tonsillar** herniation of cerebellum into foramen magnum

CEREBRAL VENOUS DRAINAGE

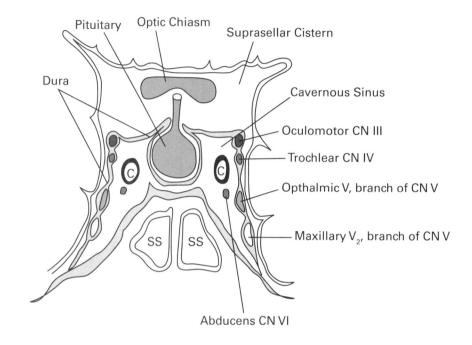

Figure 40 Cavernous Sinus Anatomy
(Adapted from *Toronto Notes*)

- A special sinus that lies around the pituitary is called the cavernous sinus.

- Structures traversing the sinus include the third, fourth, and sixth cranial nerves; the first two divisions of the fifth nerve; sympathetic fibers supplying the pupil; and the internal carotid artery.

- Wall of the cavernous sinus surrounds the sphenoid sinus and sphenoid sinusitis can result in cavernous sinus thrombophlebitis.

- Cavernous sinus syndrome can result in opthalmaplegia and maxillary sensory loss.

- Other lesions of the cavernous sinus may be caused by tumors or carotid aneurysms.

OPTHAMOLOGY

Glaucoma	Open/wide angle	Close/Narrow angle	Treatment
	Silent and painless Obstructed outflow of canal of Schlemm Associated with age, myopia	Painful!!! Obstruction between iris and lens Associated with rock hard eye, headache	Epinephrine- (Do NOT use in close angle) Beta blockers Acetazolamide Pilocarpine Physostigmine Latanoprost
Cataract	Painless opacification of lens that results in decreased vision	RF: old age, diabetes, alcoholism, exposure to sunlight	Surgery
Retinal detachment	Separated pigment epithelium from retina	Leads to vision loss RF: diabetes, trauma to eye	Surgery
Macular degeneration	Degeneration of central focal point of retina	Dry: fat deposits, gradual vision loss Wet: Neovascularization, rapid vision loss	Surgery
nternuclear opthalmoplegia	Lesion in MLF associated with MS	Medial palsy on lateral gaze, nystagmus on abducting eye	 **Figure 41**

Table 18 Venus drainage

SEIZURES

Seizures are involuntary physiological reaction caused by synchronized, high frequency firing of neurons.

Partial Seizures	Focal area of brain is affected and often proceeded by aura 1. **Simple Partial:** occurs while consciousness is intact. Can be motor, sensory and autonomic 2. **Complex Partial:** Consciousness is not intact	First line for partial seizure: Carbamezapine. Can also use: Phenytoin Lamotrigine Gabapentin Phenobarbital (first line for pregnant women and children) Valproic acid
Generalized Seizures	Diffuse area of brain is affected 1. **Absence:** petit mal, simple blank stare, no motor, sensory component. 2. **Myoclonic:** rapid, jerky movements 3. **Tonic-clonic:** shifting between movement and stiffness 4. **Tonic:** Just stiffness 5. **Atonic:** drops to floor with loss of motor control	First line for prophylaxis: Phenytoin First line for tonic-clonic: Phenytoin, carbamazepine, valproic acid First line for absence: Ethosuximide First line for status epilepticus: Benzodiazepine
Febrile seizures	Benign seizures in young children	No treatment needed

Table 19 Seizures

HEADACHES

Migraine	Throbbing unilateral pain with nausea, vomit, photo-phobia Can present with aura	NSAIDs Propanolol Sumatriptan: causes vasoconstriction
Tension Headache	Bilateral pain without any aura, photophobia Related to stress > 30 minutes in duration	NSAIDs
Cluster Headache	Young males Unilateral and associated with ipsilateral lacrimation and periorbital pain Horner's syndrome	Oxygen! Sumatriptan

Table 20 Headaches

Sumatriptan can cause coronary vasospasm! Contraindicated in patients with CAD or Prinzmetal's angina

CHAPTER 14

PHARMACOLOGY

PHARMACOKINETICS

Pharmacokinetics describes what happens to a drug as it passes through the body. The process can be separated into four entities: absorption, distribution, metabolism, and excretion. Clinically, the variability seen in drug effect from patient to patient can be attributed to differences in these processes. Pharmacokinetics is affected by disease states, especially diseases of the major organs involved in drug metabolism and excretion (kidneys and liver). Knowledge of pharmacokinetics is important in determining the dosage intervals of a drug.

Absorption

Absorption describes how the drug enters the body, either by (1) mouth (PO), usually requiring gastrointestinal (GI) absorption (beware of the first-pass effect), (2) intramuscular (IM) injection, (3) subdermal/intradermal injection, (4) inhalation, (5) sublingual, (6) buccal, (7) rectal, (8) topical, or (9) intravenous (IV) administration. The route of absorption used depends on availability, need for rapid access, and patient compliance. Some drugs may have to be given by IV because they are broken down in the GI tract. The route of administration affects the drug's **bioavailability** (percentage of drug reaching systemic circulation). By definition, IV drugs have 100% bioavailability, whereas the bioavailability of oral drugs is equal to the percentage of drug remaining after the first pass in the liver.

Drugs absorbed via the GI tract are often significantly metabolized by the liver before reaching the systemic circulation, so only a fraction of the initial amount reaches the serum (recall that venous return from the stomach and bowels travels via the portal circulation through the liver before reaching the systemic circulation). This means that an IV dose required for a particular drug may be smaller than the PO dose of the same drug. Liver disease may result in increased bioavailability of these drugs because of decreased drug metabolism by the sick liver.

Distribution

Distribution is the transfer of drug from one body compartment to another. Distribution of drugs follows the laws of thermodynamics (mass effect, equilibrium kinetics, reversibility). Many drugs distribute throughout the body, so that the body acts as a reservoir. **Volume of distribution (V_d)** is a quantitative measure of how well a drug is distributed.

Because of their increased body fat, elderly are more susceptible to overdose and side effects of fat soluble medications.

Antipsychotic medications block dopamine (D2) and serotonin receptors

Levodopa is used to treat Parkinson's disease. It easily crosses the blood-brain barrier and gets converted to dopamine

$$V_d \text{ (liters)} = D/[C_p]$$

Where D = total amount of drug in the body and C_p = concentration of drug in plasma.

In general, drugs with smaller V_d tend to remain in the blood whereas drugs with higher V_d are dispersed more outside the intravascular volume and distribute into most tissues. Of note, the V_d of drugs that are bound to plasma proteins (e.g., albumin) is affected (increased) by liver and kidney disease.

Metabolism

Metabolism is the chemical modification of drugs in the body, usually as a first step in the removal of the drug. Drug metabolism usually takes place in the liver, but it also occurs in the kidney, lungs, and bloodstream. Metabolism is particularly important for lipophilic drugs because these are absorbed rapidly and distribute well and would therefore linger and cause toxicity if they were not broken down. Metabolism usually occurs in two steps: phase I (biotransformation) and phase II (conjugation).

- **Phase I** metabolism, or biotransformation (e.g., oxidation, reduction, deamination, hydrolysis), involves the liver's **cytochrome P-450** system adding a functional group (e.g., -OH, -NH$_2$) to the drug to increase water solubility of the drug. There are multiple forms of the P-450 enzymes, each with different substrate specificities. They metabolize both endogenous molecules and exogenous drugs, and they cover a broad range of substrates, so that one drug may compete with the metabolism of another drug. Increasing the burden of drug in the body (e.g., regular consumption of valium) increases the levels of P-450 enzymes due to enzyme synthesis. These enzymes display considerable genetic variability from person to person. Older patients lose this form of metabolism.

- **Phase II** metabolism, or conjugation (e.g., glucuronidation, acetylation, sulfation), involves the addition of an organic moiety (e.g., glucuronic acid, acetate, sulfate, glutathione, glycine, methyl groups) to the drug to decrease lipid solubility so that the drug can be eliminated via the urine or bile. Older patients mainly rely on this form of metabolism.

Excretion

Excretion is the physical removal of drugs from the body. It occurs primarily in the kidney but can also occur through the GI tract and skin. Only drugs not bound to plasma proteins can be eliminated by the kidney; in other words, drugs must be hydrophilic or modified to be more hydrophilic for renal excretion. Drugs in the kidney can be passively filtered, actively reabsorbed, or actively secreted. The rate of renal excretion depends on the glomerular filtration rate. **Elimination**, or removal of active drug molecules from the body, is calculated by the following formula: Metabolism + Excretion = Elimination.

Drugs that induce P-450 system

GRAB SPC
Griseofulvin, **R**ifampin, **A**lcohol (chronic), **B**arbiturates, **S**t John's wart, **P**henytoin, **C**arbemazepine

Drugs that inhibit P-450 system

I C PACKAGES
Isoniazid, **C**iprofloxacin, **P**rotease inhibitors, **A**lcohol (acute), **C**imetidine, **K**etoconazole, **A**miodarone, **G**rapefruit juice, **E**rythromycin, **S**ulfonamides

Kinetics

Elimination, absorption, and distribution all obey the principles of thermodynamics and are described as either first-order or zero-order kinetics (Figure 1). (There are a few instances of more complicated kinetics in the body's handling of drugs.)

- **Zero-order kinetics**: Regardless of the concentration of drug, a constant amount is eliminated, absorbed, or distributed. Zero-order kinetics occur when the organ or enzyme's ability to process the drug is saturated. Common examples of drugs with zero-order kinetics include **ethanol**, **phenytoin**, and **aspirin.**

- **First-order kinetics**: In this case the rate of elimination, absorption, or distribution is directly proportional to the concentration of the drug. This produces an exponential decay in the concentration of the drug and a **half-life of elimination** that is constant regardless of drug concentration. Most drugs behave in this way in the body.

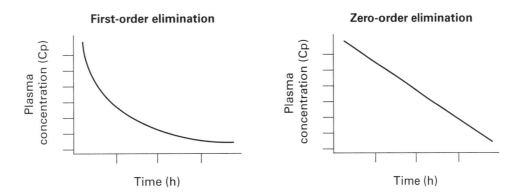

Figure 1 First-order and zero-order kinetics

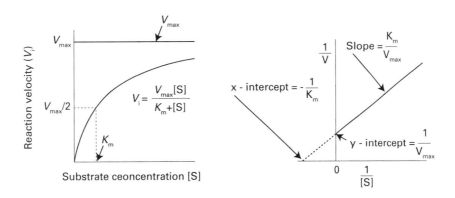

Figure 2 Michaelis-Mentin curve and Lineweaver Burk plot

Clearance: the volume of blood completely cleared of drug per unit of time.

CL = rate of elimination/concentration of drug in plasma

$CL = V_d \bullet K_c$

(Where K_c is the elimination constant)

Dosage intervals

The components of pharmacokinetics (absorption, distribution, elimination) must be considered in designing a dosing regimen for a particular drug. Here are a few key concepts:

- **Half-life**: For drugs subject to first-order kinetics, half-life is the time it takes for a given concentration of drug to be either reduced during elimination, or increased during constant infusion, by 50% of the starting concentration (e.g., after 1 half life, concentration is 50% of the original concentration; after 2 half-lives, the concentration is 25% of the original concentration; after 3 half-lives, the concentration is 12.5% of the original concentration).

$$t_{1/2} = (0.693 \bullet V_d)/CL$$

Where $t_{1/2}$ = half-life, V_d = volume of distribution, and CL = clearance

- **Therapeutic index**: This ratio (TI) of the drug concentration producing toxicity to the drug concentration required for intended therapeutic effect can be used to estimate the safety of a drug. The higher the therapeutic index, the safer the drug. Be careful with the drugs that have a narrow therapeutic index because the dose that grants the desired effect is very close to the dose that causes toxicity.

$$TI = LD_{50} / ED_{50}$$

Where LD_{50} is the median lethal dose

And ED_{50} is the median effective dose

- **Dosing interval**: The dosing interval depends on drug half-life, therapeutic index, and patient convenience. The interval should be narrow enough that drug's peak concentration is below toxic levels, while the trough levels are at or above the drug's minimum effective concentration.

- **Loading dose**: When a patient is initially given a drug, the first several doses may have to be higher than subsequent maintenance doses. This is because the initial drug doses fill the body's volume of distribution before reaching high enough levels to produce a therapeutic level in the bloodstream. Once the V_d is filled, a maintenance dose in required to offset the body's elimination of the drug, thus maintaining steady-state serum concentrations. Of note, the loading dose is not affected by liver or kidney disease.

$$Loading\ dose = C_p \bullet V_d$$

- **Maintenance dose**: The dose needed for a given dosing interval to maintain a steady-state concentration of drug of drug in the bloodstream. In contrast to the loading dose, the maintenance dose is affected (decreased) in patients with either liver or kidney disease.

$$Maintenance\ dose = Cp \bullet Clearance$$

Individual Factors

- **Age**: Hepatic drug metabolic activity decreases with increasing age. Therefore, drug doses often need to be lowered in older patients.

- **Gender**: There are likely to be differences in hepatic enzyme function and efficacy between man and women, a subject only now being investigated.

- **Disease**: Liver disease reduces drug metabolizing activity, and renal disease reduces excretion. Dosages must be altered according to the clinical situation.

- **Tolerance**: With many drugs, the degree of responsiveness (effect) diminishes with continued administration (tolerance). The mechanism may be at the receptor and cellular level (e.g., down-regulation of receptors) or the result of up-regulation of metabolic enzymes in the liver. Rapid loss of response after a drug is administered is called **tachyphylaxis**. With tolerance, larger doses are needed to achieve the same effect that was previously achieved.

- **Dependence**: Withdrawal of the drug produces symptoms and signs that are often the opposite of the drug's effects. Dependence can be psychological or physical.

- **Compliance**: Physicians must be aware of the availability and desire of patients to comply with prescribed regimens. Often, side effects are intolerable to the patient, and drugs are discontinued. A common example is β-blockers, which have side effects of general dysphoria—and in men erectile dysfunction—and may be intolerable.

- **Body weight**: Weight has an obvious effect on the dosing of a drug because a larger mass has a larger absolute volume of distribution.

PHARMACODYNAMICS

Receptors

A receptor is simply any macromolecule in the body to which a drug must bind to achieve its effects. Receptors can be soluble molecules (acetylcholinesterase), cell membrane proteins (ion channels), intracellular organelle proteins (ribosomes targeted by aminoglycoside antibiotics), or nucleic acids (many chemotherapeutic agents).

Structure-Activity Relationships

The binding of a drug to a receptor is a function of the usual intermolecular forces: hydrogen bonds, van der Waals forces, ionic bonds, and covalent bonds.

Agonists and Antagonists

Agonists are drugs that bind to receptors and stimulate their associated cellular activities. Receptor agonists activate the primary effect of binding of ligand to receptor. Agonists are classified into three types:

- **Full agonist** produces the full response when bound to the receptor.

- **Partial agonist** produces a lower response than a full agonist, even when receptors are fully bound.

- **Inverse agonist** binds a receptor and produces the opposite effect; this can be seen with beta-carbolines, which elicit anxiogenic and convulsant effects when they bind benzodiazepine receptors.

Efficacy is the maximal effect that a drug can produce at high levels (i.e., maximum receptor occupancy). Zero efficacy means that even with all the receptors bound, the drug has no effect. Partial agonists have lower efficacy than full agonists. **Potency**, on the other hand, refers to the amount of drug needed to produce an effect. It is usually denoted as EC_{50}, the concentration to achieve half-maximal effect.

Antagonists bind to receptors and block their activation. There are three subcategories:

- **Competitive antagonist**: A drug that binds reversibly to the receptor at the same site as the agonist, so that adding more and more antagonist inhibits the binding of the agonist by mass effect (i.e., it floods out the agonist). Of note, competitive agonists shift the log-dose response curve to the right, decreasing the potency of the agonist. This effect can be overcome by simply adding more agonist. There is no change in the efficacy of the agonist.

- **Noncompetitive antagonist**: A drug that binds to the receptor at a different site than the agonist. It induces a conformational change, so even if the agonist is present, it cannot bind and cannot flood out the antagonist, no matter how high the concentration. Of note, noncompetitive agonists shift the log-dose response curve downward, decreasing the efficacy of the agonist.

- **Irreversible antagonist**: Once bound to the receptor, it does not fall off. No matter how much of the agonist is available, that receptor is blocked.

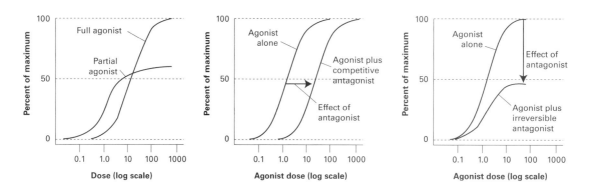

Figure 3 Dose-response curves for partial agonist, full agonist, agonist plus competitive antagonist, and agonist plus noncompetitive antagonist

Side Effects

Side effects are a key aspect of drugs, not only because physicians pledge to "do no harm," but also because the examination tests your knowledge of drug side effects. Toxic side effects are included in drug discussions throughout this chapter and the rest of the book.

AUTONOMIC NERVOUS SYSTEM PHARMACOLOGY

The autonomic nervous system (ANS) is concerned with autonomic, unconscious, and involuntary bodily activities (Figure 4). The ANS is composed of **adrenergic** (norepinephrine [NE] = primary neurotransmitter), **cholinergic** (acetylcholine [ACh] = primary transmitter), and **dopaminergic** (dopamine = primary neurotransmitter) synapses (Figure 5).

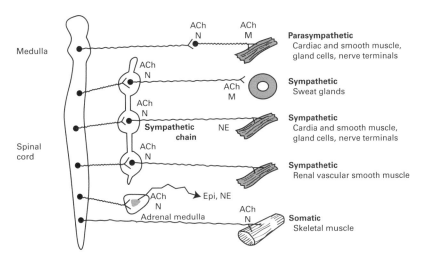

Figure 4 Sympathetic and parasympathetic nerve endings. (ACh = acetylcholine; NE = norepinephrine; Epi = epinephrine; N = nicotine; M = muscarinic

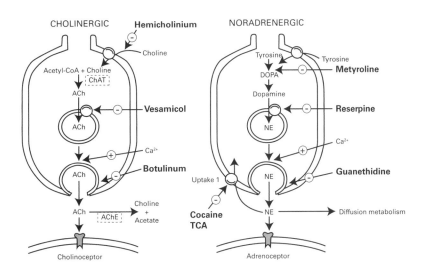

Figure 5 Cholinergic (ACh) and adrenergic (NE) nerve terminals

Adrenergic receptors are G protein coupled receptors for the catecholamines (norepinephrine, epinephrine), which are responsible for the sympathetic response. The sympathetic system is the part of the ANS that originates in thoracic and lumbar spinal cord segments (T1-L5). **Cholinergic receptors** are specific for the neurotransmitter acetylcholine (ACh), and can be divided into **muscarinic** (G protein coupled) or **nicotinic** receptors. The parasympathetic system originates in the cranial nerves and sacral spinal cord segments. Preganglionic neurons in both the sympathetic and parasympathetic nervous system synapse onto nicotinic acetylcholine (ACh) receptors, which are ligand-gated Na^+/K^+ channels. The postganglionic sympathetic neurons release NE as their primary neurotransmitter, while the postganglionic parasympathetic neurons synapse onto muscarinic acetylcholine (ACh) receptors. The effects of the ANS on different organ systems is shown in Figure 6 and described further in Table 1.

Bold type = sympathetic actions
italic type = parasympathetic actions

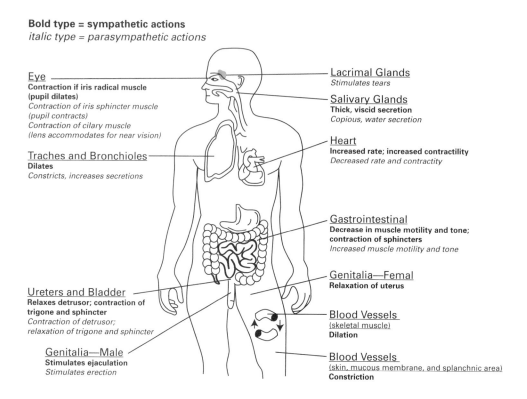

Eye
Contraction if iris radical muscle (pupil dilates)
Contraction of iris sphincter muscle (pupil contracts)
Contraction of cilary muscle (lens accommodates for near vision)

Traches and Bronchioles
Dilates
Constricts, increases secretions

Ureters and Bladder
Relaxes detrusor; contraction of trigone and sphincter
Contraction of detrusor; relaxation of trigone and sphincter

Genitalia—Male
Stimulates ejaculation
Stimulates erection

Lacrimal Glands
Stimulates tears

Salivary Glands
Thick, viscid secretion
Copious, water secretion

Heart
Increased rate; increased contractility
Decreased rate and contractity

Gastrointestinal
Decrease in muscle motility and tone; contraction of sphincters
Increased muscle motility and tone

Genitalia—Femal
Relaxation of uterus

Blood Vessels
(skeletal muscle)
Dilation

Blood Vessels
(skin, mucous membrane, and splanchnic area)
Constriction

Figure 6 Actions of the sympathetic and parasympathetic nervous system

Area	Sympathetic Receptor	Effect	Parasympathetic Receptor	Effect
Heart				
Sinoatrial node	ß$_1$	Increases firing	M$_2$	Decreases firing
Ectopic pacemakers	ß$_1$	Increases firing	None	
Contractility	ß$_1$	Increases firing	M$_2$	Decreases
Blood vessels				
Splanchnic vessels	α	Contraction	M$_3$	Relaxation
To skeletal muscle	ß$_2$	Relaxation	M$_3$	Relaxation
	α	Contraction		
	M	Relaxation		
Gastrointestinal tract				
Smooth muscle	α$_2$	Relaxation	M$_3$	Contraction
	ß$_2$	Relaxation		
Sphincters	α$_1$	Contraction	M$_3$	Relaxation
Myenteric plexus	α	Inhibition	M$_1$	Activation
Secretion	None	None	M$_3$	Increases
Lungs: bronchi	ß$_2$	Relaxation	M$_3$	Contraction
Genitourinary tract				
Bladder	ß$_2$	Relaxation	M$_3$	Contraction
Sphincter	α$_1$	Contraction	M$_3$	Relaxation
Uterus	ß$_2$	Relaxation	M$_3$	Contraction
	α	Contraction		
Penis	α	Ejaculation	M	Erection
Eye				
Radial muscle	α$_1$	Contraction	None	None
Circular muscle	None	None	M$_3$	Contraction
Ciliary muscle	ß	Relaxation	M$_3$	Contraction
Skin				
Pilomotor muscles	α	Contraction		
Sweat glands	α (apocrine)	Activation	M (thermo-regulatory)	Activation

Table 1 Autonomic nervous system effects by organ system

Most drugs that target the autonomic nervous system create their effects by acting on ion channels of nerve cells and altering ion flow. With ligand-gated ion channels, this is accomplished through binding of neurotransmitters to receptors, which are coupled to channel proteins. There are several different types of receptor-channel coupling. Some receptors act directly on the channel protein, and some are coupled to channel proteins through a G protein, with or without diffusible second messengers. **G coupling proteins** include **Gs, Gi, Gq.** Flowcharts of G proteins and their actions are depicted in Figures 7, 8, and 9. These G-protein linked 2nd messenger systems are used in association with the following receptors:

- sympathetic (α**1,** α**2,** β**1,** β**2**) receptors utilize Gq, Gi, Gs, Gs proteins, respectively. (**QIS**)

- parasympathetic (**M1,M2,M3**) receptors utilize Gq, Gi, Gq proteins, respectively. (**QIQ**)

- dopamine (**D1,D2**) receptors utilize Gs, Gi proteins, respectively. (**SI**)

- histamine (**H1,H2**) receptors utilize Gq, Gs proteins, respectively. (**QS**)

- vasopressin (**V1,V2**) receptors utilize Gq, Gs, proteins, respectively. (**QS**)

KISS, KICK, SICK, SEX = QIS, QIQ, SI, QS, QS.

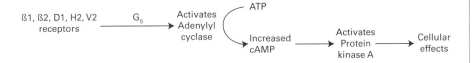

Figure 7 Gs protein activates the cAMP-dependent pathway

(β**1,** ββ2, D1, H2,V2 receptors) = **B**ig **B**oys **D**on't **H**a**V**e **2**

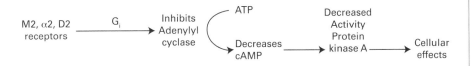

Figure 8 Gi protein inhibits the cAMP-dependent pathway

(M2, α2, D2 receptors) = **2 MAD**

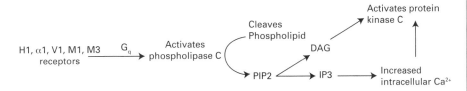

Figure 9 Gq protein activates phopholipase C, releasing DAG/IP3

(H1,α1,V1,M1,M3 receptors) = **HAV 1 M&M**

Adrenergic Agents

Sympathomimetics, or adrenergic-receptor agonists, include the catecholamines and any drugs capable of stimulating the sympathetic response. There are two general categories of sympathomimetic drugs. Some act **directly** at the adrenergic ($\alpha1$, $\alpha2$, $\beta1$, $\beta2$) receptors, while others act **indirectly** by either releasing endogenous NE from the presynaptic terminal (e.g., amphetamine), or blocking synaptic reuptake of NE (e.g., cocaine) (Figure 5). Long-term treatment with receptor or neuronal blockers leads to accommodation, whereby the postsynaptic cell increases the number of receptors and develops enhanced sensitivity to catecholamines. Therefore, abrupt withdrawal of the blocker may be dangerous. Increased catecholamines (e.g., in pheochromocytoma) and increased sympathetic tone (e.g., congestive heart failure) may lead to decreased sensitivity to catecholamines (e.g., through loss of receptors from the cell surface by internalization). Here is a list of **adrenergic receptors** and their effects:

- **$\alpha1$**: mainly smooth muscle contraction (including veno- and vasoconstriction, mydriasis, pilomotor smooth muscle contraction, salivary and sweat gland secretion); increased glyco-genolysis/gluconeogenesis; decreased GI motility.

- **$\alpha2$**: some vasoconstriction; platelet aggregation; inhibition of lipolysis and pancreatic insulin secretion; decreased release of both ACh and NE from nerve terminals.

- **$\beta1$**: increases cardiac output (HR, contractility, AV conduction); increases renin release from juxtoglomerular cells.

- **$\beta2$**: smooth muscle relaxation (including bronchodilation, vasodilation in skeletal muscle and smaller coronary arteries, decreased GI/GU motility, uterine relaxation); striated muscle tremor with increased glycogenolysis/gluconeogenesis/insulin release.

- **D1**: vasodilation in renal and splanchnic blood vessels.

- **D2**: inhibits adenylyl cyclase.

Here is a list of the **direct sympathomimetics**, the drugs which act at the adrenergic receptor, along with their selectivity and clinical applications.

- **Epinephrine**: $\alpha1$, $\alpha2$, $\beta1$, $\beta2$; used to treat hypotension, anaphylaxis, glaucoma, asthma.

- **Norepinephrine**: $\alpha1$, $\alpha2$, $\beta1$; used to treat hypotension (watch for reflex bradycardia!).

- **Phenylephrine**: $\alpha1 > \alpha2$; used to treat hypotension, papillary dilation, decongestion.

- **Clonidine**: $\alpha2 > \alpha1$; used to treat hypertension.

- **Isoproterenol**: $\beta1 = \beta2$; used to treat bradycardia, heart block.

- **Dobutamine**: $\beta1 > \beta2$; used to treat cardiogenic shock, heart failure.

- **Terbutaline**: $\beta2 > \beta1$; used as tocolytic to prevent preterm labor for 48 hours.

- **Albuterol**: $\beta2 > \beta1$; used to treat acute asthma attacks.

- **Salmeterol**: $\beta2 > \beta1$; used daily to decrease frequency/severity of asthma

- **Dopamine**: $D1 > \beta > \alpha$; used to treat renal failure associated shock, and heart failure.

(Of note, dopamine is D1 selective at low doses, β at medium doses, and α at high doses.)

Here is a list of the **indirect sympathomimetics**, the drugs which act indirectly by either releasing endogenous NE from the presynaptic terminal or blocking synaptic reuptake of NE.

- **Amphetamine**: promotes release of NE; used to treat ADHD, narcolepsy, obesity.

- **Ephedrine**: increases NE activity; used to treat nasal decongestion, urinary incontinence.

- **Cocaine**: inhibits the reuptake of NE; used for anesthesia and abused to "get high".

Antiadrenergic agents work by blocking the release of NE or by blocking post-synaptic adrenergic receptors. These can be divided into alpha-blockers and beta blockers.

Here is a list of common **alpha blockers**, which all cause orthostatic hypotension in toxicity. The orthostatic response is exaggerated with the first dose of alpha1-blockers so caution must be taken. **Epinephrine reversal** refers to a phenomenon in which epinephrine actually causes a drop in BP after administration of a nonselective alpha blocker.

- **Phenoxybenzene**: α-blocker (nonselective); used to treat pheochromocytoma.

- **Phentolamine**: α-blocker (nonselective); used for MAOI/tyramine ingestion.

(Of note, watch for reflex tachycardia with these two drugs!).

- **Prazosin, terazosin**: α1-blocker (selective); used to treat BPH, hypertension.

- **Mirtazapine**: α2-blocker (selective); used as an antidepressant.

Here is a list of common **beta blockers**, whose toxicity includes bradycardia, AV block, CHF. In addition, beta blockers should be used with caution in diabetics, as they mask the symptoms of hypoglycemia and inhibit glycogenolysis.

- **Timolol**: β-blocker (nonselective); used to treat glaucoma.

- **Nadolol**: β-blocker (nonselective); used to treat HTN, angina.

- **Propanolol**: β-blocker (nonselective); used to treat HTN, SVT, angina, acute MI.

(Of note, nonselective β-blockers cause bronchoconstriction; don't give to asthmatics!)

- **Atenolol**: β1 > β2 blocker (selective); used to treat HTN, SVT.

- **Acebutolol**: β1 > β2 blocker (selective); used to treat HTN, SVT; (partial β agonist).

- **Esmolol**: β1 > β2 blocker (selective); used to treat HTN, SVT; (given as IV drip).

- **Metoprolol**: β1 > β2 blocker (selective); used to treat HTN, SVT, angina, acute MI.

(Of note, the β1-selective blockers don't bronchoconstrict—safe to use in asthmatics).

- **Butoxamine**: β2 > β1 blocker (selective); not used clinically.

Some drugs have *both* alpha- and beta-blocking activity.

- **Labetalol**: α1, β (nonselective) blocker; used to treat HTN, CHF, pheochromocytoma.

- **Carvedilol**: α1,β (nonselective) blocker; used to treat CHF.

Cholinergics

Cholinomimetics, or cholinergic-receptor agonists, include the catecholamines and any drugs capable of stimulating the parasympathetic response. There are two general categories of cholinomimetics, those that act **directly** at the cholinergic receptors (e.g., acetylcholine), and those that act **indirectly** (anticholinesterases, e.g., neostigmine). The direct-acting drugs are further divided into **muscarinic** and **nicotinic** stimulators. Direct cholinergic stimulation has the following effects: CNS stimulation, pupillary constriction (miosis), decreased cardiac output, vasodilation, bronchoconstriction, increased GI motility, bladder contraction, sphincter relaxation, and increased glandular secretion.

Here is a list of the **direct cholinomimetics**, the drugs which act at the cholinergic receptor, along with their selectivity and clinical applications.

- **Acetylcholine**: acts on both muscarinic (M) and nicotinic (N) receptors.

- **Carbachol**: acts on M, N receptors; used for glaucoma, ophthalmic surgery.

- **Bethanochol**: acts on M receptors; used to treat bowel/bladder retention.

- **Pilocarpine**: acts on M receptors; used to stimulate tears, sweat, saliva.

- **Nicotine**: acts on nicotinic receptors to stimulate adrenal catecholamine release.

Indirect cholinomimetics (anticholinesterases) are drugs which indirectly increase cholinergic activity by inhibiting the cholinesterase enzyme and preventing breakdown of acetylcholine. They can be divided into three groups: edrophonium, the carbamates (neostigmine, physostigmine, pyridostigmine), and organophosphates (echothiophate, malathion, parathion). Their toxicity can be remembered by the mnemonic **DUMBBELS**: Diarrhea, Urination, Miosis, Bradycardia, Bronchoconstriction, Excitation, Lacrimation, Salivation, Sweating. Here is a list of the major anticholinesterases, along with their selectivity and clinical applications:

- **Edrophonium**: short-acting; used to diagnose myasthenia gravis.

- **Neostigmine**: intermediate-acting carbamate; used to treat bowel/bladder retention, myasthenia gravis, and to reverse neuromuscular blockade.

- **Pyridostigmine**: intermediate-acting carbamate; used to treat myasthenia gravis.

- **Physostigmine**: intermediate-acting carbamate; used to treat glaucoma.

- **Echothiophate**: long acting organophosphate; used to treat glaucoma.

- **Malathion**: long acting organophosphate; used as insecticide.

- **Parathion**: long acting organophosphate; used as insecticide (the most toxic!)

(Of note, the reversal agent used to treat anticholinesterase poisoning is **pralidoxime**).

Anticholinergic agents work by blocking the parasympathetic action of acetylcholine. These drugs can be divided into muscarinic and nicotinic antagonists. Here is a list of common **muscarinic antagonists**.

- **Atropine**: nonselective muscarinic antagonist used to treat symptomatic bradycardia, organophosphate poisoning; Toxicities include the opposite symptoms as DUMBBELS: decreased GI motility, decreased urgency, pupillary dilation, bronchodilation, vasodilation/flushing, decreased glandular secretion, pupillary dilation, paralyzed accommodation and delirium; (Dry as a bone, red as a beet, and mad as a hatter.)

- **Scopolamine**: used to treat motion sickness.

- **Benztropine**: used to treat parkinsonism.

- **Ipratroprium**: used to treat asthma, COPD.

- **Methoscopalamine**: used to reduce gastric acid secretion.

- **Oxybutynin**: used to reduce urinary urgency and bladder spasms.

Here is a list of common **nicotinic antagonists**:

- **Hexamethonium**: ganglion blocking agent; blocks both sympathetic / parasympathetic.

- **Turbocurarine**: nondepolarizing neuromuscular blocker.

- **Pancuronium**: nondepolarizing neuromuscular blocker.

- **Atracurium**: nondepolarizing neuromuscular blocker.

- **Vecuronium**: nondepolarizing neuromuscular blocker.

CNS PHARMACOLOGY

Alcohols

Ethanol is the most important alcohol, as it is commonly used and abused recreationally. After ingestion, ethanol is metabolized by **alcohol dehydrogenase** and a liver microsomal ethanol-oxidizing system. **Disulfiram** inhibits the enzyme alcohol dehydrogenase, resulting in accumulation of acetaldehde and severe nausea and vomiting. Several other drugs produce a similar disulfiram-like reaction, including metronidazole and some cephalosporins. Effects of ethanol include disinhibition, ataxia, and sedation. Chronic consumption leads to tolerance, dependence, liver dysfunction, peripheral neuropathy, and teratogenicity (fetal alcohol syndrome). Naltrexone can reduce craving in alcoholics, and benzodiazepines are used to treat withdrawal and delirium tremens.

Barbiturates

Barbiturates are drugs that cause CNS depression with sedative, hypnotic, anxiolytic, muscle relaxant, and anticonvulsant effects. The mechanism of action involves potentiation of GABA effects, by increasing the *duration* of GABA-stimulated chloride channel opening. These drugs have severe side effects, including cardiovascular and respiratory depression. In addition, tolerance and dependence can develop. Members of this class of drugs include:

- **Phenobarbital**: used as an epileptic.

- **Thiopental**: used for anesthesia induction.

Benzodiazepines

Benzodiazepines (BZPs) are another group of CNS depressants with sedative, hypnotic, anxiolytic, amnesic, muscle relaxant, and anticonvulsant effects. The mechanism involves enhanced action at the γ-aminobutyric acid ($GABA_A$) receptor by increasing the *frequency* of GABA-stimulated chloride channel opening. Benzos have replaced barbiturates for the most part because they cause less severe cardiovascular and respiratory depression. Continued use leads to development of tolerance and dependence. Most BZPs are metabolized by the P 450 system, and **Flumazenil** is used to treat BZP overdose. Flumazenil is effective at countering the sedative effects but not the benzodiazepine-induced respiratory depression. Benzodiazepines can be subclassified based on their duration of action.

- **triazolam, oxazepam, midazolam** (short-acting): used for status epilepticus, anesthesia.

- **lorazepam, temazepam, alprazolam** (intermediate-acting): used to treat panic disorder, anxiety, insomnia, and alcohol withdrawal.

- **flurazepam, chlordiazepoxide, diazepam** (long-acting): used to treat panic disorder, anxiety, insomnia, and alcohol withdrawal.

Anti-Epilepsy Drugs

These drugs have various mechanisms of action, but all of them suppress the continued action potentials responsible for epileptic activity. Their discontinuation must be gradual to avoid withdrawal seizures.

- **Phenytoin**: Na^+ channel blocker in neurons; used in tonic-clonic and partial seizures; toxicities include teratogenicity (fetal hydantoin syndrome, arly nystagmus, and induction of cytochrome P-450).

- **Valproate**: Na^+ channel blocker in neurons; used in tonic-clonic and partial seizures; toxicities include teratogenicity (neural tube defects), fatal hepatotoxicity. In contrast to many other antiseizure medications, valproic acid inhibits cytochrome P-450.

- **Carbamazepine**: Na^+ channel blocker in neurons; used in tonic-clonic & partial seizures; toxicities include teratogenicity (neural tube defects), hepatotoxicity, aplastic anemia, and induction of cytochrome P-450 system (CYP3A).

- **Ethosuximide**: inhibits Ca^{2+} channels in neurons; drug of choice for absence seizures; toxicities include Stevens-Johnson syndrome.

- **Phenobarbital**: barbiturate; increases Cl^- channel opening duration; drug of choice for neonatal seizures; used for all adult seizures except absence; causes sedation, dependence, and induction of cytochrome P-450 system (CYP2B).

- **Diazepam, lorazepam**: fast-acting benzos; increases Cl^- channel opening frequency; drugs of choice for status epilepticus; also causes sedation, tolerance, dependence.

- **Lamotrigine**: Na^+ channel blocker; used in tonic-clonic and partial seizures, as well as bipolar disorder (mood stabilizer); toxicity includes Stevens-Johnson syndrome.

- **Gabapentin**: GABA analog used to treat refractory seizures and neuropathic pain; toxicities include sedation, peripheral edema, and movement disorders.

- **Topiramate**: Na^+ channel blocker; used as to treat seizures and migraines; toxicities include sedation and nephrolithiasis.

Endorphins and Opiate Receptors

Opioids, both exogenous and endogenous, have diverse effects and involve almost every organ system. The opioids bind to opiate receptors on neurons, resulting in presynaptic inhibition. Opiate receptors are found in virtually all parts of the CNS. The effects of opioids include analgesia, sedation, altered consciousness, cough suppression, constipation, miosis, respiratory depression, and suppression of gonadotropin-releasing hormone release.

The **opioid receptor** is G-protein coupled and has several subtypes. The **delta** subtype prefers endogenous enkephalin, the **kappa** subtype prefers endogenous dynorphin, the **epsilon** subtype prefers endogenous β-endorphins, and the **mu** subtype prefers exogenous opiates (morphine; think "mu for morphine").

Endogenous opioid peptides are made in the body and include **beta-endorphin, met-enkephalin, leu-enkephalin,** and **dynorphin.** DNA for these proteins is found on the three genes proopiomelanocortin, proenkephalin, and prodynorphin, respectively. Proopiomelanocortin is cleaved and processed to ultimately yield several products, including β-endorphin, adrenocorticotropic hormone, and melanocyte-stimulating hormone. Exogenous opiates are not made in the body. Common examples include the following:

- **Codeine, dextromethorphan**: used as cough suppressants.

- **Loperamide, diphenoxylate**: used as anti-diarrheals.

- **Meperidine**: some pain relief; cannot be used with MAOIs or SSRIs.

- **Hydrocodone, Oxycodone**: provide good pain relief.

- **Methadone**: oral drug used to manage opiate withdrawal (longer half-life).

- **Heroin**: street drug; look for triad of lethargy, pinpoint pupils, respiratory depression.

- **Morphine**: good pain relief but watch out for respiratory suppression.

- **Dilaudid**: good pain relief but watch out for respiratory suppression.

- **Fentanyl**: can be used as an anesthetic and sedative.

Opiates have reinforcing properties, or feelings of satisfaction that accompany their use. Tolerance and physical dependence can quickly develop, resulting in significant abuse potential. Of note, patients do NOT develop tolerance to constipation, in contrast to many of the other symptoms. An **abstinence syndrome**, which includes agitation, mydriasis, lacrimation, rhinorrhea, chills, hyperthermia, and diarrhea, will occur if opiates are stopped. Treatment of opiate addiction may include detoxification (quitting cold turkey), using alternative approaches (e.g., acupuncture), incarceration, support groups, and maintenance on a surrogate opiate. **Methadone** is a long-acting opiate with a half-life of approximately 24 hours. The longer half-life reduces the abstinence syndrome and craving effect while the addict is weaned off opiates. **Opiate overdose** can produce coma, respiratory depression, and hypotension, a potentially fatal combination. If overdose is suspected, IV **Naloxone** (Narcan) and **naltrexone** can be administered to reverse coma and respiratory depression associated with opiate overdose. Opioids interact with ethanol, sedative-hypnotics, anesthetics, antipsychotic drugs, TCAs, and antihistamines to produce an additive CNS depressant effect.

Stimulants

Stimulants exhibit direct and indirect sympathomimetic actions with strong central action (more hydrophobic than catecholamines) and a long duration of action (not susceptible to breakdown by enzymes that degrade catecholamines, namely, catechol *O*-methyltransferase and monoamine oxidase). They act directly on dopamine receptors in the CNS and produce stimulation, including restlessness, insomnia, tremor, mood elevation, and increased alertness, and activity.

- **Nicotine**: stimulant found in tobacco products that creates psychological dependence, with withdrawal symptoms of headache, anxiety, and lethargy.

- **Caffeine**: stimulant found in soft drinks/tea/coffee; creates psychologic dependence, with withdrawal symptoms of headache, anxiety, and lethargy.

- **Amphetamines**: illicit or frequently-abused prescription drugs that cause anorexia and a euphoric "high" sensation that leads to abuse and dependence; overdose causes fever, tachycardia, and seizures; withdrawal causes depression and fatigue.

- **Cocaine**: illicit drug that causes anorexia and a euphoric "high" sensation that leads to abuse and dependence; overdose can cause hypertension, fatal arrhythmias, and seizures; withdrawal causes depression and fatigue.

Antidepressants

Subtypes of antidepressants include monoamine oxidase (MAO) inhibitors, tricyclic antidepressants (TCAs), and selective serotonin-reuptake inhibitors (SSRIs). According to the amine hypothesis of mood, NE and 5HT are key players, with decreased levels in the brain causing depression and increased levels in the brain causing elevated mood. Most of the antidepressants increase the levels of NE and/or 5HT to create their effect.

- **MAO inhibitors (isocarboxazid, phenelzine, selegiline, tranylcypromine)**: oldest of the antidepressant medications; inhibit the enzyme monoamine oxidase and nonselectively block metabolism of NE, 5HT, dopamine, and tyramine; not typically used as first-line agents because of the many side effects; toxicities include sympathomimetic effects, hyperthermia, agitation, seizures, hypertensive crisis (when taken together with tyramine-containing foods like wine and cheese); cannot be taken with SSRIs!

- **Tricyclic antidepressants, or TCAs (nortriptyline, amitriptyline, desipramine, clomipramine)**: older drugs that were previously the mainstay of treatment for depression; inhibit NE and 5HT reuptake; inexpensive but have numerous side effects (can be lethal in overdose!); toxicities include sympathomimetic and antimuscarinic effects, sedation, weight gain, orthostatic hypotension, withdrawal syndrome, additive CNS depression with other central depressants, coma, convulsions, and cardiotoxicity (QRS widening and QT prolongation on EKG); cannot be taken with SSRIs!

- **Heterocyclics (bupropion, trazodone, nefazodone, mirtazapine, venlaxafine)**: inhibit NE and 5HT reuptake; toxicities include sedation, seizures, and autonomic effects; bupropion induces P-450 enzymes.

- **Selective serotonin-reuptake inhibitors, or SSRIs (fluoxetine, sertraline, paroxetine, citalopram, escitalopram)**: selectively block serotonin reuptake of 5HT and have a more favorable side effect profile; safer in overdose and lack the anticholinergic effects and cardiotoxicity of TCAs; toxicities include sexual dysfunction, GI side effects, cytochrome P450 inhibition, and life-threatening **serotonin syndrome** (muscle rigidity, myoclonus, fever, seizures, and hemodynamic instability) when taken with MAOIs, TCAs, meperidine.

Mood Stabilizers

The drugs are used to treat bipolar disorder and include lithium and certain anticonvulsants. In addition, antipsychotics are sometimes used to treat manic episodes, and antidepressants can similarly be used for depressive episodes.

- **Lithium**: used as a mood-stabilizer; decreases NE release and increases 5HT synthesis; narrow therapeutic index and must be monitored carefully; toxicities include edema, acne, sedation, tremor, ataxia, nystagmus, leukocytosis, diabetes insipidus, thyroid abnormalities, and teratogenicity (cannot be taken during pregnancy!)

- **Anticonvulsants (valproic acid, carbamazepine, lamotrigine)**: as previously discussed.

Neuroleptics

The actions of antipsychotic drugs are not completely understood, but most are associated with blockade of the dopamine (D2) and/or serotonin ($5HT_{1A, 2A, C}$) receptors in the central nervous system. Neuroleptics are effective against the positive symptoms of schizophrenia, such as hallucinations and delusions, but do not reduce the negative symptoms. Because the actions of these drugs appear to be nonselective, however, a number of undesirable side effects can also occur, including sedation (histamine receptor blockade), orthostatic hypotension (alpha receptor blockade), anticholinergic side effects (muscarinic receptor blockade), hyperprolactinemia (pituitary dopamine receptor blockade), extrapyramidal symptoms (dopamine receptor blockade), and neuroleptic malignant syndrome (which can be treated with **dantrolene**). New atypical antipsychotics are believed to have better side effect profiles.

- **Phenothiazines (chlorpromazine, thioridazine, fluphenazine, prochlorperazine)**: older first-generation "typical" antipsychotics; cause significant sedation and orthostatic hypotension (watch out for elderly falls!); significant but variable extrapyramidal and autonomic side effects; thioridazine causes cardiotoxicity; prochlorperazine can be used as an antiemetic.

- **Butyrophenones (haloperidol)**: another "typical" antipsychotic commonly used for acute psychosis, agitation, and delirium; causes minimal sedation, orthostatic hypotension, and autonomic side effects; has the greatest extrapyramidal side effects.

- **Heterocyclics (risperidone, clozapine, olanzapine, quetiapine, ziprasidone)**: second generation "atypical" antipsychotics; more expensive but cause less extrapyramidal effects; clozapine toxicity includes agranulocytosis.

ANESTHESIA

Local Anesthetics

These drugs are classified as either esters or amides. Both act by blocking voltage dependent Na^+ channels, which in turn blocks membrane depolarization and action potential conduction. Small, myelinated nerve fibers are easier to block than large, unmyelinated fibers. Typically, these drugs are used in smaller surgical procedures as well as in spinal anesthesia. Of note, the pH of the tissue plays a role in the effectiveness of the drug. Local pH can be significantly lower in infected tissue, and more drug is required to achieve the desired anesthesia.

- **Esters**: include **procaine** (short acting), **cocaine** (medium), **tetracaine** (long acting); notice suffix "-aine"; all act as vasodilators except cocaine which is a vasoconstrictor; allergies are common; general toxicities include convulsion and coma; bupivicaine can cause arrhythmias; cocaine can also cause arrhythmias as well as MI and cerebral hemorrhage (secondary to hypertension).

- **Amides**: include **lidocaine** (short onset < 1 min), **prilocaine**, and **bupivacaine** (longest onset > 10 min); notice the suffix "aine" and presence of 2 "i"s in name; all act as vasodilators; toxicities include convulsions and coma; allergies are uncommon.

General Anesthetics

Anesthesia occurs in three stages: (1) **induction** (from walking until complete anesthesia), (2) **maintenance**, and (3) **recovery** (from complete anesthesia until consciousness is regained). General anesthetics can be subclassified by the route of administration (inhaled or IV).

Inhalational agents have CNS actions with an unclear mechanism. Once inhaled, these agents will equilibrate with the blood and brain at a rate that is unique for each drug. Those drugs with lower *blood solubility* will equilibrate faster and have faster induction. Drugs with higher *lipid solubility* will pass into the brain faster to achieve their effects. Lipid solubility and **oil/gas partition** coefficient are directly proportional to potency. **Minimum alveolar anesthetic concentration (MAC)** is a measure of the anesthetic's potency. MAC tells you what alveolar concentration (percentage of inspired air) of the anesthetic is required to achieve anesthesia from a standard painful stimulus in 50% of patients. Drugs with the lower MAC have higher potency.

- **Nitrous oxide**: has the lowest blood solubility and therefore the fastest induction; has the highest MAC (> 100%) and therefore the lowest potency; toxicity involves impaired oxygen uptake and resulting hypoxia.

- **Sevoflurane, isoflurane, enflurane, halothane**: these volatile liquid agents have relatively higher blood solubility and therefore slower induction; also have lower MAC and therefore higher potency; isoflurane is the most commonly used; toxicities include hypotension, respiratory depression, nephrotoxicity, **malignant hyperthermia** (treat with **dantrolene**); halothane is associated with hepatotoxicity.

Intravenous general anesthetics are comprised of several different types of drugs, including propofol, etomidate, ketamine, opioids, barbiturates, and benodiazepines.

- **Propofol**: GABA agonist that has rapid onset/recovery, and only works if administered in constant infusion; toxicity includes hypotension, respiratory depression.

- **Etomidate:** GABA agonist; toxicity includes adrenal insufficiency, myoclonus, emesis.

- **Ketamine:** glutamate antagonist that inhibits the NMDA receptor and produces a dissociative, catatonic state with amnesia; toxicity includes emergence hallucinations.

- **Opioids** (morphine, fentanyl): do not directly depress cardiac function, and are therefore useful in cardiac patients who might not tolerate otherwise tolerate general anesthesia.

- **Barbiturate** (thiopental): GABA agonist with rapid onset used for anesthesia induction; toxicity includes cardiopulmonary depression; also causes decreased intracranial pressure.

- **Benzodiazepine** (midazolam, diazepam, lorazepam): used for **conscious sedation** during smaller surgical procedures as well as for induction; toxicity is respiratory depression.

Muscle Relaxants

Neuromuscular blocking agents are used during surgery to cause muscle and respiratory paralysis, to allow for easier ventilation and surgical manipulation. They can be subclassified as either nondepolarizing or depolarizing, based on their mechanism of action.

Nondepolarizing blockade is caused by pure antagonists of nicotinic receptors at the skeletal muscle endplate. The nondepolarizing neuromuscular blocking drugs compete with ACh and bind its receptors, thereby preventing sodium channel opening, subsequent depolarization, and muscle fasciculation. The effects can be overcome with high doses of acetylcholine through administration of **cholinesterase inhibitors** (neostigmine, pyridostigmine). Nonpolarizing agents can be subclassified by the duration of their action.

- **Atracurium, mivacurium**: short duration; give slowly or massive histamine release.

- **Vecuronium, rocuronium**: Intermediate duration; watch for arrhythmias/AV block.

- **Tubocurarine, pancuronium**: long duration; tubocurarine causes bronchospasm.

Depolarizing blockade is caused by agonists of nicotinic receptors at the skeletal muscle endplate. The depolarizing neuromuscular blocking drugs bind ACh receptors and cause depolarization and an initial muscle fasciculation. However, the depolarization is continuous (as long as the drug is infused) and there is no opportunity for repolarization until muscles become desensitized to ACh. By that point the block is achieved and muscles are paralyzed. Addition of cholinesterase inhibitors *before* repolarization will only worsen the paralysis. In contrast, cholinesterase inhibitors *given after* repolarization will reverse the paralysis.

- **Succinylcholine** is a commonly used depolarizing agent that is made up of two connected acetylcholine molecules. It is relatively resistant to breakdown by acetylcholinesterase, and is metabolized by plasma cholinesterase. Succinylcholine is often used for induction of paralysis prior to surgery, with subsequent administration of a nondepolarizing agent for maintenance of effects. Toxicity includes muscle pain, autonomic ganglia stimulation, and lethal hyperkalemia. Hyperkalemia, either due to rhabdomyolysis (in muscular dystrophy) or upregulation of Ach receptors (in burns, upper/lower motor denervation, muscle trauma), can cause fatal ventricular dysrhythmias. Succinylcholine is rapidly hydrolyzed by plasma pseudocholinesterase rather than acetylcholinesterase. Patients with a congenital deficiency of plasma pseudocholinesterase are slow metabolizers of succinylcholine, and may experience prolonged paralysis when given this drug.

AUTACOIDS AND ERGOT ALKALOIDS

Autacoids are endogenous substances that include **histamine** and **serotonin** (5-HT), both products of amino acid modification (histidine and tryptophan, respectively). These compounds have various effects throughout the body, depending on the location of their receptors. Several common drugs block histamine receptors to produce their actions:

- **H1** receptors: found in smooth muscle; involved in vasodilation and bronchoconstriction; H1 blockers (e.g., **diphenhydramine**) can be used for IgE-mediated allergic reactions; toxicity of H1 blockers includes sedation.

- **H2** receptors: found in mast cells, heart, and stomach; involved in gastric acid secretion; H2 blockers (e.g., **cimetidine**) can be used in peptic ulcer disease, Zollinger-Ellison syndrome, and gastroesophageal reflux disease; toxicity of H2 blockers includes inhibition of drug metabolism by the liver.

- **H3** receptors: found in the CNS and PNS; involved in modulation of neurotransmitters; H3 blocker is **thioperamide.**

Serotonin (5-HT) also plays a role in the CNS, as well as the enteric nervous system. Here is a list of the serotonin receptors, along with their respective antagonists and their clinical uses.

- **5-HT$_{1D}$** receptors: found in the brain; involved in smooth muscle contraction, migraines; 5-HT$_{1D}$ agonists (**sumatriptan**) are helpful in treatment of migraine headaches.

- **5-HT$_2$** receptors: found in smooth muscle; involved in flushing, diarrhea, and bronchoconstriction associated with carcinoid tumor; 5-HT$_2$ antagonists (**ketanserin**).

- **5-HT$_3$ receptors:** found in the CNS vomiting center; 5-HT$_3$ antagonists (**odansetron**) are very common and effective anti-emetic.

Ergot alkaloids are a group of biologically active molecules derived from a fungus (*Claviceps purpurea*) that act as partial agonists at α-adrenoreceptors and 5-HT receptors. They can be divided into three categories, based on whether they act in the CNS, vascular smooth muscle, or uterine smooth muscle. Below are common examples from these groups.

- **LSD:** acts in CNS to produce hallucinogenic effects.

- **Bromocriptine** acts in the pituitary as a competitive inhibitor of dopamine receptors, causing suppression of prolactin secretion; also used to treat Parkinson's disease.

- **Ergotamine:** acts on vascular smooth muscle to produce α-adrenergic receptor-mediated vasoconstriction. The cerebral vasculature is most sensitive to these agents, which is why they are used to treat acute migraines. Ergotamines also cause uterine smooth muscle contraction, which can be taken advantage of to help control postpartum bleeding.

- **Ergonovine:** acts on uterine and cerebrovascular smooth muscle to produce vasoconstriction, used for migraine prophylaxis and to control postpartum bleeding.

- **Methysergide:** also acts on cerebrovascular smooth muscle to produce vasoconstriction, but only used for migraine prophylaxis (not acute attacks).

GLAUCOMA DRUGS

Various drugs used to decrease intraocular pressure, including alpha agonists, beta blockers, cholinomimetics, diuretics, and prostaglandin (ABCD and P). All of these agents affect either the synthesis, outflow, or secretion of aqueous humor.

- **Epinephrine:** nonselective α agonist that increases outflow; causes mydriasis.

(Of note, epinephrine can only be used with open angle glaucoma!)

- **Brimonidine:** selective α$_2$ agonist that decreases synthesis.

- **Timolol:** nonselective β blocker that decreases secretion.

- **Pilocarpine, carbachol:** direct cholinomimetics that decrease outflow; causes miosis.

- **Physostigmine, echothiophate:** indirect cholinomimetics; decrease outflow; cause miosis.

- **Acetazolamide:** diuretic/carbonic anhydrase inhibitor that decreases secretion.

- **Latanoprost:** prostaglandin that increases outflow; may cause darkening of iris.

DIURETICS

Diuretic agents are a group of drugs that increase sodium and water excretion in the urine. Figure 10 illustrates the sites of action of diuretic drugs.

- **Acetazolamide:** diuretic and carbonic anhydrase inhibitor that acts in the proximal convoluted tubule and causes diuresis of sodium bicarbonate; used to treat idiopathic intracranial hypertension, glaucoma and metabolic alkalosis; toxicity includes sulfa allergy, hypochloremic metabolic acidosis.

- **Mannitol**: osmotic diuretic that remains (not reabsorbed) in the collecting tubules and osmotically "holds onto" water, mainly in the proximal convoluted tubule; used to treat elevated intracranial pressure, acute glaucoma, drug overdose; toxicities include hyponatremia, pulmonary edema.

- **Hydrochlorothiazide**: thiazide diuretic that acts in the distal convoluted tubule and inhibits reabsorption of sodium chloride; used mainly in treatment of mild HTN. Toxicities include sulfa allergy, hypokalemic metabolic alkalosis, hyperglycemia, hyperlipidemia.

- **Furosemide**: loop diuretic that acts in the thick ascending limb of the loop of Henle by inhibiting a $Na^+/K^+/2Cl^-$ transporter and decreasing NaCl reabsorption; used to treat moderate to severe HTN, as well as fluid overload in CHF, ascites, nephrotic syndrome; toxicities include sulfa allergy, hypokalemic metabolic alkalosis, hypocalcemia, dehydration, ototoxicity.

- **Ethacrynic acid**: loop diuretic similar to furosemide, with the exception that it is not a sulfonamide and is safe to use in patients with sulfa allergies.

- **Spironolactone**: potassium-sparing diuretic that acts in the collecting tubules by decreasing Na^+/K^+ ATPase; used to treat aldosteronism and HTN in patients with intractable hypokalemia; toxicity includes significant hyperkalemia.

- **Triamterene, amiloride**: potassium-sparing diuretics that act in the collecting tubules by blocking Na^+ channels; used to treat HTN in patients with intractable hypokalemia; toxicity includes significant hyperkalemia.

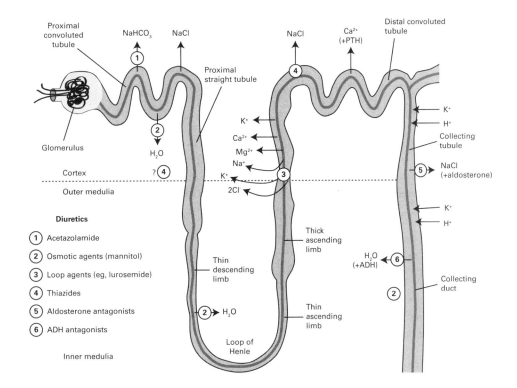

Figure 10 Diuretic agents and their sites of action

CARDIOVASCULAR PHARMACOLOGY

Below is a review of the major drugs used to treat hypertension, angina, CHF, and arrhythmias. In addition there is a discussion about hyperlipidemia medications.

Antihypertensives

Major classes of these agents include ACE inhibitors, ARBs, Beta blockers (and other sympathoplegics), Calcium channel blockers (and other vasodilators), and Diuretics (ABCD). Some patients have good blood pressure control with monotherapy while others do well on a combination of drugs. Here is a list of commonly used antihypertensive drugs, along with their respective mechanisms, clinical applications, and toxicities.

- **ACE inhibitors (lisinopril, enalapril, captopril)**: increase vasodilating bradykinin and decrease aldosterone, angiotensin II by inhibiting angiotensin-converting enzyme; these drugs are known to be renal protective; used in treatment of HTN, CHF, diabetic nephropathy; toxicities include cough, angioedema, fetal nephrotoxicity. Unlike many of the other antihypertensives, ACE inhibitors do not cause erectile dysfunction.

- **Angiotensin II receptor blockers, or ARBs (losartan, valsartan, irbesartan)**: cause vasodilation, decrease aldosterone by inhibiting the angiotensin II receptors in the heart and on blood vessels; used to treat HTN, CHF; toxicities are similar to ACE inhibitors except ARBs are not associated with cough or angioedema.

- **Beta blockers (propanolol, metoprolol)**: decrease blood pressure, heart rate, contractility, AV conduction and juxtaglomerular cell renin release; used to treat HTN, SVT, angina, and glaucoma; toxicities include bradycardia, AV block, and CHF.

- **Clonadine**: sympathoplegic/$\alpha 2$ agonist that inhibits both ACh and NE release, but has a net effect of decreased sympathetic tone; used to treat HTN; toxicities include hypotension as well as rebound hypertension when the drug is discontinued.

- **Prazosin**: sympathoplegic/$\alpha 1$ antagonist that prevents vasoconstriction; used to treat HTN, BPH; toxicity includes orthostatic hypotension.

- **Calcium channel blockers (nifedipine, verapamil, diltiazem, amlodipine)**: decrease smooth muscle/cardiac contractility, which in turn leads to vasodilation and a decrease in heart rate, AV conduction, and total peripheral resistance; used to treat HTN, SVT, angina; toxicities include AV block, CHF, peripheral edema.

- **Hydralazine**: vasodilator that acts by increasing cGMP levels which leads to decreased phosphorylation of smooth muscle myosin light chains; only used to treat severe HTN; toxicity includes compensatory tachycardia and SLE-like syndrome.

- **Minoxidil**: vasodilator whose metabolite opens K^+ channels and hyperpolarizes smooth muscle cells; this drug is also only used to treat severe HTN; toxicities include hirsutism and pericardial effusion.

- **Nitroprusside**: short-acting vasodilator that works by releasing nitric oxide and causing increased cGMP levels; used to treat hypertensive emergency; toxicities include hypotension, tachycardia, and cyanide poisoning.

- **Diazoxide**: longer-acting vasodilator that opens K^+ channels and hyperpolarizes smooth muscle cells; used to treat hypertensive emergency; toxicities include hypotension, hyperglycemia, and Na^+ retention.

- **Hydrochlorothiazide (HCTZ)**: thiazide diuretic that acts in the distal convoluted tubule and inhibits reabsorption of sodium chloride; used mainly in treatment of mild HTN. Toxicities include sulfa allergy, hypokalemic metabolic alkalosis, hyperglycemia, hyperlipidemia.

- **Furosemide**: loop diuretic that acts in the thick ascending limb of the loop of Henle by inhibiting a $Na^+/K^+/2Cl^-$ transporter and decreasing NaCl reabsorption; used to treat moderate to severe HTN; toxicities include sulfa allergy (**ethacrynic acid** can be used in these patients), hypokalemic metabolic alkalosis, hypocalcemia, dehydration, ototoxicity.

Antianginal Drugs

Because angina pain is the result of inadequate oxygen delivery to meet the needs of the myocardium, antianginal drugs work by either increasing delivery of oxygen or decreasing the myocardial oxygen consumption (MVO_2). MVO_2 is determined by blood volume (end-diastolic), venous tone, peripheral resistance, heart rate, contractility, and ejection time. Anti-anginal drugs which decrease these parameters include nitrates (decrease preload), calcium channel blockers (decrease preload), and beta blockers (decrease afterload).

- **Nitrates (nitroglycerin, isosorbide dinitrate)**: vasodilators (such as venodilation) that act by releasing nitric oxide and causing increase in cGMP levels; there is a decrease in EDV, BP, and ejection time, with a reflex increase in HR and contractility; net effect is a decrease in MVO_2; used to treat acute angina and pulmonary edema; toxicities include headache, tachycardia, and orthostatic hypotension (can be life-threatening if taken together with sildenafil!).

- **Beta blockers (propanolol, metoprolol)**: there is a decrease in BP but increase in EDV, ejection time, *without* the reflex increase in HR, contractility (both are decreased); net effect is a decrease in MVO_2; used for anginal prophylaxis (note the prophylaxis is for exercised induced but not vasospastic angina); often used together with nitrates to negate their reflex effects.

- **Nifedipine:** calcium-channel blocker that acts more like nitrates because of the greater vasodilation and reflex tachycardia compared to the other Ca^{2+} blockers.

- **Verapamil, diltiazem**: calcium-channel blockers that act more like beta blockers.

CHF Medications

Drugs used in the treatment of congestive heart failure target the body's natural responses to the decreased contractility and cardiac output seen in CHF—specifically the compensatory increases in HR, peripheral vascular resistance, NaCl retention, and cardiomegaly. Goals of therapy include increasing HR and contractility while decreasing preload, afterload, and salt/water retention.

Cardiac glycosides (digoxin, digitalis): increase contractility by inhibiting Na^+/K^+ ATPase and increasing intracellular calcium via reduced Na^+/Ca^{2+} exchange; used to treat CHF with systolic dysfunction, as well as in treatment of atrial fibrillation/flutter; watch for toxic accumulation (worsened with quinidine, furosemide, HCTZ, amiodarone, verapamil, and in renal failure) which can lead to hypokalemia, arrhythmias and even cardiac arrest—treatment for digitalis toxicity includes K^+ supplementation, antiarrythmics (lidocaine) and **Digoxin immune FAB.**

Many of the other drugs in CHF treatment are the same ones used in treating HTN and angina. For **acute CHF**, ACE inhibitors, β1 agonists (dobutamine, dopamine), loop diuretics (furosemide) and **phosphodiesterase inhibitors (amrinone, milrinone)** are also beneficial, with vasodilators (nitroprusside, nitroglycerine) reserved for severe cases. For **chronic CHF**, ACE inhibitors are first line agents (decrease morbidity/mortality), but certain β-blockers (carvedilol, labetalol, metoprolol), diuretics (furosemide, hydrochlorothiazide, spironolactone), and vasodilators (hydralazine, isosorbide dinitrate) are beneficial as well.

Antiarrythmics

Arrythmias are irregular heartbeats that range from clinically benign to life threatening. Common examples of more significant arrhythmias include atrial flutter, atrial fibrillation, ventricular tachycardia, and ventricular fibrillation. Drugs used to treat arrhythmias are grouped into four classes, based on their mechanism of action—they all have effects on the action potential. Normally, there is a series of predictable ionic currents, beginning with the sodium influx (I_{Na}) causing rapid depolarization in phase 0. This is followed by a transient potassium efflux and repolarization to 0mV in phase 1. In the plateau of phase 2 there is both a potassium efflux (I_{Kr}) and calcium influx (I_{Ca}). Phase 3 involves rapid repolarization due to unopposed potassium efflux (I_{Kr}). The resting phase 4 is the start of a new cycle, with three simultaneous currents (I_{Kr}, I_{na}, I_{Ca}) slowly depolarizing the cell during diastole. The transmembrane ionic gradients required for normal function are maintained by the Na^+/K^+ ATPase and Na^+/Ca^+ exchanger. Figure 11 depicts the electrical activity of the cardiac cell.

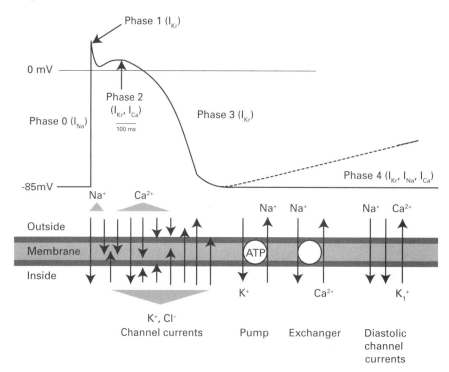

Figure 11 Ionic currents in the cardiac cell

Class I Antiarrythmics: these local anesthetics are Na^+ channel blockers that act on phase 0 and phase 4 to preferentially depress conduction and abnormal pacemakers in depolarized cells (e.g., during tachycardia or in hypoxic state).

- **Class IA (quinidine, procainamide, amiodarone, disopyramide)**: act in atrial, Purkinje, and ventricular tissue to increase QRS duration, QT interval, AP duration, and effective refractory period; used to treat both atrial and ventricular arrhythmias; quinidine toxicity includes cinchonism; procainamide toxicity includes SLE-like syndrome, particularly in "slow acetylators."

- **Class IB (lidocaine, mexiletine, tocainamide, phenytoin)**: act in Purkinje and ventricular tissue to decrease AP duration but also slow recovery of Na$^+$ channels; there are no EKG changes; used to treat ventricular arrhythmias with ischemia (after MI), and atrial arrhythmias secondary to digitalis, toxicity includes convulsions and arrythmias; Lidocaine has extensive first-pass metabolism and can be cardiotoxic if given orally.

- **Class IC (flecainamide, encanaide, moricizine, propafenone)**: act in atrial and ventricular tissue to significantly slow the sodium current and conduction velocity; no effect on AP duration or QT interval; used to treat refractory ventricular tachycardias and intractable SVTs; toxicity includes arrhythmias.

Class II Antiarrythmics (esmolol, propanolol, metoprolol, atenolol): these beta blockers cause a decrease in cAMP levels and a subsequent decrease in both Na$^+$ and Ca^{2+} currents, which blocks abnormal pacemakers; act in the AV node to increase the PR interval; esmolol is used to treat acute arrhythmias; propanolol, metoprolol, and atenolol are used for prophylaxis after MI; toxicities include bradycardia, AV block, CHF, and bronchoconstriction.

Class III Antiarrythmics (sotalol, ibutilide, dofetilide, amiodarone): these drugs are potassium channel blockers that decrease the repolarizing Kr current in phase 3, prolong AP duration, and increase both QT interval and effective refractory period (ERP); used to treat refractory arrhythmias; major toxicity includes torsades de pointes and bradycardia; amiodarone toxicity includes pulmonary fibrosis, thyroid dysfunction, and hepatotoxicity

Class IV Antiarrythmics (verapamil, diltiazem): these drugs are calcium channel blockers that decrease the calcium current during the action potential and phase 4; act in the AV node to decrease conduction velocity and increase PR interval and effective refractory period (ERP); used to convert AV nodal reentry back to sinus and prevention of recurrence; toxicity includes AV block, CHF, peripheral edema.

Hyperlipidemia Medications

Elevated blood cholesterol levels are associated with development of atherosclerosis and an increased risk of heart disease and stroke. For this reason lipid-lowering agents are commonly prescribed. These drugs have various effects on the fat transporters: low-density lipoprotein (LDL), high-density lipoprotein (HDL), and triglycerides (TG). Figure 11 illustrates the metabolism of lipoproteins. LDL carries cholesterol from the liver to the rest of the body and is known as "bad cholesterol." HDL carries cholesterol in the opposite direction, from the body cells to the liver, and is known as "good cholesterol." Here is a list of lipid-lowering agents

- **Statins (atorvastatin, fluvastatin, lovastatin, simvastatin, pravastatin)**: HMG-CoA reductase inhibitors that decrease cholesterol biosynthesis; have the greatest effect on LDL (significant decrease); also increase HDL and decrease TG; toxicities include teratogenicity and hepatotoxicity.

- **Fibrates (gemfibrozil, fenofibrate, clofibrate)**: bind PPAR-α protein that causes increased lipoprotein lipase activity as well as decreased cholesterol biosynthesis; have the greatest effect on TG (significant decrease); also decrease LDL and increase in HDL; toxicities include nausea and cholesterol gallstones.

- **Bile acid resins (cholestyramine, colestipol)**: bind intestinal bile acids and prevent their absorption as well as decreasing amount of hepatic cholesterol used to make lipids (used to replace lost bile acids instead); decrease LDL and cause small increase in HDL and TG; toxicity includes bad taste.

- **Niacin**: decreases hepatic VLDL secretion and cholesterol synthesis; has the greatest effect on HDL (significant increase) and also decreases LDL and TG; causes cutaneous flushing which improves with aspirin pretreatment; also causes hepatotoxicity.

- **Ezetimibe**: newer drug that decreases intestinal absorption of cholesterol; decreases LDL but has no effect on HDL or TG; toxicities include steatorrhea, myositis, transaminitis.

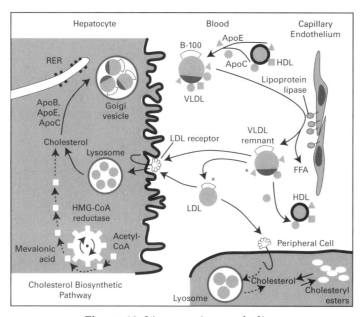

Figure 12 Lipoprotein metabolism

ANTICLOTTING DRUGS

The three major classes of drugs used to treat the various coagulation disorders include thrombolytics, anticoagulants, and antiplatelet drugs. Figure 13 illustrates the coagulation cascade as well as the degradation of clots.

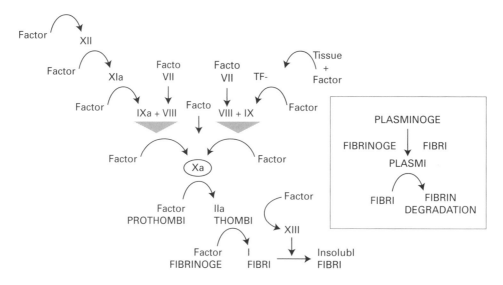

Figure 13 Blood coagulation cascade and clot dissolution

Thrombolytics (tPA, alteplase, urokinase, streptokinase, anistreplase): result in conversion of plasminogen to plasmin, and subsequent breakdown of existing clot; used to treat acute coronary artery thrombosis (MI) and ischemic stroke if given in timely fashion; main toxicity is hemorrhage, especially cerebral hemorrhage (always rule out hemorrhagic stroke before giving the drug!); **aminocaproic acid** can be used as an antidote for thrombolytic toxicity.

Anticoagulants decrease clot formation through several mechanisms. Members of this class of drugs include heparin, low-molecular-weight heparin, factor Xa inhibitors, direct thrombin inhibitors, and warfarin.

- **Heparin**: binds and activates antithrombin III, which in turn deactivates thrombin and factor X; given intravenously; works immediately, short-acting duration; affects the intrinsic pathway and increases aPTT (must be carefully monitored); used to treat DVT, PE, Afib, angina, MI, stroke; safe during pregnancy; toxicity includes hemorrhage and heparin-induced thrombocytopenia (HIT); **protamine sulfate** can be used as an antidote for heparin toxicity.

- **Low-molecular-weight heparin (enoxaparin)**: similar to heparin with greater bioavailability and greater duration of action, allowing for once daily dosing, subcutaneous administration, and no lab draws.

- **Factor Xa inhibitors (fondaparinux)**: derivative of heparin that binds antithrombin III with high affinity and inactivates factor Xa (not thrombin); given subcutaneously; no lab monitoring necessary; decreased risk of major bleeding or heparin-induced thrombocytopenia.

- **Direct thrombin inhibitors (lepirudin, argatroban)**: can be used in patients with heparin-induced thrombocytopenia (HIT); must monitor PTT; lepirudin has renal metabolism and argatroban has hepatic metabolism.

- **Warfarin**: interferes with vitamin K-dependent modification of clotting factors II, VII, IX, X, and proteins C and S; given orally; takes days to work; longer duration of action; affects the extrinsic pathway and affects PT, INR (must be carefully monitored); used to treat DVT, PE, Afib, angina, MI, stroke; *not* safe during pregnancy; toxicity includes hemorrhage, teratogenicity, dermal vascular necrosis and drug interactions (warfarin is metabolized by cytochrome P450); inhibited by vitamin K-rich leafy green vegetables; **vitamin K** and **fresh frozen plasma** (FFP) are slow and fast reversal agents, respectively.

Antiplatelet agents inhibit platelet aggregation through reversible and irreversible effects on ADP, glycoprotein IIb/IIIa receptor, and thromboxane A2. Important drugs in this group include ADP receptor inhibitors, glycoprotein IIb/IIIa receptor inhibitors, aspirin, and other NSAIDS.

- **Clopidogrel, ticlopidine**: irreversible ADP-receptor inhibitors that prevent platelet aggregation; effect lasts for days; commonly used to prevent ischemic stroke/heart attack (especially in patient who cannot tolerate aspirin), as well as thrombosis in patients with coronary stents; toxicities include hemorrhage, neutropenia, TTP.

- **Abciximab, eptifibatide, tirofiban**: reversible glycoprotein IIb/IIIa receptor inhibitors that prevent activation of platelets and binding to fibrinogen; used in acute coronary syndromes and to prevent restenosis after coronary angioplasty; toxicity includes hemorrhage and thrombocytopenia.

- **Aspirin**: salicylate that irreversibly inactivate cyclooxygenase 1,2 and inhibit conversion of arachadonic acid to prostaglandin, prostacyclin, and thromboxane A_2; effect lasts for days; used to treat fever, pain, inflammation, and to prevent heart attack and stroke; toxicities include hemorrhage, tinnitus, Reye's syndrome.

- **Ibuprofen, indomethacin, naproxen**: **nonselective NSAIDS** that reversibly inactivate cyclooxygenase 1,2 and inhibit conversion of arachadonic to prostaglandin, prostacyclin, and thromboxane A_2; used to treat fever, pain, and inflammation; toxicity includes GI mucosal ulceration, bleeding; ibuprofen has nephrotoxicity.

- **Celecoxib, rofecoxib**: selective **COX-2 inhibitors** that have no effect on cyclooxygenase 1 and therefore, a decreased risk of GI mucosal irritation; however, there is an increased risk of thrombosis, MI, stroke.

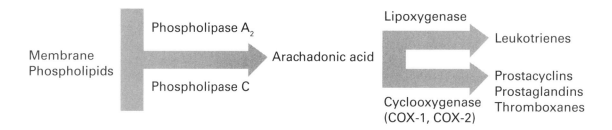

Figure 14 Biosynthesis of the four families of eicosanoids (leukotrienes, prostacyclins, prostaglandins, and thromboxanes)

GOUT MEDICATIONS

Drugs used to treat gout target the central issues of painful joint inflammation and uric acid accumulation.

- **Acetaminophen**: reversible cyclooxygenase inhibitor with analgesic but *no* anti-inflammatory effects; hepatic metabolism; toxicity includes hepatic necrosis; antidote for overdose is **N-acetylcysteine.**

- **Aspirin**: as previously discussed, used for analgesia and anti-inflammation.

- **Nonselective NSAIDS (Ibuprofen, indomethacin, naproxen)**: as previously discussed, used for analgesia and anti-inflammation in acute gout (mainly indomethacin).

- **COX-2 inhibitors (celecoxib, rofecoxib)**: analgesia and anti-inflammation.

- **Corticosteroids (dexamethasone, prednisone, triamcinolone, hydrocortisone)**: powerful anti-inflammatory drugs that inhibit phospholipase and production of arachadonic acid; used for acute gout but not long-term because of the significant side effect profile (Cushing's syndrome, osteoporosis); always rule out septic joint first!

- **Colchicine**: binds tubulin and inhibits microtubule assembly, decreasing leukocyte migration; used for acute gout.

- **Probenecid**: uricosuric drug that inhibits reabsorption of uric acid; used only in chronic gout; toxicity includes precipitation of acute gout (can be avoided by coadministration of colchicines or indomethacin).

- **Allopurinol**: inhibits xanthine oxidase and conversion of xanthine to uric acid; used for chronic gout; toxicity includes peripheral neuritis and precipitation of acute gout.

ASTHMA MEDICATIONS

Drugs used to treat asthma target the central issues of bronchospasm and airway inflammation. The major drugs with bronchodilating effects include beta-agonists, methylxanthines, muscarinic antagonists, and leukotriene modulators. Corticosteroids address the inflammatory issues. Figure 15 illustrates the pathophysiology of asthma.

- **Nonspecific β agonists (isoproteranol)**: stimulate adenylyl cyclase to increase cAMP levels and cause bronchodilation; may cause tremor, tachycardia, and arrhythmias.

- **Specific, short-acting β2 agonists (albuterol, terbutaline)**: bronchodilators used for acute asthma attacks but not prophylaxis; causes tremor, minimal tachycardia.

- **Specific, long-acting β2 agonists (salmeterol, formoterol)**: bronchodilator used for asthma prophylaxis but not acute attacks; causes tremor, minimal tachycardia.

- **Methyxanthines (caffeine, theophylline, theobromine)**: phosphodiesterase inhibitors that decrease cAMP conversion to AMP and cause brochodilation; may cause GI irritation and arrhythmias.

- **Muscarinic antagonists (ipratropium)**: block vagal-mediated bronchoconstriction; used mainly in COPD, but also useful for some asthmatics; no tremor or arrhythmias.

- **Leukotriene modulators (zileuton, zafirlukast, montelukast)**: zileuton inhibits 5-lipoxygenase conversion of arachadonic acid to leukotrienes, while zafirlukast and montelukast are leukotriene receptor antagonists; used only for prophylaxis against bronchospasm secondary to exercise, aspirin, or allergy.

- **Mast cell stabilizers (cromolyn)**: decrease release of leukotrienes from mast cells; used only for asthma prophylaxis.

- **Inhaled corticosteroids (Beclomethasone, budesonide, dexamethasone, flunisolide, fluticasone)**: anti-inflammatory drugs that inhibit phospholipase and production of arachadonic acid; used in moderate to severe asthma and considered the most effective long-term control; toxicity includes oropharyngeal candidiasis and growth retardation.

- **Systemic corticosteroids: Corticosteroids (dexamethasone, prednisone)**: powerful anti-inflammatory drugs that inhibit phospholipase and production of arachadonic acid; used only for severe acute asthma attack or status asthmaticus.

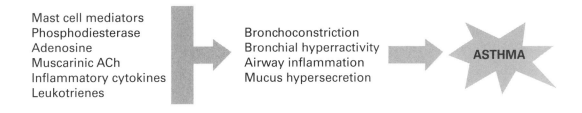

Figure 15 Pathophysiology of asthma

ANTIDIABETIC AGENTS

Drugs used in the treatment of diabetes target the central issues of decreased insulin production or insulin resistance. Exogenous insulin can be administered by subcutaneous injection, but there are also many oral medications available as well, including the insulin secretagogues, biguanides, thiazolidinedinones, and alpha-glucosidase inhibitors.

- **Insulin**: binds to its own tyrosine kinase receptor, which results in increased glucose transport, glycogen synthesis, protein synthesis, and triglyceride storage; also causes increased cellular uptake of potassium; required for type I diabetics but also used to treat diabetes and hyperkalemia; can be given in ultra-rapid onset/short-acting form, rapid onset/short-acting form, intermediate onset/intermediate-acting form, or slow onset/long-acting form; main toxicity is hypoglycemia (treat with **glucose** or **glucagon**).

- **Insulin secretagogues (glyburide, glipizide, tolbutamide, chlorpropamide)**: these sulfonylureas are oral hypoglycemic agents that close pancreatic B cell membrane K^+ channels and stimulate release of insulin; only used in type II diabetes; main toxicity is hypoglycemia; chlorpropamide can cause SIADH.

- **Biguanides (metformin)**: oral hypoglycemic agents that suppress hepatic gluconeogenesis and stimulate peripheral glycolysis; can be used in *both* type I and II diabetes; major toxicity is lactic acidosis.

- **Thiazolidinediones (rosiglitazone, pioglitazone, troglitazone)**: these glitazones increase insulin sensitivity; only used in type II diabetics; toxicity includes edema, anemia, and P450 induction; troglitazone causes hepatotoxicity.

- **α-glucosidase inhibitors (acarbose, miglitol)**: these carbohydrate analogs inhibit the intestinal enzyme α-glucosidase and prevent breakdown and absorption ingested sugars; side effects are GI upset and flatulence from fermentation of undigested sugars in colon.

ANTIBIOTICS

Antibiotics are probably one of the hardest things to study for the Step 1 examination because of the sheer number of organisms and drugs that cover them, not to mention resistance. We recommend that you learn the classic toxicities and coverage of each class of antibiotics, without spending too much time on details. You are not expected to know dosages.

Antimicrobials That Damage DNA

Nitrofurantoin is a bactericidal drug that is renally excreted and gets reduced to destructive metabolites by bacterial flavoproteins. Toxicities include GI upset and hemolysis in G6PD deficiency. Nitrofurantoin is used in treatment of simple UTI and prophylaxis for recurrent UTI.

Metronidazole is a bactericidal drug that reacts with ferredoxin and forms toxic metabolites that interact with DNA. Resistance is low, but can be achieved through decreased reduction efficiency, decreased drug uptake, active drug efflux or inactivation of drug. Toxicity is also rare, but includes peripheral neuropathy, leukopenia/neutropenia, and disulfiram-like reaction when taken together with alcohol. Metronidazole is effective against obligate anaerobes (*Clostriudium, Bacteroides*), facultative anaerobes (*Gardnerella vaginalis*), protozoa (*Giardia, Entamoeba, Trichomonas*), and the microaerophilic *H.pylori*. Common indications for this drug are trichomoniasis, *C.Diff* colitis and intraabdominal infections.

DNA Synthesis Inhibitors

Sulfonamides are bacteriostatic competitive analogues of para-aminobenzoic acid (PABA) that inhibit DNA synthesis by preventing the synthesis of folic acid. Sulfonamides inhibit the first step in folic acid synthesis by blocking the enzyme **dihydropteroate synthetase**, preventing the synthesis of dihydropteroic acid from PABA. Bacterial resistance to sulfonamides develops through 1) reduced drug uptake, 2) increased intracellular PABA, or 3) decreased sensitivity of the dihydropteroate synthetase enzyme. Toxicities include allergic reactions, Stevens-Johnson syndrome, nephrotoxicity, hemolysis in G6PD deficiency, and blood dyscrasia.

- **Silver sulfadiazine**: a topical cream used in burn infections.

- **Sulfamethoxazole**: often used in combination with trimethoprim.

Trimethoprim is another bacteriostatic antifolate drug that also blocks DNA synthesis by inhibiting a separate, downstream reaction in folic acid synthesis. This drug inhibits **dihydrofolate reductase**. Bacterial resistance develops through decreased sensitivity of the dihydrofolate reductase. Toxicity is mainly hematologic.

- **Trimethoprim/sulfamethoxazole (TMP/SMX)** these two drugs are often used together (bactericidal) because of their synergism; used to treat UTIs and MRSA infections, as well as for *Pneumocystis carinii* pneumonia (PCP) treatment/prophylaxis.

Fluoroquinolones are bactericidal drugs that inhibit bacterial **topoisomerase II (DNA gyrase)** and **IV**. The mechanism involves prevention of coiled DNA relaxation, which is normally a prerequisite to transcription and replication. Bacterial resistance is developed through alterations in binding site or decreased permeation of drug. Toxicities include GI distress, tendinopathy, and pediatric cartilage abnormalities. Children and pregnant women should not use these drugs.

- **Ciprofloxacin**: second generation; good gram negative coverage; used to treat UTIs and intestinal infection; also used in combination with metronidazole for intraabdominal infection; there is significant resistance today due to overuse and misuse.

- **Levofloxacin**: third generation; same as above, with gram positive and some anaerobic coverage; also used for community acquired pneumonia in certain populations.

- **Moxifloxacin, gatifloxacin**: fourth generation; same as above with less resistance.

Cell Wall Synthesis Inhibitors

Penicillins are bactericidal beta lactam antibiotics that interfere with cell wall synthesis, resulting in bacterial cell lysis. **Penicillin-binding proteins (PBPs)** are bacterial proteins used in cell wall manufacture that bind penicillin and contribute to the bactericidal effect of penicillin. Bacterial resistance is usually due to presence of β-**lactamases (penicillinases)**, which break the beta-lactam ring found in penicillin. **Clavulinic acid** is a penicillinase-inhibitor that can be given together with penicillins (ampicillin, amoxicillin) to broaden the spectrum and increase drug activity. **Tazobactam** is another β-lactamase inhibitor that is given together with penicillins (piperacillin). Penicillin toxicity includes allergic reactions.

- **Penicillin G,V**: used to treat GPC, GPR, GPR, spirochetes (first line for syphilis).

- **Ampicillin, amoxicillin**: second-generation; wider spectrum; coverage against PHLEM (*Proteus mirabilis, Haemophilus influenzae, Listeria monocytogenes, Escherichia coli, Moraxella catarrhalis*); used to treat otitis media, sinusitis; may cause *C. Diff* colitis.

- **Ticarcillin, carbenicillin**: third generation; have additional *Pseudomonas* coverage.

- **Piperacillin, mezlocillin**: fourth generation; used for *Pseudomonas*, resistant gram(-); **Piperacillin/tazobactam** is a "big gun" that is often used empirically in critically ill patients with peritonitis, hospital-acquired pneumonia, or neutropenia fevers.

- **Methicillin, nafcillin, dicloxacillin:** used for β-lactamase producing gram(+) bugs; today the use of methicillin is reserved for laboratory identification and differentiation of methicillin-resistant *Staph aureus* (MRSA) from methicillin-sensitive Staph aureus (MSSA).

(Good Protection, **PECK**)

Cephalosporins are similar to penicillins in that they are bactericidal beta-lactam drugs that bind PBPs and inhibit cell wall synthesis. Bacterial resistance develops through β-lactamases, alterations in PBP, and decreased membrane permeability (there has been a recent spread in **extended spectrum beta-lactamase (ESBL)** producing organisms). Toxicity includes allergic reactions.

- **Cefazolin, cephalexin**: first generation; work against GPCs, *Proteus, E.Coli, Klebsiella*.

- **Cefoxitin, cefaclor**: second generation; less gram(+) but better gram(-) coverage.

- **Ceftriaxone, ceftazadime**: third generation; extended gram negative coverage; cross BBB and treats meningitis; ceftriaxone is first-line for gonorrhea.

- **Cefipime**: fourth generation; good gram positive and gram negative coverage.

Carbapenems have beta-lactams which are relatively resistant to breakdown by bacterial β-lactamases. These drugs have broad spectrum coverage (GPC, GNR, anaerobes) and are typically reserved for inpatient resistant ESBL organisms (*Klebsiella, Enterobacter, EColi*).

- **Imipenem**: usually given together with **cilastatin** to prevent renal metabolism.

- **Meropenem, Ertapenem**: not susceptible to renal degradation and don't need cilastin.

Aztreonam is another example of a bactericidal beta-lactam that is resistant to breakdown by some bacterial β-lactamases. This drug binds to PBP3 and inhibits cell wall synthesis. Aztreonam provides good coverage against GNRs, and is commonly used in penicillin-allergic patients as well as renal patients who can't tolerate aminoglycosides. Toxicity is minimal.

Bacitracin is not a beta-lactam, but does inhibit cell wall synthesis. The mechanism involves inhibition of dephosphorylation of lipid pyrophosphate. Bacitracin is mainly effective against GPCs and is typically applied topically because of nephrotoxicity.

Vancomycin is another example of a bactericidal drug outside the beta-lactam group that inhibits cell wall synthesis in gram-positive organisms. The mechanism involves binding D-Ala D-Ala and blocking elongation and crosslinking of polymers that ultimately form the cell wall. Bacterial resistance is recent issue (e.g. VRE) that is due to replacement of D-ala with D-lactate, preventing binding of the antibiotic. Toxicities include red-man syndrome, ototoxicity, nephrotoxicity (RON). Vancomycin is used to treat methicillin-resistant *Staphylococcus aureus* and *epidermidis* (**MRSA, MRSE**), as well as severe *Clostridium difficile* (**C.Diff**) infections (given PO for the latter).

Protein Synthesis Inhibitors

This is a heterogenous group of drugs that all act through inhibition of either the **30s** ribosomal subunit (aminoglycosides, tetracyclines), or the **50S** ribosomal subunit (macrolides, lincosamides, linezolid, chloramphenicol).

Aminoglycosides are bactericidal drugs that bind the bacterial **30S** ribosomal subunit to inhibit protein synthesis. The mechanism involves prevention of formation of the initiation complex, misreading of mRNA, and inhibition of translocation. Aminoglycosides are **synergistic** with **beta-lactam antibiotics**, which allow for increased uptake of the antibiotic. Bacterial resistance develops due to development of enzymatic deactivation of the antibiotic by **group transferases**. Toxicities include nephrotoxicity and ototoxicity.

- **Gentamycin, tobramycin, amykacin, neomycin**: mainly used against aerobic GNRs (e.g., *Pseudomonas, E.Coli, Klebsiella—PEcK*).

- **Streptomycin**: used against TB and plague.

- **Neomycin**: used in bowel preps for surgery.

Tetracyclines are older, broad-spectrum, bacteriostatic drugs that bind the **30S** ribosomal subunit to inhibit protein synthesis. The mechanism involves blocking attachment of aminoacyl tRNA to ribosomes. Resistance can develop through decreased uptake by energy-dependent transporters or through the development of a protein "pump" that actively excretes the drug. Toxicities include tooth enamel dysplasia, bone growth abnormalities, photosensitivity, hepatotoxicity, and Fanconi's syndrome.

- **Tetracycline**: used against *Mycoplasma pneumonia, Chlamydia* (drug of choice), *Rickettsia* (Rocky Mountain spotted fever), *Borrelia burgdorferi* (Lyme disease); acne.

- **Doxycycline**: same indications as above, plus malaria prophylaxis; cannot be taken with dairy, antacids, iron products, calcium supplements, or laxatives with magnesium.

Macrolides are bacteriostatic drugs that bind the **50S** ribosomal subunit (the 23s portion) and inhibit protein synthesis. The mechanism involves inhibition of peptidyl transferase and early dissociation of tRNA from the ribosome during elongation. Bacterial resistance is developed through alteration of the ribosomal binding site or formation of esterases that degrade macrolides. Toxicities include GI upset and acute cholestatic hepatitis.

- **Erythromycin**: used to treat pneumonia because of coverage against GPCs (S. pneumonia), some GNRs (H. influenza, M. catarrhalis), and atypicals (Mycoplasma pneumonia, Legionella, Chlamydia); acts as motilin analogue to promote GI motility.

- **Azithromycin**: even better coverage against above pathogens (given as Z-pack).

- **Clarithromycin**: used against H.Pylori and Mycobacterium avium complex (MAC).

Lincosamides (e.g., **clindamycin**) are bacteriostatic drugs that bind the **50S** ribosomal subunit (the 23s portion) and inhibit protein synthesis. The mechanism involves early dissociation of tRNA from ribosomes and inhibition of chain elongation. Bacterial resistance is developed through alteration of the ribosomal binding site or formation of enzymes that inactivate lincosamides. Toxicity includes **pseudomembrane colitis**, an overgrowth of *Clostridium difficile* causing an invasive colitis after prolonged antibiotic use (classic drug is clindamycin).

- **Lincomycin**: older drug no longer used because of toxicity.

- **Clindamycin**: used against GPCs (including MRSA) and anaerobes (*Bacteroides, Clostridium*); given to PCN-allergic patients for endocarditis prophylaxis.

Chloramphenicol is a bacteriostatic drug that binds the bacterial **50S** ribosomal subunit (the 23s portion) to inhibit protein synthesis. The mechanism involves inhibition of ribosomal peptidyl transferase, which prevents peptide bond formation. Bacterial resistance is developed through alteration of the ribosomal binding site, inactivation of the drug by acetyltransferases, or decreased membrane permeability to prevent crossing of the drug. Toxicity is severe, and includes aplastic anemia, bone marrow suppression, and grey baby syndrome. Because of significant risk, the drug is rarely used outside of staphylococcal brain abscesses and meningitis (crosses BBB and has good coverage against *H. influenzae, N. meningiditis,* and *S. pneumoniae*)

Linezolid is a newer bacteriostatic drug that binds the bacterial **50S** ribosomal subunit (the 23s portion) to inhibit protein synthesis. The mechanism involves prevention of initiation complex formation. Bacterial resistance is extremely low at this point in time. Toxicities include transaminitis, pancreatitis, neuropathies, bone marrow suppression, and lactic acidosis. Linezolid can be used against any gram positive organisms, including MRSA and VRE, but cost is high.

Antimycobacterial Drugs

Important members of the mycobacteria family include *Mycobacterium tuberculosis, Mycobacterium leprae,* and *Mycobacterium avium-cellulare* (MAC). These organisms are responsible for causing tuberculosis, leprosy, and opportunistic infections, respectively. All three are notoriously difficult to treat, and require prolonged multidrug therapy.

Tuberculosis treatment has several obstacles to overcome. Mycobacteria are slow growing, and granulomatous lesions are often difficult to penetrate with drugs. In addition, emerging resistance is a major issue for anti-TB drugs, and to prevent this they must be used in combination. The gold standard treatment is a six-month course of **R**ifampin, **I**soniazid, **P**yrazinamide, **E**thambutol (**RIPE**), which raises issues of compliance. Below is a list of anti-TB drugs (re**SPIRE**), with a brief description.

- **Streptomycin** is an aminoglycoside that can be used against TB.

- **Pyrazinamide** is a bacteriostatic/bactericidal drug used against TB. The drug is activated by mycobacterial pyrazinamidase. Like other anti-TB drugs, resistance develops quickly if pyrazinamide is used alone. Toxicity includes arthralgias and hyperuricemia.

- **Isoniazid (INH)** is a bacteriostatic/bactericidal drug that inhibits synthesis of mycolic acids that are required to make cell walls. Like other anti-TB drugs, resistance develops quickly if INH is used alone. Toxicities include hepatotoxicity, P450 inhibition, neurotoxicity (improved with Vitamin B6), SLE-like syndrome, and hemolysis in G6PD deficiency. Isoniazid is used to treat tuberculosis, as well as prophylaxis (used alone for 9 months).

- **Rifampin** is a bactericidal drug that inhibits RNA polymerase. Like other anti-TB drugs, resistance develops quickly if the drug is used alone. Toxicities include hepatotoxicity, light chain proteinuria, and cytochrome P450 induction. Rifampin is used against *Mycobacterium* to treat tuberculosis and leprosy. It is also used for meningococcal prophylaxis.

- **Ethambutol** is a bacteriostatic drug that inhibits arabinosyl transferase and blocks cell wall synthesis. Resistance occurs quickly if the drug is used alone. Toxicity includes visual abnormalities. Ethambutol is only used for TB.

Leprosy can be treated with a prolonged course of dapsone and rifampin. **Dapsone** is a bacteriostatic drug that competes with PABA for dihydropteroate synthetase and blocks synthesis of folic acid. Toxicity includes hemolysis in G6PD deficiency. Rifampin is typically given together with dapsone to prevent development of resistance. Similar to the other myobacterial infections, **MAC infection** also requires prolonged (12 months) multidrug treatment, usually including some combination of macrolides, rifampin, and ethambutol.

ANTIVIRALS

By definition viruses require living cells in order to replicate. Most of the antiviral drugs interfere with this replication cycle by attacking its different steps. In order, the steps of viral infection include attachment, penetration, uncoating, early protein synthesis, DNA synthesis, late protein synthesis, protein packaging/assembly, and viral shedding.

- **Amantadine**: prevents penetration/uncoating by binding viral matrix protein (M2) and raising endosomal pH; used against rubella and influenza A (prophylaxis/treatment); helps Parkinson's by causing dopamine release; toxicities include ataxia, slurred speech.

- **Zanamivir, Oseltamivir**: prevent viral shedding by inhibiting neuraminidase; used against influenza A and B; there is no significant toxicity.

- **Interferons**: cytokines that interfere with RNA and DNA synthesis; used to treat chronic hepatitis B/C infection and Kaposi's sarcoma; main toxicity is neutropenia.

- **Ribavirin**: inhibits IMP dehydrogenase (prevents guanine nucleotide synthesis), RNA capping, and RNA polymerase; used against RSV, HCV; toxicity includes teratogenicity.

Herpesviridae are a family of large DNA viruses that include the common members HSV-1, HSV-2, VZV, CMV, HHV6, HHV7, EBV, and Kaposi's sarcoma-associated viruses. All of the antiherpes drugs are **nucleoside analogs** that inhibit DNA synthesis.

- **Acyclovir**: a guanosine analog that gets phosphorylated by thymidine kinase, then inhibits viral DNA polymerase; used against HSV, VZV for treatment, as well as prophylaxis in immunocompromised patients; toxicities include encephalopathy and nephrotoxicity.

- **Ganciclovir**: another guanosine analog that gets phosphorylated by thymidine kinase, then inhibits viral DNA polymerase; used for CMV treatment/prophylaxis; main toxicity is bone marrow suppression.

- **Foscarnet**: pyrophosphate analog (does *not* require phosphorylation by thymidine kinase) that inhibits viral DNA polymerase; used for CMV treatment/prophylaxis; main toxicity is nephrotoxicity.

- **Vidarabine**: an adenine analog that gets phosphorylated by kinases, then inhibits viral DNA polymerase; used against HSV,VZV, CMV; toxicities include GI upset, leukopenia, thrombocytopenia.

Human immunodeficiency virus (HIV) is a retrovirus that infects cells of the immune system and use the enzyme reverse transcriptase to convert its RNA genome into DNA. The final stage of HIV disease is known as AIDS. Anti-HIV drugs consist of three major categories, which include both nucleoside and non-nucleoside reverse transcriptase inhibitors (NRTIs/NNRTIs, or "nukes"/"non-nukes"), as well as protease inhibitors. Current guidelines recommend that all patients with either CD4<500, an AIDS-defining illness, or pregnancy should be on an antiretroviral regimen. In an effort to prevent resistance, these drugs are currently administered in combination, which is known as **highly active antiretroviral therapy (HAART)**. Typically two NRTIs are used together with either one non-NRTI or a protease inhibitor.

Nucleoside reverse transcriptase inhibitors (NRTIs) : anti-HIV drugs that require host cell kinase activation before competitively inhibiting reverse transcriptase (and DNA synthesis).

- **Zidovudine (AZT)**: thymidine analog/NRTI; toxicity includes bone marrow suppression that is additive with other myelosuppressants (e.g., TMP-SMX, which is often used for PCP prophylaxis).

- **Stavudine (d4T)**: thymidine analog/NRTI; toxicity includes peripheral neuropathy.

- **Zalcitabine (ddC)**: cytosine analog/NRTI; toxicity is pancreatitis, peripheral neuropathy.

- **Lamivudine (3TC)**: cytosine analog/NRTI; toxicity includes pancreatitis.

- **Didanosine (ddI)**: adenosine analog/NRTI; toxicity is pancreatitis, peripheral neuropathy.

- **Abacavir**: a guanosine analog and NRTI; toxicity includes fatal hypersensitivity.

Non-nucleoside reverse transcriptase inhibitors (NNRTIs) : anti-HIV drugs that also prevent DNA synthesis by noncompetitively inhibiting reverse transcriptase, but in contrast to NRTIs, have different binding sites and do not require phosphorylation activation.

- **Nevirapine**: NNRTI; prevents vertical transmission; toxicity is severe hypersensitivity.

- **Delavirdine**: NNRTI; toxicity includes drug interactions; contraindicated in pregnancy.

- **Efavirenz**: NNRTI; toxicities include insomnia, depression; contraindicated in pregnancy.

Protease inhibitors (PIs): anti-HIV drugs that block cleavage of Gag-Pol polyproteins into functional enzymes and structural proteins, thereby preventing new viral offspring from assembling and maturing.

- **Indinavir**: inhibits HIV-1 protease; toxicities include nephrolithiasis/nephrotoxicity.

- **Ritonavir**: inhibits HIV-1 protease; toxicity includes GI upset.

- **Saquinavir**: inhibits HIV-1 protease; toxicity includes neutropenia.

- **Nelfinavir**: inhibits HIV-1 protease; toxicity includes diarrhea.

- **Amprenavir:** inhibits HIV-1 protease; toxicity includes Stevens-Johnson syndrome.

ANTIFUNGAL AGENTS

Superficial fungal infections (skin, hair, nails) by dermatophytes can be treated with **griseofulvin**, a drug that accumulates in keratin and interferes with fungal microtubule formation. Major toxicities include teratogenicity and carcinogenesis. **Terbinafine** is another drug that accumulates in keratin and is effective in nail infections.

Systemic fungal infections are treated by drugs that target ergosterol, which is found in the fungal cell membrane.

- **Nystatin**: fungicidal drug that binds ergosterol, causing formation of pores in the cell membrane that allow electrolytes to leak; used topically against *Candida*.

- **Amphoteracin B**: wide spectrum, fungicidal drug with similar mechanism as nystatin; IV form used to treat serious systemic fungal infections (*Blastomyces, Candida, Coccidioides, Cryptococcus, Histoplasma, Mucor, Aspergillus*); intrathecal form is used to treat fungal meningitis; toxicities include fever, hypotension and renal tubular acidosis, arrhythmias.

Azoles are relatively newer drugs that inhibit a fungal cytochrome P450 enzyme required for ergosterol synthesis. They offer similar protection against systemic fungal infections compared to amphoteracin B, but with a better side effect profile. Azoles also treat superficial fungal infections (dermatophytes). Toxicity of azoles includes hepatotoxicity.

- **Fluconazole**: *Candida, Cryptococcus* (including cryptococcal meningitis)

- **Ketoconazole**: *Coccidiodes, Histoplasma*; inhibits cytochrome P450 and can cause life-threatening cardiotoxicity if taken together with cisapride.

- **Itraconazole**: *Blastomyces, Histoplasma, Sporothrix*

- **Voriconazole**: *Aspergillus*

ANTIPROTOZOAL AGENTS

Here is a list common antiparasitic agents that target vital enzymes.

- **Quinine, Chloroquine, Mefloquine**: antimalarial treatment/prophylaxis.

- **Primaquine**: antimalarial used against liver stages of *Plasmodium vivax* and *P. ovale*.

- **Metronidazole**: amoebicide for *Giardia, Gardnerella, Entamoeba, Trichomonas*.

- **Pentamidine:** used for prophylaxis for *Pneumocystis* pneumonia.

- **TMP-SMX**: used in treatment/prophylaxis for *Pneumocystis carinii* pneumonia.

- **Pyrimethamine/sulfadiazine**: used against *Toxoplasma gondii*.

- **Nifurtimox**: used against *Trypanosoma cruzi* (American trypanosomiasis).

- **Suramin**: used against *Trypanosoma brucei* (African trypanosomiasis).

- **Sodium stibogluconate**: used against *Leishmania*.

ANTHELMINTIC AGENTS

Here is a list of drugs commonly used to treat infection by nematodes (roundworms).

- **Albendazole**: broad spectrum agent used against *Ascaris* (roundworm), *Necator* (hookworm), *Ancylostoma* (hookworm), *Trichuris* (whipworm), *Strongyloides* (threadworm), *Enterobius* (pinworm), and larva migrans.

- **Diethylcarbamazine**: used against *Wuchereria bancrofti, Brugia malayi* (filariasis).

- **Ivermectin**: used against *Strongyloides* and *Onchocerca* (river blindness).

- **Mebendazole**: used against *Ascaris, Necator, Ancylostoma, Trichuris, Enterobius.*

- **Thibendazole**: used against larva migrans.

- **Pyrantel pamoate**: used against *Ascaris, Necator, Ancylostoma, Enterobius.*

Here is a list of drugs commonly used to treat infection by trematodes (flukes).

- **Praziquantel**: used against Schistosoma, Paragonimus.

- **Bithionol**: used against Fasciola.

Here is a list of drugs commonly used to treat infection by cestodes (tapeworms).

- **Praziquantel**: used against *Diphyllobothrium, Taenia*—(not cysticercosis).

- **Niclosamide**: used against *Diphyllobothrium, Taenia*—(not cysticercosis).

- **Albendazole**: drug of choice for *Taenia solium* cysticercosis and *Echinococcus granulosus* hydatid disease.

IMMUNOSUPPRESSANTS

There are several situations in which the immune response can have adverse effects, and suppression of that undesirable response would be beneficial, such as autoimmune disease and organ transplant rejection. Here are some important immunosuppressive agents.

- **Antithymocyte globulin (ATG)**: binds to T-cells and preventing antigen recognition by causing complement destruction of the T-cells; used for maintenance in solid organ transplantation and to prevent GVHD in bone marrow transplantation; toxicities include anaphylaxis and serum sickness.

- **Cyclosporine**: binds to cyclophilin, inhibits calcineurin, and prevents IL-2 expression, thereby inhibiting T-cell proliferation/differentiation as well as cytokine production; used for solid organ transplantation, GVHD, and autoimmune disease; toxicity includes nephrotoxicity and neurotoxicity.

- **Corticosteroids (prednisone)**: anti-inflammatory effects; used in organ transplantation and autoimmune diseases; toxicities include Cushing's syndrome and osteoporosis.

- **Azathioprine**: cytotoxic drug that destroys proliferating lymphoid cells (T > B); used in autoimmune disease and solid organ transplant (kidney); toxicity includes bone marrow suppression.

- **Cyclophosphamide**: cytotoxic drug that destroys proliferating lymphoid cells (B > T); used in autoimmune disease and bone marrow transplantation; toxicities include pancytopenia and hemorrhagic cystitis.

- **Tacrolimus (FK506)**: binds to FKBP, inhibits calcineurin, and prevents IL-2 expression, thereby inhibiting T-cell proliferation/differentiation as well as cytokine production; used for solid organ transplantation (liver, kidney); may cause nephro- and neurotoxicity.

- **Sirolimus**: binds to FKBP but is *not* a calcineurin inhibitor; inhibits T-cell response to cytokines as well as B-cell proliferation; used for solid organ transplantation (kidney, heart); may cause nephro- and neurotoxicity.

- **Mycophenolate mofetil**: inhibits inosine monophosphate dehydrogenase and blocks purine synthesis, which suppresses activation of T- and B-cells; used for solid organ transplantation (kidney, liver, heart); toxicity includes GI irritation.

ANTINEOPLASTIC DRUGS

The underlying rationale for the use of chemotherapy is that cancers are made up of rapidly dividing cells. Therefore, drugs that disrupt various aspects of **cell division** have been the primary modality of most chemotherapy drugs. The most chemo-responsive tumors are usually those with a high **growth fraction** (most childhood tumors, acute lymphoblastic leukemia, Hodgkin's disease, and testicular/ovarian germ cell cancers).

Specific chemotherapeutic agents have particular side effects that must be monitored, but most are the result of disruption of normally dividing cells. Commonly affected areas include hair follicles (alopecia), GI cells (stomatitis, nausea, vomiting, and diarrhea), marrow/lymphoid cells (pancytopenia), and germinal cells of the testis/ovary (infertility). Other general side effects to be aware of during chemotherapy include the following:

- **Tumor lysis syndrome**: when bulky tumors are effectively killed by chemotherapy, many cells die and lyse. These dead cells flood the body with a load of intracellular debris, which can be fatal if not treated.

- **Hyperuricemia**: Urate is released and can cause renal failure by plugging up the kidneys. Treatment is with allopurinol and aggressive hydration with IV fluids.

- **Hyperkalemia**: This can lead to arrhythmias. Prophylaxis is achieved with IV fluids. Treatment includes calcium gluconate (cardioprotection), kayexalate (chelates K^+ in the gut), bicarbonate (drives K^+ intracellularly), a β-agonist (drives K^+ intracellularly), glucose/insulin (drives K^+ intracellularly), or furosemide (increases K^+ excretion).

Clinically, most cancers are treated with combination therapy. There are many different types of drugs including antimetabolites, plant alkaloids, alkylating agents, antibiotics, hormones, and monoclonal antibodies. These can be classified as either cell cycle-specific or cell cycle-nonspecific. **Cell cycle-specific drugs** only target actively cycling tumor cells that are in either the G_1, S, G_2, or M phase. They have no effect on resting cells in the G_0 phase. In contrast, the **cell cycle-nonspecific drugs** target all tumor cells, whether resting or cycling.

Antimetabolites are cell cycle-dependent drugs and analogues of normal metabolites that act during the **S phase** of the cell cycle to block DNA synthesis.

- **Methotrexate**: folate analog that inhibits dihydrofolate reductase and dTMP production; commonly used for leukemia, lymphoma, osteosarcoma, ectopic pregnancy, abortion; toxicity includes bone marrow suppression (reduced with **leucovorin** coadministration).

- **Mercaptopurine (6-MP)**: purine analog activated by HGPRTases to inhibit purine synthesis; commonly used for leukemia, non-Hodgkin's lymphoma; toxicities include bone marrow suppression and hepatotoxicity.

- **Fluorouracil (5-FU)**: pyrimadine analog that is transformed to 5F-dUMP, which inhibits thymidilate synthase and dTMP production; commonly used for colon and pancreatic cancer; toxicities include bone marrow suppression and mucositis.

- **Cytarabine (Ara-C)**: pyrimadine analog that inhibits DNA polymerase; commonly used to treat acute leukemias, non-Hodgkin's lymphoma; toxicities include bone marrow suppression, neurotoxicity.

Alkylating agents are cell cycle-nonspecific drugs (most active during G_0 resting phase) that damage DNA by attaching alkyl groups to guanine bases at the N7 position.

- **Cyclophosphamide**: activated by P-450 enzyme; commonly used to treat neuroblastoma, leukemia, non-Hodgkin's lymphoma, breast/ovarian cancer; toxicities include bone marrow suppression and hemorrhagic cystitis.

- **Mechlorethamine**: spontaneously self-activated after administration; commonly used to treat leukemia and both Hodgkin's and non-Hodgkin's lymphoma; toxicities are severe and include anaphylaxis, chemical burns, carcinogenicity, teratogenicity.

- **Cisplatin, Carboplatin**: platinum containing drugs; commonly used to treat solid tumors, including testicular cancer, sarcoma, small cell lung cancer, ovarian cancer; toxicities include nephro- and neurotoxicity.

- **Procarbazine**: activated by the liver to form hydrogen peroxide; commonly used to treat Hodgkin's lymphoma, brain tumors; toxicity includes disulfiram-like reaction.

Plant alkaloids are cell cycle-specific drugs that interfere with either microtubule or topoisomerase function.

- **Vinblastine, vincristine**: bind tubulin to prevent microtubule polymerization and mitotic arrest during metaphase; commonly used to treat leukemia, lymphoma, Wilm's tumor, choriocarcinoma; toxicity for vinblastine includes bone marrow suppression; toxicity for vincristine includes neurotoxicity.

- **Paclitaxel, docetaxel**: spindle poisons that prevent microtubule disassembly during metaphase/anaphase transition; commonly used to treat breast and ovarian cancers; toxicity for paclitaxel includes neutropenia, peripheral neuropathy; toxicities for docetaxel include neurotoxicity, myelosuppression.

- **Etoposide, Teniposide**: inhibit topoisomerase II during S and G_2 phases to cause DNA damage; commonly used against Kaposi's sarcoma, Ewing's sarcoma, lung cancer, testicular cancer; toxicity is typical (bone marrow suppression, alopecia, GI effects).

Antibiotics are cell cycle-nonspecific drugs (except bleomycin) that can: intercalate between DNA base pairs, generate DNA damaging free radicals, or inhibit key enzymes involved in DNA synthesis.

- **Doxorubicin, daunorubicin**: widely used drug that intercalates between DNA base pairs, generates free radicals, and inhibits topoisiomerase II; commonly used to treat sarcomas, breast/ovarian/endometrial cancer, lung cancer, thyroid cancer; toxicities include cardiotoxicity (reduced by **dexrazoxane**).

- **Bleomycin**: intercalates between DNA base pairs and creates free radicals; commonly used to treat testicular cancer, Hodgkin's lymphoma; toxicity includes pulmonary fibrosis.

- **Dactinomycin**: binds DNA and inhibits RNA synthesis; commonly used to treat melanoma and Wilm's tumor; toxicity is typical (myelosuppression, alopecia, GI upset).

Antineoplastic hormones/antihormones act by stimulating or blocking, respectively, hormone receptors found on tumor cells, relying on the principle that cell tumor growth is regulated by these hormone receptors.

- **Prednisone**: used to treat leukemias and lymphomas, including Hodgkin's disease; toxicities include Cushing's syndrome and osteoporosis.

- **Tamoxifen**: estrogen antagonist commonly used to treat hormone receptor-positive breast cancer; toxicity includes hot flashes, cataracts, DVT/PE, stroke, and increased risk of endometrial carcinoma (acts as a partial agonist in the endometrium).

- **Anastrozole:** aromatase inhibitor used to treat hormone receptor-positive breast cancer in post-menopausal women; toxicity includes osteoporosis, hot flashes, DVT/PE.

- **Flutamide**: androgen receptor antagonist commonly used to treat prostate cancer; toxicities include gynecomastia and hepatotoxicity.

- **Leuprolide**: gonadotropin-releasing hormone agonist used to treat prostate cancer.

Monoclonal antibodies are newer drugs that bind to cancer-cell specific antigens.

- **Bevacizumab**: VEGF-A inhibitor that slows angiogenesis.

- **Cetuximab, Panitumumab**: EGFR inhibitors used only if KRAS is normal.

- **Rituximab**: binds CD20 on B cells, causing their destruction; used in lymphoma.

- **Trastuzamab**: HER2 receptor antagonist used to treat HER2+ breast cancer.

TOXICOLOGY

Toxicology is an important part of pharmacology. There are almost 1 million ER visits for poisoning each year in the U.S., with some 30,000 deaths annually. The majority of these are unintentional, but a significant number are involved in suicide attempts as well. Almost any therapeutic drug can be toxic in high doses, but in addition physicians must be familiar with the toxic potential of street drugs, gaseous toxins, heavy metals, insecticides, solvents, and industrial compounds.

This can be a bit overwhelming, but in terms of management of a poisoned patient, we start with the basic "**ABCs**" (airway, breathing, circulation). Basic vitals should be taken along with appropriate supportive measures. History and physical may be limited but are critical nevertheless. Labs should always be drawn. There are also a couple knee-jerk actions that have little downside. **Oxygen, glucose, thiamine,** and **naloxone** can quickly treat patients whose symptoms are due to hypoxia, hypoglycemia, alcoholism/malnutrition, or opioid overdose, respectively.

Once laboratory values are obtained, calculating the **anion gap** may provide additional information, as a number of toxic substances cause anion gap acidosis. The anion gap is calculated by subtracting the chloride and bicarbonate laboratory values from the sodium value. A normal gap is 8-12 mEq/L. If the value is *greater than 12*, the patient has an increased anion gap. This gap may be caused by certain disease states (e.g., lactic acidosis or diabetic acidosis) or by the ingestion of poisonous substances, as a result of unmeasured anions (e.g., phosphate, sulfate) in the plasma that accompany metabolic acidosis. A mnemonic for the causes of anion gap acidosis is **MUDPILES**:

- Methanol

- Uremia (it's really the inorganic anions, not the urea nitrogen)

- Diabetic ketoacidosis

- Paraldehyde

- Intoxication (ethyl alcohol, isopropyl alcohol)

- Lactic acid

- Ethylene glycol

- Salicylates

Common Toxicities

It is worthwhile to learn the syndromes associated with certain toxicities.

- **Antimuscarinic toxicity**: fever, ↑HR, ↑BP, CNS excitation, seizure, pupillary dilation, urinary retention, ileus.

  - Treatment involves physostigmine, thermal control.

- **Cholinomimetic toxicity**: perspiration, ↑secretion, ↑GI motility, pupillary constriction, seizure, coma, paralysis.

  - Treatment includes atropine/pralidoxime, respiratory support.

- **Opioid toxicity**: ↓HR, ↓BP, lethargy/coma, respiratory depression, pupillary constriction.

  - Treatment includes naloxone/naltrexone, respiratory support.

- **Salicylate toxicity:** fever, ↓K$^+$, anion gap metabolic acidosis, lethargy/coma, seizure.

  - Treatment includes bicarbonate, dialysis.

- **Sedative-hypnotic toxicity**: lethargy/coma, nystagmus, ↓muscle tone, hypothermia.

  - Treatment includes respiratory support (flumenazil for benzos).

- **Stimulant toxicity**: fever, ↑HR, ↑BP, arrhythmia, agitation, seizure, pupillary dilation.

  - Treatment includes control of fever, seizure, and HTN.

- **Tricyclic antidepressants toxicity**: fever, ↑HR, ↑BP, cardiotoxicity, coma, convulsions.

  - Treatment includes IVF, bicarbonate, ventilation, and control of fever and seizure.

Antidotes

Removal and elimination of poison from the body are mainstays of treatment once poisoning is confirmed, but in some cases there are specific antidotes that can be given. We suggest that you memorize these antidotes, as they are commonly tested items.

- **Aminocaproic acid**: used for tPA and streptokinase poisoning.

- **Atropine**: used for cholinesterase inhibitor/organophosphate poisoning.

- **Deferoxamine**: chelator used for iron poisoning.

- **Digoxin immune FAB**: used for digitalis toxicity.

- **Dimercaprol (BAL)**: chelator used for arsenic/mercury/lead/gold poisoning.

- **EDTA**: chelator used in lead poisoning.

- **Ethanol**: used for methanol or ethylene glycol poisoning.

- **Glucagon**: used for β-blocker poisoning.

- **Flumenazil**: used to reverse benzodiazepines.

- **Hydroxocobalamin**: used for cyanide poisoning.

- **Fresh frozen plasma (FFP)**: used to reverse warfarin.

- **Methylene blue:** used for methemoglobin poisoning.

- **N-acetylcysteine**: used in acetaminophen overdose.

- **Naloxone/naltrexone:** used to reverse opioids/opiates.

- **Nitroprusside:** used to treat ergot alkaloid toxicity.

- **Nitrite (amyl nitrite)**: used for cyanide poisoning.

- **Oxygen, 100%:** used for carbon monoxide poisoning.

- **Penicillamine:** chelator used as first line agent for copper poisoning.

- **Physostigmine:** used for overdoses of anticholinergics.

- **Pralidoxime:** used for organophasphate cholinesterase inhibitor poisoning.

- **Protamine**: used to reverse heparin.

- **Succimer**: used in lead toxicity.

- **Vitamin K**: used to reverse warfarin.

DRUG REACTIONS AND OFFENDING AGENTS

- **Agranulocytosis**: carbemazepine, clozapine, colchicine, chloramphenicol, methimazole, mebendazole, mirtazapine, propythiouracil

- **Anticholinergic effects**: antipsychotics, TCAs, muscle relaxants, antihistamines

- **Aplastic anemia**: antimalarials, benzene, chloramphenicol, dapsone, antiepileptics (carbemazepine, phenytoin, valproate), methimazole, propylthiouracil (**ABCD AMP**)

- **Cinchonism**: quinine, quinidine

- **Coronary artery spasm**: cocaine, amphetamine, sumatriptan (Coronary Artery Spasm)

- **Cough**: ACE inhibitors

- **Cutaneous flushing**: vancocmycin, adenosine, niacin, Ca^{2+} channel blockers (**VANC**)

- **Cardiomyopathy (dilated):** doxorubicin, danorubicin (Dilated double **D**s)

- **Diabetes insipidus:** lithium, demeclocycline, methoxyflurane

- **Disulfram-like reaction with ETOH:** metronidazole, cephalosporins, griseofulvin, tolbutamide

- **Fanconi's syndrome:** tenofovir, expired tetracycline

- **Gingival hyperplasia:** phenytoin, verapamil

- **Gout:** cyclosporine, furosemide, thiazides, niacin, pyrazinamide

- **Grey baby syndrome:** chloramphenicol

- **Gynecomastia:** spironolactone, digitalis, cimetidine, alcohol (chronic), ketoconazole (SACKED: Spironolactone, Alcohol (chronic), Cimetidine, Ketoconazole, Estrogen, Digitalis)

- **Hemolysis in G6PD-deficiency**: INH, sulfa drugs, primaquine, aspirin, ibuprofen, nitrofurantoin (Hemolysis IS PAIN)

- **Hemorrhagic cystitis**: cyclophosphamide, ifosfamide

- **Hepatitis**: isoniazid, rifampin

- **Hepatic necrosis**: valproate, acetaminophen, halothane (**V**ery **A**ngry **H**epatocytes)

- **Hot flashes**: tamoxifen

- **Hypothyroidism**: amiodarone, lithium

- **Hyperglycemia**: steroids, diuretics, atypical antipsychotics, niacin, protease inhibitors

- **Interstitial nephritis**: diuretics, NSAIDS, penicillins (methicillin)

- **Lactic acidosis**: metformin, isoniazid, nucleoside reverse transcriptase inhibitors

- **Megaloblastic anemia**: phenytoin, methotrexate, sulfa drugs (Mega **PMS**)

- **Myopathies**: fibrates, colchicines, cocaine, zidovudine, glucocorticoids, antimalarials, statins, penicillamine, antipsychotics, interferon α, niacin, zidovudine (**FCC Z GAS PAIN**)

- **Osteoporosis**: corticosteroids, heparin

- **Ototoxicity**: aminoglycosides, vancomycin, cisplatin, carboplatin, furosemide, ASA

- **Parkinsonism:** antipsychotics, metoclopramide

- **Positive Coombs test, aka Coombs' test:** penicillin, methyldopa, quinidine

- **Photosensitivity:** sulfonamides, amiodarone, tetracycline (**SAT** for a photo)

- **Pulmonary Fibrosis:** bleomycin, busulfan, amiodarone, nitrofurantoin, cyclophosphamide, methotrexate

- **Red man syndrome**: vancomycin

- **Seizures:** buproprion, venlaxafine, INH, antipsychotics, stimulants, ETOH withdrawal

- **SIADH:** carbamazepine, chlorpropamide, cyclophosphamide, thiazides, antipsychotics, TCAs, MAOIs

- **SLE-like syndrome**: hydralazine, isoniazid, procainamide (HIP)

- **Sulfa allergy**: celecoxib, acetazolamide, trimethoprim/sulfamethoxazole, dapsone, glyburide, glipizide, furosemide, sumatriptan), hydrochlorothiazide. (CATS DGG FSH)

- **Stevens-Johnson syndrome**: phenytoin, phenobarbital, lamotrigine, ethosuximide, allopurinol, sulfa drugs

- **Tardive dyskinesia**: long term antipsychotics

- **Tendon damage**: fluoroquinolones

- **Thrombocytopenia**: PCN, quinidine, furosemide, NSAID, gold, ranitidine, sulfonamides

- **Tinnitus:** excessive aspirin

- **Torsades de pointes**: quinidine, sotalol, erythromycin

- **Venous Thromboembolism**: oral contraceptives

Regulatory Issues

Most new drugs are found by one of the following methods: screening of natural products, rational drug design based on known physiologic mechanisms, or chemical alteration of a known drug molecule. The goal of drug investigation is to produce a "lead molecule," which is a front runner for a possible usable drug. Initial studies include the following:

- Pharmacologic profiles, which use molecular studies, such as receptor binding and enzyme activity studies.

- Cellular studies of the effects on cell function.

- Systems and disease models, often using animal models.

Preclinical safety testing is performed to evaluate the potential side effects of a new drug (done in the laboratory). This testing encompasses the following areas: acute toxicity, chronic toxicity, teratogenicity, carcinogenicity, mutagenicity, and investigative toxicity.

An attempt is also made to determine the **no-effect dose**, the maximal dose at which no toxic effect is seen; the **minimum lethal dose**, the smallest dose needed to kill any animal; and the LD_{50} (lethal dose, 50%), the dose that kills half of the experimental animals.

There are several limitations to human trials. First, the variable natural course of most diseases confounds results. Second, the presence of comorbid conditions is difficult to control and eliminate. In addition, one must always be mindful of subject and observer bias, including the placebo response. Ideally, this factor is controlled with double-blind studies.

Some drugs designed to treat rare diseases are known as **orphan drugs**. An amendment in 1983 provides incentives for the development of these drugs. Before a new drug is approved by the U.S. Food/Drug Administration (FDA), it must undergo three phases of clinical testing.

- **Phase I trials**: drug is given to healthy volunteers in varying doses to determine safety.

- **Phase II trials**: drug is given to patients with the disease and compared to an older, gold-standard drug or a placebo. Safety and efficacy of the drug is evaluated.

- **Phase III trials**: drug is given to hundreds to thousands of patients while compliance, side effects, and other factors are measured.

- **Phase IV trials**: after FDA approval, the drug is monitored in actual clinical use and rare side effects are found (e.g., the diet drug dexfenfluramine was pulled from the market because it caused rare but potentially fatal pulmonary HTN and heart valve damage.

Common Suffixes Found in Drug Names

Ending	Type of drug	Examples
-zosin	α_1 antagonist	prazosin, terazosin, tamsulosin
-olol	β antagonist	propanolol, timolol, sotalol
-terol	β_2 agonist	albuterol, salmeterol, formoterol
-barbital	barbiturates	phenobarbital, allobarbital, amobarbital
-azepam	benzodiazepines	clonazepam, diazepam, lorazepam
-zolam	benzodiazepines	alprazolam, midazolam, estazolam
-etine	SSRIs	paroxetine, fluoxetine, dapoxetine
-triptyline	TCAs	amitriptyline, nortriptyline, protriptyline
-ipramine	TCAs	clomipramine, desipramine, imipramine
-azine	antipsychotics	chlorpromazine, thioridazine
-idone	antipsychotics	risperidone, ziprasidone, lurasidone
-operidol	antipsychotics	haloperidol, droperidol
-caine	local anesthetics (esters)	cocaine, procaine, tetracaine ("i" × 1)
-caine	local anesthetics (amides)	lidocaine, bupivicaine, mepivicaine ("i" × 2)
-ane	inhaled anesthetics	halothane, isoflurane, sevoflurane
-pril	ACE inhibitors	lisinopril, enalapril, captopril
-oxin	cardiac glycoside	digoxin, digitoxin, acetyldigoxin
-afil	erectile dysfunction meds	sildenafil, tadalafil, vardenafil
-tidine	H_2 antagonists	famotidine, ranitidine, cimetidine
-triptan	migraine meds	sumatriptan, rizatriptan, naratriptan
-cillin	penicillins	penicillin, amoxicillin, methicillin
-ithromycin	macrolides	erythromycin, clarithromycin, azithromycin
-mycin	aminoglycosides	gentamicin, tobramycin, neomycin
-cycline	tetracyclines	tetracycline, doxycycline, minocycline
-floxacin	fluoroquinolones	ciprofloxacin, levofloxacin, moxifloxacin
-azole	antifungals	fluconazole, ketoconazole, voriconazole
-navir	antiviral protease inhibitors	saquinavir, ritonavir, indinavir

CHAPTER 15

PSYCHIATRY

DIAGNOSIS OF MENTAL DISORDERS

The standard basis for classification in the United States is the **Diagnostic and Statistical Manual of Mental Disorders, Fifth Edition Text Revision (DSM-IV-TR).** This is a 5-level, multiaxial diagnostic approach that takes into account all the factors that impact the patient's mental health. Table 1 lists the five axes. Each disorder has a descriptive categorization according to symptoms. Many disease entities overlap and patients can have multiple DSM diagnoses.

GAF (70–100): mild or minimal symptoms
GAF (< 50): serious impairment (e.g., suicidal ideation)

Axis I	Lists major mental disorders, learning disorders, substance abuse disorders
Axis II	Lists any personality disorders (e.g., histrionic) or mental retardation
Axis III	Includes any general medical conditions (e.g., diabetes, hypertension)
Axis IV	Lists any psychosocial or environmental factors (e.g., unemployment)
Axis V	The global assessment of functioning (GAF) on a scale of 1 to 100

Table 1 DSM Multiaxial Diagnostic System

NEUROTRANSMITTERS

Recent research in psychiatry has focused on neurotransmitters, or chemical messengers in the brain. For example, the actions of monoamines (dopamine, serotonin, and norepinephrine) in the CNS, and imbalances in their levels are believed to be responsible for many psychiatric disorders. While these compounds play different roles in the CNS, all three are removed from the brain by the enzyme monoamine oxidase. The **monoamine hypothesis of depression** attributes the symptoms to depleted levels of these neurotransmitters in the brain.

Antipsychotic medications block dopamine (D2) and serotonin receptors

Levodopa is used to treat Parkinson's disease. It easily crosses the blood-brain barrier and gets converted to dopamine

Cholinergic effects
SLUDGEM
Salivation/**S**weating,
Lacrimation,
Urination,
Defecation, **G**I upset,
Emesis, **M**iosis

Anticholinergic
effects
**Dry as a bone, Red
as a beet, Blind as a
bat, Mad as a hatter,
Hot as a hare.**
(Decreased
sweating/salivation/
lacrimation,
along with urinary
retention, ileus,
cutaneous
vasodilation/flushing,
mydriasis, sedation,
delirium, hallucination,
seizure)

Dopamine acts via 5 receptor subtypes (D1-D5) and gets metabolized by the enzyme monoamine oxidase (MAO). Dopaminergic pathways include nigrostriatal, mesolimbic, mesocortical, periventricular, and hypothalamic. Mesolimbic dopaminergic neurons are believed to play a crucial role in reward seeking and reinforcement, including drug addiction. The **dopamine hypothesis of schizophrenia** implicates abnormal dopaminergic neurotransmission in the pathogenesis of schizophrenic psychosis. Dopamine is also believed to play a role in depression, mania, and ADHD. Parkinson's disease results from the death of dopamine-producing neurons.

Serotonin (5-HT) acts via multiple receptor subtypes and also gets metabolized by monoamine oxidase. Serotonergic pathways include the median and dorsal raphe, locus coeruleus, and pineal body. According to the **monoamine hypothesis of depression**, abnormally low levels of serotonin (along with norepinephrine and dopamine) are responsible for depression. Medications used to treat depression target and block the metabolism and reuptake of serotonin. Abnormal serotonin levels have also been implicated in bipolar disorder and mania.

Norepinephrine (NE) and Epinephrine act via alpha- and beta-adrenergic receptors, and are also metabolized by the enzyme monoamine oxidase. CNS pathways include the locus coeruleus and lateral tegmental neurons. Underactivity of NE (as well as serotonin) may lead to depression, whereas overactivity may be related to mania. Tricyclic antidepressants and MAO inhibitors potentiate the actions of NE by inhibiting its reuptake and blocking its removal, respectively.

Acetylcholine (ACh) acts via cholinergic (muscarinic and nicotinic) receptors, and then gets rapidly destroyed by the enzyme **acetylcholinesterase (AChE)**. CNS pathways include corpus striatum, nucleus accumbens, motor cortex, and thalamus. Cholinergic stimulation by ACh results in salivation, lacrimation, micturition, defecation, GI motility, emesis, and miosis. Anticholinergic drugs act through muscarinic or nicotinic blockade, and have opposite effects (decreased sweating, decreased salivation, decreased lacrimation, urinary retention, ileus, hyperthermia, flushing, meiosis, sedation, delirium, hallucination, seizure, and reduction of parkinsonism symptoms). Many medications used to treat depression and schizophrenia have these anticholinergic side effects. Ach also plays a role in memory, and dysfunction has been implicated in Alzheimer's dementia.

Glutamate is an excitatory neurotransmitter that has 4 receptor subtypes, including the NMDA receptor, which can be blocked by alcohol, nitrous oxide, ketamine, and phencyclidine (PCP).

GABA is an inhibitory neurotransmitter that acts via 2 receptor subtypes (A and B). $GABA_A$ receptors are influenced by alcohol, barbiturates, benzodiazepines, and gamma-hydroxybutyrate (GHB).

SLEEP DISORDERS

Circadian rhythm refers to a biological process that follows a 24-hour cycle. While the rhythm is endogenous, it can be modified by external cues such as the light-dark cycle. Sleeping patterns are driven in part by circadian rhythms. Sleep itself consists of REM (rapid eye movement) and NREM (non rapid eye movement) sleep that alternates at 90-minute intervals. The duration of REM sleep increases as the night goes on.

Sleep Stage	Percentage total sleep	Characteristics of EEG pattern	Comments
Awake	—	Low amplitude, high frequency beta waves (NO sawtooth waves)	—
Relaxed wakefulness	—	Rhythmic alpha waves	—
Stage 1 (light sleep)	5%	Low amplitude, mixed frequency theta waves	Usually short duration (1–7 min)
Stage 2	45%	Slower waves with bursts of rapid **sleep spindles and K comple**xes	—
Stage 3–4 (deep sleep)	25%	High amplitude, low frequency (slow) **delta waves**	Sleepwalking, night terrors, and bedwetting occur here; depression and benzodiazepines decrease deep sleep
REM sleep	25%	Low amplitude, high frequency beta waves AND sawtooth waves (similar to awake state)	Dreams, nightmares, rapid extraocular movements, loss of motor tone, and penile/clitoral tumescence occur here; ACh is main neurotransmitter, but NE decreases REM

Table 2 Sleep cycle

Narcolepsy is a sleep disorder characterized by daytime sleep attacks, episodes of cataplexy (collapse from paralysis of muscles), sleep paralysis, trouble sleeping, and hallucinations. Different types of hallucinations include visual, auditory, tactile, olfactory, and gustatory. **Hypnagogic hallucinations** occur when falling asleep. **Hypnopompic hallucinations** occur when waking up from sleep. The treatment for narcolepsy is amphetamines. Both types are often associated with the sensation that someone else is present in the room. The treatment for narcolepsy is amphetamines.

Parasomnias refer to a group of sleep disorders that involve disturbing events that occur while sleeping. Examples include nightmares, sleepwalking, and sleep terrors. **Nightmares** involves sudden awakening from REM sleep with fear and recollection of bad dream. **Sleep terrors** refer to sudden awakening from NREM delta sleep with fear and inconsolable screaming, but no recollection of any dream. **Sleepwalking** also occurs during NREM delta sleep, and may involve sitting up, opening eyes, ambulating, talking, and other complex activities with no recollection afterwards.

Restless Legs Syndrome is characterized by abnormal sensations of the lower legs and uncontrollable kicks just before falling asleep. The symptoms may be worsened with stress and may cause insomnia, irritability, and depression.

AMNESIA

Amnesia refers to the loss of one's memory. **Anterograde amnesia** is a type of memory loss in which there is an impaired ability to form new memories, but established memories are intact. **Retrograde amnesia** is a type of memory loss in which preexisting memories are lost, but the ability to form new memories is intact.

NORMAL INFANT DEVELOPMENT

Apgar Score

The Apgar score is a commonly used but seldom useful scoring system for newborns, evaluated at one and five minutes after birth. Score ranges from 0 to 10, with 10 being a perfect score. The 5-minute score correlates best with long-term outcome.

APGAR = **A**ppearance, **P**ulse, **G**rimace, **A**ctivity, **R**espiration

Feature	0 Points	1 Points	2 points
Color	Blue-gray	Pink trunk only	Pink all over
Heart rate	0	< 100	> 100
Reflex irritability	No grimace or cough	Grimace only	Grimace and cough
Muscle tone	limp	Some activity	Moving limbs, crying
Respiratory effort	0	Rhythmic alpha waves	Regular

Table 3 Apgar score

Maternal Emotional Deprivation

René Spitz did empirical research on infants to study the effects of maternal emotional deprivation. Several physical changes were noted, including decreased weight and muscular tone as well as an increase in physical illness. In addition, language development and socialization skills were impaired, and those infants did not develop basic trust. **Anaclitic depression** refers to the depression seen in young children after being deprived of maternal affection for a prolonged period of time. The condition was noted to be reversible if the child was reunited with the mother in less than six months, but irreversible after that.

Motor and Language Development

A typical USMLE question will list a number of tasks a child can do and test your ability to gauge whether the child is age-appropriate. Be sure you know the developmental milestones.

At birth: Babinski, Moro, palmar, rooting reflexes (all disappear within 1 year)

2 months: moves extremities, coos, looks at faces, tracks moving objects, turns to sound

4 months: holds head up, rolls over tummy to back, hands to mouth, social smile

6 months: sits assisted, grasps objects, rolls over both directions, responds to name/sounds

9 months: sits alone, crawls, pulls to stand, transfers objects, mama/dada, stranger anxiety

12 months: cruises, picks up objects with thumb and forefinger, shakes/bangs objects

18 months: walks, drinks from cup, scribbles, points, uses single words, separation anxiety

2 years: runs, climbs, kicks ball, can build a 4-block tower, can draw lines and circles, object permanence

3 years: tricycle, conversation, core gender identity, parallel play

4 years: can hop on one foot, simple drawing, cooperative play, can name colors

5 years: uses fork and spoon, toilet-trained, can count to 10, wants to be like friends

6-11 years: same-sex friends, identifies with same-sex parent, develops conscience

Tanner Stages of Sexual Development

Tanner Stages (Girls)
Stage 1: Prepubertal; elevated papilla but no breast development; vellus hair but no pubic hair
Stage 2: Palpable breast bud below nipple; sparse straight pubic hair along labia
Stage 3: Enlarging cone of breast and areola; increased darker, curled pubic hair over mons pubis
Stage 4: Secondary mound of areola/papillae above breast; adult type pubic hair across mons
Stage 5: Mature adult breast, recessed areola; triangular distribution of pubic hair to medial thigh

Tanner Stages (Boys)
Stage 1: Prepubertal; testes/scrotum/penis similar to childhood; vellus hair but no pubic hair
Stage 2: Enlargement of reddened scrotum/testes; sparse straight pubic hair at base of penis
Stage 3: Increased length of penis and growth of testes/scrotum; increased dark curly pubic hair
Stage 4: Enlarged penile length/circumference with a developed glans penis and darkened scrotum; pubic hair is increased in distribution but does not yet reach the medial thigh
Stage 5: Mature adult size/shape genitalia; triangular distribution of pubic hair to medial thigh

CHANGES IN THE ELDERLY

There are a number of age-related physiological changes seen in the elderly, including a general decline in function of all systems. For example, there are decreases in cardiac output, gas exchange, creatinine clearance, muscle mass, and bone density. There is an increase in the incidence of both medical and psychiatric pathology, especially depression. Sleep patterns are altered as well, with a decrease in both REM and slow-wave sleep, and an increase in frequency of awakenings. In terms of sexual function, men may have decreased sperm production, erectile dysfunction, and longer refractory periods. Women similarly have decreased estrogen which results in the thinning of vaginal walls and decreased vaginal lubrication. Considering all these negative changes it may not be surprising that suicide rates in the elderly are elevated.

PHYSIOLOGIC CHANGES DURING STRESS

Stress typically causes a "fight or flight" response in the body, to prepare us for potential physical dangers. Specific effects include stimulation of the pituitary-adrenal axis, resulting in increased release of glucocorticoids, catecholamines, vasopressin, and growth hormone. There is also a decrease in insulin, thyroid hormone, and gonadotropins.

DEVELOPMENTAL THEORIES

Cognitive Development (Jean Piaget)

Sensorimotor phase (0–2 years): Child explores environment through physical actions and assimilation and develops object permanence (knowing things exist even when hidden from view).

Preoperational phase (2–7 years): Language acquisition and symbolic thinking begins. The child has magical thinking as well as egocentrism (is only aware of his or her own point of view).

Concrete operational phase (7–11 years): Logical thinking begins, as well as awareness of other points of view, and child begins to understand concepts of conservation of mass and volume.

Formal operation phase (11 to adolescence): Child now has abstract reasoning, and there is increased flexibility, awareness of one's own thoughts.

Psychosocial Development (Erik Erikson)

Infancy (0–18 months): Children learn to develop trust if their daily needs are met.

Early childhood (18 months–3 years): Children try to assert independence. If encouraged, they become more confident. If discouraged, they develop shame and self-doubt.

Play age (4–6 years): Children make plans and initiate activities with others. If discouraged, they may develop guilt and become followers.

School age (6–13 years): Children develop pride in accomplishments. If discouraged (e.g., at school) they may develop sense of inferiority.

Adolescence (11–20 years): Adolescents form their sense of identity based on the results of their exploration. If discouraged, they may develop confusion about who they are.

Young adulthood (20–35 years): Young adults explore relationships with others. If discouraged, they may develop fear of intimacy and commitment, leading to isolation.

Middle adulthood (35–65 years): Adults begin to make a contribution to society through work and child-rearing. If discouraged, they develop a sense of stagnation.

Late adulthood (65 and older): Older adults start to reflect on life accomplishments to achieve a sense of satisfaction. If life was unproductive, they may develop a sense of despair.

Psychoanalysis (Sigmund Freud)

Freudian theory is a structural theory in which three parts of the psychic apparatus explain human development, emotions, and illness. The three parts are the ego, the id, and the superego. **Id** represents a collection of the raw impulses and drives, such as sex, fear, and aggression. **Superego** is the conscience of the mind, telling us what we "should do." **Ego** is the rational mediator between the desires of the id and the expectations of the superego. According to Freudian theory, the psychosexual stages of development must be completed or else patients develop a fixation at a particular point. The "Oedipus complex" refers to repressed sexual feelings towards a child's opposite-sex parent, as well as a rivalry with the same-sex parent.

Oral stage (0–18 months): Child obtains oral pleasure by putting things in his or her mouth. If there is an abnormal amount of gratification, the child may develop an oral fixation.

Anal stage (18–36 months): Child obtains pleasure through anal stimulation while attaining bowel control. Anal fixation, as a result of inappropriate parental responses (e.g., strict training or shaming with accidents) may lead to a preoccupation with cleanliness and control (anal retentive personality).

Phallic stage (3–5 years): Children obtain pleasure from genitals and develop an Oedipus complex. Fixation here can result in abnormal sexuality.

Latency period (6–puberty): Children play with same sex peers as sexuality is repressed.

Genital stage (after puberty): Develop interest in opposite gender with reawakened sexual urges.

CONDITIONING

Classical Conditioning

Classical conditioning is a type of behavior modification (learning) in which a previously neutral stimulus (e.g., bell) becomes capable of eliciting a desired involuntary response (e.g., salivation) after being repeatedly presented together with an unconditioned stimulus (e.g., food) that normally elicits that response.

Operant Conditioning

Operant conditioning is a type of behavior modification (learning) in which consequences are used to affect voluntary behavior in the future. Reinforcement increases the likelihood and strengthens a desired behavior. Positive reinforcement introduces a pleasant stimulus (reward), whereas negative reinforcement removes an unpleasant stimulus. Punishment involves the use of a consequence to decrease the likelihood of a desired behavior. Positive punishment introduces an unpleasant stimulus, whereas negative punishment removes a pleasant stimulus. Note that positive refers to the addition of a stimulus and negative refers to the removal of a stimulus. Extinction involves the gradual weakening of a conditioned response after the consequence is removed.

Reinforcement schedule refers to the frequency of the consequence used in operant conditioning. In continuous reinforcement, the consequence is used every time the desired behavior occurs. It is associated with faster learning as well as faster extinction once the consequence is removed. In contrast, partial reinforcement (e.g., the variable ratio schedule) entails the use of a consequence only part of the time. This option is associated with slower learning and slower extinction once the consequence is removed.

EARLY ONSET DISORDERS

Motor skill and Learning Disorders

Developmental coordination disorder: Motor skill disorder in which motor coordination in daily activities is way below average, given age and intelligence. There are marked delays in motor milestones and a general clumsiness that interferes with achievement.

Reading disorder: Learning disorder characterized by impaired reading accuracy, speed, or comprehension that impairs achievement.

Mathematics disorder: Learning disorder in which a child's math ability is way below average for age, intelligence, and education.

Disorder of written expression: learning disorder in which writing abilities, as measured by standardized tests, are way below average for age, intelligence, and education.

Communication Disorders

Expressive language disorder: Child has trouble expressing himself or herself with speech but understands well. Of note, the child has no trouble pronouncing words, unlike phonologic disorder.

Mixed receptive-expressive language disorder: Child has problems both expressing himself and understanding others. There is no difficulty pronouncing words, unlike phonologic disorder.

Phonologic disorder: Child fails to develop all of the speech sounds appropriately for age.

Stuttering: Child may have "classic" stuttering, in which sounds and syllables are repeated or last longer than normal. The problem may worsen with time to include words and phrases, and the child's speech may have a struggling quality and forced sound. Other symptoms include pauses and circumlocutions (word substitutions to avoid potentially problematic words).

MENTAL RETARDATION

Mental retardation is defined as an IQ below 70. Mentally retarded persons experience significant delay in developmental and social milestones. Mental retardation is associated with early fetal insults, such as congenital infections and alcohol exposure. Certain genetic syndromes, such as Down syndrome, are also associated with mental retardation.

Level of Mental Retardation	Intelligence quotient (IQ)	Proportion of MR population
Mild	50–55 to70	85%
Moderate	35–40 to 50–55	10%
Severe	20–25 to 35–40	3%
Profound	< 20–25	2%

Table 4 Classification of Mental Retardation

PERVASIVE DEVELOPMENTAL DISORDERS

Autistic disorder is characterized by markedly impaired language and social interaction, along with restricted, repetitive and stereotyped patterns of behavior, interests, and activities. For example, these children often have delayed and limited speech, with difficulty starting and sustaining conversation. They often have inflexible routines and rituals, with abnormal interest in only a few things, and may exhibit repetitive hand movements. Taken together these symptoms make it impossible to develop age-appropriate peer relationships.

Asperger's disorder is like a milder form of autism, with impaired social skills and communication, but normal early language skills. Another key feature is extreme interest and preoccupation with a single topic.

Rett's disorder mainly affects females and is characterized by normal early development until age 6–18 months, when development and growth become delayed, and there is loss of speech and purposeful hand movement. They exhibit stereotyped hand movement like wringing or patting.

Childhood disintegrative disorder is also characterized by normal early development, but after 3–4 years there is a loss of previously acquired motor language, and social skills, as well as bladder/bowel control. By age 10 the level of impairment is quite severe.

IMPULSE-CONTROL DISORDERS

In these disorders patients are unable to resist impulses to perform certain actions that result in negative consequences. They may experience significant anxiety leading up to the action as well as relief and gratification afterwards.

Intermittent explosive disorder is characterized by unpredictable episodes of excessive anger and aggression. In contrast to conduct disorder and antisocial personality, the behavior is completely absent between episodes.

Pathological gambling is characterized by a persistent pattern of gambling that is disabling.

Kleptomania is characterized by compulsive stealing of objects that are not needed.

Pyromania is characterized by compulsive fire-setting done out of fascination with fire. In contrast with conduct disorder and antisocial personality, there is no malicious intent.

Trichotillomania is characterized by compulsive hair-pulling, resulting in noticeable hair loss.

Autistic disorder features impaired language skills.

Asperger's disorder has normal language skills.

DISRUPTIVE BEHAVIOR DISORDERS

Attention-deficit/hyperactivity disorder (ADHD): These children develop a problem with inattention, impulsivity, and sometimes overactivity. To make this diagnosis onset must occur before age 7 and symptoms must last for 6 months. A classic example is the schoolboy who can't sit still, has a short attention span, and blurts out answers rather than waiting his turn. Many of these children also have **conduct disorder** or **oppositional defiant disorder**. Medication with amphetamines (e.g., dextroamphetamine or methylphenidate) has been shown to be helpful.

Conduct disorder: These children develop a persistent pattern of rule-breaking behavior that violates the rights of others (e.g., destroying property, lying, stealing, fighting, and committing other crimes). Symptoms must last for more than 6 months. There is an association with ADHD and an increased risk of developing antisocial personality in adulthood.

Oppositional defiant disorder (ODD): These children develop a pattern of negative, argumentative, and hostile behavior towards authority figures, but without seriously violating the rights of others. Typically, the behavior problems are milder than those seen with conduct disorder and legal violations are not characteristic. There is an association with ADHD and an increased risk of developing conduct disorder.

Children have
Conduct disorder.
Adults have
Antisocial
personality disorder.

OTHER CHILDHOOD DISORDERS

Encopresis: > 3 months of involuntary defecation in an inappropriate setting, after age 5.

Enuresis: > 3 months of involuntary or intentional urination, after age 5.

Feeding disorder: > 1 month of failure to eat enough to gain weight and grow normally.

Pica: > 1 month of craving and eating non-nutritive substances (e.g., dirt).

Reactive attachment disorder: lifelong condition where child cannot make healthy bonds with caregivers, typically seen in abused or neglected children.

Rumination: Potentially fatal disorder of intentional regurgitation and rechewing of food.

Selective mutism: > 1 month of inability to speak only in certain situations (e.g., school).

Separation anxiety disorder: > 1 month of excessive worry about separation from parents.

Stereotypic movement disorder: > 1 month of repetitive, purposeless movements, often self-injurious (examples include biting, hitting, and headbanging). May see with mental retardation.

Tourette's disorder: > 1 year of uncontrolled **tics** (recurrent, sudden, rapid vocalizations or movements). Examples include throat clearing, shouting obscenities, shoulder shrugging, and blinking. Males are affected more than females.

Transient tic disorder: > 1 month but less than 1 year of uncontrolled tics.

EATING DISORDERS

Anorexia nervosa is characterized by a refusal to maintain 85% of expected weight, leading to amenorrhea and signs and symptoms of starvation. These patients have an intense fear of gaining weight as a result of distorted body image, and are typically in denial of their low weight and its impact on their health. Prevalence is highest in female teens, especially those involved with activities that require thin body types. There is also an association with depression, anxiety, and OCD. Most patients will eventually recover, but some will develop chronic anorexia, and others may succumb to fatal cardiac arrhythmias or suicide.

Bulemia nervosa is characterized by recurrent episodes of binge eating followed by a compensatory behavior which can be subclassified as purging or non-purging. The purging subtype is characterized by either self-induced vomiting or the use of laxatives and diuretics after an eating binge. The nonpurging subtype is characterized by fasting or extreme exercise after an eating binge. Again, the majority of these patients are females preoccupied with their weight and body image, and concurrent depression is common. In contrast to anorexia, patients may have normal weight. Watch for abrasions to back of hands and poor dentition from self-induced vomiting. Patients may need hospitalization to correct electrolyte disturbances.

Of note, **body mass index** (BMI = mass (kg) / (height (m))^2) is frequently used by health professionals to evaluate a patient's need for weight loss or gain. For example a BMI between 18.5 and 25 indicates optimal weight, whereas a BMI less than 18.5 means the patient is underweight, and a BMI greater than 25 means the patient is overweight. A major limitation of the body mass index is that it doesn't account for the distribution of fat or muscle.

SEXUAL DYSFUNCTION

Sexual dysfunction refers to any problem during the normal sexual response cycle, including difficulty with desire, arousal, or orgasm, as well pain disorders. Common examples in men include decreased libido, erectile dysfunction, and premature ejaculation. Common examples in females include decreased libido, anorgasmia, dyspareunia, and vaginismus. In the evaluation of any patient with suspected sexual dysfunction, it is important to always consider medication side effects, medical illness, and psychological factors as potential contributing factors.

PARAPHILIAS

Paraphilias are a group of disorders characterized by recurrent, intense, and deviant sexual urges and fantasies. The symptoms must be present for 6 months, and the patients must either act on the urges, or experience distress as a result of them.

Exhibitionism: fantasy and urge to expose one's genitals to strangers.

Voyeurism: fantasy and urge to observe an unsuspecting person disrobing or engaging in sexual behavior.

Frotteurism: fantasy and urge to touch or rub against an unsuspecting person.

Fetishism: fantasy and urge involving a nonliving object as source of sexual excitement.

Transvestic fetishism: heterosexual male with fantasy and urge to cross-dress.

Pedophilia: fantasy and urge to have sexual relations with prepubescent child.

DISSOCIATIVE DISORDERS

Dissociative amnesia: Inability to recall a significant period of time, usually after a stressful event.

Dissociative fugue: Sudden, unexpected travel, and memory loss with confusion about identity.

Dissociative identity disorder is characterized by at least two distinct states or personalities that can each take control, while the other(s) have no awareness or recollection of what happens.

Depersonalization: Persistent feeling of detachment, as if the subject is in a dream.

DEMENTIA VS. DELIRIUM

Dementia is a gradual, insidious, constant, and nonreversible global deterioration in cerebral function (memory loss, cognitive decline, personality change, sensorimotor decline) with normal consciousness and lack of hallucinations. **Alzheimer's disease**, the most common cause of dementia, is characterized by an insidious onset and slow deterioration. There is impaired executive function, personality, speech, and motor function. Other systemic, psychiatric, and neurologic causes must be excluded for this diagnosis. **Vascular dementia** is often caused by multiple infarcts or generalized small vessel disease, usually in the presence of vascular risk factors (DM, HTN, arteriosclerosis, smoking). It often presents with a more sudden onset and stepwise deterioration in cognitive function with or without language and motor dysfunction. Other causes of dementia include head trauma, alcoholism, malnutrition, and HIV/AIDS. Regardless of cause, management of dementia entails treatment of the underlying disorder and supportive care.

Delirium is also characterized by global decline in memory, cognition, personality, and sensorimotor function, but in contrast with dementia there is a more acute onset, fluctuating course, altered consciousness, and hallucinations. Another key distinction is the fact that delirium is reversible. The differential diagnosis is broad. Causes of delirium include drug intoxication/withdrawal, electrolyte disturbances, infection, sleep deprivation, trauma, stroke, urinary/fecal retention, cardiopulmonary disease. "ICU psychosis" is a transient form of delirium that may include multiple psychiatric symptoms (e.g., anxiety, agitation, paranoia, delusions, and psychosis). Frequently, the symptoms are worse at night, a phenomenon known as "sundowning." The etiology is usually

Causes of
DELERIUM(S)

Drugs (benzos/opioids), Drug withdrawal (ETOH, benzos)

Elderly/Emotional

Low O_2 states (MI, CHF, PE, COPD, ARDS)

Infection (sepsis, encephalitis, meningitis)

Retention (urinary, fecal)

Ictal states (Ex: seizures, strokes), Intestinal obstruction/perforation/inflammation

Underhydration, Undernutrition
Metabolic (electrolytes, acidosis, glucose, thyroid)

Subdural hemorrhage or hematoma, sleep deprivation

multifactorial, including many of the stressors commonly found in the ICU like critical illness, metabolic disturbances, dehydration, polypharmacy, sleep deprivation, loss of light-dark cycles, and constant stimulation with light, noise, and pain. Treatment involves addressing any underlying medical causes, minimizing polypharmacy, regulating sleep cycles, and frequent reorientation. Haloperidol and quetiapine are also helpful.

SUBSTANCE USE DISORDERS

The following definitions are useful in understanding substance disorders:

Formication: Tactile hallucinations and paresthesias seen with cocaine and amphetamine use that result in sensation of bugs crawling on skin. May lead to compulsive scratching and skin picking.

Intoxication: A reversible symptom caused by use of a drug, resulting in "maladaptive behavior."

Drug abuse: A pattern of recurrent substance use for the purpose of personal pleasure that interferes with and leads to failure at work, home, school, and other areas.

Psychological dependence: A pattern of compulsive drug-seeking behavior and use despite knowledge of adverse effects and risks.

Physiological dependence: When these patients stop using their drug of abuse, they experience real signs and symptoms, typically the opposite of what they experience while using.

Tolerance: Progressive need for greater amounts of a drug to achieve the same effect. This is due to a decreased response to the drug over time.

Withdrawal: A substance-specific syndrome of symptoms that develops after cessation of use. Typically the withdrawal syndrome has opposite effects compared to the intoxication (e.g., withdrawal from CNS stimulants like cocaine causes exhaustion and depression).

The following are various substances of abuse, along with their symptoms of intoxication and withdrawal.

Caffeine is found in coffee and many carbonated drinks. Intoxication may cause tremor, insomnia, nervousness, flushing, diuresis, tachycardia, cardiac arrhythmias. Withdrawal symptoms include severe headache, lethargy, and irritability.

Nicotine is found in tobacco products. Intoxication may cause tremors, insomnia, nervousness, decreased appetite. Withdrawal symptoms include dysphoria, insomnia, irritability, anxiety, and difficulty concentrating.

Alcohol is one of the oldest recreational drugs. Consumption can result in intoxication, with resulting slurred speech, ataxia, reduced inhibition, impaired judgment, reduced inhibition, and sedation. Withdrawal symptoms include hyperactivity, tremor, nausea, vomiting, anxiety, insomnia, tachycardia, hypertension, hallucinations, seizures, and delirium tremens.

Delirium tremens can be life threatening and peaks 3–5 days after abstaining from alcohol (ETOH). Look for tachycardia, agitation, tremors, confusion and psychosis. DTs are managed with benzodiazepines.

Screening for alcoholism: CAGE = subject has felt need to **C**ut down, **A**nnoyed when asked, **G**uilty about drinking, **E**ye-opener drink in the morning

Blood alcohol content (BAC), measured in g/100mL of blood BAC > 0.08% impaired motor skills; legal limit BAC > 0.12% drunkenness BAC > 0.30% loss of consciousness BAC > 0.50% death

Look for "track marks" in IV drug abusers—the users may eventually destroy their veins and resort to subcutaneous injections ("skin popping") that can lead to abscesses.

Always suspect heroin/opioid intoxication in a patient with pinpoint pupils, lethargy, and respiratory depression.

Barbiturates are sedative-hypnotic drugs with CNS-depressive effects. Intoxication may cause slurred speech, ataxia, drunken behavior, reduced inhibition, coma, respiratory depression, cardiovascular depression, death. Withdrawal symptoms include hyperactivity, tremor, nausea, vomiting, anxiety, insomnia, seizures, and death.

Benzodiazepines are sedative-hypnotic drugs that have largely replaced barbiturates because of increased safety. Examples include alprazolam, lorazepam, diazepam, and flunitrazepam. Intoxication may result in slurred speech, ataxia, drunken behavior, reduced inhibition, coma, respiratory/cardiovascular depression, death. Withdrawal symptoms include hyperactivity, tremor, nausea, vomiting, anxiety, insomnia, seizures, and death.

Amphetamines are stimulants that create a sensation of euphoria. Examples include methamphetamine ("speed," "crystal meth") and MDMA ("ecstasy"). Intoxication may result in fever, tachycardia, hypertension, perspiration, agitation, pupillary dilation, formication, seizure, arrhythmias, and death. Withdrawal symptoms include dysphoric mood, fatigue, nightmares, and increased appetite. Methamphetamine abusers can have multiple skin ulcerations ("speed bumps") due to compulsive scratching and picking from formication. Also look for poor oral hygiene ("meth mouth").

Cocaine ("crack") is another powerful stimulant with similar effects to amphetamines. Intoxication may result in fever, tachycardia, hypertension, perspiration, agitation, pupillary dilation, formication, seizure, arrhythmias, heart attack, stroke, death. Withdrawal symptoms include dysphoric mood, fatigue, paranoia, nightmares, increased appetite. Snorting may lead to nosebleeds and septal necrosis as a result of vasoconstriction.

Heroin and other opioids (morphine, hydromorphone, fentanyl, oxycodone, hydrocodone) are all derived from the opium poppy. Many are used in healthcare setting for their analgesic properties, but tolerance and dependence can develop quickly. Intoxication can result in pupillary constriction (miosis), constipation, respiratory depression, drowsiness, coma, and death. Withdrawal syndrome can be extremely unpleasant, with nausea, vomiting, diarrhea, muscle jerks/aches, sweating, yawning, pupillary dilation (mydriasis), lacrimation, and rhinorrhea.

Marijuana and **Hashish** are psychoactive drugs derived from the Cannibis plant. Intoxication may result in euphoria or anxiety, slowed sense of time, altered perception, impaired judgment, increased appetite, tachycardia, social withdrawal. There is no withdrawal.

Hallucinogens such as LSD, mescaline, and psilocybin (from certain mushroom spores) can cause altered perception that may be pleasant or unpleasant, leading to panic attacks. Withdrawal symptoms include paranoia, psychosis, flashbacks.

Phencyclidine (PCP), also known as "angel dust", is another dangerous hallucinogen and is also neurotoxic. Intoxication may cause nystagmus, psychosis, violent behavior, seizures, and death. Withdrawal may cause agitation and depression.

Ketamine has several uses in human medicine, including pain management and pediatric anesthesia. It is also a dissociative anesthetic commonly used by veterinarians. Intoxication may result in hallucination, dissociative effect, paresthesia, emergence reactions, disorientation, and amnesia. Withdrawal symptoms include insomnia, agitation, and depression.

Gamma-hydroxybutyric acid (GHB) is a CNS depressant that has been used in treatment of narcolepsy. Intoxication may cause nausea, vomiting, loss of consciousness, respiratory depression, seizures, and death. Withdrawal symptoms include insomnia, anxiety, tremor, and delirium.

Inhalants such as nitrous oxide and industrial solvents are frequently abused by children and adolescents due to their easy accessibility and low cost. Common household examples are aerosol cans, glue, markers, paint, cleaning fluids, and gasoline. Solvents are among the most dangerous of substance abuse, as they can cause asphyxia, loss of consciousness, multiorgan damage, and death.

PSYCHOTIC DISORDERS

Psychosis is a general term used to describe a state of lost contact with reality, during which the patient may have disorganized thoughts, delusions, and or hallucinations. Hallucinations are typically auditory or visual perceptions that occur in the absence of any true external stimulus. Delusions are false beliefs that are not shared by others and persist despite abundant evidence that they are not true. The different types of delusions include paranoid delusion, religious delusion, grandiose delusion, ideas of reference, thought broadcasting, and delusions of being controlled. Psychosis may occur as a result of general medical conditions, dementia, delirium, drugs, personality disorders, mood disorders, and psychotic disorders.

Schizophrenia is a deteriorating mental disorder characterized by disturbed thought, emotion, and behavior and a variable combination of "positive" and "negative" symptoms. Positive symptoms include hallucinations (auditory more common than visual), delusions, and bizarre behavior. Negative symptoms include social withdrawal, emotional blunting, cognitive deficits, demotivation, self neglect, reduced emotion, poverty of speech and motor activity. DSM-IV-TR diagnostic criteria were established to make the diagnosis of schizophrenia. The patient must have 2 or more of the above symptoms, each for 1 month, along with significant functional impairment. The total duration of the disturbance must be greater than 6 months, and all other causes must be excluded. Onset may be sudden or gradual, and usually occurs in the second or third decade of life. There is a genetic basis, although environment and family play important roles in its development. Treatment involves neuroleptics (antipsychotic drugs) and psychosocial support. See Table 5 for a list of antipsychotic medications.

Remember that children can abuse inhalants, which have high risk of morbidity and mortality.

Ketamine, Rohypnol, and GHB are sometimes used as date-rape drugs.

Methamphetamine overdose treatment: supportive care, temperature control

Benzodiazepine overdose treatment: flumazenil

Benzodiazepine withdrawal treatment: long acting benzodiazepines

Alcohol withdrawal treatment: benzodiazepines

Opioid overdose treatment: naloxone

Opioid withdrawal treatment: methadone

4A's of schizophrenia: Ambivalence, Autism, Affect blunting, Associative loosening

Antipsychotic agent	Toxicities and other information
Chlorpromazine	the most toxic of all; acute dystonia, tardive dyskinesia, neuroleptic syndrome, antiadrenergic effects, endocrine effects, orthostatic hypotension
Thioridazine	Possible cardiotoxicity; fewer extrapyramidal effects
Prochlorperazine	Can be used as an antiemetic
Haloperidol	Used for acute psychosis, has severe extrapyramidal side effects
Atypical antipsychotics (clozapine, olanzapine, risperidone, quetiapine, ziprasidone, aripiprazole)	More effective and less toxic than the older drugs; lower risk of extrapyramidal symptoms and tardive dyskinesia, but greater risk of weight gain and variable anticholinergic effects

Table 5 Neuroleptics

The actions of neuroleptics are not completely understood, but most are associated with blockade of the dopamine and serotonin receptors in the central nervous system. Because the actions appear to be nonselective, however, a number of undesirable side effects can occur, including sedation, anticholinergic effects and extrapyramidal symptoms. Older first-generation antipsychotics include phenothiazines such as chlorpromazine, thioridazine, haloperidol. Second generation antipsychotics, also known as atypical antipsychotics, have better side effect profiles but cost more. Below is a list of side effects from neuroleptics.

Sedation is more common with the older drugs, but also occurs with newer atypical antipsychotics as a result of histamine receptor blockade.

Anticholinergic effects such as dry mouth, urinary retention, constipation, dilated pupils, visual disturbances, tachycardia, and decreased sweating are a result of muscarinic receptor blockade. Postural hypotension may result from alpha adrenoreceptor blockade. Impotence is also common.

Endocrine effects such as hyperprolactinemia, gynecomastia, and infertility.

Neuroleptic malignant syndrome is a rare but acute, life-threatening, hyperthermic illness caused by the use of neuroleptics. Patients experience fever, impaired sweating, muscle rigidity, autonomic dysfunction, and delirium. The neuroleptic should be immediately withdrawn, and the patient should receive dantrolene, bromocriptine (dopamine agonist) and supportive care.

Extrapyramidal symptom (EPS) describes a diverse group of movement disorders, from acute dystonia, to akathisia, parkinsonism, and tardive dyskinesia.

Acute dystonia: Sustained muscle contractions that cause stiffness, abnormal postures, and twisting and repetitive movements. May occur hours to days after starting meds. Treatment is with anticholinergics.

Akathisia: Extreme restlessness and inability to remain motionless. Occurs days to weeks after taking medications.

Parkinsonism is characterized by tremor, bradykinesia, impaired speech and muscle rigidity that occurs days to weeks after neuroleptics, and can be reversed with anticholinergics.

Tardive dyskinesia is characterized by irreversible, involuntary choreoathetoid movements of the mouth and extremities that occurs months to years after long-term use of neuroleptics. There is no effective treatment (anticholinergics actually worsen the symptoms!).

Schizophreniform disorder is similar to schizophrenia, but while the symptoms last for more than 1 month, they do not last beyond 6 months. Treatment is also with neuroleptics.

Brief psychotic disorder is characterized by psychosis that lasts for less than 1 month. The psychosis may occur following a stressful event, delivery of a baby, or without any identifiable precipitant. It is treated with neuroleptics, anxiolytics, and therapy.

Schizoaffective disorder is a mixture of schizophrenia and concurrent mood disorder, either major depression or a manic episode. It is classified as either bipolar type (with manic symptoms) or depressive type (with depressive symptoms). Treatment involves a combination of neuroleptics with either mood stabilizers for the bipolar type, or antidepressants for the depressive type.

Delusional disorder is characterized by persistent nonbizarre delusions lasting for more than 1 month. There are no hallucinations or disorganized speech and behavior.

GRIEF

Normal grief (bereavement): natural response to a loss that lasts 6 months to 1 year. There may be intense, but intermittent feelings of sadness and loneliness, interspersed with periods of normal feeling. Suicidal ideation, particularly with a plan, is not a part of the grieving process, although the individual may express a desire to join the deceased. Self-blame and feelings of guilt are usually focused on the deceased. In contrast, depression features continuous sadness and loneliness, with feelings of guilt and worthlessness centered around the self, not just in regard to the deceased. The grieving welcome emotional support and feel better after sharing or discussing their feelings, whereas those suffering from major depression tend to withdraw from support.

Duration of psychosis:

Acute psychotic disorder < 1 month

Schizophreniform disorder > 1 and < 6 months

Schizophrenia > 6 months

Kubler-Ross stages of grief:
Denial, Anger, Bargaining, Grieving, Acceptance
(Note that these do not necessarily occur in this sequence, and reversion to a previous stage may also occur.)

Pathological grief can manifest as **absent grief** or **delayed grief**, in which the feelings of grief are repressed and denied, only to come back later as a more prolonged and distorted grief. Individuals who experience delayed grief are at greater risk for developing major depression.

Distorted grief occurs when a facet of the grieving process becomes disproportionately prolonged or overshadows the others. Disabling "survival guilt" is one example. Another example is the individual who over-identifies with the deceased to the point where he/she may forsake his/her own interests to pursue those of the deceased. Other examples of distorted grief include **conversion disorder**, in which the individual develops symptoms identical to those of the deceased, and denial of loss, in which the individual attempts to leave the room previously occupied by the deceased and/or their possessions completely unchanged.

MOOD DISORDERS

Depression is a general term used to describe episodes of low mood, decreased energy, and loss of interest and enjoyment. The extent of the depression is variable. Mild to moderate depression is characterized by depressive symptoms and some functional impairment. Major depression is more serious and disabling, and severe depression is characterized by additional agitation or psychomotor retardation with marked somatic symptoms. Depressive episodes can be further characterized as catatonic, melancholic, psychotic, or atypical. **Melancholic depression** is the most common form (60%) where patients have decreased levels of interest, pleasure, appetite, and sleep. **Psychotic depression** is the next most common form, and these patients experience delusions or hallucinations. **Atypical depression**, the third subtype, is characterized by increased levels of sleep and appetite, along with a fear of rejection.

Major depressive disorder (MDD) is a common syndrome comprised of 1 or more major depressive episodes defined by strict DSM-IV-TR criteria, with no history of mania or hypomania. A major depressive episode must last at least 2 weeks, and include either depressed mood or decreased ability to experience pleasure, as well as 4 or more of the following symptoms; fatigue, difficulty concentrating, weight change, sleep disturbance, psychomotor disturbance, anhedonia, feelings of worthlessness or guilt, and recurrent suicidality. MDD has a lifetime prevalence of 10–20%, with women being affected twice as often as men. Approximately 50% of affected individuals will have recurring symptoms. Patients with depression often have a family history of depression (and substance abuse), and the monoamine hypothesis suggests that low levels of NE, 5HT, and dopamine are responsible for the symptoms. Treatment primarily consists of psychotherapy and pharmacologic antidepressants, with electroconvulsive therapy reserved for severe refractory cases.

Subtypes of antidepressants include monoamine oxidase (MAO) inhibitors, tricyclic antidepressants (TCAs), and selective serotonin-reuptake inhibitors (SSRIs). **MAO inhibitors** are the oldest of the antidepressant medications, but are not typically used as first-line agents

Signs of depression
SIG E CAPS =
Suicidal ideation,
Interest decrease,
Guilt, **E**nergy decrease,
Concentration decrease,
Appetite change,
Psychomotor change,
Sleep disturbances

because of their many side effects. By inhibiting the enzyme monoamine oxidase, they block metabolism and therefore increase levels of NE, 5HT, and dopamine. **Hypertensive crisis** can occur when these drugs are taken together with tyramine-containing foods. **Tricyclic antidepressants (TCAs)** are also older drugs that were previously the mainstay of treatment for depression. Their mechanism involves inhibition of norepinephrine and serotonin reuptake. TCAs are inexpensive but have numerous side effects, including sedation, weight gain, orthostatic hypotension, withdrawal syndrome, and cardiotoxicity in overdose. Today TCAs have largely been replaced by **selective serotonin-reuptake inhibitors (SSRIs)**, drugs that only block the reuptake of serotonin and have a more favorable side effect profile. While SSRIs cause more sexual dysfunction and GI side effects, they are safer in overdose and lack the anticholinergic effects and cardiotoxicity. **Serotonin syndrome** is a life-threatening interaction between SSRIs and MAO inhibitors, characterized by muscle rigidity, myoclonus, fever, seizures, and hemodynamic instability.

TCAs can have lethal cardiotoxicity in overdose.

Agent	Mechanism	Side effect/Toxicity
Monoamine oxidase (MAO) inhibitors Isocarboxazid Phenelzine Selegiline Tranylcypromine	Blocks metabolism of monoamines (e.g., norepinephrine, serotonin, dopamine) by enzyme inhibition	Hypotension, hyperthermia, agitation, seizures, hepatotoxicity, hypertensive crisis when taken with foods containing tyramine (e.g., wine, cheese)
Tricyclic Antidepressants (TCAs) Nortriptiyline Amitriptyline Desipramine Clomipramine	Blocks reuptake of serotonin and norepinephrine at receptor	Sedation, dry mouth, weight gain; orthostatic hypotension, overdose cardiotoxicity; additive CNS depression with other drugs
Selective serotonin-reuptake inhibitors (SSRIs) Fluoxetine Sertraline Paroxetine Citalopram Escitalopram	Selectively blocks reuptake of serotonin at receptor	Nausea, vomiting, diarrhea, dizziness, insomnia, headache, decreased libido, male impotence
Miscellaneous agents Bupropion	Unknown	Induces P-450 enzymes; seizures, minimal anticholinergic effects

Table 6 Antidepressants

Dysthymic disorder is a chronic condition lasting more than 2 years in which patients experience continuous symptoms of depressed mood, poor self-esteem, and additional symptoms of depression that do not meet criteria for major depressive disorder. Treatment involves psychotherapy.

Adjustment disorder is a much less specific condition where an excessive emotional or behavioral response occurs after a stressful life event (divorce, loss of job, medical illness). Symptoms must occur within 3 months of the stressful event and disappear within 6 months of the end of the stressor. Note that the stressor in adjustment disorder is less severe than that of PTSD and acute stress disorder.

Mania symptoms
DIG FAST
Distractibility, **I**ndiscretion, **G**randiosity, **F**light of ideas, **A**ctivity increase, **S**leep change, **T**alkativeness

Mania is characterized by a period of elevated, expansive, or irritable mood, during which patients may have increased energy, decreased need for sleep, flight of ideas, and pressured speech. They often have feelings of increased productivity and creativity, and may experience euphoria, increased self-esteem, delusions, and hallucinations. As a result they often engage in dangerous activities. Manic episodes last more than 1 week and cause significant disability. Treatments include lithium and valproic acid.

Hypomania is a shorter manic episode that lasts less than 4 days and typically does not cause disability. Treatment is lithium as well.

Bipolar Disorder is characterized by marked mood swings between mania (mood elevation) and depression that result in significant personal distress or social dysfunction. Onset is usually in adolescence and early adulthood, and there is an increased risk of disability and suicide. To make the diagnosis, medical illness, other psychiatric disorders, and substance abuse must be ruled out. **Bipolar Type I disorder** is diagnosed when episodes of depression are interspersed with mania or mixed episodes. **Bipolar Type II disorder** is diagnosed when depression is interspersed with less severe episodes of elevated mood that do not lead to dysfunction or disability (hypomania). **Rapid cycling bipolar disorder** is characterized by 4 episodes of any combination of mania and depression within a 1 year period. Treatment for bipolar disorder includes hospitalization and first line mood stabilizing medications such as lithium and certain anticonvulsants (valproic acid, carbamazepine, lamotrigine). Several atypical antipsychotics and antidepressants are used as well. The mechanism of lithium is not completely understood, but it decreases the symptoms of mania, as well as frequency and severity of mood swings. Adverse side effects are common and include edema, tremor, sedation, ataxia, aphasia, leukocytosis, diabetes insipidus, and teratogenicity. Antidepressant medications are associated with a high risk of **antidepressant induced mania (AIM)** and rapid cycling. For this reason they should only be taken in conjunction with a mood stabilizer.

Lithium levels need to be monitored regularly because of the many side effects (edema, tremor, sedation, ataxia, aphasia, leukocytosis, diabetes insipidus, and teratogenicity).

Watch out for opposite mood swing after administration of medication.

Cyclothymia is a chronic, blunted version of bipolar disorder, lasting at least 2 years, in which the patient experiences short cycles of mild depression and hypomania. There is usually no significant impairment in functioning, but euthymia does not last greater than 2 months. Treatment for this condition is with lithium and antidepressants.

ANXIETY DISORDERS

Anxiety disorders are characterized by generalized uncomfortable emotional states (anxiety) or persistent or irrational fears (phobias). They are believed to be multifactorial, with components of genetic predisposition, learned responses, and environment. Abnormalities in the GABA receptor have been implicated because many effective anxiolytics (benzodiazepines) work at this site.

Phobias: The list is quite long, but some important ones are mentioned below. Treatment includes psychotherapy, behavior modification, and drugs for somatic symptoms.

Agoraphobia entails a fear of being caught in a situation in which one cannot escape, leading to embarrassment and panic. Common examples of such situations include elevators and supermarkets. Often there is an associated feeling of being closed in and crowded by other people.

Social phobia is characterized by a persistent fear of scrutiny, embarrassment, and humiliation in social situations. Common examples include parties or public speaking.

Specific phobia entails a fear of a very specific thing, such as blood, heights, or animals.

Panic disorder is characterized by recurrent, unpredictable panic attacks that consist of episodes of fear and anxiety accompanied by feelings of impending doom. Physical symptoms include palpitations, tachycardia, trembling, dizziness, nausea, and chest pain. General medical conditions, other mental disorders, and drugs must be ruled out. Patients will have at least 1 month of persistent worry about having another panic attack, and may even change their behavior to avoid them. This disorder is more common in women, and frequently begins in adolescence and early adulthood. Treatment is with anxiolytics (benzodiazepines).

PANIC disorder
Palpitations,
Anxiety,
Nausea,
Impending doom,
Chest pain

Generalized anxiety disorder (GAD) is characterized by persistent and excessive anxiety or worry over many different activities and events that occurs on most days for at least 6 months and interferes with daily activities. These patients may complain of difficulty concentrating, trembling, restlessness, fatigue, muscle tension, insomnia, tachycardia, dry mouth, and increased vigilance. As with panic disorder, incidence is higher in women. Treatment includes buspirone, antidepressants (SSRIs), anxiolytic (benzodiazepines), and cognitive behavioral therapy (exposure, relaxation, cognitive restructuring).

Post-traumatic Stress Disorder (PTSD) is characterized by recurrent nightmares, vivid recollections, and flashbacks of a psychologically traumatic event (war, assault, rape) that lead to hypervigilance, irritability, emotional numbing, and avoidance behavior. The symptoms are disabling and must last for more than 1 month after the event. Of note, many of these patients will self-medicate with substance abuse. Treatment includes cognitive behavioral therapy (desensitization) and antidepressants (SSRIs).

Acute stress disorder is similar to PTSD, but this diagnosis can only be given within the first month after a major traumatic event. There's also more emphasis on symptoms of dissociation, such as emotional numbing, reduced awareness, and depersonalization. Many but not all of these patients will go on to have PTSD. Treatment is also with psychotherapy and antidepressants (SSRIs).

Obsessive-compulsive disorder involves repetitive obsessions (unwanted thoughts, ideas, or feelings) that cause anxiety and result in the patient performing compulsions (repetitive mental acts or behaviors) that relieve the anxiety. Common examples include checking, counting, and fear of germs with excessive washing. Symptoms cause significant distress or interfere with daily activities, and are not due to medical illness or drug use. The patient is usually aware that the behavior is abnormal. Onset typically occurs in adolescence to the 30s, and treatment includes cognitive behavioral therapy and antidepressants (SSRIs).

SOMATIZATION

Somatization is a process where patients will consciously or unconsciously use physical illness for some personal gain. **Primary gain** refers to an internal benefit, such as relief from emotional conflict or unpleasant feelings. For example an injury may prevent the patient from having to face a fear at home or work. **Secondary gain** refers to more tangible benefits, such as attention, affection, financial gain, or access to drugs.

Somatoform Disorders

These disorders all have in common an unconscious use of physical illness for personal gain. Patients are completely unaware they are doing this and may be quite resistant to such suggestion.

Somatization disorder is characterized by recurrent complaints of multiple vague symptoms, beginning before age 30, lasting for several years, and causing significant impairment. The symptoms often involve 2 or more GI symptoms, 4 pain symptoms in different sites, and GU as well as neurological complaints. This disorder is much more common in women and may lead to frequent trips to the doctor. Medical disease and substance abuse must be ruled out prior to making the diagnosis. Management includes establishing continuity of care, to limit the number of unnecessary tests and eventually help the patient develop insight as to the problem.

Conversion disorder is characterized by neurologic dysfunction (sensorimotor deficits) with no identifiable organic pathology after appropriate evaluation. Common symptoms include paralysis, blindness, deafness and seizures. This disorder is also more common in women, often occurring after an acute stress. Treatment is supportive, and symptoms usually resolve quickly.

Hypochondriasis is characterized by an abnormal preoccupation with minor symptoms and fear of the possibility of serious disease. Physical symptoms may be accompanied by signs of anxiety or depression. This disorder occurs equally in men and women, and tends to begin in middle age or later. Establishing a good therapeutic alliance is important.

Body dysmorphic disorder is characterized by persistent preoccupation with a perceived physical defect. There is an underlying fear of rejection and humiliation. These patients will frequently surface in plastic surgery clinics.

Factitious Disorders and Malingering

In contrast to somatiform disorder, these disorders involve the voluntary faking of physical symptoms or illness for some primary or secondary gain. The patients are well aware of what they are doing.

Factitious disorder is characterized by the faking of symptoms in order to assume the "sick role." It is more common in younger adults, with a female predominance. The classic example is a health care worker who secretly self injects insulin to become hypoglycemic. These patients are at increased risk for unnecessary procedures and operations. They require psychiatric evaluation because they are unable to control their behavior.

Munchausen syndrome by proxy is characterized by a caretaker faking or creating illness in the person for whom they are caring. The classic example is a young mother with a "sick" child.

Malingering is characterized by intentional faking of symptoms for secondary gain. Common examples are falsely made up work injuries used to obtain disability benefits.

PERSONALITY DISORDERS

Personality disorders (Axis II) are inflexible and maladaptive personality traits that cause significant impairment in social or occupational functioning. They usually manifest in adolescence and continue throughout adulthood. These disorders are divided into 3 different clusters based on similar traits. Treatment involves psychotherapy, and is often unsuccessful.

Cluster A

Subtypes in this group feature suspicious, odd or eccentric behavior that interferes with social functioning. There is a genetic link to schizophrenia.

Paranoid personality disorder is characterized by a pattern of pervasive mistrust and suspicion of others, with no real basis.

Schizoid personality disorder is characterized by a pattern of detachment from social relationships and limited range of emotional expression. Patients usually have cold, introverted personalities and are self-absorbed loners with no desire for friendship. In contrast to schizotypal personality disorder there is no abnormal thought content.

Schizotypal personality disorder is characterized by impaired social interaction, "magical thinking," eccentric appearance, and odd behavior.

Cluster B

Subtypes in this group feature hostile, unstable, emotional, and self-entitled behaviors. There is a genetic link to mood disorders.

Antisocial personality disorder: disregard for the rights of others, beginning in childhood. It is more common in males, those in lower socioeconomic circles, and among prison inmates.

Borderline personality disorder is characterized by unstable relationships and self-image, along with impulsivity and inappropriate anger. These patients are preoccupied with abandonment.

Histrionic personality disorder is characterized by excessive emotionality and attention-seeking behavior, accompanied by dysphoria with loss or rejection. Examples include sexually provocative dress and seductive behavior.

Narcissistic personality disorder is characterized by a grandiose sense of self-importance, need for admiration, sensitivity to criticism, and lack of empathy. These individuals tend to be high achievers.

Cluster C

Subtypes in this group feature fearful, anxious, and clinging behavior. There is a genetic link to anxiety disorders.

Avoidant personality disorder is characterized by social discomfort, fear of rejection, and marked timidity that may lead to depression, anger, anxiety, and failure to develop relationships.

Dependent personality disorder is characterized by an excessive need to be taken care of that leads to submissiveness, clinging behavior, and fear of separation.

Obsessive-compulsive personality disorder is characterized by a preoccupation with orderliness, perfectionism, and interpersonal control. This is different from Obsessive Compulsive Disorder (OCD), where obsessions and compulsions are not necessarily related to neatness and disorder).

EGO DEFENSES

Ego defenses are ways that everyone, including normal people, deal with reality. They are classified based on the stage of development in which they are used.

Narcissistic Defenses

Narcissistic defenses are the earliest defense mechanisms, typically used by young children to preserve their idealized sense of self and avoid painful feelings.

Denial is characterized by a refusal to acknowledge a negative event, such as a fatal medical diagnosis. In psychotic patients denial may be replaced by fantasy.

Distortion is characterized by extreme reshaping or reinterpretation of events. This may accompany wish-fulfilling delusions.

Primitive idealization and **splitting** involve the classification of things as either all good or all bad. Splitting is frequently seen in patients with borderline personality disorder.

Projection is characterized by the transfer of unacceptable traits or feelings to an outside source—for example, an unfaithful husband accusing his wife of infidelity.

Immature Ego Defenses

Acting out involves the expression of unconscious or unacceptable wishes by immediate action. Typically this takes the form of extreme immediate misbehavior.

Blocking entails the inhibition of a feeling. Blocking is similar to repression, but involves more feelings of tension.

Hypochondriasis is characterized by transference of feelings of reproach and shame towards others into personal complaints of somatic pain. May coexist with depression or anxiety disorders.

Identification and **introjections** are characterized by feelings of similar identity with another person, out of guilt or love. For example, a victim of domestic abuse may begin to identify with her spouse.

Passive-aggressive behavior is characterized by passivity and indirect behavior instead of open confrontation of reality. For example, an employee may make a poor effort instead of telling his boss he refuses to do an assigned task.

Regression involves reverting back to an earlier developmental stage. A classic example is bedwetting in older children during periods of stress.

Schizoid fantasy is characterized by the use of isolated fantasy to avoid conflict resolution.

Somatization is characterized by the conversion of unresolved conflicts into somatic symptoms. This is not the same as somatization disorder.

Turning against self involves the redirection of unacceptable urges away from the original target and towards oneself—for example causing injury to oneself instead of hurting others.

Neurotic Defenses

Neurotic defenses are seen in OCD and persons with mild personality disorders. They are also used by normal adults under stressful conditions.

Controlling is characterized by excessive management to avoid anxiety. Examples include tight scheduling and over-planning of treatment.

Displacement involves the unconscious shifting of feelings to another object. For example, feelings of anger towards a boss can instead be displaced onto a family member.

Doing and undoing entail taking a symbolic, unacceptable action, and then taking the opposite action.

Inhibition describes a limitation of actions to avoid anxiety or conflict.

Intellectualization uses overanalysis to achieve emotional control—for example, thinking about and mentally defending actions to avoid feelings.

Isolation entails the separation of feelings from ideas. This may involve repression or displacement as well.

Rationalization is characterized by the use of justification with reasons for actions performed that would otherwise be unacceptable—for example, arguing that special treatment for a friend would have happened anyway.

Reaction formation is when an unacceptable impulse is transformed into its opposite and becomes a character trait—for example, a person is very nice to someone with whom she is angry.

Repression describes the unconscious withholding of an idea or feeling—for example, forgetting the anniversary of a loved one's death. Contrast with the more conscious suppression.

Sexualization is when sexual significance is attributed to someone to avoid personal impulses— for example, calling someone "promiscuous" to avoid dealing with attraction to him or her.

Mature Defenses

Mature defenses are considered normal adaptive functioning.

Altruism is characterized by spontaneous generosity to others, resulting in relief of guilt.

Anticipation entails overconcern about the future to allay anxiety. In this situation a person may dwell obsessively on all the positive and negative outcomes.

Asceticism involves the elimination of pleasurable activities, objects, and states of being. For example, a person may achieve gratification by renouncing riches, fame, and sexuality.

Humor is characterized by making light of difficult situations to avoid feelings of pain—for example, joking about a seriously ill patient.

Sublimation is used to obtain gratification of an inappropriate impulse through a more acceptable channel. For example, feelings of competitiveness with classmates can be redirected to sports.

Suppression is the conscious decision to not focus on a stressful idea or feeling—for example, trying not to think about an upcoming test in an effort to enjoy a party. Contrast with unconscious repression.

TRANSFERENCE AND COUNTERTRANSFERENCE

Transference is a phenomenon where a patient unconsciously redirects feelings to the physician/therapist. **Countertransference** refers to a similar phenomenon where the physician/therapist redirects feelings to the patient. For example, the therapist may remind the patient of his mother.

ABUSE

Child abuse is a general term that refers to child neglect (intentional failure to provide basic necessities) as well as physical, sexual, psychological, or emotional mistreatment of children. It is a grossly underreported problem, and over 1000 children in the U.S. die each year. In cases of **physical abuse**, children may have a history of multiple ER visits and typically present with multiple injuries and vague explanations. Examples include retinal detachment, suspicious burn injuries, multiple bruises, and multiple fractures of different ages. In cases of **sexual abuse**, the offender, who is typically known to the victim, uses the child for sexual stimulation. Many children will deny abuse out of fear of repercussions. Look for sexually transmitted disease and genitoanal trauma as possible evidence. Any suspected child abuse MUST be reported to local authorities.

Spousal abuse is another common and underreported problem. Domestic abuse is the leading cause of injury to women. Every 9 seconds in the US a woman is assaulted. Approximately half of injured women seen in the ER are victims of abuse. The abuse may be part of a chronic maladaptive relationship between partners. The abusing spouse may have an accompanying substance abuse problem, and it is not uncommon for victims to blame themselves for "rocking the boat," which leads to underreporting. Look for a pattern of repetitive, unexplained injuries, sometimes concentrated in areas of the body that are hidden by clothing. Try to document with photos if possible. Most states require reporting to the police. In addition, offer support services and shelter information, whenever the victim is ready.

Elder abuse usually takes the form of neglect rather than trauma, and is also an underreported problem. Look for signs of neglect such as dehydration and malnourishment. If you have a suspicion, you MUST report it to the authorities.

SUICIDE

Suicide is the intentional taking of one's life. There are over 1 million suicides per year in the US. The risk is highest in teens and young adults, with whites being the most affected race. Women attempt suicide more than men, but often use methods that are not very effective (e.g., swallowing pills). In contrast, men actually commit suicide more often by using more definitive methods (e.g., guns). There are many risk factors, but hopelessness is a key feature. Always ask depressed patients about suicidal ideation and whether they have a plan or not. If you believe someone is a threat to themselves, admit them to the hospital, even against their will.

MEDICAL ETHICS

Medical ethics refers to the application of moral principles to the practice of medicine. The four major principles include respect for patient autonomy, beneficence, non-maleficence, and justice. **Patient autonomy** refers to the fact that the patient has the ultimate say in his or her healthcare, provided he or she is informed, has decision-making capacity, and is able to communicate that decision. Some people may choose to use **advance directives** to guide their care in the event of a serious medical illness. **Living wills** specify the individual's desire to withhold care in the event of terminal illness. **Durable power of attorney** specifies who the decision-maker will be in the event of an illness that prevents the patient from making their own decisions. **Beneficence** refers to the physician's responsibility to always keep the patient's best interests in mind. **Non-maleficence** refers to the physician's responsibility to do no harm to the patient. Finally, **justice** refers to fair distribution of health resources.

There are many ethical dilemmas where is not always possible to adhere to all four principles, but every effort must be made nonetheless. **Informed consent** refers to the physician's obligation to ensure the patient's understanding of risks and benefits prior to major medical decisions. In these cases, a patient may agree to a procedure despite risks of harm. **Confidentiality** refers to the physician's obligation to respect the patient's privacy and not disclose personal information without the patient's permission. In some cases, this confidentiality can be violated by the physician (e.g., if a patient says he's going to kill himself or another). It is legally allowed and required for the physician to warn others (Tarasoff v. Regents of the University of California, 17 Cal. 3d 425, 551 P.2d 334, 131 Cal. Rptr. 14 (Cal. 1976)).

SAD PERSONS
S: sex (male)
A: age (elderly or adolescent)
D: depression
P: previous attempt
E: ethanol abuse
R: rational thinking loss
S: social supports lacking
O: organized plan
N: no plan
S: sickness

CHAPTER 16

PUMONOLOGY & RESPITORY SYSTEM

ANATOMY

The Upper Airway

Along the path that air travels from the nose and mouth down to the lungs are several distinct regions that form a continuum (Figure 1):

- After hairs in the nose filter dust particles, air travels back to the **nasopharynx**. Important structures are pharyngeal tonsils and the openings for the eustachian (auditory) tubes.

- The **oropharynx** is continuous with the oral cavity and the nasopharynx at the level of the soft palate and hard palate. The palatine tonsils and uvula are found here.

- The **oral cavity** includes mainly the tongue and teeth.

- The **hypopharynx** (laryngopharynx) starts below the oropharynx, at the level of the epiglottis, leading directly into the larynx.

- The **epiglottis** is cartilage that closes off the trachea during swallowing (to prevent aspiration).

- The **vallecula** is the nook in front of the epiglottis and behind the tongue. It is medically important because it is the landmark for placing the blade of a laryngoscope when performing intubations.

- The vocal cords and arytenoids are found in the **larynx**, which continues down to the **cricoid cartilage**.

- The **cricothyroid membrane** is the anteromedial space below the thyroid cartilage (Adam's apple) and above the cricoid cartilage. This is where a catheter, scalpel, or even a hollow ballpoint pen shaft (as seen on TV) can be inserted to establish an emergency surgical airway.

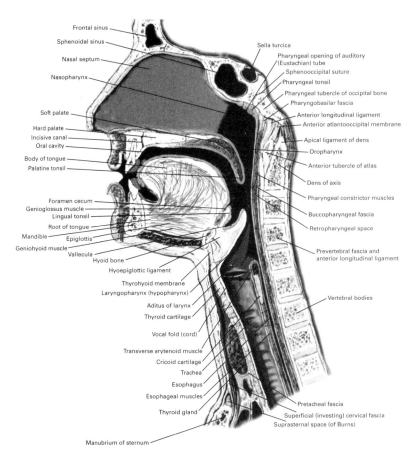

Frontal sinus
Sphenoidal sinus
Nasal septum
Nasopharynx
Soft palate
Hard palate
Incisive canal
Oral cavity
Body of tongue
Palatine tonsil
Foramen cecum
Genioglossus muscle
Lingual tonsil
Root of tongue
Mandible
Epiglottis
Geniohyoid muscle
Vallecula
Hyoid bone
Hyoepiglottic ligament
Thyrohyoid membrane
Laryngopharynx (hypopharynx)
Aditus of larynx
Thyroid cartilage
Vocal fold (cord)
Transverse arytenoid muscle
Cricoid cartilage
Trachea
Esophagus
Esophageal muscles
Thyroid gland
Manubrium of sternum

Sella turcica
Pharyngeal opening of auditory (Eustachian) tube
Sphenooccipital suture
Pharyngeal tonsil
Pharyngeal tubercle of occipital bone
Pharyngobasilar fascia
Anterior longitudinal ligament
Anterior atlantooccipital membrane
Apical ligament of dens
Oropharynx
Anterior tubercle of atlas
Dens of axis
Pharyngeal constrictor muscles
Buccopharyngeal fascia
Retropharyngeal space
Prevertebral fascia and anterior longitudinal ligament
Vertebral bodies
Pretacheal fascia
Superficial (investing) cervical fascia
Suprasternal space (of Burns)

Figure 1 Anatomy of the upper airway
(Adapted from *Atlas of Human Anatomy*)

- The tracheal cartilage rings are C-shaped and open in the back, except the **cricoid cartilage**, which is the only ring that completely encircles the trachea.

- **Trachea**: Below the cricoid cartilage, the larynx becomes the trachea proper (Figure 2).

- **Mucociliary escalator**: Traps and propels phlegm back up.

- **Carina**: The bifurcation of the trachea into the right and left main stem bronchi, takes place approximately at the level of the 4th Thoracic vertebrae (T4) and the angle of Louis (the palpable junction manubrium and body of the sternum). Can be used as a point of reference on a CT scan.

- **Bronchi**: The left main stem bronchus branches off at a sharp angle and sits above the heart. The right main stem bronchus is almost a straight shot downward compared to the left main stem. Aspiration is therefore more common on the right, specifically in the right upper lobe, because it's the dependent lobe in supine patients. For the same reason, inadvertent right main stem intubation is a common error.

- **Bronchioles and terminal bronchioles**: Further bifurcations of the bronchi, which lead eventually to the lung's functional unit, the terminal respiratory unit. Smooth muscle in the walls reacts to irritation.

- **Terminal respiratory unit**: Contains terminal bronchioles and their associated alveoli, like a bunch of grapes on a stem.

- **Alveolus**: The little air sac responsible for gas exchange; up to the alveoli, the whole system is a big air conduit (dead space) or a set of pipes to transport air.

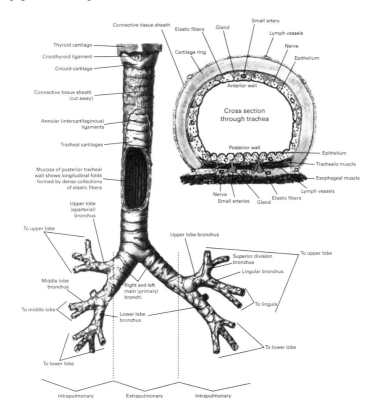

Figure 2 Trachea and major bronchi

It takes approximately **16 generations** of bifurcations in the bronchial tree to reach terminal bronchioles and the respiratory exchange units.

Lung Anatomy

- The right lung has three **lobes**; the left has two (think of it as the heart taking up the space of the left lung's third lobe) (Figure 3).

- In the left lung, the **major** or **oblique fissure** divides the upper and lower lobes. The left upper lobe has a **lingula** (literally, tongue).

- In the right lung, the **major fissure** divides the lower lobe from the other two lobes. The **horizontal** or **minor fissure** divides the right upper and middle lobes.

- Each lung can then be further divided into 10 segments. The names and locations of these are beyond the scope of the USMLE but are important clinically. For instance, a pulmonologist can localize a lung mass to a specific segment via bronchoscopy to guide surgical resection.

On chest X-ray, extra pleural fluid (e.g. CHF, interstitial lung disease) can sometimes be seen tracking into these fissures. Interstitial fluid in the segmental fissures produce **Kerley B lines** on chest X-ray.

- Each lung is anchored at the **hilum** (plural = hila), which is where all the lung's plumbing comes in and out (this is a common anatomic theme: nerves, arteries, veins, lymphatics, and other conduits conveniently tend to travel together). Lymph nodes are found here, too.

- Like most other internal organs, the lung is encased in **visceral pleura**, which is contiguous with the **parietal pleura** that lines the chest wall. The pleural space is a potential space between the two pleural layers. This is the space that pathologically fills with air (in a pneumothorax), or fluid (in CHF).

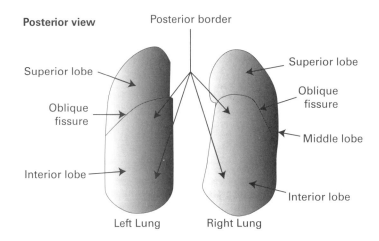

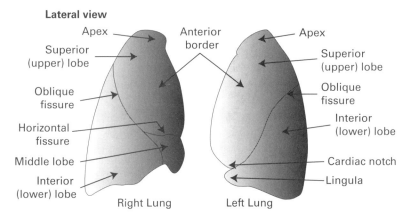

Figure 3 Lobes and fissures of the lungs

Vasculature

- **Pulmonary circulation**: Pulmonary arteries carry deoxygenated blood through the lungs for air exchange in the capillary bed, after which it leaves through the pulmonary veins. Unlike most other arterial vessels, the pulmonary arterial system is thin walled and more elastic than muscular. This quality, along with the vast branching of pulmonary arteries into capillaries, makes for a low-resistance circuit.

- **Bronchial circulation**: The bronchial arteries are small branches that come directly off the aorta to supply oxygenated blood to the pleura and airway walls. Some of this blood returns to the heart via the pulmonary veins, so some deoxygenated blood is dumped into the systemic circulation, resulting in a **shunt** (described later, under "Physiology").

- **Lymphatics**: Important for staging cancers of the lung because most lung tumors spread via lymphatics.

EMBRYOLOGY

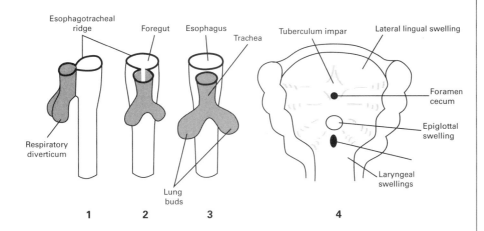

Figure 4 Early lung development

Development

The respiratory system develops from the ventral wall of the primitive **foregut** (Figure 4). The epithelium of the larynx, trachea, bronchi, and alveoli derive from **endodermal** tissue, whereas the cartilaginous and muscular tissue comes from the **mesoderm**. At 4 weeks of development, the **esophagotracheal septum** forms, dividing the lungs and trachea from the foregut. The larynx is formed from tissues of the fourth and sixth pharyngeal arches. Abnormalities in development can lead to the formation of **tracheoesophageal (T-E) fistulas**, which present with non-bilious vomiting, polyhydramnios, abdominal distention, and aspiration.

The lung buds form into three lobes on the right and two on the left (Figure 5). After about 17 weeks, the alveolar epithelial cells begin to form. Gas exchange is possible after about 32 weeks' gestation. Alveoli continue to develop during this period and even up to 10 years of age!

Type C T-E fistulas are the most common type, in which the proximal esophagus ends as a blind pouch, while the distal esophagus comes off the trachea.

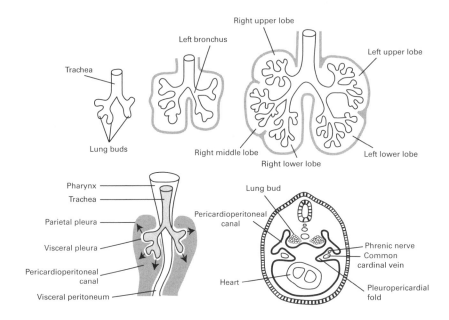

Figure 5 Later lung development

Fetal Maturation and Perinatal Changes

In the developing fetus, blood flow through the pulmonary vessels is minimal because the collapsed lungs form a high-resistance circuit. **Surfactant**, the substance that decreases surface tension and prevents collapse of the alveoli, is not produced until approximately 24–26 weeks' gestation. Babies born earlier than this develop **neonatal respiratory distress syndrome** (RDS), discussed later in the chapter.

In the newborn, clamping the umbilical cord (containing the umbilical artery and veins) leads to dramatic changes in the circulation. Blood flow increases markedly in the pulmonary circulation, which now becomes a low-resistance circuit after lung expansion and the baby's first breaths.

HISTOLOGY

The upper airway is characterized by the presence of tall, pseudostratified columnar, ciliated cells (larynx, trachea) required for the mucociliary escalator that is responsible for removing foreign material and debris. There is then a gradual transition to simple cuboidal cells (terminal bronchioles). Finally the types of cells found in the respiratory exchange units (alveoli) are as follows:

- **Type I pneumocytes**: The alveolar lining cells that form part of the gas diffusion barrier.

- **Type II pneumocytes**: Thicker, granulated cells that secrete surfactant. These cells also possess mitotic activity, replacing both Type I and Type II cells after damage.

- **Fenestrated endothelial cells** of the capillary wall.

- **Alveolar macrophages (dust cells)**: These cells, like other monocyte-derived cells, phagocytize debris nearby.

- **Smooth muscle**: Found in the mucosal layer, it becomes more prominent as the airway diameter decreases. It is thought that spasm in the smooth muscle is a major factor in **reactive airway disease** (RAD), asthma, and **chronic obstructive pulmonary disease** (COPD).

- Sympathetic tone (e.g., during stress or exercise) activates b-adrenergic receptors in these cells, leading to smooth muscle relaxation and airway opening for greater air movement. This is why inhaled b-agonists, such as albuterol, are given to wheezing asthmatics and patients with COPD.

- Cholinergic activity induces smooth muscle constriction; therefore, inhaled anticholinergic drugs (e.g., ipratropium) open airways and dry out secretions.

Hemosiderin-laden macrophages can be visualized with a Prussian-blue stain in patients with left-sided heart failure (often called "heart failure cells")

PHYSIOLOGY

Diffusion in the Lung

Air moves by bulk flow from the nose to terminal bronchioles. After that, air moves by diffusion **Fick's law** (Figure 6) can be used to calculate the rate of this process:

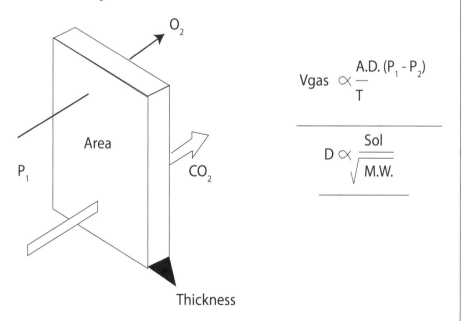

$$Vgas \propto \frac{A.D. (P_1 - P_2)}{T}$$

$$D \propto \frac{Sol}{\sqrt{M.W.}}$$

Figure 6 Representation of Fick's Law
(Adapted from *Respiratory Physiology—The Essentials*, 4th Edition)

In the lung, the total surface area is huge (50–100 m^2) and the thickness is very small, optimizing diffusion. The diffusion constant, D, depends on the solubility and molecular weight of a particular gas. Even though CO_2 and O_2 have similar molecular weights, CO_2 diffuses 20 times faster than O_2 because it is much more soluble.

Once an oxygen molecule arrives at an alveolus, it must pass through the gas exchange interface (Figure 7), which includes:

- Surfactant fluid layer

- Alveolar epithelium

- Interstitial space

- Capillary endothelium

- Blood plasma

- Erythrocyte membrane

After all this, the O_2 finally reaches the hemoglobin molecule The **interstitial space** is drained via lymphatics. Thickening of this space by either fluid (e.g., CHF) or fibrosis (e.g., interstitial lung disease) increases the gas diffusion barrier

Note that during resting conditions the normal inspiration-to-expiration ratio is greater than 1 : 2.

The innervation of the diaphragm is the phrenic nerve (from the roots of C3, C4, and C5) "C3, C4, C5 keeps the diaphragm alive"

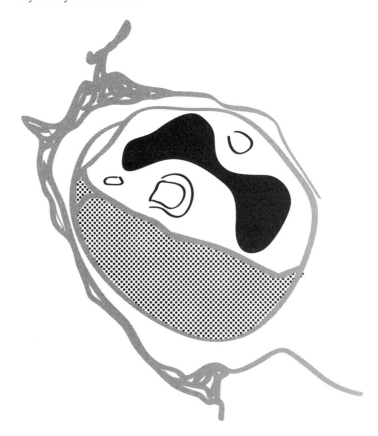

Figure 7 The alveolar gas exchange interface
(Adapted from *Respiratory Physiology—The Essentials*, 4th Edition)

Mechanics of Breathing

The lung is an elastic entity that expands during **inspiration** as a result of the negative pressure gradient generated by diaphragmatic contraction. **Expiration** is a passive event at rest. During exercise and stress, expiration is in part active, with the abdominal muscles and internal intercostal muscles taking part.

The components of chest wall mechanics include:

- **Diaphragm**: innervated by the phrenic nerve

- **Intercostal muscles**: stiffen the chest wall, preventing collapse of the chest wall during inspiration

- **External intercostals**: assist in inspiration

- **Internal intercostals**: assist in expiration

- **Accessory muscles** of respiration: scalene and sternocleidomastoid muscles, observed in patients in respiratory distress.

Other important concepts include the following:

- **Elastic recoil**: The rubbery nature of the lung (think of blowing up a balloon) creates resistance to lung expansion during inspiration, as does the resistance to airflow of the airways themselves.

- **Compliance**: How much the lung volume changes for a given change in pressure.

  o High compliance means that for a relatively small increase in inspiratory pressure, the lung volume expands a lot.

  o Low compliance implies "stiff" lungs that requires relatively large increases in inspiratory pressure for a given degree of expansion.

- **Surfactant**: The law of Laplace describes the effect of alveolar surface tension as a function of radius. Surfactant is an amphipathic phospholipid that helps decrease this surface tension. Without surfactant, surface tension between larger and smaller alveoli would be the same, causing smaller alveoli to experience greater pressures and collapse.

- **Hysteresis**: As in Figure 8, the lung's pressure-volume curve is different for inspiration than for expiration. On expiration, at any given pressure, the lung volume is greater than on inspiration, implying that more alveoli are open. This is a result of surfactant's effect on reducing surface tension.

- Airway resistance peaks in the segmental bronchi (about the fifth generation of divisions).

Emphysematous lungs, with lots of interstitial tissue loss, are highly compliant, whereas the fibrotic lungs of interstitial lung disease have low compliance.

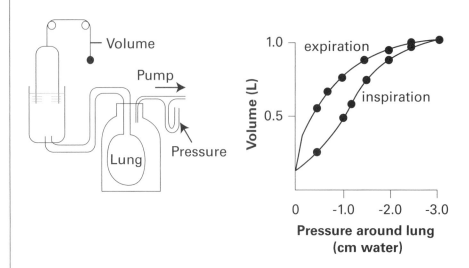

Figure 8 Pressure-volume relationship
(Adapted from *Respiratory Physiology—The Essentials*, 4th Edition)

Lung Volumes

$PaCO_2$ = arterial CO_2 (an approximation of $PACO_2$, alveolar CO_2)

$PECO_2$ = CO_2 in expired air.

$PECO_2$ is always less than $PaCO_2$

- **Tidal volume** (V_T): The volume of air inspired and expired during a normal breath, approximately 6–8 ml/kg body weight at rest (Figure 9).

- **Dead space** (V_D): The fraction of tidal volume taken up by dead space (and not involved in ventilation. About 150 ml, or 2 ml/kg body weight. Can be calculated using the **Bohr equation**:

$$V_D/V_T = (PaCO_2 - PECO_2)/(PaCO_2)$$

- **Anatomic dead space:** including air in the conducting airways that does not reach the alveoli.

- **Alveolar dead space:** the air which is used to ventilate alveoli which are not being perfused (in healthy individuals, this volume is negligible).

- **Inspiratory reserve volume** (IRV): After a normal inspiration, the amount of additional air that can be sucked in.

- **Expiratory reserve volume** (ERV): The volume that can be expired after a normal expiration, usually about 1,100 ml.

- **Residual volume** (RV): After exhaling all that can be exhaled, the volume of air remaining in the lungs. This volume cannot be measured directly by spirometry; a helium dilution technique or plethysmography must be used.

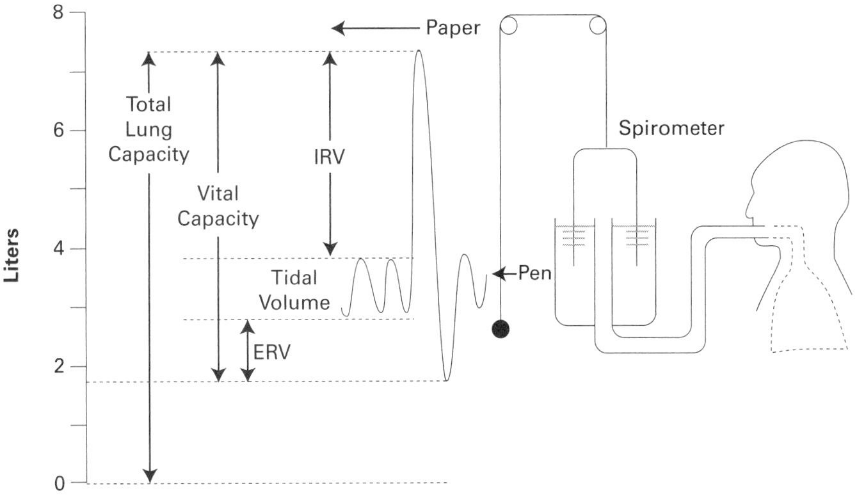

Figure 9 Representation of lung volumes
(Adapted from *Respiratory Physiology—The Essentials*, 4th Edition)

Lung Capacities

The term capacity refers to the sum of two or more volumes.

- **Functional residual capacity** (FRC): FRC = ERV + RV. The volume left in the lungs after normal expiration.

- **Inspiratory capacity** (IC): IC = V_T + IRV. The amount of air that can be sucked in after a normal expiration.

- **Vital capacity** (VC): VC = ERV + V_T + IRV.

- **Total lung capacity** (TLC): The whole shebang. TLC = RV + ERV + IRV + V_T.

Respiratory rate (RR) is usually described as breaths per minute (normal: 8–12). Minute ventilation (V_E) = RR × V_T is the total volume of air exchanged per minute (normal, 4–6 liters/minute).

Pulmonary Function Tests

Pulmonary function tests (PFTs) are done to measure lung volumes and are used clinically to diagnose a variety of pulmonary diseases, including obstructive, restrictive, and reactive airway disease. Because the lung cannot completely empty its air (the RV remains after complete exhalation), **spirometry**—in which the patient sucks and blows into a tube—cannot be used alone to calculate any capacity that includes RV (i.e. FRC & TLC). Instead, one of two techniques must be used:

- **Helium dilution technique** (Figure 10): The patient is hooked up to a spirometer. A known concentration of helium is introduced at the end of expiration (remember, the remaining volume is the FRC) and is breathed in by the patient (helium is not absorbed into the bloodstream, so the given quantity is constant). The helium mixes with the air in the patient's lungs and is diluted. The following equation, with the old and new concentrations of helium (C_1, C_2), gives the volume (V_2) in the patient's lungs:

$$C_1 \times V_1 = C_2 \times (V_1 + FRC)$$

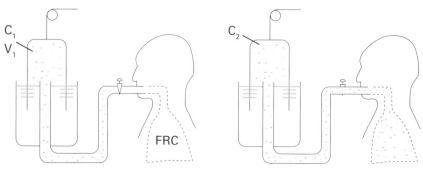

Before equilibration   After equilibration

$$C_1 \times V_1 = C_2 \times (V_1 + FRC)$$

Figure 10 Helium dilution technique
(Adapted from *Respiratory Physiology—The Essentials*, 4th Edition)

- **Body plethysmography** (Figure 11): Remember **Boyle's law**? It states that in a closed system, pressure (P) times volume (V) is a constant: $P_1 \times V_1 = P_2 \times V_2$. In this technique, the patient sits in an airtight booth and takes in a big breath against a closed mouthpiece. The lungs expand slightly, increasing lung volume and decreasing lung (intrapleural) pressure. As a result, the pressure increases as the volume of air in the box decreases slightly. These changes can be measured and plugged into Boyle's law, giving us the lung volume.

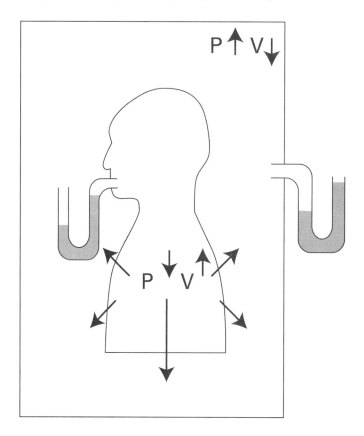

Figure 11 Body plethysmography
(P = pressure; V = volume; K = constant.)
(Adapted from *Respiratory Physiology—The Essentials*, 4th Edition)

Other PFTs are used to determine various characteristics of ventilation:

- **Forced expiration**: The subject inhales maximally and then exhales as hard as possible. The **forced expiratory volume** in one second (FEV_1) is then measured. The ratio between the FEV_1 and the **forced vital capacity** (FVC) (usually slightly less than the actual VC) is then calculated.

- A normal FEV_1/FVC is 0.8–1.0.

- In **restrictive** lung disease, both FEV_1 and FVC are decreased, so the ratio is normal or slightly increased (often with smaller volumes, it's easier to blow all the air out in 1 second)

- In **obstructive** lung disease, the FEV_1 is markedly reduced because the airway's resistance is increased (from the obstruction), whereas the FVC is decreased to a lesser extent. This makes the FEV_1-to-FVC ratio low in obstructive disease.

Obstructive lung disease	Restrictive lung disease

• Chronic obstructive pulmonary disease
 	
• Asthma
 	
• Obliterative bronchiolitis
 	
• Bronchiectasis
 	
• Cystic fibrosis
 	
• Upper airway obstruction
	• Parenchymal disease, including
	  o Interstitial lung disease
	  o Pulmonary edema
	  o Pneumonia
	  o Sarcoidosis (can also be obstructive)
	  o Pleuritis
	
	• Chest wall disease, including
	  o Neuromuscular disease (e.g., paralysis)
	  o Thoracic cage defects (e.g., scoliosis)
	  o Obesity

Table 1 Differential diagnosis of obstructive and restrictive lung diseases

Disease pattern	FEV_1	FVC	FEV_1/FVC	$FEF_{25–75\%}$	TLC
Normal	—	—	–0.8	—	—
Restrictive	↓	↓	— or ↑↑	↓	↓↓
Obstructive	↓↓	↓	↓↓	↓↓	— or ↑

FEV_1 = forced expiratory volume in 1 second; FVC = forced vital capacity; $FEF_{25–75\%}$ = forced expiratory flow mid-expiratory loop; TLC = total lung capacity.

Table 2 Lung volumes in obstructive and restrictive lung states

- **Flow-volume curves** provide a way to assess lung disease during PFTs (Figure 12). Inspiration and expiration are measured and plotted as flow versus lung volume. In restrictive disease, the flow pattern shows small flows and volumes, whereas in obstructive disease, the overall lung volume is large (due to chronic air trapping), but expiration ends prematurely. In addition, a scalloped appearance (coving) of the non-effort-dependent portion of expiration is usually seen. The forced expiratory flow in the middle of the expiratory loop ($FEF_{25-75}\%$) can also be measured. A decrease in the $FEF_{25-75}\%$ is a more sensitive indicator of obstructive disease (Table 2).

- Another important component of PFTs is bronchodilator response. Reactive airway disease (RAD) responds to bronchodilators, and as airways open up in response to bronchodilators, FEV_1 increases, thereby raising the FEV_1-to-FVC ratio. Values before and after bronchodilator use are then compared.

> Specifically, reactive airway disease is defined by a > 12% increase in FEV1/FVC ratio after giving a bronchodilator.

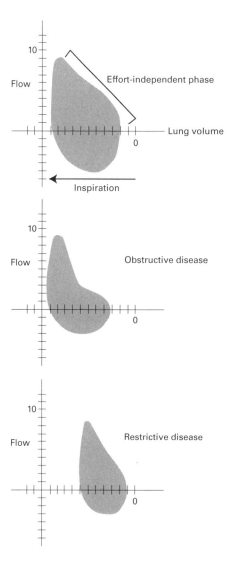

Figure 12 Flow-volume curves

- **Diffusion capacity**: The normal transit time for an RBC through the pulmonary capillaries is about 0.75 seconds.

- CO_2 rapidly diffuses between the alveoli and the bloodstream, so its transfer is limited by how fast the blood gets pumped through the capillaries (**perfusion-limited**)

- Carbon monoxide (CO) slowly equilibrates with the bloodstream, so its transfer is **diffusion-limited**.

- In PFTs, diffusion of carbon monoxide (DL_{CO}) is often measured to assess the diffusion capacity of the lungs.

- Oxygen is normally perfusion-limited, but in disease states that impair diffusion (e.g., interstitial pulmonary edema) O_2 transfer becomes diffusion-limited.

Alveolar Gas Exchange

Room air at sea level has a barometric pressure of 760 mm Hg. Air is 21% O_2, and the partial pressure of O_2 (PO_2) is simply this percentage multiplied by the barometric pressure after water vapor pressure has been subtracted. Because the lungs exchange both O_2 and CO_2 through the same airways and alveoli, the oxygen-rich inspired air mixes with the CO_2-rich air already in the alveoli at the end of expiration. Also, the air is humidified with H_2O, taking up space that O_2 cannot occupy (the partial pressure of H_2O [PH_2O] at body temperature is 47 mm Hg). With all these compounding factors, the **alveolar gas equation** determines how much O_2 actually ends up in the alveoli:

$$PAO_2 = (\text{Atmospheric pressure} - PH_2O) \times [FIO_2 - (PACO_2/RER)] = (760 - 47) \times [FIO_2 - (PACO_2/RER)$$

Where FIO_2 = fraction of inspired air that is oxygen, and RER (respiratory exchange ratio) = VCO_2/VO_2 which basically says that given normal metabolism, there is a constant ratio between the amount of O_2 consumed and CO_2 produced by the body, which is factored into the amount of CO_2 found in the alveoli. The RER depends on the primary fuel being used for metabolism; if the fuel source is carbohydrate, the RER is 1.0; if the fuel source is fat, the RER is 0.7. The RER on a typical Western diet pattern is estimated to be 0.8.

If we know the inspired O_2 content, the PAO_2, and if we simultaneously measure arterial O_2, the PaO_2 (via an arterial blood gas measurement), we can calculate the **alveolar-arterial O_2 gradient**—(A–a) O_2. This gradient, normally less than 15 mm Hg, is used clinically to determine how well a patient is able to deliver oxygen to the bloodstream.

Perfusion

The pulmonary circulation is a low-resistance circuit, in contrast to the systemic circulation. With the exception of the bronchial arteries, vessels are thin walled and elastic and not particularly muscular. Mixed venous blood (low O_2, high CO_2) from the right ventricle pumps into the pulmonary arterial system, eventually to a large capillary network. The blood then drains into the four pulmonary veins, which dump into the left atrium.

The pulmonary circulation is a **low-pressure system**. Note that the pulmonary vascular resistance (PVR) is normally markedly lower than the **systemic vascular resistance** (SVR). The lower afterload facing the right heart explains why the right ventricle is normally thinner and smaller than the left ventricle (LV).

The low pressure and low resistance of the right side mean that if the LV fails (fluid overload, myocardial infarction, valvulopathy), the pulmonary circulation "backs up" with fluid, and the increased hydrostatic pressure gradient causes fluid leak into the interstitium (Starling's equation). This leads to interstitial pulmonary edema, which can evolve into alveolar pulmonary edema, impairing pulmonary gas exchange.

There are several determinants of pulmonary vascular resistance:

- **Recruitment**: As pressures increase, capillary beds that are normally under-perfused start filling, which lowers the resistance.

- **Lung volume**: As the alveoli distend with more and more air, the capillaries imbedded within the alveolar walls are pulled taut, resulting in increased transmural pressures and therefore increased resistance to blood flow.

- **Hypoxia**: The lung vasculature is unique in that local hypoxia (reduction in PAO_2) in a particular area of the lung triggers constriction of that region's small arterioles, termed **hypoxic vasoconstriction**. This effectively draws blood flow away from areas of the lung that are not able to supply adequate O_2. In other words, the lung is always trying to maximize ventilation and perfusion $\dot{V}/\dot{Q}$ matching (discussed later). The mechanism is likely to be a local mediator acting on the smooth muscles of the arterioles.

Blood flow distribution is uneven throughout the lungs, and it depends on three pressures: alveolar air pressure (PA), arterial pressure (Pa), and venous pressure (Pv). Because gravity causes flow to be greater in the dependent portions of the lung, and aeration is also greater in the dependent portions of the lung, the relationship between these three pressures varies from top to bottom in the lung. The lung can therefore be divided into three distinct zones of perfusion (Figure 13):

Zone 1: Alveolar pressure dominates, blood flow is low: (PA > Pa > Pv).

Zone 2: Alveolar pressure is in the middle, therefore blood flow is determined by the difference between arterial and alveolar pressures: (Pa > PA > Pv).

Zone 3: Alveolar pressure is small compared to both arterial and venous pressures: (Pa > Pv > PA).

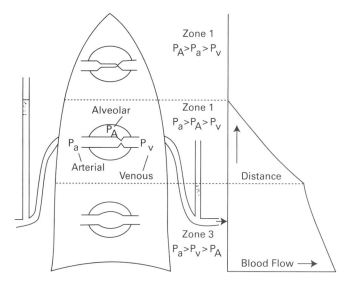

Figure 13 Zones of perfusion
(Adapted from *Respiratory Physiology—The Essentials,* 4th Edition)

To measure pulmonary blood flow, the **Fick method** can be used:

$$Q = \frac{VO_2}{(CaO_2 - Cv_{O2})}$$

where Q = blood flow VO_2 = O_2 consumption, CaO_2 = arterial O_2 concentration, and Cv_{O2}= mixed venous O_2 concentration.

A **shunt** is defined as blood flow through parts of the lung that are not ventilated. There are two important normal physiologic shunts (Bronchial and Thebesian vessels) in addition to a variety of pathological processes:

- **Bronchial vessels**: These supply the bronchi and pleura with blood but don't participate in gas exchange.

- **Thebesian vessels**: Coronary venous blood that directly dumps into the left ventricle.

  o Abnormal sources of shunt include the following:

  o Anatomic intracardiac shunts (e.g., atrial or ventricular septal defects)

- Intrapleural shunts (atrioventricular malformations, unventilated but perfused lung due to disease)

In the clinical setting, the differential diagnosis of a low PaO_2 (hypoxemia) found on arterial blood gas (ABG) includes hypoxia (low delivery of O_2 to the blood) and a shunt that prevents some blood from reaching the alveoli. These two possibilities can be distinguished by having the patient breathe 100% O_2. With pure hypoxia, the hypoxemia can be corrected, whereas in a significant shunt, the hypoxemia cannot be completely corrected (the shunted blood never sees the 100% O_2).

A clinically important concept is the ratio between ventilation and perfusion in the lung. The lungs are constantly trying to maintain an ideal ratio of ventilation/perfusion. If V/Q is too high, it implies that blood flow to ventilated lung is inadequate (i.e. in situations with increased dead space, such as a pulmonary embolus), whereas a V/Q that's too low indicates underventilated yet well-perfused lung (shunt). The V/Q ratio also depends on the region of lung being examined. Note that both blood flow and ventilation decrease toward the top of lung, but blood flow changes more rapidly with lung position, resulting in a higher V/Q ratio at the lung apex and a lower V/Q at the bases (Figure 14).

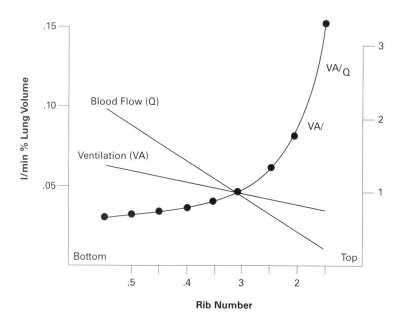

Figure 14 V/Q based on lung position
(Adapted from *Respiratory Physiology—The Essentials*, 4th Edition)

Gas Transport and the Bloodstream

Oxygen is transported in two forms: dissolved and bound to hemoglobin. The contribution of dissolved oxygen to total blood oxygen is very small. The relationship of oxygen bound to hemoglobin is described by the **O_2 dissociation curve** (Figure 15). Remember, the PO_2 can decrease to approximately 60–70 mm Hg while the O_2 saturation remains greater than 90%.

Note that most portable devices cannot distinguish between Hb bound to CO and Hb bound to O_2. Therefore, falsely elevated readings may be observed in carbon monoxide poison.

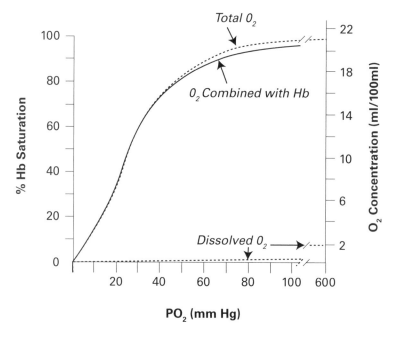

Figure 15 Oxygen-hemoglobin dissociation curve

A right shift in the curve implies that at any given PO_2, less O_2 is bound to hemoglobin, whereas a left shift implies that hemoglobin binds more tightly to O_2 at any given PO_2. A right shift occurs in the setting of increased temperature, increased 2,3- diphosphoglycerate, increased PO_2, or decreased pH (Figure 16).

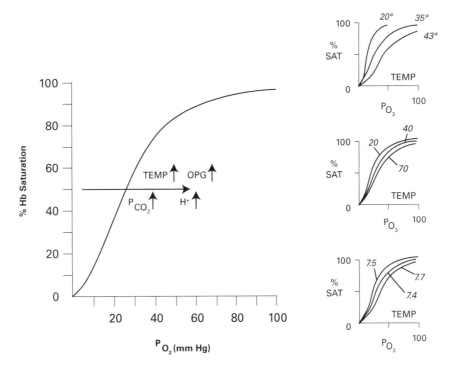

Figure 16 Factors influencing oxygen-hemoglobin dissociation curve
(Adapted from *Respiratory Physiology—The Essentials*, 4th Edition)

Essentially, the hemoglobin prefers to unload its O_2 more easily to the peripheral tissues in stressful situations (e.g., exercise, fever, chronic hypoxia).

The concentration of oxygen in the blood can be calculated as follows:

O_2 content of blood = $(1.39 \times Hg \times O_2\,sat/100) + 0.003 \times PO_2$

where Hb = hemoglobin concentration, O_2 sat = percentage of hemoglobin bound to O_2 (as measured by ABG or pulse oximetry), $PO_2 = O_2$ partial pressure (in mm Hg), 0.003 = solubility of O_2 in blood, and 1.39 = a correction factor.

A **pulse oximeter** is a simple little Band-Aid–like sensor attached to the patient's finger that reads out O_2 saturation and pulse rate. It uses two wavelengths of infrared light, which are modified by the amount of oxygenated or deoxygenated hemoglobin and used to calculate the O_2 saturation.

CO_2 is transported in three forms: dissolved, as bicarbonate, and bound to proteins.

- CO_2 is 20 times more soluble than O_2; therefore, 10% of CO_2 is found in dissolved form.

- Bicarbonate production is catalyzed by carbonic anhydrase via the following reaction

$$CO + H_2O \rightarrow H_2CO_3 \rightarrow H^+ + HCO_3^-$$

- Deoxygenated hemoglobin can chelate H^+ ions, thereby allowing more bicarbonate to form from CO_2; in other words, decreased O_2 facilitates the blood's CO_2^- carrying capacity. This is known as the **Haldane effect**.

Acid-Base Equilibrium

No discussion about CO_2 in the body is complete without reference to acid-base status. Because bicarbonate is the primary buffer system in the blood, blood pH is largely determined by the balance between PCO_2 and bicarbonate concentration, as expressed in the **Henderson-Hasselbalch equation** (pK_a = negative log of the equilibrium constant):

$$pH = pK_a + \log[HCO_3^-/0.03/PCO_2)]$$

Arterial Blood Gas Analysis

Some general principles of ABG analysis are as follows:

- In addition to the pH and pCO_2, PaO_2 is also measured in ABG analysis and is quite useful for evaluating hypoxia or the presence of a shunt.

- Two organ systems account for the maintenance of acid-base status in the body: the **lungs** and the **kidneys**.

- The lungs can breathe off or retain CO_2 by increasing or decreasing minute ventilation, respectively. This ultimately affects systemic pH through the titration of CO_2 with bicarbonate. When the lung is compensating for a systemic pH disturbance, it is most effective in acute (minutes to hours) situations.

- The kidneys can excrete more or less bicarbonate to maintain body pH. The kidney's compensation for acid-base disturbances is largely a chronic (hours to days) process.

- Normal pH is 7.40. The body tries to maintain this pH in the face of metabolic and or respiratory disorders that may force the pH from normal. A normal pH is necessary for maintaining cellular metabolic functions.

Changes in the various acid-base disorders are described in Table 3.

Condition	pH	PCO$_2$	Bicarbonate
Normal	7.40 (7.38–7.42)	40 (35–45)	24 (22–26)
Respiratory acidosis	< 7.40	> 4 0	Compensated ↑
Metabolic alkalosis	< 7.40	Compensated ↓	< 24
Respiratory alkalosis	> 7.40	< 40	Compensated ↓
Metabolic alkalosis	> 7.40	Compensated ↑	> 24

Table 3 Arterial blood gas analysis in acid-base disorders

Simultaneous acid-base disorders can coexist in one patient (up to three because respiratory acidosis and alkalosis cannot coexist). The algorithm for evaluating an ABG is as follows:

1. **Look at the pH**: This determines the primary disorder (< 7.40 means acidemia, > 7.40 means alkalemia).

2. **Look at the CO_2**: Is the primary disorder respiratory? For respiratory acidosis, $PaCO_2$ > 40 because CO_2 is retained; for respiratory alkalosis, $PaCO_2$ < 40 because CO_2 is blown off. Otherwise, the primary process is metabolic.

3. **Look for compensation**: There should be reciprocal changes in bicarbonate concentration or PCO_2 as a result of the primary disorder. However, a pH of 7.40 in the presence of an abnormal CO_2 or bicarbonate implies multiple acid-base disorders because the body cannot completely compensate and bring pH back to normal.

Acute respiratory acidosis can be caused by anything that decreases ventilation, including the following:

- Obstruction

- Aspiration

- Central nervous system (CNS) injury

- Narcotic overdose

- Suffocation

Chronic respiratory acidosis may be a result of COPD or chronic lung disease. Hyperventilation of any sort, leads to **respiratory alkalosis**.

If a metabolic acidosis is suggested **look at the anion gap** (AG):

$$AG = Na^+ - (Cl^- + HCO_3^-)$$

Normal anion gap is less than 12. Increased anion gap implies an **anion gap metabolic acidosis**. The way to remember causes of metabolic acidosis with an anion gap is with the mnemonic MUDPILES:

- **M**ethanol

- **U**remia

- **D**iabetic ketoacidosis

- **P**ara-aldehyde

- **I**ntoxication (ethanol)

- **L**actate (tissue hypoxia)

- **E**thylene glycol (antifreeze)

- **S**alicylates (aspirin)

If there's no increased anion gap in the presence of metabolic acidosis, then it's a **non-gap metabolic acidosis**. It can be caused by

- Diarrhea (lost HCO_3^-)

- Overzealous administration of normal saline (which is hyperchloremic and displaces HCO_3^-)

- Renal tubular acidosis

Finally, **metabolic alkalosis** may be caused by

- Vomiting (lost H^+)

- Overzealous bicarbonate administration

- Contraction alkalosis (with diuresis, distal tubule tries to compensate for lost volume by actively reabsorbing excreted Na^+ via an Na^+/H^+ exchanger, so H^+ is lost in the urine)

These determinations are made frequently on the wards, especially in the intensive care unit (ICU), and they factor into treatment decisions, so it's a real help to have a systematic approach to ABG analysis.

Physiologic Response to Exercise, Stress, and High-Altitude Physiology

Minute ventilation increases from 4–6 liters/minute at rest up to 100 liters/minute at maximal exertion on exercise, an increase of nearly 20 times! As a result, $PaCO_2$ usually decreases slightly, PaO_2 stays about the same, and pH stays the same or falls slightly from anaerobic lactate production.

With increased cardiac output, there is decreased transit time for the blood passing through the pulmonary circulation. Unless pulmonary disease is present, this shortened transit time is still adequate for maximal oxygenation.

REGULATION OF RESPIRATORY FUNCTION

Control of Respiration

There are both local and central controls of respiration:

- **Local**: Hypoxia promotes pulmonary vasoconstriction to optimize the V/Q ratio.

- **Central**: The brain stem contains the respiratory centers, where respiratory drive is thought to originate, specifically in the **reticular formation** of the medulla. The pneumotaxic center in the **pons** is thought to fine-tune the respiratory rate and tidal volume. Voluntary control from cortical input is possible, however limited.

- For example, it is easy to induce voluntary hyperventilation but much harder to induce voluntary hypoventilation (try holding your breath as long as possible!) because central stimuli to breathe related to hypercarbia and hypoxia take over.

Sensors of Respiration

There are both central and peripheral sensors of respiration:

- **Central chemoreceptors**: These are located in the medulla, surrounded by cerebrospinal fluid (CSF), and highly sensitive to H^+ con- centration (i.e., pH). Increased blood CO_2 allows CO_2 to cross the blood-brain barrier (via diffusion), lowering CSF pH as the CO_2 is converted to H^+ and HCO_3. This increased H^+ concentration is sensed at the central chemoreceptors, which stimulate the drive to breathe. With chronic hypercarbia, as seen in COPD, this central chemoreceptor can shift its "set point" so that increased respiratory drive occurs at higher blood CO_2 concentrations.

- **Peripheral chemoreceptors**: The carotid body (as opposed to the carotid sinus, which senses carotid artery pressure) and the aortic body sense PaO_2 and $PaCO_2$, leading to increased minute ventilation with hypoxemia, and to a lesser extent, in response to hypercarbia and acidemia.

Pulmonary Mechanoreceptors

- **Stretch receptors**: Located in smooth muscle, stretch receptors respond to lung parenchymal distention. The signal travels via the vagus (X) nerve. Inflation leads to decreased respiratory rate and increased expiratory time (the Hering-Breuer reflex).

- **Irritant receptors**: Stimulated by noxious substances (e.g., smoke, gases, dust, cold air). These impulses also travel via the vagus nerve. They cause bronchoconstriction and hyperpnea (increased depth of breathing).

- **J-receptors** (juxtacapillary): Stimulated by pulmonary capillary engorgement, leading to rapid, shallow breathing. They are likely responsible in large part for the sensation of dyspnea in CHF and pulmonary edema patients.

Integrated Responses

- **CO_2**: Normally, $PaCO_2$ is the most important factor in determining minute ventilation. Reducing $PaCO_2$ below normal effectively diminishes the drive to breathe. Sleep, age, chronic hypercapnia, and drugs (e.g., opiates, barbiturates) suppress the CNS response to $PaCO_2$.

- **O_2**: PaO_2 can be reduced markedly (down to ~50 mm Hg) without stimulating the respiratory drive. The exception is in chronic CO_2 retention (e.g., COPD). As discussed earlier, the central CO_2 (more accurately H^+) chemoreceptors of these patients have been reset to higher CO_2 levels, so that PaO_2 becomes their primary stimulus to breathe. This is why COPD patients on high oxygen concentrations can become apneic.

Overall: Central chemoreceptors respond more to $PaCO_2$, whereas peripheral chemoreceptors respond more to PaO_2.

- **pH**: Can be a strong stimulus to breathe, as seen in patients with diabetic ketoacidosis who undergo Kussmaul breathing (rapid, deep breaths).

Additional Lung Functions

The lung does much more than exchange gases. Some other functions include the following:

- **Immune**: protection against inhaled toxins and pathogens; IgA secretion; protection by pulmonary alveolar macrophages

- **Fibrinolytic system**: clot lysis

- **Metabolic and synthetic function**: Converts angiotensin I to angiotensin II, the active form via angiotensin converting enzyme (ACE). Inactivates bradykinin, serotonin, prostaglandin E, prostaglandin F, norepinephrine, and possibly histamine. Synthesis of factor VIII. Synthesis of surfactant.

- **Filter**: filters debris from venous return and prevents CNS and end-organ embolic events

- **Blood reservoir**: as a low-resistance circuit, the pulmonary circulation acts as a blood reservoir

DISORDERS OF THE UPPER RESPIRATORY TRACT

Otitis Externa

Otitis externa (OE) is infection of the external auditory canal. OE usually begins as a pustule or folliculitis. Common organisms include skin flora, including Staphylococcus and Streptococcus. OE is also associated with hot tubs (where it is usually caused by Pseudomonas) giving it the nickname "swimmer's ear".

Diabetics are at risk for **malignant otitis**, an aggressive form due to Pseudomonas. If not treated early, malignant otitis can rapidly invade the surrounding bone, soft tissue, and even brain, leading to death.

Signs and Symptoms

Ear pain, which can be severe, and itching

Diagnosis

Otoscopic examination

Treatment

Topical antibiotics if there is no associated cellulitis; systemic antibiotics (e.g., dicloxacillin, erythromycin) are required if there is. Malignant otitis requires surgical debridement.

Otitis Media

Otitis media (OM) is an infection of the middle ear. It is often caused by common upper respiratory tract infection (URI) pathogens, with plugging of the Eustachian canals, leading to inflammation of the middle ear. Preschoolers are at greatest risk for OM because the anatomy of the Eustachian tube is more horizontal, which prevents drainage.

Common organisms include Streptococcus pneumoniae, Haemophilus influenzae, Moraxella catarrhalis, and viruses. Complications include mastoiditis, meningitis, and brain abscess. Chronic OM can cause tympanic membrane (TM) scarring and diminished hearing.

Signs and Symptoms

Ear pain, fever, vertigo, and tinnitus. In young kids, there may not be localizing symptoms, just irritability.

Diagnosis

Otoscopic eaxmination shows an inflamed TM. Decreased mobility of the TM with air insufflation is the most sensitive and specific test.

Treatment

Antibiotics. Good choices are amoxicillin or trimethoprim-sulfamethoxazole (TMP/SMX). Kids with recurrent OM can have drainage tubes placed to open the Eustachian tubes.

Rhinitis

Rhinitis is a very common disorder that involves inflammation or infection of the nasal cavity. The most common pathogens are viral and may be associated with pharyngitis or conjunctivitis. Rhinitis can also be caused by hypersensitivity states, such as allergic rhinitis (hay fever), which can predispose patients to developing sinusitis.

Signs and Symptoms

Itchy, red nose with watery discharge. Patients with allergic rhinitis often have a horizontal skin crease at the bridge of the nose caused by repeated rubbing of the nose. With trauma or CNS surger, a runny nose may indicate a CSF leak, not nasal inflammation.

Diagnosis

Wet preparation of nasal secretions shows eosinophils in allergic rhinitis but not in infectious rhinitis. It is rarely performed.

Treatment

Because of the viral etiology, infectious rhinitis should not be treated with antibiotics. Patients may get subjective relief with symptomatic cold medications, such as decongestants and antihistamines.

Sinusitis

Infection of the normally air-filled sinuses in the skull is called sinusitis. Common organisms include S. pneumoniae and H. influenzae. Anaerobes are less common. Complications include meningitis, brain abscess, and subdural empyema.

Signs and Symptoms

Headache, stuffiness, pain, and pus in the turbinates

Diagnosis

Transillumination of the sinuses shows opacity. Sinus X-rays or computed tomography (CT) scan show opacification and air-fluid levels.

Treatment

Antibiotics, such as amoxicillin or TMP/SMX, and nasal decongestants

Stomatitis

Stomatitis is inflammation of the mouth, and it can have a variety of etiologies. **Thrush** is caused by Candida and is seen in infants, immunocompromised patients (e.g., cancer, AIDS), and patients receiving broad-spectrum antibiotics. **Aphthous stomatitis** (canker sores) consists of painful, discrete, flat ulcers. These sores are benign and are treated symptomatically. **Herpes simplex virus (HSV-1)** causes lesions on the vermilion border of the lips and oral mucosa. It is treated with acyclovir. Finally, **vitamin deficiencies** may cause stomatitis and angular cheilosis.

Pharyngitis

Pharyngitis, or "sore throat," is an extremely common disease and is often caused by respiratory viruses (e.g., rhinovirus, influenza, parainfluenza, Epstein-Barr virus [EBV]) or Streptococcus pyogenes, with most cases occurring in winter. Complications of infection with Group A Beta-Hemolytic Streptococcus pyogenes include post-infectious glomerulonephritis and acute rheumatic fever.

Signs and Symptoms

Usually associated with cold symptoms: rhinorrhea, fever, myalgias, and cough. EBV may cause infectious mononucleosis, with enlarged lymph nodes and pharyngeal erythema.

Diagnosis

Based on clinical symptoms. Streptococcus must be ruled out because of the potential complications (rheumatic fever). Rapid Streptococcus antigen test kits are quickly replacing the throat culture. The monospot test for EBV antibodies is also available.

Treatment

Symptomatic. Strep throat responds to penicillin (or erythromycin if patient is allergic to penicillin).

Epiglottitis

Consider H. influenza epiglottitis in a patient with negative or questionable history of vaccinations.

Epiglottitis is a potential emergency usually seen in young children and is caused by H. influenzae. Infection of the epiglottis leads to upper airway obstruction, stridor, and potentially death. Young children in contact with known cases should receive rifampin prophylaxis.

Signs and Symptoms

Sore throat with difficult swallowing, copious secretions, severe throat pain, and stridor. These patients characteristically lean forward to prevent complete obstruction of the epiglottis.

Diagnosis

Examination (patient is kept sitting up to minimize laryngospasm), lateral X-rays of the neck, and indirect laryngoscopy.

Treatment

Antibiotics. Airway management (intubation) if necessary. This disease has become exceedingly rare thanks to widespread H. influenzae vaccinations.

DISORDERS OF THE LOWER RESPIRATORY TRACT

Infectious Bronchiolitis

Infectious bronchiolitis is most often seen in young children and is probably the most common reason for admission to a pediatrics ward. It is often seen in winter months and must be differentiated from pneumonia or URI.

The most common causative pathogen is respiratory syncytial virus (RSV), but it is also caused by parainfluenza, influenza, and adenovirus. It is usually seen in 6 month olds to 3 year olds: At that size, the bronchioles are more likely to obstruct with secretions when infected. There is an increased rate of infection in premature infants, particularly those with bronchopulmonary dysplasia (discussed later).

Signs and Symptoms

Cough, fever, irritability, and audible wheezes

Diagnosis

Wheezes on examination; CXR shows hyperinflation, air bronchograms, and patchy, migrating atelectasis, with possible consolidation.

Treatment

Bronchodilators, supplemental O_2, and chest therapy to mobilize secretions. Antibiotics are not needed. Intubation with mechanical ventilation is used in severe cases, and ribavirin may be beneficial.

Pneumonia

Pneumonia is a huge part of internal medicine, accounting for about 10% of adult medicine admissions. It is caused by pathogens (viruses, rickettsiae, mycoplasmas, chlamydiae, bacteria, protozoa, fungi, parasites) entering the lung by either (1) inhalation of aerosolized particles, (2) aspiration of oropharyngeal secretions—the most common cause, (3) hematogenous spread, or (4) local spread of infection.

Signs and Symptoms

History is crucial. Determine whether the pneumonia is community acquired or nosocomial, the age group, possible unique exposures, and time course. Viral, pneumococcal, and mycoplasmal pneumonia are usually acute (hours to days), whereas tuberculosis (TB), anaerobes, and fungi take longer to evolve. A URI prodrome suggests mycoplasma or viral pneumonia. Diarrhea is associated with Legionella.

Common symptoms include cough, fever, tachypnea, tachycardia, and sometimes pleuritic pain. Respiratory distress (increased tachypnea, use of accessory muscles, cyanosis) indicates severe disease. Chest examination shows signs of consolidation: rales, bronchial breath sounds, or decreased breath sounds if pleural effusion is present. Egophony and tactile fremitus may be elicited.

Diagnosis

CXR is warranted. CXR in Mycoplasma pneumonia classically looks much worse than the patient appears clinically, with significant, bilateral patchy opacities. Pneumyocystis carinii infection is the opposite: The CXR often looks better than the patient. Realize that a "negative" CXR does not rule out pneumonia because radiographic signs may lag behind the infection by many hours. Bacterial pneumonia classically demonstrates lobar consolidation. Chronic lung disease patients often show no radiographic signs of pneumonia. Interstitial involvement may suggest a viral etiology. TB can look like absolutely anything on CXR but is classically seen as an upper lung nodule or tiny disseminated (military) nodules. A pleural effusion is common.

On laboratory tests, the CBS shows an elevated WBC with left shift. Sputum smear and culture are an essential part of the diagnosis and management. A sputum specimen is considered adequate if it has (1) none to few epithelial cells and (20) polymorphonuclear neutrophils (PMNs).

Treatment

The general treatment principle for suspected pneumonia is initial broad empiric treatment based on clinical judgment about the likely organism. Antibiotics are then tailored to the organism, as determined from the sputum. Mycoplasma is usually treated on an outpatient basis, but the majority of pneumonia patients require hospitalization. Issues of importance include oxygenation status (provide supplemental O_2), systemic complications (sepsis), and management of secretions.

Persistent infection suggests antibiotic resistance, whereas recurrent infections in the same part of the lung suggest **postobstructive pneumonia**. **Empyema** is simply pus that gest into the pleural cavity. Pleural effusion in a febrile patient must be examined via thoracentesis. Pneumococcal and influenza pneumonia can be prevented in susceptible patients (e.g., immune-compromised, postplenectomy, elderly) with vaccination.

Tuberculosis

The causative organism is Mycobacterium tuberculosis, an acid-fast bacillus. Until the advent of antibiotics, patients were sent to sanitoriums, and as recently as 40 years ago, patients were subjected to such desperate measures as pleuroplasty, where the chest and lung were permanently surgically collapsed in an effort to starve the organisms of oxygen. Today, TB is on an upsurge after decades of control in the United States (both clinically and on board examinations), mainly because of immigration from endemic parts of the world and the association of TB with AIDS.

- **Primary infection**: Results from an exposure to an actively contagious host, spread via aerosolized particles. It is usually self-limited, with the only manifestation being a conversion to positive purified protein derivative (PPD). Sometimes primary infection leads to respiratory symptoms (cough, fever), and CXR may show patchy infiltrates. Hematogenous dissemination can seed all over the body, leading to sites that can become sources of latent reactivation. About 5–15% of infections lead to active disease. Risk factors include immunosuppression, older age, infancy, diabetes, and other pre-existing parenchymal lung disease. Progressive primary TB occurs when the disease progresses at an early stage, often leading to hematogenous spread, or **miliary TB**, in which the lung is full of many tiny TB foci, resembling millet seeds.

- **Reactivation** is the most common presenting form of the disease. After the bugs have remained dormant in some part of the body, the patient begins to experience fever, night sweats, and hemoptysis. CXR shows cavitary lesions with consolidation classically in the posterior segment of the upper lobes or in the superior segments of the lower lobes.

- **Extrapulmonary TB**: Important entities include genitourinary TB, bone and arthritic TB, and meningeal TB. HIV patients often present with disseminated TB, and patients are often PPD-nonreactive (controls are also unreactive, due to overall anergy).

Diagnosis

The diagnosis relies on (1) history, (2) PPD (may be false-positive in those who received bacillus Calmette-Guerin (BCG) vaccination, an ineffective vaccine), (3) positive CXR, and (4) sputum samples for smear and culture (culture takes 4–6 weeks). With high clinical suspicion, bronchoscopy is indicated if the sputum smears are negative. Smears reveal acid-fast bacilli (red snappers).

Treatment

Because of public health concerns, the first step is respirator isolation for patients with active disease. Given the possibility of resistant strains, drug therapy uses multiple drug regimens. The standard full-course treatment is four-drug therapy: isoniazid (INH), rifampin, ethambutol, and pyrazinamide for 2 months, and then only isoniazid and rifampin for another 4 months, for a total of 6 months of treatment. Treatment may be longer if resistant strains are suspected.

Household and intimate contacts of actively infected patients must be treated with isoniazid prophylaxis for 6–12 months (or full treatment if they also have disease).

Obstructive Lung Diseases

This class of respiratory disease encompasses bronchitis and emphysema (collectively called COPD), asthma, bronchiectasis, and cystic fibrosis (CF). These diseases are characterized by increased airway resistance, which is the result of several (overlapping) pathologic mechanisms:

	COPD	Asthma	Bronchiectasis	CF
Loss of elastic recoil	✔	—	—	—
Smooth muscle constriction	✔	✔	—	—
Inflammation	✔	✔	✔	—
Mucus plugs	—	—	—	✔

Table 4 Obstructive lung diseases

The common result is increased airway resistance and obstruction which leads to decreased peak expiratory flow rates, decreased flow volumes, air trapping, and increased TLC, RV, and FRC. The hyperinflation that develops helps to keep the overly collapsible airways open, a physiologic compensatory mechanism. Subsequently, the altered mechanics and parenchyma results in $\dot{V}/\dot{Q}$ mismatch and decreased oxygenation. The impaired ventilation leads to CO_2 retention. Eventually, the CO_2 set point in the medulla shifts to accept higher baseline $PaCO_2$ values.

Asthma

Asthma is characterized by airway obstruction that results from hyper-reactivity of the inflammatory response of the airways, leading to bronchospasm. The disease is subdivided into several categories, listed in Table 5. The classification is important in patient education so as to avoid substances that might trigger future attacks.

Classification	Etiology
Extrinsic	Extermal allergens leading to mast cell degranulation
Instrinsic	Unknown
Exercise or humidity induced	Mediator release triggered by alterations in airway temperature
Adult onset	Unknown
Aspirin sensitive	Aspirin and nonsterodial anti-inflammatory drugs
Occupational	Various triggers (e.g., dust)
Allergic aspergilosis	Hypersensitivity to Aspergilus

Table 5 Categories of asthma

Signs and Symptoms

Intermittent dyspnea, wheezing, and sometimes dry cough may be the only symptoms. Symptoms are often worse at night, possibly due to circadian variations. Specific triggers can often be identified (e.g., exercise, cold, URI).

Diagnosis

CXR shows hyperinflation when symptomatic: PFTs show obstruction with significant bronchodilator response. Alternatively, the asthma may be triggered by administering histamine, cold air, or methacholine.

Treatment

Inhalers, including beta-agonists and anticholinergics for smooth muscle hyperreactivity, cromolyn for mast cell stabilization, and steroids for inflammation. Methylxanthines (theophylline, aminophylline) are bronchodilators with an uncertain mechanism of action; uses is controversial given potential toxicity (anxiety, tremor, arrhythmias, seizures). Avoidance of triggers is crucial, and in severe cases, systematic desensitization (allergy shots) to stimulants may be beneficial.

Status asthmaticus is an acute, severe asthma attack that is unresponsive to routine therapy. It is a medical emergency. PaO_2 progressively fails, and $PaCO_2$ initially falls with hyperventilation but then gradually rises with impaired ventilation. Intubation may be necessary, along with aggressive bronchodilator and steroid treatment.

Chronic Obstructive Pulmonary Disease

COPD is a progressive disease that results in airway obstruction, dyspnea, and hypoventilation. The tempo of the disease is one of slow progression, often punctuated by acute exacerbations requiring hospitalization. Classically, this is a disease of middle-aged to elderly smokers. Worsening disease is accompanied by increased hypoventilation, increased pulmonary vascular resistance (a result of hypoxic vasoconstriction leading to vascular remodeling and parenchymal tissue destruction) leading to right heart failure, and acute respiratory failure.

Classically, COPD has been subclassified as emphysema (thin, cachectic patients—**pink puffers**) or chronic bronchitis (edematous, cyanotic patients— **blue bloaters**). With the current understanding, the disease is thought to encompass three overlapping components: emphysema, chronic bronchitis, and reactive airway disease (RAD). A particular patient has some combination of the three entities (Figure 17).

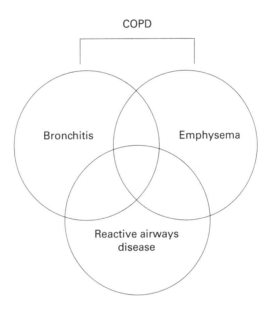

Figure 17 Schematic representation of COPD

- **Emphysema**: Destruction of the alveolar walls, possibly by overactive proteases, leads to enlargement of the air spaces. There is a loss of elastic recoil and increased compliance. Cigarette smoke is thought to trigger this cascade by increasing the neutrophil and macrophage inflammatory response. Laboratory findings peculiar to emphysema include hyper-lucency on CXR that corresponds to bullae and increased airways space, attenuation of pulmonary vasculature secondary to the destructive process, and decreased DL_{CO} on PFTs, a result of destruction of pulmonary capillaries.

- **Chronic bronchitis**: Persistent cough with sputum production. Cigarette smoke is the major cause of disease, leading to bronchospasm, mucus plugging, and associated emphysema. Chronic bacterial colonization occurs, commonly with S. pneumoniae, H. influenzae, and Moraxella.

- **RAD**: Small airways are irritated, with smooth muscle hyper-reactivity and eventual fibrosis leading to obstruction.

COPD exacerbations are usually triggered by an infection, as the altered airway immunoprotection (cough, impaired clearance of secretions, hypoxia) leads to colonization of the airways by pathogens.

Signs and Symptoms

Presenting symptoms include dyspnea on exertion, wheezing, and productive cough. Tobacco use is often associated.

Diagnosis

Examination may demonstrate wheezing. CXR shows hyperinflation (increased anterposterior diameter, flattened diaphragm, increased diaphragmatic excursion), loss of pulmonary vasculature, and perhaps an enlarged right heart. In severe disease, bullae (large air spaces left after destruction of the lung parenchyma) may be seen. Electrocardiography (ECG) and echocardiography may show right heart enlargement, consistent with increased pulmonary artery pressures. PFTs are characteristic. Bronchodilator response is usually modest.

Treatment

The armamentarium is similar to that for asthma: beta-agonsists, anticholinergics, steroids, cromolyn, and methylxanthines. Patients with documented chronic hypoxemia ($PAO_2 < 55$ mm Hg) require home supplemental oxygen. In COPD exacerbations, empiric antibiotic treatment is often initiated. Smoking cessation is obvious preventative measure.

Chronic Bronchiolitis

Chronic bronchiolitis is an inflammation of the small airways leading to fibrosis. Two general processes are seen: (1) Inflammation and scarring leads to luminal narrowing, producing an obstructive disease process, such as constrictive bronchiolitis, and (2) the inflamed small airways plug up, and the inflammation spreads into adjacent parenchyma, resulting in **bronchiolitis obliterans with organizing pneumonia (BOOP)**. BOOP shows parenchymal consolidation on CXR and a restrictive pattern on PFTs. Bronchiolitis is a pulmonary end point of several disease processes, including recurrent or severe infection, toxin inhalation, and connective tissue disease (particularly rheumatoid arthritis). Chronic rejection in lung transplantation may result in BOOP, and graft-versus-host disease in bone marrow transplant patients is also a cause. Treatment is with bronchodilators. Recurrent infections are treated with antibiotics and pulmonary hygiene.

a1-Antitrypsin Deficiency

a1-Antitrypsin deficiency is an autosomal inherited disorder characterized by destruction of elastic components in the lung as well as the liver. The normal gene for a1-antitrypsin is the PiM, the mutant gene is PiZ; whereas heterozygotes (MZ) exhibit attenuated disease. The loss of this inhibitory enzyme leads to destruction of lung parenchyma and emphysematous changes. The approach to treatment is similar to that for emphysema.

Bronchiectasis

Bronchiectasis is widening of the bronchi with loss of structural integrity, usually the result of severe or recurrent bouts of infection, especially severe necrotizing infection. Predisposing factors include immune deficiency states, CF, and defective ciliary motility (e.g., Kartagener's, Young's syndromes). Chronic colonization usually occurs, with S. pneumoniae, Pseudomonas, H. influenzae, Staphylococcus, or atypical mycobacteria.

Signs and Symptoms

Persistent cough, sometimes hemoptysis and foul-smelling sputum. Examination may show cyanosis, clubbing, and crackles over the affected lung area. CXR may be unremarkable or may show linear atelectasis and bronchial thickening. Patients may present with massive hemoptysis.

Diagnosis

Made with CT scan, demonstrating widened, thickened bronchi. PFTs are consistent with obstructive disease, although a restrictive component may also be present.

Treatment

Antibiotics are used for acute exacerbations and sometimes prophylactically. Chest physical therapy (vigorous percussion) is also helpful.

Cystic Fibrosis

CF is an autosomal recessive disorder occurring in about 1 in 2,500 live births in Caucasians with a particular associated gene that has been localized to the long arm of chromosome 7, Mutations in this **chloride transporter** gene result in defective exocrine gland secretory function. This results in thick mucus plugs in the respiratory and gastrointestinal (GI) tracts, impaired mucociliary transport, recurrent infections, bronchiectasis, and inflammation. Staphylococcus aureus in childhood and Pseudomonas aeruginosa (and to a lesser extent H. influenzae or Pseudomonas cepacia) in adulthood colonize the respiratory tract, leading to recurrent infection. The resultant inflammation and damage leads to progressive respiratory failure.

Signs and Symptoms

CF usually presents in childhood with a broad range of symptoms, from recurrent respiratory infection and irritation, to GI symptoms (e.g., steatorrhea, constipation pancreatic insufficiency) from mucus plugs.

Diagnosis

Made with sweat chloride test, in which chloride is elevated.

Treatment

Supportive care throughout childhood has imporoved mean survival to 29 years. Antibiotics for infections, frequent pulmonary toilet, and bronchodilators are used. Newer approaches include gene therapy to introduce the CF gene into the respiratory epithelial cells and treating with viscosity-reducing substances. Advanced disease necessitates evaluation for lung transplantation.

RESTRICTIVE & PARENCHYMAL LUNG DISEASES

These diseases include alveolar and interstitial disorders and the pneumoconiosis. Although the etiology of many of these diseases remains obscure, the pathologic mechanism may be due to one or more of the following factors:

1. Direct toxicity (gases, radiation)

2. Damage secondary to an inflammatory response

3. Immune-mediated injury (e.g., Ag-Ab complex deposition, complement activation)

Some of the more common examples of such diseases are:

- **Pneumoconiosis**: Inhalation of substances as a result of occupational or environmental exposure.

- Asbestos exposure, seen in construction/shipyard workers or plumbers, can cause pulmonary fibrosis but is also associated with bronchogenic carcinoma and malignant mesothelioma.

- Coal worker's pneumoconiosis ("black lung") causes interstitial fibrosis.

- Silicosis, seen in sandblasters and silica miners, increases the risk of TB infection.

- Berrylliosis, seen in individuals in nuclear or aerospace industries, increases the risk of lung cancer.

- **Hypersensitivity pneumonitis**: An abnormal sensitivity to an extrinsic allergen leads to an allergic alveolitis with eosinophils. Reticulonodular infiltrates are seen on CXR. Resolution occurs with removal of the offending agent.

- **Sarcoidosis**: An enigmatic disease characterized pathologically by noncaseating, noninfectious granulomas. The disease predominantly affects the lung (appearing as **bilateral hilar lymphadenopathy** on radiography) but can also involve the liver, spleen, lymph nodes, joints, muscles, skin, eyes, and CNS. Classically, the disease presents in the third or fourth decade of life in women more than men, in African-Americans more frequently than others. Hypercalcemia and hypercalcuria may be present.

- **Idiopathic pulmonary fibrosis (IPF)**: A diagnosis of exclusion. Patients are usually middle-aged and present with progressive dyspnea. The disease course can be rapid, culminating in death within months, or progress more slowly. Treatment usually results in a moderate response to steroids, and lung transplantation is the definitive therapy in severe disease. In untreated patients, death usually occurs within 2 years. IPF is also known as usual interstitial pneumonitis, to differentiate it from desquamative interstitial pneumonitis.

- **Desquamative interstitial pneumonitis (DIP)**: an interstitial pneumonitis in which the primary pathology involves mononuclear aggregation in the alveoli, presumably from a desquamation process. The cause is unknown, and many patients respond to steroids. The current belief is that DIP may be an early stage of IPF rather than a distinct disease entity.

- **Connective tissue disease**: Many of the collagen-vascular diseases have pulmonary manifestations. Most commonly, a chronic interstitial fibrosis process (e.g., IPF) is seen. Pulmonary manifestations of **rheumatoid arthritis** include pleurisy, interstitial lung disease, intrapulmonary nodules, Caplan's syndrome (an association between rheumatoid nodules with coal worker's pneumoconiosis), pulmonary hypertension, bronchiolitis obliterans, and upper airway obstruction. In systemic lupus erythematosus (SLE), the most common pulmonary manifestation is pleuritis with or without effusion. In Sjögren's syndrome, patients may have lymphocytic interstitial pneumonitis and bronchiolitis obliterans.

Signs and Symptoms

Progressive dyspnea, cough with or without sputum, fever, occasionally hemoptysis, and systemic symptoms if the disease is part of a systemic disease (e.g., SLE). It is critical to elicit the patient's work history, home situation, medication history, and medical history to document possible exposures and associated risks. The onset is usually insidious.

Diagnosis

Lung examination reveals dry crackles, often bibasilar. Look for systemic signs of disease: skin changes, arthropathy, ocular changes. CXR is normal in more than 10% of patients. The classic appearance is diffuse reticulondular opacities, often with upper lung zone predominance. Hair lymphadenpath, pleural involvement, increasing lung volumes, clacifications, or even pneumothorax may be evident, depending on the particular disease. CT scan is extremely informative in characterizing the process. PFTs often deomonstrate a restrictive pattern with reduced compliance (the lungs become more snappy with the parenchymal disease). DL_{CO} may be decreased because of the loss of air exchange surface area and V/Q mismatch. Some diseases (e.g., sarcoidosis, hypersensitivity pneumonitis, eosinophilic lung disease) can also show a superimposed obstructive process with airway involvement. Bronchoscopy is performed to rule out infection or malignancy and to make a diagnosis. Lung biopsy (fiberoptic bronchoscopy, thoracoscopy, or open lung biopsy) usually makes the diagnosis.

Diffuse Alveolar Hemorrhage

Diffuse alveolar hemorrhage is bleeding into the alveolar airspace secondary to damage to the pulmonary capillary epithelium. Causes include the following:

- Immune-mediated damage: Goodpasture's syndrome, SLE, other vasculitides

- Direct chemical- or radiation-induced damage

- Physical trauma (contusion)

- Coagulopathy

- Increased capillary pressure (e.g., CHF, mitral stenosis) Presentation includes hemoptysis, dyspnea, and abnormal CXR with diffuse, patchy opacities. Diagnosis is made with bronchoscopy, which demonstrates frank bleeding that persists. The treatment involves correcting the underlying disorder and usually steroids.

Eosinophilic Pneumonias

The eosinophilic pneumonias are as follows:

- **Acute eosinophilic pneumonia**: due to an inhaled antigen.

- **Löffler's syndrome**: A transient form of eosinophilic pneumonia in response to parasitic infections.

- **Churg-Strauss**: a systemic eosinophilic disease, with a polyarteritis picture in which small- to medium-sized vessels are affected. Asthma and rhinitis are seen.

- **Pulmonary eosinophilic granuloma** (histiocytosis X): a disease with a benign course and diffuse reticulonodular pattern on CXR. Signs and symptoms include: dyspnea, fever, night sweats, and weight loss. Asthma occurs concomitantly in 50% of cases. CXR shows peripheral interstitial opacification—the "photographic negative" of pulmonary edema (this is pathognomonic). CBC shows eosinophilia, high erythrocyte sedimentation rate, and anemia. Bronchoalveolar lavage shows eosinophils. Treatment is with steroids, often long term.

Disorders in the Control of Breathing

This is a class of diseases in which either a peripheral (mechanical) or central mechanism (CNS) causes a decrease in the ability to ventilate properly. It includes the following:

- **Neurologic disease**: Lesions in the brain stem can result in abnormal breathing patterns, including neurogenic hyperventilation, apneustic breathing (sustained pauses in the inspiratory part of the respiratory cycle), and Cheyne-Stokes breathing (regular cycles of rapid breathing separated by periods of apnea). Central sleep apnea can also occur (described later).

- **Neuromuscular disease**: Ineffective use of the diaphragm or accessory muscles of breathing. Causes include stroke, inflammatory neuropathies, amyotrophic lateral sclerosis, myasthenia gravis, and polio.

- **Bellows dysfunction**: Includes diaphragmatic disease and chest wall anatomic defects that can impair proper chest wall bellows motion, including kyphoscoliosis, obesity, respiratory muscle fatigue (as seen in chronically ill patients or recently extubated patients), and thoracotomy.

- **Flail chest** occurs when trauma to the chest wall results in a part of the chest wall that moves freely away from the rest of the chest wall (Figure 18). As a result, that part of the chest wall moves paradoxically during respiration.

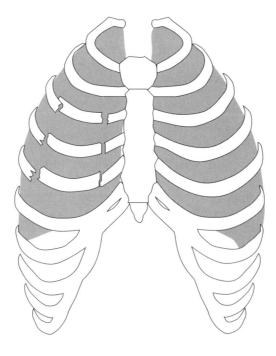

Figure 18 Flail chest

Sleep Apnea

Sleep apnea syndrome is defined as repeated episodes of apnea (i.e., no air flow in the nose and mouth for at least 10 seconds) and hypopnea during sleep. Severe obstructive sleep apnea can result in hundreds of such episodes a night. The sequelae include daytime fatigue, irritability, and falling asleep at work and on the road. The syndrome is classified as either:

1. **Obstructive sleep apnea** (OSA), in which the diaphragm contracts but cannot move air because of an upper airway obstruction.

2. **Central apnea**, the result of dysfunction of the respiratory drive center.

3. **Mixed apnea**, a combination of the two. OSA is the most common form.

The most common points of obstruction in OSA are the velopharynx (behind the soft palate) and the hypopharynx, as a result of muscle relaxation during sleep. Obesity contributes to the obstruction with increased soft tissue in the upper airways.

Central sleep apnea used to be called **Pickwickian syndrome** after Pickwick, the Dickens character, who has the typical body habitus of the patient with central apnea: obese, male, and often short in stature. It is now clear that not all patients with central apnea have this habitus. Dysfunction of the central respiratory drive center results in apnea during sleep.

Signs and Symptoms

Most often seen in obese, older males but also seen on postmenopausal women. Much of the sleep history can be obtained from the patient's spouse. Patients present with daytime somnolence, disturbed sleep, and excessively loud snoring. The inadequate sleep leads to poor job performance, automobile accidents and deterioration of relationships. The continued apnea and associated hypoxia leads to hypoxic vasoconstriction of the pulmonary vasculature and pulmonary hypertension. Hypoxia can also lead to arrhythmias and stroke.

Diagnosis

A sleep study is performed to diagnose sleep apnea syndrome. The patient's sleep patter, O_2 saturation, airflow, and ECG are monitored overnight, and the episodes of apnea and desaturation are monitored.

Treatment

The first step is encouraging weight loss, but success with this strategy is predicatably low. Nasal decongestants (including mechanical devices such as "Breathe Right" nasal dilating adhesive strips have variable benefit. Patients should avoid sedative-hypontics and alcohol at bedtime. With severe daytime somnolence, cardiovascular manifestations, and frequent apnea, the next step in intervention is continuous positive airway pressure (CPAP) during sleep. Positive pressure throughout the respirator cycle keeps the airways open, but it's not well tolerated by patients. The final step in intervention is surgery.

DISEASES

Pneumothorax

Pneumothorax is a potentially life-threatening condition. Air can get to the pleural space by several routes: (1) direct injury of the chest wall, (2) damage to alveoli, leading to air in the interstitial space (pulmonary interstitial emphysema, seen often in mechanically ventilated patients, especially newborns with neonatal RDS), which can rupture through into the pleural space. Air enters the mediastinum, tracking into the interstitium, and then into the pleural space.

Causes of pneumothorax can be classified as follows:

- **Spontaneous**: Emphysema, interstitial lung disease, granulomatous disease, CF, asthma, cancer, or idiopathic. Idiopathic pneumothorax is often seen in tall, thin, Caucasian males. Regardless of etiology, spontaneous pneumothorax is characterized by a collapse of lung tissue, which characteristically shifts the mediastinal compartment to the ipsilateral side.

- **Traumatic**: Penetrating chest trauma, non-penetrating trauma, esophageal perforation, and iatrogenic causes. A pneumothorax should be evacuated if it consists of greater than 15% of air-space on chest X-ray, causes significant dyspnea or respiratory compromise, causes hypoxemia, recurs, is secondary to pulmonary disease, or is a tension pneumothorax.

- In a **tension pneumothorax**, enough air gets into the pleural space to produce positive pressure, leading to displacement of the mediastinal compartment to the contralateral side (mediastinal shift). This is a true emergency because this air pressure can reduce blood return to the heart and lead to hemodynamic collapse.

Pleural Effusion

There is normally an undetectable, very small amount of fluid in the pleural space. Anything more than 200 ml of fluid (which is abnormal) can be detected on CXR as blunting of the costophrenic angle. Pleural fluid is classified as either transudate or exudate (Table 6).

- **Transudates** results from increased net pressure for fluid to "filter" out of the vasculature into the pleural space, according to Starling's law (due to increased hydrostatic pressure or decreased oncotic pressure). As a result, transudate has the characteristics of an "ultrafiltrate" of plasma.

- **Exudates** results from loss of integrity of the vascular barrier or from frank production of fluid locally within the pleural space. An exudate has chemical characteristics closer to blood.

Transudates	Exudates
Congestive heart failure	Infection
Nephrotic syndrome	Malignancy (primary or metastatic)
End-stage liver disease	Rheumatologic diseases
Abdominal fluid leakage (ascites,	Pulmonary embolism
postperitoneal dialysis)	Abdominal processes (pancreatitis)

Table 6 Causes of transudates and exudates

Pleural fluid can be classified according to overall fluid composition.

- A **hydrothorax** is just fluid (Table 7).

- A **hemothorax** is frank blood, with a hematocrit of the fluid greater than 20; it implies cancer, trauma, or pulmonary embolism (PE) with infarction.

- A **chylothorax** is chylous lymph that appears milky, with high triglyceride content.

Pleural fluid	Transudate	Exudate
Protein	< 3 g/dl	> 3 g/dl
Ratio of pleural protein to serum protein	< 0.5	> 0.5
LDH	< 200 IU/Liter	> 200 IU/liter
Ratio of pleural to serum lactate dehydrogenase	< 0.6	> 0.6

Table 7 Fluid composition of transudates and exudates

Treatment

An effusion that affects ventilation or oxygenation needs to be evacuated. This can be done by one-time thoracentesis or chest tube placement. Parapneumonic effusions may require antibiotics and thoracentesis drainage. Loculated fluid (pockets of fibrin-bound fluid) requires chest tube placement and instillation of thrombolytics.

PULMONARY VASCULAR DISEASE

Pulmonary Hypertension

Pulmonary hypertension is persistent elevation of the pressures in the pulmonary circulation (mean PAP >20 mm Hg). Pulmonary hypertension can be caused by intracardiac shunts, left ventricular failure, obliteration or obstruction of the vasculature, or prolonged hypoxia.

Persistently elevated pressures lead to many hemodynamic changes:

- **In the heart**: Increased afterload on the right heart leads to right ventricular hypertrophy, right atrial enlargement, and eventually signs of right heart failure (elevated jugular venous pressure, pedal edema).

- With severe hypertension, the right ventricle fills more than normal, pushing the interventricular septum into the LV and thereby impairing left ventricular function (septal bulge).

- **In the lungs**: With persistent hypertension, remodeling of the pulmonary vasculature occurs, leading to thick-walled vessels. Mild hypoxemia is seen secondary to loss of the capillary circulation andQ worsened V/Q match.

Pulmonary Embolism

Pulmonary embolism (PE) can occur from the embolization of clot, fat, marrow, air, or other materials into the pulmonary vasculature. The most common cause of PE is the embolism of a deep venous thrombosis (DVT), most commonly found in the calf. The embolus can then act as a nidus for clot extension, which can be fatal if massive or left untreated. Postsurgical and postpartum patients are at increased risk for developing PE.

Signs and Symptoms

Patients may experience sudden dyspnea and hypoxia.

Diagnosis

Made by V/Q scan, which can often have ambiguous results. Doppler ultrasound of the legs is done to search for a likely source. The gold standard is pulmonary angiography, in which dye is squirted into the main pulmonary arteries and X-rays are taken. The risks are significant, including nephrotoxicity from dye, dye anaphylaxis, and bleeding.

Treatment

The mainstay of therapy is anticoagulation. Remember that anticoagulation prevents new clot formation and does not dissolve old clot, but anticoagulation shifts the balance between clot formation and lysis toard lysis. Proven DVTs are treated with 6 weeks of anticoagulation if the result of a known brief insult (e.g., surgery, trauma), and 6 months or longer otherwise. Heparin is started first, with the goal of a partial thromboplastin time (PTT) at 1.5–2.5 times normal. Warfarin is then overlapped to achieve an international normalized ration (INR) of 2.0–3.0. The two are overlapped because of the theoretical consideration that warfarin first depletes proteins C and S before depleting factor VII, then factors II, IX, and X, and persons with protein C and S deficiency will then be in a hypercoagulable state. The recent trend has been toward treating with low-molecular-weight heparin because, with it, PIT does not need to be checked. Severe PE with hemodynamic compromise or significant respirator compromise may require thrombolysis (e.g., with streptokinase or tissue-type plasminogen activator). Massive PE is usually fatal, but experimental therapeutic strategies include surgical thrombectomy. Recurrent embolism from known DVT may be prevented by installation of a caval interruption filter, which is placed percutaneously in the inferior vena cava, with the intent of catching floating emboli before they get to the lungs. Inferior vena cava are also an option for patients with contraindications to anticoagulation (e.g., CNS bleed, recent surgery, severe GI bleed).

ASPIRATION

Suspect aspiration pneumonia with enteric bacteria species (such as Klebsiella) in an alcoholic patient with right lobar pneumonia.

Aspiration refers to a solid or liquid entering the airways. Aspiration can cause a chemical pneumonitis (gastric secretions), pneumonia (oral or GI flora), or airway obstruction with foreign objects. Obstruction with foreign objects is important in children, who tend to inhale hot dogs, grapes, peanuts, and various small objects. Risk factors include chronic illness, loss of gag reflex, vomiting, and altered mental status. Treatment is supportive, with endoscopic removal of foreign objects and appropriate antibiotic coverage if pneumonia is expected.

Trauma

Remember that airway and breathing are the A and B of the ABCs of resuscitation. Maintaining a patent airway and ventilating a patient are perhaps the most useful skills to have in managing a code situation (usually the job of the anesthesiologist). Airway can be maintained with several maneuvers, including

- Positioning

- Clearing the airway

- Mask ventilation

- Oral airway insertion

- Laryngeal mask airway

- Endotracheal tube

- Cricothyrotomy or tracheostomy

NEOPLASMS

Nose, Sinus, and Nasopharyngeal Neoplasms

These include lymphoid tumors (plasmacytomas), olfactory neuroblastomas—highly malignant papillomas (occurs in the nose and paranasal sinuses, benign but locally invasive), and carcinomas (squamous cell carcinoma is the most common). Nasopharyngeal squamous cell carcinoma is associated with EBV infection, is particularly common in Southeast Asians, is locally invasive, and metastasizes rapidly. It is highly radiosensitive, however, and the 5-year cure rate is up to 80%.

Oral Cavity Neoplasms

Leukoplakia is a white raised plaque with up to a 15% transformation rate to malignancy. **Erythroplasia** is red, velvety, and not raised; it has up to a 50% transformation rate to malignancy. **Hairy leukoplakia** is associated with HIV infection and is seen on the lateral surface of the tongue. It is associated with human papillomavirus (HPV) and EBV; it usually contains a Candida superinfection and is not precancerous.

Squamous cell carcinoma comprises 95% of all oral cavity tumors. Alcohol, smoking, and chewing tobacco are all risk factors. It spreads via the submandibular nodes to distant sites. The 5-year survival rate is 85–90% for lip cancers, 25–65% for floor of the mouth cancers, with the difference due to earlier metastasis in the latter. It is treated by surgical resection.

Laryngeal Neoplasms

Benign laryngeal polyps are smooth, round, sessile polyps often found on the vocal cords. The polyps can ulcerate, leading to a strong inflammatory response. They occur mostly in males, and in smokers. Papillomas are small (< 1 cm), friable, stratified squamous epithelium surrounding a fibrous core. They may be multiple and rarely transform to malignant form.

Squamous cell carcinoma accounts for 95% of all laryngeal carcinomas. It is more common in males than females, and there is increased incidence in smokers, older age, and people with asbestos exposure. They are usually found directly on vocal cords. Patients present with hoarseness, stridor, odynophagia, and hemoptysis.

Diagnosis

Laryngoscopy and biopsy

Treatment

Surgical excision with radiation therapy. The 5-year survival rate exceeds 50%. Tumor spreads directly, can invade vital structure (airway, major vessels), and then spread via lymphatics.

Lung Neoplasms

Benign lung neoplasms include:

- **Bronchial adenoma**: the most common centrally located benign tumor of the lung.

- **Hamartoma**: the most common peripherally located benign tumor of the lung. On CXR, it typically shows up as a popcorn-shaped calcification.

Carcinoma of the lung is currently the leading cause of cancer deaths in the United States in both men and women (having surpassed breast cancer in women). The primary risk factor is tobacco exposure. Lung cancer rarely affects patients younger than 35 years of age and is most common in the fourth and fifth decades of life.

Clinically, it is appropriate to think of lung carcinoma in terms of **small cell** versus **non-small cell** because this is the primary determinant of prognosis and management. Lung carcinoma is divided into four major histologic classifications:

- Small cell carcinoma (20–25%)

- Adenocarcinoma, including bronchoalveolar carcinoma (32–40%)

- Squamous cell carcinoma (20–25%)

- Large cell carcinoma (8–16%)

A general rule is that non–small cell carcinoma is evaluated for resectability (surgical intervention), and small cell carcinoma is primarily managed with chemotherapy. This is because non–small cell carcinoma often presents as a distinct parenchymal lung mass with or without lymph node involvement, whereas small cell carcinoma usually presents as diffuse lung disease with or without metastases, and small cell carcinoma often metastasizes early.

Signs and Symptoms

Patients often present with an asymptomatic abnormal CXR, or they may present with symptoms related to the tumor's effect on the airways, including dyspnea, cough, hemoptysis, or recurrent infection. Sometimes patients present with symptoms or paraneoplaastic syndrome, Pancoast tumor, or Horner's syndrome (described later).

- **Paraneoplastic syndrome**: Because lung carcinoma cells are dyplastic, they often secrete abnormal hormones, leading to unusual symptoms and signs.

- **Pancoast tumor**: Lung tumors located in the apices of the lung may lead to compression of the brachial plexus. Involvement of the inferior cervical ganglion may lead to **Horner's syndrome** (ptosis, miosis, anhidrosis).

Obstruction of a bronchus may lead to recurrent infections in the affected segment or lobe, called postobstructive pneumonia. Compression of the superior vena cava leads to facial and upper extremity edema, headache, and other symptoms associated with increased intracranial pressure. Involvement of the recurrent laryngeal nerve, which loops under the aorta by the ligamentum arteriosum, leads to hoarseness. Spread to the pleura leads to pleural effusion.

Diagnosis

The key is obtaining tissue for diagnosis. Start with a CXR, and compare it to old CXRs to assess interval changes. A CT scan is useful for (1) assessing the details of the primary lesion—calcifications, spiculations, satellite lesions—all of which point to malignancy, (2) determining the presence of additional intrapulmonary lesions, (3) staging—evaluating the presence of hilar, mediastinal, or distant lymphadenopathy; pleural effusion; and involvement of the pleura or chest wall. Remember that the advantage of CT scan over CXR is not resolution (plain films have better resolution) but contrast enhancement. Sputum samples can be evaluated for cytology, although sensitivity is low (50%). The next step is obtaining tissue. Bronchoscopy with or without transbroncial biopsy is indicated for centrally located lesions. One option for evaluation or peripheral lesions is fine-needle aspiration under CT guidance. Most clinicians agree to proceed directly to surgery if the patient is a reasonable candidate.

Treatment

Treatment options include surgery, chemotherapy, and, to a limited extent, radiation therapy. The general rule is that non-small cell carcinoma is treated with surgery (if feasible), and small cell carcinoma is treated with chemotherapy. A small number of small cell carcinoma patients present with limited lung involvement and may benefit from combined modality therapy: chemotherapy plus radiation to shrink the tumor followed by surgery. Unfortunately, overall 3-year survival for small cell carcinoma is less than 5%.

Other Tumors of the Lung and Thorax

- **Carcinoid of lung**: Bronchial carcinoid makes up about 1–5% of all lung tumors. Histologically, the cells contain dense secretory granules. Patients present with wheezing, dyspnea, cough, hemoptysis, and obstructive pneumonia. Many carcinoid tumors secrete vasoactive substances, particularly **serotonin**, leading to signs and symptoms of **carcinoid syndrome**: warmth, flushing, cyanosis, and diarrhea. Carcinoids rarely metastasize and are therefore amenable to resection. The 5- to 10-year survival is 50–95%.

- **Lymphoma**: Non-Hodgkin's lymphoma and Hodgkin's disease may present with mediastinal or hilar lymphadenopathy. These diseases are described in more detail in chapter 9.

- **Benign mesothelioma**: Also known as a pleural fibroma, it can be very large, but it is always confined to the pleural surface. There is no association with asbestos exposure.

- **Malignant mesothelioma**: These are fortunately rare tumors but are associated with asbestos exposure. In shipping and industrial areas, up to 90% of mesotheliomas have associated asbestos expo- sure. There is a long latency to development of mesothelioma after exposure (20–50 years), and there is no increased risk with concomitant smoking. Note that in asbestos-related bronchogenic carcinoma, there is a markedly increased risk of cancer when a patient is both a smoker and has asbestos exposure. Prognosis is poor.

CRITICAL CARE MEDICINE

Respiratory Failure

Respiratory failure is defined as one of the following:

- Poor oxygenation: $PaO_2 < 55$ mm Hg

- Poor ventilation: $PaCO_2 > 55$ mm Hg

These criteria are based on normal individuals. Patients with chronic, partially compensated respiratory disease (e.g., COPD, pulmonary hypertension, shunt) may have relatively poor oxygenation and ventilation as a baseline.

Respiratory failure is an indication for intubation and mechanical ventilatory support. Other indications include altered mental status with inability to protect the airway, apnea, neuromuscular paralysis, pulmonary hemorrhage, and therapeutic hyperventilation for increased intracranial pressure.

Neonatal Respiratory Distress Syndrome

Premature newborns born before week 24 of gestation cannot adequately produce surfactant. As a result, their lungs cannot expand, pulmonary vascular resistance remains high, and respiratory failure ensues. Pregnant women who appear to be at risk of premature labor are given corticosteroids because these appear to hasten lung development. After birth, treatment consists of mechanical ventilatory support until the baby can make its own surfactant as well as the use of a new, artificial surfactant.

Common complications resulting from high pressures of mechanical ventilators include pulmonary interstitial emphysema and pneumothorax. With eventual recovery, a significant portion of patients develop **bronchopulmonary dysplasia**, characterized by abnormal CXR, showing areas of bronchiectasis and fibrous scarring, a tendency to recurrent RSV infection, and RAD.

Adult Respiratory Distress Syndrome

Pathologically, it is believed that a primary event somewhere in the body leads to the release of systemic factors, including cytokines, which then lead to leaky capillary membranes. This results in interstitial edema, hypoxemia, and respiratory distress—adult RDS (ARDS). This entity was first described in 1967 by physicians treating Vietnam War soldiers in various states of trauma and infection leading to respiratory failure. Respiratory failure occurs, usually in a hospitalized patient, necessitating mechanical ventilation.

Major criteria for ARDS are as follows:

- Opacities in all four quadrants of the lung fields on CXR

- Poor oxygenation (defined as $PaO_2/FIO_2 < 200$)

- Normal pulmonary capillary wedge pressure (PCWP) (to rule out cardiogenic causes)

Minor criteria for ARDS are as follows:

- Reduced lung compliance

- Clinical picture of sepsis or multi-organ failure syndrome

- Large amount of PEEP required (PEEP is positive end-expiratory pressure, which keeps the alveoli open and improves oxygenation.)

Mortality with ARDS approaches 40–50%. Treatment options are limited. Support in the ICU is necessary. Investigational treatments, including specific alterations in the means of delivering mechanical ventilation, delivering antibodies to various inflammatory mediators, giving inhaled nitric oxide (to improve oxygenation via vasodilation), and placing the patient in a prone position (because ARDS affects dependent portions of the lung more, and so the prone position may improve $\dot{V}/\dot{Q}$ match in the relatively disease-free zones of lung).

PHARMACOLOGY

Table 8 lists drugs commonly used in the treatment of respiratory disorders.

Agent	Mechanism	Use	Toxicities
Antihistimines **Diphenhydramine** Chlorpheniramine Loratadine Fexofenadine Astemizole Cetrizine	Histamine-receptor antagonist	Allergic rhinitis, urticaria, anaphylaxis	Sedation, antimuscarinic effects (dry mouth, blurred vision)
Cough suppressants Codeine Dextromethorphan	Central cough suppression	Symptomatic relief of cough	Sedation, tolerance, and dependence with codeine Tremor, tachycardia, palpitations, arrhythmias
Beta-agonists Albuteral Terbutaline Metaproterenol	Selective for 2 receptors, causing smooth muscle relaxation	Acute asthma attacks, COPD maintenance and exacerbations	Tremor, tachycardia, palpitations, arrhythmias
Anticholinergics Ipratropium	Reverses acetylcholine-induced bronchoconstriction	Acute asthma attacks, COPD maintenance and exacerbations	Dry mouth, urinary retention, tachycardia, agitation
Cromolyn	Stabilizes mast cells and prevents degranulation, inhibiting histamine release	Asthma and COPD	Dry mouth, throat irritation
Methylxanthines Theophylline Aminophylline Theobromine	Unclear; appears to inhibit phosphodiesterase, leading to increased cellular cAMP Increases respiratory drive, mucociliary clearance, and diaphragm contractility	Asthma and COPD	Mild: anorexia, nausea and vomiting, headache, anxiety, gastrointestinal distress Severe: arrhythmias and seizures Levels must be checked regularly
N-Acetylcysteine	Reduces sulfur bridges in proteinaceous secretions	Also used for acetaminophen overdose	Increases respiratory tract mucus

Table 8 Drugs used in respiratory disorders

CHAPTER 17

RENAL SYSTEM

ANATOMY

The urinary system consists of a pair of kidneys and ureters connected to a bladder and a urethra (Figure 1).

The **kidneys** are located in the retroperitoneum and lie in the L1–L4 distribution. Remember that the right kidney is usually lower than the left because the liver pushes the right kidney downward.

The **ureters** are also retroperitoneal and travel along the psoas muscle. The ureters can be obstructed by renal calculi at three frequent sites of constriction: (1) the ureteropelvic junction, which is the most common, (2) the crossing of the pelvic brim, and (3) the ureterovesicular junction. The ureter has a muscular wall that propels urine to the bladder by a peristaltic wave.

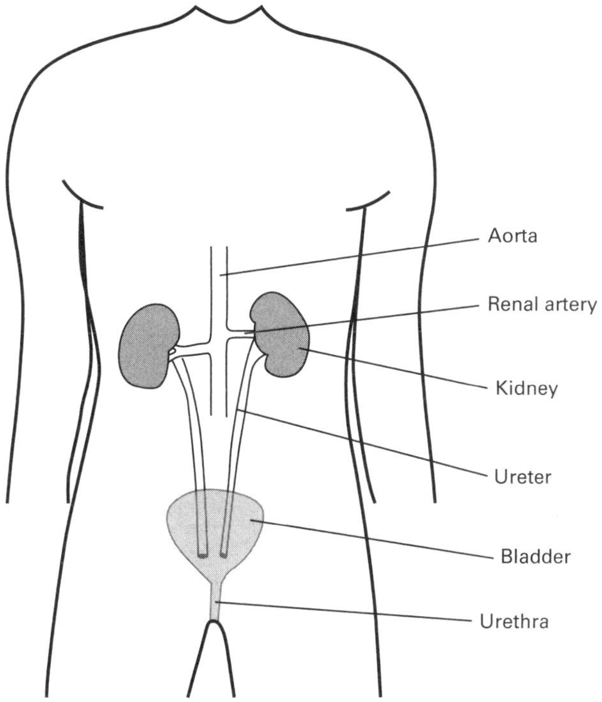

"Water under the bridge"
Water = ureter
Bridge = renal arteries

Figure 1 The urinary system
(Adapted from *Functional Histology: A Text and Colour Atlas*)

The **detrusor** muscle of the bladder squeezes urine into the urethra when stimulated by parasympathetic signals to void.

The **renal arteries** lie just inferior to the superior mesenteric artery (Figure 2). Because the aorta lies slightly to the left of center, the right renal artery must travel further to reach the right kidney than the left. In contrast, the inferior vena cava (IVC) lies just to the right of center, so the left renal vein travels further than the right. The renal veins pass in front of the arteries. The testicular and ovarian arteries arise from the aorta and cross the ureters anteriorly.

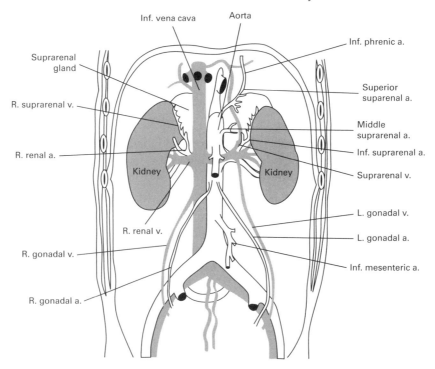

Figure 2 Location of kidneys, ureters, and associated vasculature

The **urethra sphincter** muscle lies within the urogenital diaphragm and helps keep urine from leaking out (Figure 3). In addition to autonomic innervations, the urethra sphincter can be controlled voluntarily, which is especially helpful on long road trips.

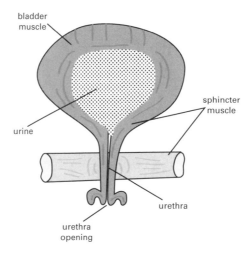

Figure 3 Location of kidneys, ureters, and associated vasculature

In men, the **prostate** sits between the bladder and the sphincter urethrae muscle. As men get older, many develop benign prostatic hyperplasia (BPH), in which the prostate gets larger and compresses the urethra, making it difficult to urinate.

Women have significantly shorter urethra than men and are more prone to frequent **urinary tract infections** (UTIs). Women may develop **stress incontinence** resulting in involuntary urine leaking when coughing or laughing. Stress incontinence often occurs after childbirth because the levator ani and muscles of the urogenital diaphragm are stretched and weakened as the baby passes through the vaginal canal.

EMBRYOLOGY

During the fourth and fifth week of development, nephrotomes develop from intermediate mesoderm (Figure 4) and later give rise to the **pronephric**, **mesonephric**, and **metanephric** systems.

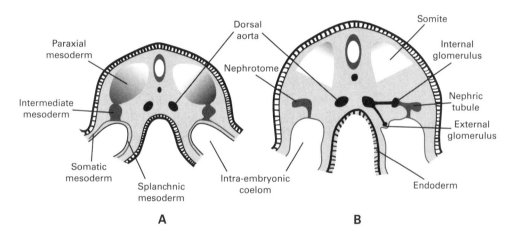

Figure 4 Origin of the kidney and collecting system.
A. Nephric tubule at 21 days. **B.** At 25 days.

The **pronephros** appear in the cervical region during week 4 (Figure 5A). Pronephros gives rise to the pronephric ducts, which interact with the mesonephric system and form the mesonephric tubules.

The **mesonephros** stimulates the formation of the müllerian or paramesonephric ducts, which is critical in the development of female sex organs. In men, the mesonephric duct transforms into the ejaculatory system (Figure 5B).

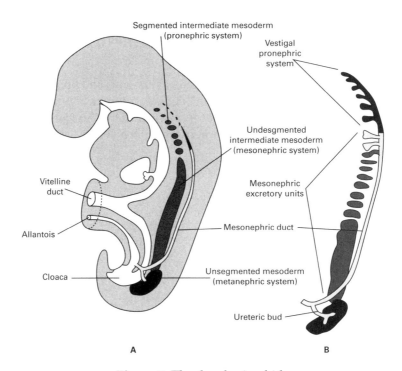

Figure 5 The developing kidney
A. Relationship of pronephric, mesoephric, and metanephric systems
B. Development of the mesonephros

The **metanephros** is called the permanent kidney and becomes the eventual kidney, beginning in week 4 and continuing through week 32–36. The **ureteric bud** grows from the bottom of the mesonephric duct and is encompassed by the metanephric blastema (Figure 6). The ureteric bud goes through multiple divisions and extensions to form the ureter, pelvis, major and minor calyces and the collecting tubules (Figure 7). Malformation of the ureteric bud and metanephric mesenchyme can lead to **Potter's Syndrome**.

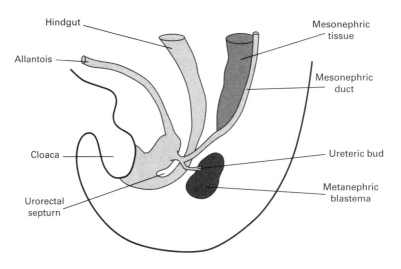

Figure 6 Origin of the permanent kidney, from interactions between the ureteric bud and metanephric blastema

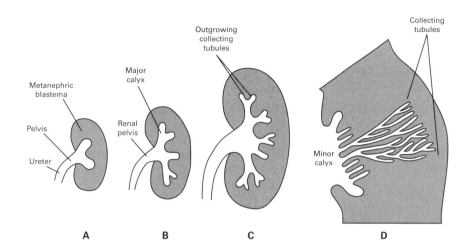

Figure 7 Development of the excretory system **A.** 6 weeks
B. End of sixth week **C.** 7 weeks **D.** Newborn

The rise of collecting tubules stimulates the metanephric tissue to form renal tubules for the rest of the nephron. The proximal part of the metanephric tubule forms **Bowman's capsule.** Eventually, Bowman's capsule will invaginate, engulfing the glomerulus. The metanephric tubules extend to form the proximal convoluted tubule, the loop of Henle, and the distal convoluted tubule. The distal part of the metanephric tubules fuses with the collecting tubules to form a patent conduit for urine to flow (Figure 8).

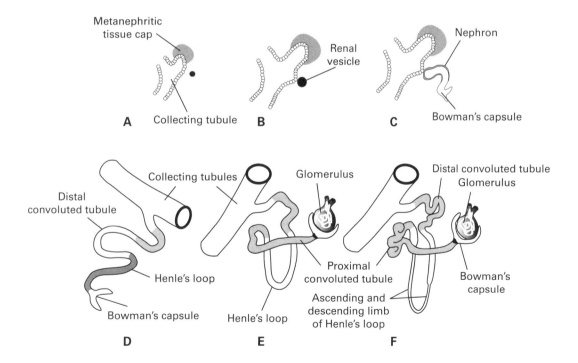

Figure 8 Development of the renal corpuscle and tubules
A. Metanephric tissue caps cover collecting tubules
B, C. Cells of tissue caps form renal vesicles, which become small tubules
C, D. Proximal tubule develops into Bowman's capsule, which indents. **E, F.** Excretory tubule
lengthens to become the proximal and distal convoluted tubules and the loop of Henle

The cloaca is divided by the urorectal septum to form the primitive urogenital sinus and anorectal canal. The **urinary bladder** then develops from the urogenital sinus and remains attached to the umbilicus by the urachus, the final remnant of the allantois (Figure 9). The urethra is derived from the definitive urogenital sinus.

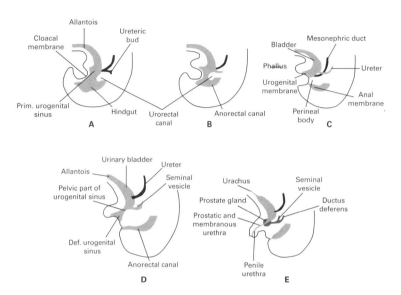

Figure 9 Origin of the urinary bladder. Development of urogenital sinus and anorectal canal at the end of **A**. the fifth week **B**. 7th week ,and **C**. 8th week **D**. Development of urinary bladder and **E**. penile urethra from urogenital sinus

During fetal development, kidneys rise superiorly, above the pelvis, while the gonads descend (Figure 10). The kidneys start to excrete urine into the amniotic cavity by the middle of the pregnancy. Although the kidneys produce urine, they are not yet responsible for removing waste products from the fetus. Prior to birth, the placenta will excrete waste products and fetal urine remains dilute.

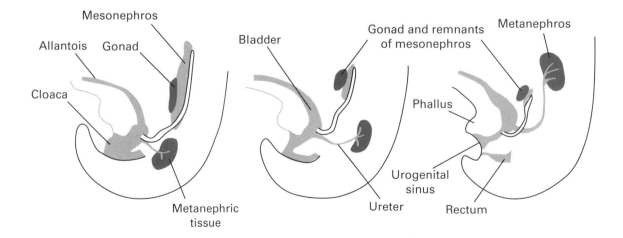

Figure 10 Development of the urinary bladder. Relative development of kidneys and gonads during development

HISTOLOGY

The Kidney

All vessels to and from the kidney are located at the **hilum**. These vessels include the renal artery, renal vein, and ureter. The kidney is divided into an outer **cortex** and an inner **medulla** (Figure 11).

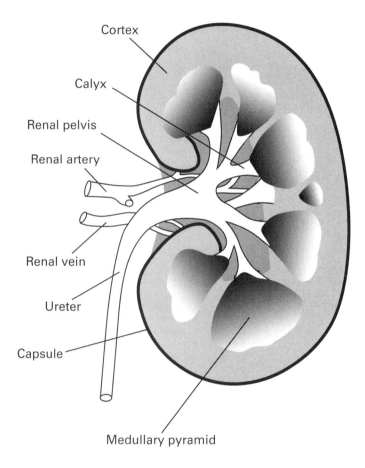

Figure 11 Anatomy of the kidney
(Adapted from *Functional Histology: A Text and Colour Atlas*)

The medulla consists of multiple medullary pyramids. The cortex surrounds the outer base if pyramids and the apex of the medulla is called the **renal papilla**. Urine passes from renal papilla, minor calyx, major calyx to renal pelvis and finally, into the ureter. Portions of the cortex consisting of the renal columns extend between the pyramids. A fibrous capsule as well as a thick layer of fat cover the kidney and protect against traumatic injuries.

The Nephron and Collecting System

The nephron consists of two major units, the renal **corpuscle** and renal **tubule** (Figure 12). The renal corpuscle is the filtering system, which consists of the **glomerulus** and the **Bowman's capsule** (Figure 13). The renal tubule carries the filtrate to the collecting duct and consists of the **proximal convoluted tubule** (PCT), **loop of Henle**, **distal convoluted tubule** (DCT), and the **collecting tubule**.

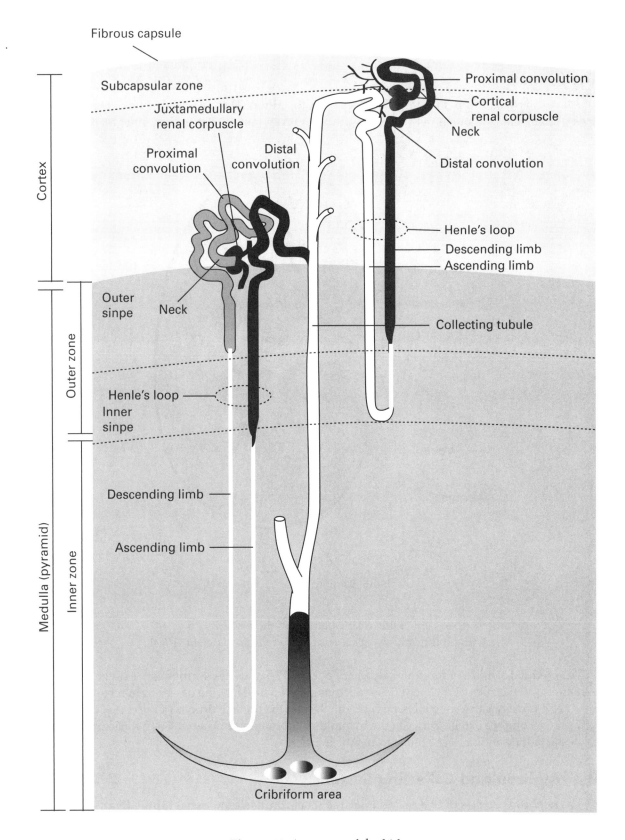

Figure 12 Anatomy of the kidney
(Adapted from *Functional Histology: A Text and Colour Atlas*)

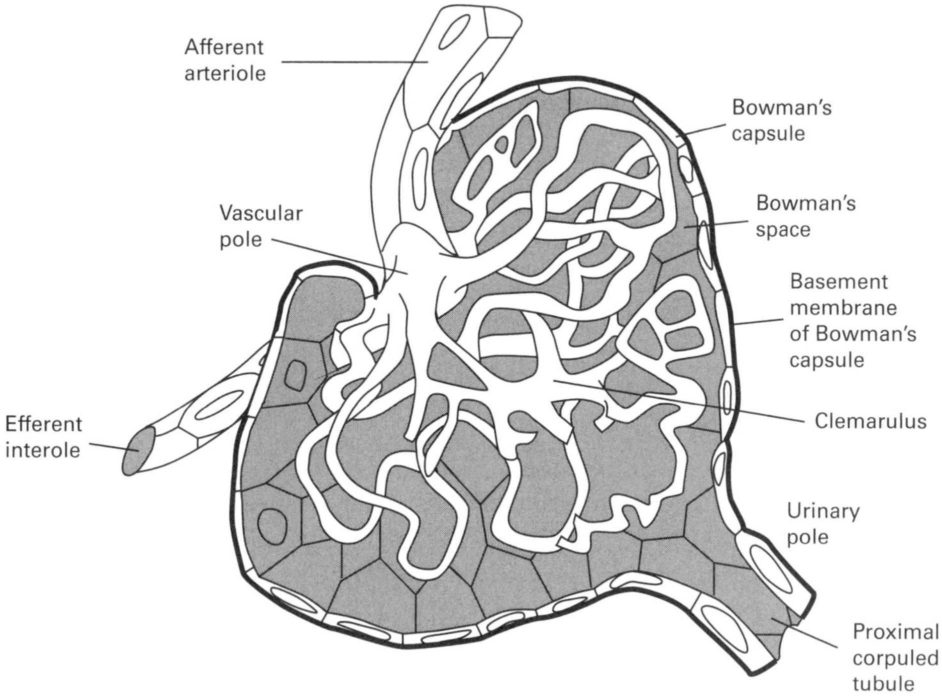

Afferent
arteriole

Bowman's
capsule

Vascular
pole

Bowman's
space

Basement
membrane
of Bowman's
capsule

Efferent
interole

Clemarulus

Urinary
pole

Proximal
corpuled
tubule

Figure 13 The glomerulus
(Adapted from *Functional Histology: A Text and Colour Atlas*)

Juxtaglomerular apparatus is a very important structure that plays a key role in blood pressure regulation. Notice that the juxtaglomerular cells are located in the wall of the afferent arteriole, whereas the macula densa is located in the wall of the DCT (Figure 14). A specialized, multilayered transitional epithelium lines the urinary system.

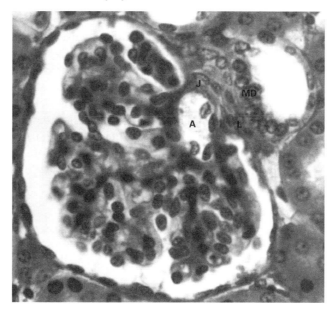

Figure 14 Light microscopy of the juxtaglomerular apparatus.
(MD = macula densa; A = afferent arteriole; J = juxtaglomerular cells; L = lacis cells.)
(Adapted from *Functional Histology: A Text and Colour Atlas*)

PHYSIOLOGY

Glomerular filtration and Hemodynamics

Renal Clearance

Clearance measures kidney's excretion ability. More specifically, renal clearance measures how fast a certain substance is removed from the blood and excreted in the urine. It can be calculated using the following formula:

$$C = (U.V)/P$$

Where C = clearance (ml/min), U = concentration in urine (mg/ml), V = volume of urine made per minute (ml/min), and P = concentration in plasma (mg/ml).

Clearance is affected by how easily a substance is filtered at the glomerulus then secreted or reabsorbed by the tubules. The clearance formula is important because it can be used to determine the **glomerular filtration rate** (GFR).

Inulin is an excellent substance used to calculate GFR because it is filtered without being secreted or reabsorbed in the tubules. Now you can apply the GFR formula with inulin as the substance:

$$C = GFR = (U_{inulin}.V)/P_{inulin}$$

For example, U_{inulin} = urine concentration of inulin (mg/ml), V = volume of urine in 24 hours (ml/24 hr), P_{inulin} = plasma concentration of inulin (mg/ml), and GFR = (ml/24 hr), which can then be converted to ml/min.

Besides inulin, **mannitol** and **sorbitol** are commonly used to determine GFR. Now that you have the inulin clearance as a standard, you can compare the clearance of any other substance to see if it's freely filtered, secreted, or reabsorbed.

In the hospital, **blood urea nitrogen (BUN)** and **creatinine** are used to estimate GFR. Creatinine clearance is only an approximate measurement of GFR as creatinine is secreted by the tubules. Therefore, creatinine clearance slightly overestimates GFR. BUN is measured amount of nitrogen in the blood and reflects metabolism of protein by the liver, whereas creatinine measures nitrogen from muscle breakdown. If GFR decreases, excretion decreases and therefore, the BUN and creatinine will both increase. As we get older, GFR decreases, but the creatinine level doesn't change because our bodies usually also have less muscle mass and less nitrogen from muscle breakdown. However, it is important to note that the rate of drug excretion decreases in older patients with decreased GFR. Therefore, it is important to renally dose medications in elderly patients.

Another way to determine GFR is by using the **Starling equation**:

$$GFR = K_f[(P_{glom} - P_{BS}) - (\neq_{glom} - \neq_{BS})]$$

Where K_f = filtration coefficient, Pglom = hydrostatic pressure in the glomerular capillary, PBS = hydrostatic pressure in Bowman's space, $\neq$glom = oncotic pressure in the glomerular capillary, and $\neq_{BS}$ = oncotic pressure in Bowman's space.

Therefore, GFR increases with constriction of the efferent arteriole or dilation of the afferent arteriole (P_{glom} increases).

Renal Blood Flow

Blood flow to the kidneys follows the same general principles discussed in chapter 4. The same formula can be used to determine renal blood flow (RBF):

$$Q = \Delta DP/R$$

Where Q = RBF, DP = Prenal artery – Prenal vein = renal perfusion pressure, and R = resistance. RBF decreases if R increases or DP decreases; RBF increases if R decreases or DP increases.

Although the systemic blood pressure may vary, the kidney keeps its blood pressure relatively constant by a process called **autoregulation**. The kidneys adjust renal vascular resistance by constriction of its arterioles in response to systemic arterial pressures fluctuations between 100 and 200 mm Hg (Figure 15).

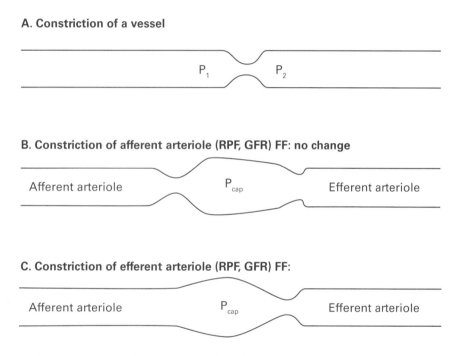

Figure 15 Alterations in renal plasma flow (RPF), glomerular filtration rate (GFR), and filtration fraction (FF) with constriction of afferent and efferent arterioles. (Pcap = pressure within glomerular capillary; P1 = pressure proximal to constriction; P2 = pressure distal to constriction.)

For example, exercise increases sympathetic tone, which causes constriction of the afferent arteriole, decreasing RBF and shunting blood to active muscles. RBF is determined indirectly by calculating the renal plasma flow (RPF). Instead of using inulin, **para-aminohippuric acid** (PAH) is used to estimate RPF. PAH is both filtered and excreted in the PCT. Because the hematocrit (Hct) measures the percentage of blood volume taken up by RBCs, and plasma is the blood "fluid" without RBCs:

$$RBF (1 - Hct) = RPF$$
$$RBF = RPF/(1 - Hct)$$

Filtration fraction (FF) refers to how much RPF is filtered through the glomerular capillary membrane. It can be calculated by the following equation:

$$FF = GFR/RPF$$

In general, normal FF is 20%, which means that 80% of the RPF passes into the efferent arterioles. Table 1 shows how constriction and dilation of the afferent and efferent arterioles affect GFR, RPF, and FF. Increased resistance leads to constriction, while decreased resistance leads to dilation.

Think through each scenario to make sure it makes sense!

Renal arteriolar vascular resistance		RPF (ml/min)	GFR (ml/min)	FF	Examples
Afferent	Efferent				
↑	—	↓	↓	—	NSAIDS
↓	—	↑	↑	—	Prostaglandins
—	↑	↓	↑	↑	Angiotensin
—	↓	↑	↓	↓	Ace inibitors

Table 1 Effects of changes in renal vascular resistance with a constant renal perfusion

Note that the glomerular filtration rate and renal plasma flow exhibit parallel shifts with changes in afferent arteriolar resistance, but exhibit divergent shifts with changes in efferent arteriolar resistance. Increases in vascular resistance always lead to a decline in renal plasma flow, and decreases in arteriolar resistance always lead to an increase in renal plasma flow. In the first two columns, upward arrows denote the effect of vasoconstriction, and downward arrows denote the effect of vasodilation.

Tubular Mechanisms for Reabsorption and Secretion

Reabsorption and Secretion Rates

The filtered load describes how much a substance was filtered per minute; the excretion rate describes how much substance was excreted in the urine per minute.

$$GFR \text{ (ml/min)} \times P \text{ (mg/dl)} = \text{Filtered load}$$

$$U \text{ (mg/dl)} \times V \text{ (ml/min)} = \text{Excretion rate}$$

If the excretion rate is greater than the filtered load, then tubular secretion has occurred. If the excretion rate is less than the filtered load, then reabsorption has occurred.

Titration Curves

The reabsorption and secretion of substances can also be represented graphically (Figure 16). First, let's use glucose as an example of a substance that is reabsorbed.

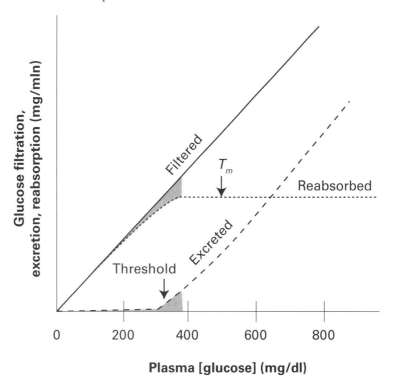

Figure 16 Titration curve for a substance that is reabsorbed (T_m = transport maximum.)

Glucose is reabsorbed in the PCT by a **sodium-glucose cotransporter**. The sodium-glucose cotransporters can reabsorb most of the glucose that is delivered to PCT, as long as the glucose concentration is less than 300 mg/dL. If the concentration of glucose is greater than 300 mg/dL, cotransporters become saturated and are unable to reabsorb all of the glucose, leading to excretion of urine. The **transport maximum** (Tm) is the point at which the cotransporters are maximally saturated with glucose. Therefore, the extra glucose that is delivered to the PCT above Tm gets excreted at a rate that is directly proportional to the plasma concentration of glucose.

Now let's consider another substance, PAH. The filtration curve for PAH is exactly the same as the one for glucose, except that the Tm curve is shifted to the left. PAH is also secreted by carriers in the PCT. However, as the concentration of PAH increases, the secretion increases accordingly. Because PAH is filtered as well as secreted, the excretion is the sum of the filtration and secretion. Once the concentration of PAH reaches a certain level, the carriers are working at full capacity, and the secretion rate cannot increase any further. This point is referred to as the Tm for PAH. After the Tm is reached, the excretion rate follows the slope of the filtration curve and is directly proportional to the plasma concentration of PAH.

Take a look at Figure 17 to compare various substances and their relative tubular fluid-to-plasma concentration ratios along the tubules of the kidney.

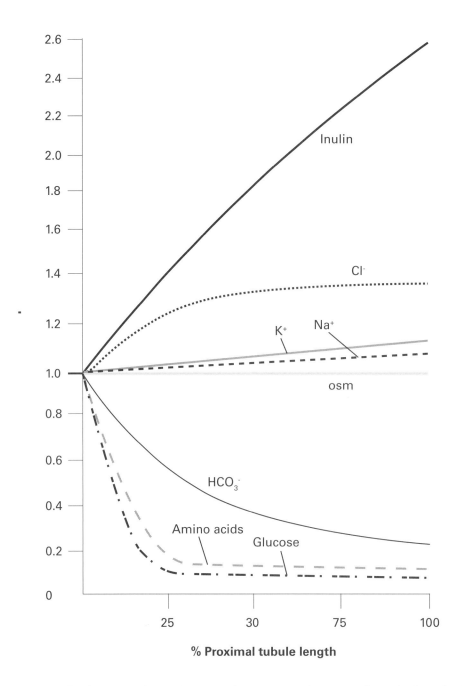

Figure 17 Tubular fluid (TF) to plasma (P) ratios for various substances along the length of the kidney (Adapted from *Ganong's Review Physiology*, 23rd Edition)

Sodium Management

Two-thirds of all filtered Na^+ is reabsorbed at the PCT (Figure 18). The early PCT use **cotransporters** to reabsorb Na^+ along with glucose, phosphate, amino acids, and lactate. The cotransporter uses the energy derived from Na^+ moving down its concentration gradient to drive the active reabsorption of the other molecules against their concentration gradients. Moreover, another cotransporter exchanges Na^+ from the tubular lumen with H^+ from the cell, which depends on the amount of filtered HCO_3^-. The favorable Na^+ gradient is maintained by a **Na^+/K^+ adenosine**

triphosphatase (ATPase), which uses ATP to pump Na⁺ out of the cell, as it pumps K⁺ into the cell. In the middle and late PCT, Cl– is reabsorbed with Na⁺ (Figure 19).

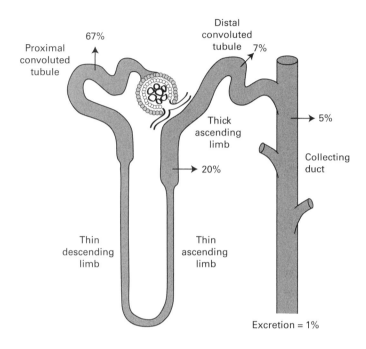

Figure 18 Reabsorption of NaCl

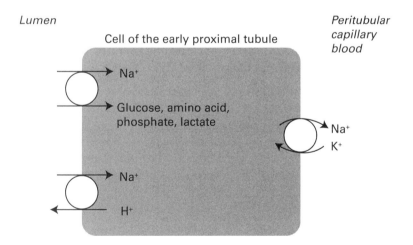

Figure 19 Na⁺ transporters in the cells of the proximal convoluted tubule

Glomerulotubular balance refers to the PCT's ability to maintain the reabsorption rate of Na⁺ no matter how much fluid is delivered. Glomerulotubular balance can be explained by the Starling forces. For example, if extracellular (ECF) volume decreases by dehydration, the

Carbonic anhydrase inhibitors work on the PCT.

peritubular capillary fluid will have a lower hydrostatic pressure, Pcap, and a higher protein concentration, which increases pcap. Both forces increase the movement of fluid from tubules to blood and enhance reabsorption. On the other hand, if ECF volume increases by overzealous water ingestion, Pcap increases and pcap decreases, which both decrease reabsorption.

Some 20% of filtered Na+ is reabsorbed by the **thick ascending limb of the loop of Henle (a-loop)** (Figure 20). The cells use a **Na$^+$/K$^+$-2Cl$^-$ cotransporter**, in which Na$^+$ is passively absorbed while providing the energy for active K$^+$ absorption. Although Na$^+$ and Cl$^-$ are both absorbed, the cells of the a-loop are impermeable to water.

Loop diuretics
(e.g., furosemide)
act on a-loop

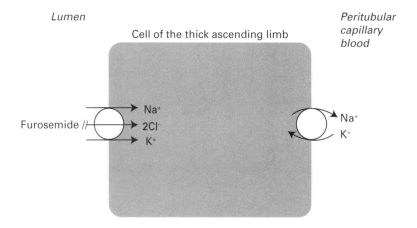

Figure 20 The Na$^+$/K$^+$/2Cl$^-$ cotransporter in the cells of the a-loop

Some 12% of filtered Na$^+$ is reabsorbed in the DCT and collecting ducts. The early distal tubule has a Na$^+$/Cl$^-$ cotransporter and is impermeable to water. **Thiazide** have their main diuretic action in the DCT.

The late DCT and the collecting duct have **principal cells** and **intercalated cells**. The principal cells reabsorb Na$^+$ and secrete K$^+$ by action of **aldosterone** and **antidiuretic hormone** (ADH), resulting in increased water reabsorption. The late DCT and collecting duct is the site of action for the **K$^+$ sparing diuretics**, such as spironolactone. The intercalated cells are also stimulated by aldosterone, which increases K$^+$ reabsorption and H$^+$ secretion.

Potassium Management

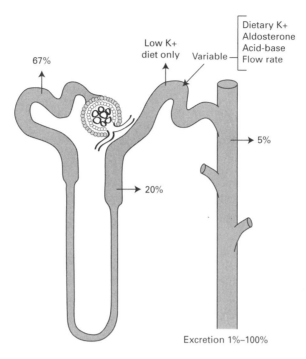

Figure 21 K⁺ management

K⁺ is freely filtered at the glomerulus. K⁺ reabsorption is similar to that of Na⁺ in that two-thirds is reabsorbed at the PCT, along with Na⁺ and water and 20% is reabsorbed at the a-loop by the Na⁺/K⁺-2Cl⁻ cotransporter (Figure 21). K⁺ is also reabsorbed or secreted at the DCT and collecting tubules depending on the following factors:

- Amount of K⁺ in diet

- Level of aldosterone

- Acid-base status

- Diuretics

- Anions in tubules

K⁺ is reabsorbed in the intercalated cells of the DCT by the **H⁺/K⁺-ATPase**. H⁺/K⁺-ATPase also plays a major role in acid-base balance.

K⁺ secretion can be initially confusing (Figure 22). First, the Na⁺/K⁺ ATPase makes sure that there's a higher concentration of K⁺ inside the cell and higher concentration of Na⁺ outside of the cell. Then, K⁺ is passively secreted into the tubular lumen depending on the number of factors, such as alkalotic state, hyperaldosteronism, and use of diuretics.

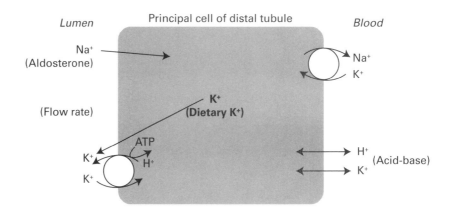

Figure 22 K⁺ secretion by cells of the distal convoluted tubule

When more K⁺ is consumed in the diet, the concentration of K⁺ in the principal cell increases, leading to a stronger K⁺ gradient. Hence, K⁺ inside the cell is greater than K⁺ concentration inside the lumen and more K⁺ is passively secreted (Figure 23). A diet low in K⁺ is just the opposite: The K⁺ gradient is smaller, so less K⁺ is secreted and more is retained in the cell.

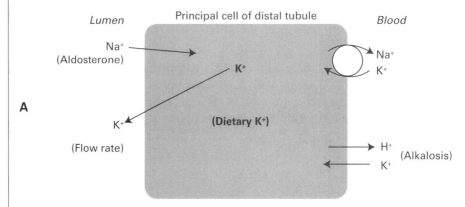

Figure 23 **A.** K⁺ secretion in the setting of high dietary K⁺, hyperaldosteronism, or alkalotic states

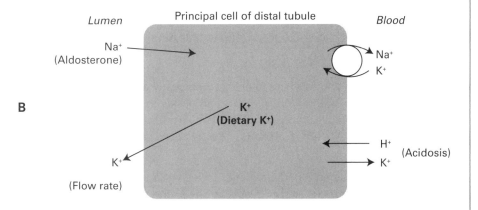

Figure 23 B. K$^+$ secretion in the setting
of low dietary K$^+$, hypoaldosteronism, or acidotic states

High aldosterone
→ low K$^+$

Low aldosterone
→ high K$^+$

Aldosterone increases the amount of Na$^+$ that enters the cell and stimulates the Na$^+$/K$^+$-ATPase to increase the amount of K$^+$ pumped into the cell. Again, because there's more K$^+$ inside the cell than outside, K$^+$ secretion increases. If the aldosterone level is too high (**hyperaldosteronism**), hypokalemia can occur. On the other hand, if the aldosterone level is too low (**hypoaldosteronism**), the K$^+$ gradient is smaller than normal, less K$^+$ is secreted, and hyperkalemia can occur.

If a patient is acidotic, the excess H$^+$ gets pulled into the cell in exchange for K$^+$ out of the cell. Less K$^+$ in the cell means a smaller gradient, less K$^+$ secretion, and hyperkalemia can ensue. In alkalosis, there's too little H$^+$ in the blood. Now, H$^+$ is kicked out of the cell in exchange for K$^+$ moving into the cell. This generates a higher K$^+$ gradient and more K$^+$ is secreted leading to hypokalemia.

Loop diuretics and thiazides increase the flow rate of urine to the distal tubule. This effectively decreases the K$^+$ concentration in the lumen and increases the K$^+$ gradient (Figure 24). As a result, K$^+$ secretion increases and hypokalemia can occur.

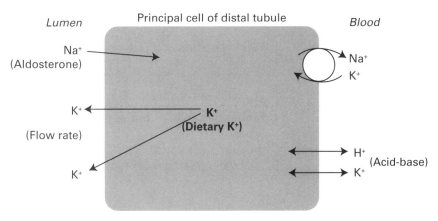

Figure 24 Effects of loop diuretics on K$^+$ secretion

Hypokalemia can be prevented by using a K^+ sparing diuretic, such as spironolactone or amiloride. Spironolactone prevents K^+ secretion indirectly as an aldosterone antagonist, while amiloride works directly on the DCT to prevent K^+ secretion.

K^+ secretion may also increase if there are excess anions in the tubular lumen (opposites attract!).

Calcium

Only 60% of Ca^{+2} in the plasma is filtered across the glomerular membrane and 90% of the filtered Ca^{+2} is reabsorbed in the PCT and the a-loop. Ca^{+2} is absorbed passively along with Na+ reabsorption. Because loop diuretics block Na^+ reabsorption, Ca^{+2} reabsorption is also inhibited. **Loop diuretics** are therefore helpful in treating **hypercalcemia.** About 9% of Ca^{+2} is actively reabsorbed by the DCT and collecting duct.

Parathyroid hormone (PTH) is released when blood Ca^{+2} levels are low and stimulates the DCT to increase Ca^{+2} reabsorption. **Thiazides** also increase Ca^{+2} reabsorption in the DCT. Therefore, patients who have renal stones precipitated by **hypercalciuria** may benefit from treatment with thiazides.

Magnesium

Mg^{+2} is reabsorbed by the PCT, DCT, and the a-loop. Mg^{+2} and Ca^{+2} compete for the same transporters in the ascending limb. Excess Ca^{+2} in the renal tubules will overpower the Mg^{+2} and be absorbed at the expense of Mg^{+2}, leading to excretion of Mg^{+2} in urine. However, the tables are turned if there is excess Mg^{+2} in the blood. Hypermagnesemia will lead to Ca^{+2} excretion.

Phosphate

About 85% of phosphate is reabsorbed by the PCT by Na^+ cotransport. Because the rest of the renal tubules cannot reabsorb phosphate, 15% of the phosphate is naturally excreted! Phosphate reabsorption is inhibited by PTH.

Urea

The PCT reabsorbs 50% of the filtered urea. Urea is also reabsorbed by the inner medullary collecting ducts with ADH. Urea is then used to help concentrate urine in hypovolemic states, such as dehydration or hemorrhage.

	Hypo-	**Hyper-**
Na^+	Lethargy, confusion, coma, muscle twitches, irritability, seizures, nausea, vomiting	Lethargy, confusion, coma, muscle twitches, irritability, seizures, stupor
K^+	Muscle weakness, cramps, tetany, polyuria, polydipsia U waves, flat T waves	Weakness, flaccid paralysis, confusion Peaked T waves, wide QRS
Ca^{2+}	Hypertension, peripheral and perioral paresthesia, abdominal pain and cramps, lethargy, irritability in infants	**Stones** (renal colic), **bones** (osteitis fibrosa), **moans** (constipation), and **groans** (neuropsychiatric symptoms—confusion)

Cl⁻	**Rare** Metabolic alkalosis, hypokalemia, hypovolemia, hyperaldosteronism	Non-anion gap acidosis
Mg^{2+}	Weakness, muscle twitches, asterixis, vertigo	Mild: Nausea, vomiting, hypotension, ↓ reflexes Moderate: Weakness, drowsiness, quadraparesis Severe: Coma, bradycardia, respiratory failure
PO_4^{3-}	Bone loss, muscle weakness + cardiac, respiratory and CNS issues.	Tetany, renal stones, metastatic calcifications

Table 2 Summary of electrolyte disturbances

Urinary Concentration and Dilution

Concentration of Urine

Urine is concentrated by a countercurrent multiplier system (Figure 25). It's countercurrent because the three limbs have flow of urine in alternating directions.

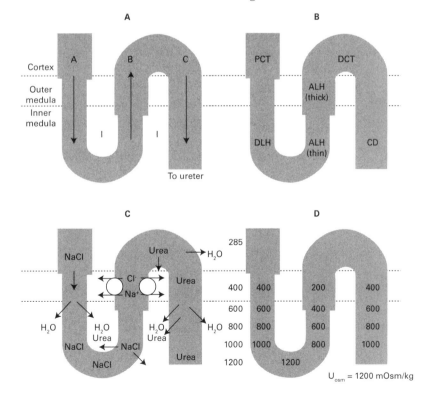

Figure 25 The countercurrent multiplier system **A.** Direction of fluid flow.
B. Location of tubule segments **C.** Movement of NaCl, H_2O, and urea.
D. Osmolarity inside and outside tubules (PCT = proximal convoluted tubule;
DLH = descending loop of Henle; ALH = ascending loop of Henle;
DCT = distal convoluted tubule; CD = collecting duct; Uosm = urine osmolarity)

As you travel deeper into the medulla, the osmotic gradient becomes progressively higher. This corticopapillary gradient derived mostly from NaCl and urea is what allows efficient water retention.

Just like Na^+, two-thirds of the water is reabsorbed in the PCT.

In the **descending limb of the loop of Henle (d-loop)**, water moves from the tubule to the interstitium, which has a much higher osmolarity. Because this portion of d-loop concentrates the tubular fluid, it's called the **concentrating segment**. The d-loop is fairly impermeable to NaCl and urea, so most of NaCL and urea stays within the tubule.

In the a-loop, urea moves down its concentration gradient and into the lumen. NaCl gets pumped out of the lumen and into the interstitium. The NaCl in the interstitium is one source of the high corticopapillary osmotic gradient. Because the a-loop is impermeable to water, and more NaCl leaves than urea enters, leaving the tubular fluid more dilute. This is why the a-loop is called the **diluting segment**.

The early DCT is also impermeable to water, diluting the tubular fluid even further. However, water and urea can be reabsorbed in the late DCT, especially when ADH is around.

In the collecting ducts, urea passively moves down its concentration gradient into the interstitium. This movement is encouraged by the presence of ADH, which increases urea and water permeability in the collecting ducts. As the collecting ducts extend into the inner medulla, water and urea are both reabsorbed. Some of the urea enters the a-loop as mentioned previously, but most gets stuck in the interstitium and adds to the strong corticopapillary osmotic gradient.

The **vasa recta** are the countercurrent exchangers (Figure 26). They follow the tubules into the medulla and are permeable to water and solutes. As blood passes into the descending limb of the vasa recta, the osmotic gradient causes NaCl and urea to move into the capillaries while water moves into the interstitium. After flowing through the vasa recta, the plasma is super concentrated. Therefore, NaCl and urea return to the interstitium and water moves back into the capillaries. To summarize, solutes are trapped in the interstitium, maintaining the osmotic gradient and water is returned to the circulation. Figure 27 describes how the body retains water in a water deprivation state.

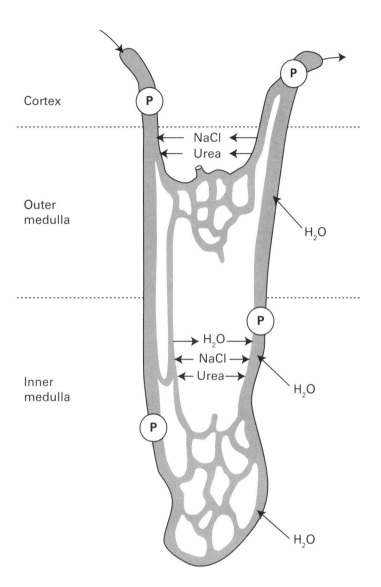

Figure 26 The importance of vasa recta in preserving the osmotic gradient. (P = plasma concentration; the larger the P, the higher the concentration.)

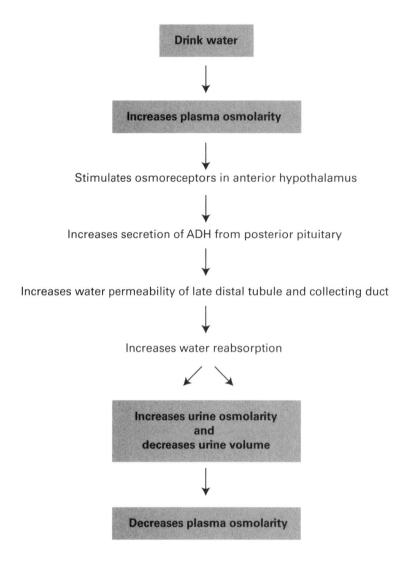

Figure 27 Physiologic response to water deprivation

Dilution of Urine

Over-consumption of water can occur in psychogenic polydipsia. In cases of water intoxication, dilution of urine can occur. Again, two-thirds of the water is reabsorbed at the PCT. The tubular fluid is also diluted in the a-loop and early DCT, where NaCl is actively removed. However, without the presence of ADH, the late DCT and collecting ducts remain impermeable to water. No matter what the osmotic gradient is, water is stuck within the tubules and is excreted as dilute urine without ADH (Figure 28).

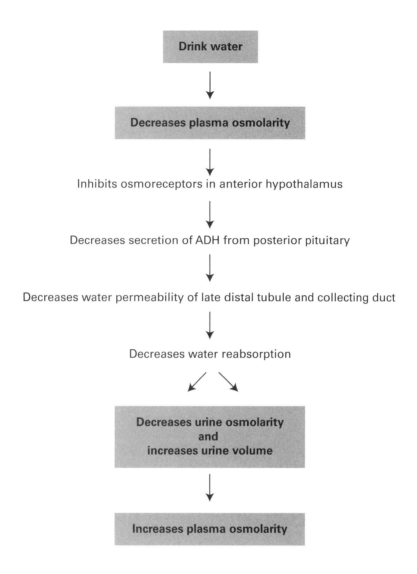

Figure 28 Physiologic response to water overload

Free Water Clearance

Free water clearance (FWC) calculates how much water is excreted or reabsorbed. When ADH is present, water is reabsorbed and FWC is negative. When ADH is absent, water is excreted and FWC is positive. To calculate the FWC, you need to know the urine flow rate (V), and the osmolar clearance (Cosm).

$$\text{FWC} = V - C_{osm}$$

Remember, $C_{osm} = (U_{osm} - V)\,/\,P_{osm}$

The C_{osm} describes how many osmoles are cleared from the urine each minute. For example, if there's a low concentration of osmoles in the urine, or if C_{osm} is low, urine must be dilute. A high osmolar clearance can only occur when the urine is well concentrated. Hence, water is reabsorbed and reflected as a negative FWC. The clinical examples listed in Table 3 should reinforce this concept.

	Serum ADH	Serum osmolarity/[Na+]	Urine osmolarity	Free water clearance
1⁰ polydipsia	↓	↓	Hypo	+
Central DI	↓	↑	Hypo	+
Nephrogenic DI	↑	↑	Hypo	+
Water deprivation	↑	↑ (high-normal)	Hyper	-
Syndrome of inappropriate ADH	↑↑	↓	Hyper	-

ADH = Antidiuretic hormone.

Table 3 Processes affecting urine and serum osmolarity and free water clearance

Body Fluid Compartments

Distribution of Body Water

Total body water (TBW) is about 60% of the body weight and can be allocated into intracellular and extracellular fluids.

Intracellular fluid (ICF) is about two-thirds of TBW. K^+ and Mg^{+2} are the major cations, whereas protein and organic phosphates, such as ATP are the major anions. **Exracellular fluid** (ECF) is the one-third remainder of TBW. Na^+ is the major cation, whereas Cl^- and HCO_3^- are the major anions. ECF can be further divided into interstitium and plasma. About three-fourths of the ECF is located in the interstitium, and the other one-fourth is found in plasma (Figure 29). Albumin and immunoglobulins comprise the major plasma proteins. Because interstitial fluid is almost identical to plasma, except that it lacks proteins, it is also called an **ultrafiltrate**.

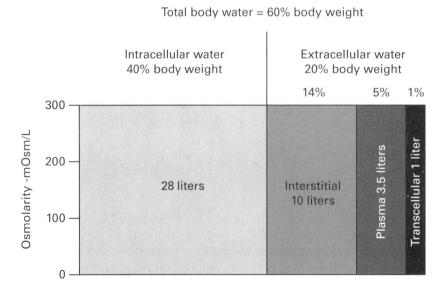

Figure 29 Distribution of body water

Specific markers can be used to measure the amount of fluid in each compartment, or volume of distribution (VD). The markers used are listed in Table 4. After a certain amount of marker is injected into the blood, it is allowed to equilibrate, and the resulting concentration is measured according to each compartment.

V_D (liters) = Marker (mg)/concentration {mg/liter}

For example, mannitol is a large molecule and cannot cross into cells. Therefore, it is a perfect marker for measuring the ECF.

Compartment	Marker
Total body water (TBW	Tritiated H_2O or D_2O
Extracellular fluid (ECF)	Inulin
	Mannitol
	Sulfate
Intracellular fluid	ECF minus plasma volume
Plasma volume	Radiolabeled albumin
	Evans blue
Interstitial	TBW minus ECF

Table 4 Markers used for evaluation of fluid compartments

Water Shifts

In general, water moves between the ECF and ICF to maintain an equal osmolarity in both compartments. The scenarios described in Figure 30 and Table 5 describes different effects on ICF and ECF.

Type	Key examples	Extracellular fluid volume	Intracranial fluid volume	Extracellular fluid osmolarity	Hematocrit, serum [Na⁺]
Isosmotic volume expansion	Isotonic NaCl infusion	↑	-	-	↓ Hct - [Na⁺]
Isotonic NaCl infusion	Diarrhea	↓	-	-	↑ Hct - [Na⁺]
Hyperosmotic volume expansion	High NaCl intake	↑	↓	↑	↓ Hct ↑ [Na⁺]

Hyperosmotic volume contraction	Sweating Fever DI	↓	↓	↑	- Hct ↑ [Na⁺]
Hyposmotic volume expansion	SIADH	↑	↑	↓	- Hct ↓ [Na⁺]
Hyposmotic volume contraction	Adrenal insufficiency	↓	↑	↓	↑ Hct ↓ [Na⁺]

Table 5 Changes in volumes and osmolarity of body fluids

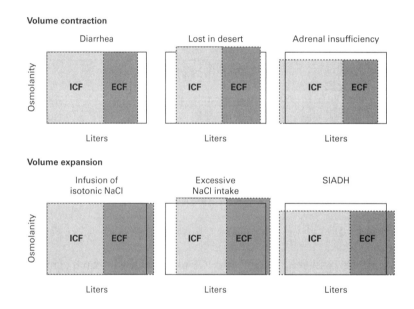

Figure 30 Alterations in extracellular fluid (ECF) and intracellular fluid (ICF) under different physiologic stressors. (SIADH = syndrome of inappropriate antidiuretic hormone)

Volume expansion states can be achieved in hyperosmotic (fluid osmolality > plasma osmolality), **isosmotic** (fluid osmolality = plasma osmolality), or **hyposmotic** (fluid osmolality < plasma osmolality) conditions.

- Excessive NaCl ingestion, or infusion with hypertonic saline can lead to **hyperosmotic over-hydration**. ECF osmolarity increases directly and draws water out of the ICF. The result is increased ECF volume as ICF volume decreases. Therefore, ICF osmolarity increases in order to equilibrate with the ECF.

- **Isosmotic overhydration** occurs with isotonic NaCl infusion. Although ECF volume increases, there's no change in osmolarity, so no water shifts out of the ICF. Extra fluid in the ECF dilutes plasma proteins and RBCs, which lowers the hematocrit.

- Syndrome of inappropriate ADH (SIADH) is an example of **hyposmotic overhydration**. Excess water is retained, which increases ECF volume and lowers ECF osmolarity. Water then shifts from ECF to ICF, thereby expanding ICF volume and lowering ICF osmolarity until it equilibrates with the ECF. One would think that the hematocrit would decrease due to dilutional effects, as in isosmotic overhydration. However, the hematocrit stays the same because the water also shifts into RBCs!

Volume contraction states, such as dehydration can also be the result of hyperosmotic, isosmotic, or hyposmotic fluid loss:

- **Hyperosmotic dehydration** can be caused by profuse sweating. ECF volume decreases, and because sweat is hyposmotic, ECF osmolarity increases. Water then shifts from ICF to ECF, which lowers ICF volume and increases ICF osmolarity until it equilibrates with the ECF. The hematocrit remains unchanged because water shifts out of the RBCs to maintain RBC concentration.

- **Diarrhea** is one way to lose isotonic fluid and lower ECF volume, while maintaining ECF osmolarity. As a result, no water shift occurs between the ECF and ICF. Hence, ICF volume remains the same. Hematocrit increases because the RBCs are also concentrated from volume loss and there is no water shift out of or into the RBCs.

- **Hyposmotic dehydration** can occur with adrenal insufficiency. If there is no aldosterone release, the DCT cannot reabsorb NaCl at a normal rate and NaCl is lost in the urine. As a result, ECF volume decreases along with drop in ECF osmolarity. Water then shifts from the ECF to ICF, increasing ICF volume but decreasing ICF osmolarity until equilibration occurs. The RBCs become more concentrated from decreased ECF volume and become larger as lower ECF osmolarity causes water to shift into the RBCs. Therefore, hematocrit increases.

Acid Base Balance

Buffer Systems

Buffers help to prevent pH changes. HCO_3^- is the major extracellular buffer, whereas proteins and organic phosphates are the major intracellular buffers. In general, a buffer pair system works the best when the pH range is within 1.0 pH unit of the pK (dissociation constant). You can calculate pH by using the **Henderson-Hasselbalch** equation:

$$pH = pK + \log [A-]/[HA]$$

$pH = -\log_{10}[H+]$, $pK = -\log_{10}K$, $[A-]$ = concentration of base, and $[HA]$ = concentration of acid.

You can also graph a titration curve to show how the concentrations of acid and base change, as H^+ increases. The concentration of acid equals the concentration of base when pH equals pK.

Winter's formula calculates expected PCO_2 of metabolic acidosis patients following respiratory compensation:

$$PCO_2 = (1.5 \ HCO_3^-) + \text{or} - 2$$

If actual = expected, respiratory compensation is adequate

If actual > expected, respiratory acidosis is also present

If actual < expected, respiratory alkalosis is also present

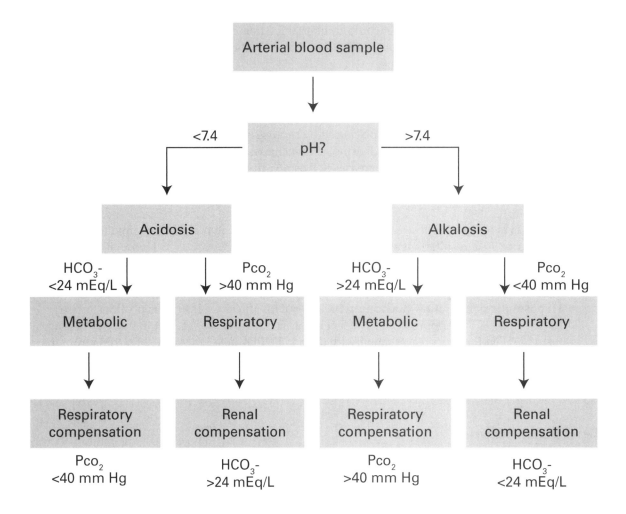

Figure 31 Flowchart of acid/base physiology

Causes

METABOLIC ACIDOSIS

↑ Anion gap (MUDPILES)

Methanol (formic acid)

Uremia

DKA

Paraldehyde or **p**henformin

Iron tablets or **INH**

Lactic acidosis

Ethylene glycol (oxalic acid)

Salicylates

Normal anion gap (8-12 mEq/L)

Diarrhea

Pancreatic or biliary drainage

Type 1 and 2 RTA

Respiratory Acidosis

Respiratory center inhibition (e.g. opiates, myxedema, oxygen therapy in chronic hypercapnia)

Neuromuscular disorders (e.g. Guillain-Barre, myasthenia gravis, botulism, hypokalemia)

Chest wall disorders

Airway obstruction

Acute and chronic lung disease

Metabolic Alkalosis

Vomiting

Gastric drainage

Diuretics

Post-hypercapnic

Bartter and Gitelman syndromes

Severe K^+ depletion

Hyperaldosteronism

Exogenous mineralocorticoid

Respiratory Alkalosis

CNS catastrophe (e.g. subarachnoid hemorrhage)

Hypoxia

Stimulation of pulmonary receptors (e.g. asthma, pulmonary edema, pulmonary embolus)

Anxiety

Aspirin

Gram negative sepsis

End-stage cirrhosis

HCO_3^- Regulation

HCO_3^- is produced from the following reaction:

$$CO_2 + H_2O \leftrightarrow H_2CO_3 \leftrightarrow H^+ + HCO_3^-$$

The formation of H_2CO_3 from CO_2 and H_2O is catalyzed by carbonic anhydrase (CA). Most of the HCO_3^- is reabsorbed in the PCT. Intracellular CA produces H^+, which is secreted into the tubular lumen by the Na^+/H^+ exchanger. The H^+ combines with filtered HCO_3^-, and gets converted to CO_2 and H_2O by CA within the brush border of the PCT cell. The CO_2 and H_2O diffuse into the cell and are subsequently used by the intracellular CA to make H^+ and HCO_3^-. In the end, a molecule of HCO_3^- is reabsorbed in the blood and H^+ returns to lumen (Figure 32).

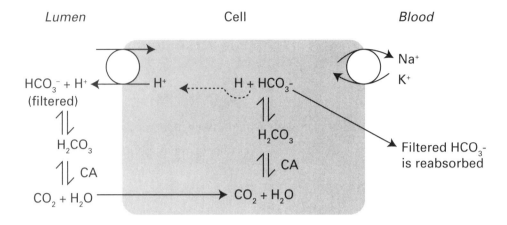

Figure 32 Reabsorption of HCO_3^- in the proximal collecting tubule

In metabolic alkalosis, as the amount of filtered HCO_3^- increases, reabsorption will also increase. However, eventually the mechanism will be saturated, and any excess HCO_3 is excreted.

In respiratory acidosis, as PCO_2 increases, more CO_2 is delivered to the PCT, leading to more intracellular CO_2, increased H^+ production, and therefore, more HCO_3^- reabsorption. The exact opposite occurs in the setting of respiratory alkalosis.

Titratable Acid ($H_2PO_4^-$)

When H^+ is pumped into the lumen by H^+-ATPase, it can also encounter a filtered HPO_4^{-2} and form $H_2PO_4^-$. This alternative combination can be excreted as titratable acid, leading to increased H^+ secretion in urine and therefore, increased HCO_3^- reabsorption (Figure 33).

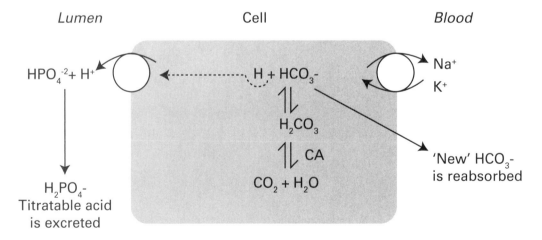

Figure 33 Formation and excretion of titratable acid

NH_4^+

H^+ may also combine with NH_3 in the tubular lumen to produce NH_4^+. Remember, H^+ is pumped into the lumen by H^+ ATPase. NH_3 is derived from glutamine as a result of protein degradation and follows its concentration gradient into the lumen (Figure 34). Once NH_4^+ is produced, the H^+ is excreted in a process called **diffusion trapping**. The HCO_3^- is now available to be reabsorbed in the blood. This process is essential for responding to acidosis because NH_3 diffusion into the lumen can reach 10 times normal!

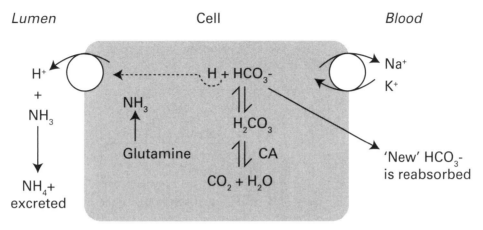

Figure 34 Formation and excretion of NH_4^+ (CA = carbonic anhydrase.)

Renal Oxygen Consumption

After the heart, the kidney is ranked second for oxygen consumption. The difference between arteriovenous oxygen concentrations is extremely small in the kidneys. Such small difference in oxygen concentration increases the effectiveness of blood shunting through the renal capillaries and results in higher oxygen content in blood returning to the IVC compared to superior vena cava.

Oxygen consumption is fairly proportional to RBF and depends on how much Na^+ is actively reabsorbed. If RBF decreases, GFR decreases, therefore, less Na^+ is filtered and the kidneys require less oxygen.

Hormones

The juxtaglomerular cells of the juxtaglomerular apparatus produce **renin**. Renin plays a crucial role in blood pressure control.

Erythropoietin (EPO) is secreted by the extraglomerular mesangial cells. EPO acts on bone marrow precursors to stimulate RBC production.

1,25-Dihydroxycholecalciferol is the active form of **vitamin D** and facilitates the absorption of Ca^{+2} from the gastrointestinal tract.

These hormones are discussed in more detail in chapters 4 and 6. See Table 6 for information about other hormones and their effect on the kidney.

Hormone	Stimulus for secretion	Actions on kidneys	Location
PTH	↓ Plasma[Ca^{2+}]	↓ Phosphate reabsorption ↑ Ca^{2+} reabsorption Stimulates 1α-hydroxylase	Proximal and distal tubules
ADH	↑ Plasma osmolarity ↓ Blood volume	↑ H_2O permeability	Distal tubule and collecting duct

Aldosterone	↓ Blood volume (via renin-angitensin II)	↑ Na+ reabsorption	Distal tubule
		↑ K+ secretion	
	↑ Plasma [K+]	↑ H+ secretion	
Atrial natri-uretic factor	↑ Atrial pressure	↑ GFR	
		↓ Na+ reabsorption	
Angiotensin II	↓ Blood volume (via renin)	↑ Na+/H+ exchange and HCO_3^- reabsorption	Proximal tubule

Table 6 Summary of hormones that act on the kidney

Normal Micturition

Micturition, or urination, is a result of complex physiological processes, which must be tightly coordinated. Initially, the detrusor muscle is innervated by **parasympathetic fibers** via the pelvic nerves from S2 and S3. The **urogenital diaphragm**, which contains the external bladder sphincter, has **somatic innervation** via the pudendal nerve. The ureters have both sympathetic and parasympathetic innervation. Urine accumulating in the pelvis triggers a peristaltic wave of innervations, contractions and relaxation of sphincters, propelling urine into the bladder. The ureters join the bladder obliquely at the trigone. This unusual angle is important for preventing urine reflux into the ureters during detrusor contraction.

As the bladder fills with urine, the bladder wall stretches, which is sensed by the sensory arm of the parasympathetic fibers. This stimulates a reflex contraction of the detrusor muscle increasing the pressure within the bladder long enough to expel the urine. The reflex eventually fatigues, and the detrusor relaxes.

Of course, the brain ultimately has the final word on when micturition occurs. The brain keeps the external bladder sphincter clamped down even when micturition reflexes occur. Once ready to void, the brain can not only relax the external sphincter but also facilitate a micturition reflex. 'Bearing down' also enhances these responses.

GENETIC AND CONGENITAL DISORDERS

Polycystic Kidney Disease

There are two forms of polycystic kidney disease.

Autosomal recessive polycystic kidney disease (ARPKD), previously called infantile polycystic kidney disease, is a recessively inherited disorder characterized by cystic dilations of the renal collecting ducts and congenital hepatic fibrosis. Ultrasound will reveal bilaterally large and echogenic kidneys. ARPKD is associated with oligohydramnios and Potter's syndrome and can lead to poorly controlled hypertension and severe renal insufficiency as adults.

Autosomal dominant polycystic kidney disease (ADPKD), previously called adult polycystic kidney disease, is a dominantly inherited disorder characterized by cystic dilatations in all parts of the nephron. ADPKD is associated with berry aneurysm and mitral valve prolapse. Cysts in the liver, pancreas and other organs are also common in ADPKD. The dominant form of polycystic kidney disease is caused by mutations of either PKD1 or PKD2 genes.

ADult form = ADPKD

Signs and Symptoms

For ARPKD, clinical manifestations often include massively enlarged kidneys, respiratory distress from pulmonary hypoplasia and clinical features of Potters syndrome, such as cranial abnormalities and clubbed feet.

For ADPKD, patients present with hypertension, hematuria, renal insufficiency, or flank pain secondary to renal hemorrhage, calculi, or frequent urinary tract infection.

Diagnosis

The large kidneys and cysts can be visualized with an ultrasound or intravenous urogram.

Treatment

There are no definitive treatments to prevent or delay the progression of polycystic disease.

For ARPKD, supportive therapy for respiratory distress may be necessary.

For ADPKD, treatment with ACE inhibitors and ARBs may slow rate of progression to ADPKD, in addition to lowering blood pressure.

Renal Agenesis

Renal agenesis results from a major error in metanephric development at an early stage. This is most commonly unilateral and accounts for 5% of all renal malformations. The majority of unilateral RA is asymptomatic and found incidentally.

In the case of bilateral agenesis, oligohydramnios develop, as the fetus cannot excrete the amniotic fluid that it swallows. The fetus can still develop because the placenta excretes waste products prior to birth. However, most infants that are born with bilateral agenesis have very poor prognoses.

Pelvic Kidney

If the kidney fails to ascend into the abdomen properly, it will often remain in the pelvis near the common iliac artery (Figure 35A). The adrenal gland on the affected side is in its normal position.

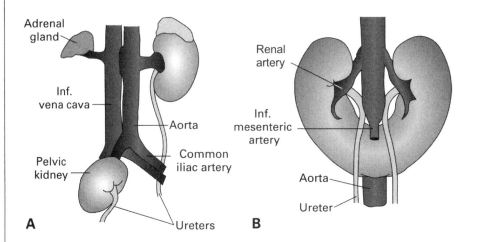

Figure 35 Pelvic (A) and horseshoe (B) kidneys. (Adapted from *TW Sadler. Langman's Medical Embryology,* 5th ed).

Horseshoe Kidney

Occasionally, as the kidneys ascend, they travel so close together that the lower poles fuse, resulting in a horseshoe shape kidney (Figure 35B). The kidneys can only travel to the lower lumbar region because the bottom of the horseshoe gets caught on the inferior mesenteric artery. This abnormality occurs in 1 in 600 people. The kidney is able to function normally.

Urachal Fistula and Cyst

Normally, the allantois is obliterated and a fibrous cord, called the urachus, takes its place. If the lumen of the allantois persists, urine can drain directly from the bladder out the umbilicus, resulting in an urachal fistula. If only a small portion of the allantois lumen persists, it can continue its secretory activity, resulting in an urachal cyst.

Cystinuria

COLA—cystine, ornithine, lysine, arginine

The basic amino acids, cystine, ornithine, arginine, and lysine are moved into the cell against their concentration gradient by a specific transport system known as the g-glutamyl cycle. These amino acids form a dipeptide with glutathione, which is then transported into the cytoplasm. A defect in this system, such as the autosomal recessive defect in amino acid transporter in PCT, leads to the excretion of all four amino acids in the urine. Treatment for cystinuria is acetazolamide to alkalinize the urine. Excess cystine in urine can lead to cysteine kidney stones or staghorn calculi.

INFLAMMATORY AND INFECTIOUS PROCESSES

Urethritis

Neisseria gonorrhoeae (gonococcal urethritis) and Chlamydia trachomatis (nongonococcal urethritis) are the most likely culprits in the sexually transmitted urethritis. Remember that gonorrhea and chlamydia infections coexist in 50% of cases.

Signs and Symptoms

Gonorrhea presents with purulent discharge, dysuria, and increased frequency of urination. Chlamydia may also cause a mucopurulent discharge, but many patients are asymptomatic.

Diagnosis

The diagnosis of gonorrhea is made by presence of gram-negative diplococci or a positive Thayer-Martin culture. Chlamydia can be detected by immunofluorescence stain. New detection systems can also check for presence of gonorrhea and chlamydia in urine.

Treatment

Ceftriaxone is the first line agent for gonorrhea. Doxycycline is the first line agent for Chlamydia. Erythromycin may be used as a substitute for doxycycline in pregnant women with chlamydia. Often, both ceftriaxone and doxycycline are given due to high co-infection rate.

Cystitis

Cystitis, or infection of the bladder, is commonly known as a urinary tract infection (UTI). Cystitis is more common in women than men due to women having significantly shorter urethras. Escherichia coli is the most common etiology in all patients. Staphylococcus saprophyticus can be seen in sexually active women, resulting in its nickname of 'honeymooner's UTI'. Risk factors for UTI in women include recent sexual intercourse, recent spermicide use and previous history of urinary tract infection.

The majority of UTIs in males occur in infancy or in the elderly. Male UTIs have a high association with urologic abnormalities, such as bladder outlet obstruction due to BPH.

No WBC casts
(unlike pyelonephritis)

Signs and Symptoms

UTI often present with dysuria, increase in urinary frequency, urgency, nocturia, and suprapubic pain.

Diagnosis

Diagnosis of UTI can be made with a "clean catch" midstream urine specimen revealing WBCs and bacteria count greater than 105. Presence of leukocyte esterase, an enzyme released by leukocytes, is indicative of pyuria. Nitrite reflects the presence of Enterobacteriaceae, which convert urinary nitrate to nitrite. A urine culture may be used to check for antibiotic sensitivities.

Treatment

Trimethoprim-sulfamethoxazole is adequate in uncomplicated UTI.

Prostatitis

The same gram-negative gastrointestinal bacteria, such as E. coli that cause cystitis, can infect the prostate. Prostatitis can be secondary to reflux of contaminated urine into the prostatic ducts.

Signs and Symptoms

Prostitis symptoms include dysuria, increase in urinary frequency, urgency, nocturia with perineal or low back pain. On digital rectal examination, the prostate is tender and 'boggy'.

Diagnosis

A sample of the seminal fluid usually shows high bacterial counts and WBCs.

Treatment

Trimethoprim-sulfamethoxazole

Pyelonephritis

Pyelonephritis is an infection of the renal parenchyma. It is usually caused by E. coli that extends from a lower UTI.

Signs and Symptoms

In addition to the symptoms for cystitis, the patient present with flank pain, fever, chills, nausea, and vomiting. Costovertebral angle tenderness is elicited on the side of the affected kidney.

Diagnosis

The urinalysis may demonstrate WBC casts, which distinguish pyelonephritis from cystitis.

Treatment

Hospitalization with intravenous antibiotics can be required. A third-generation cephalosporin or a fluoroquinolone is appropriate and treatment can last 2 weeks.

IMMUNOLOGIC DISORDERS

Nephritic Syndrome

The nephritic syndrome is characterized by proteinuria less than 3.5 grams per day and often present with oliguria, azotemia, hypertension, hematuria and edema. Nephritic syndrome can be due to an inflammatory process or due to multiple immunologic glomerulopathies.

Acute poststreptococcal glomerulonephritis occurs after an infection with certain group A β-hemolytic streptococci. Immune complexes formed between antibodies and streptococcal antigens and get lodged in the glomeruli, causing an acute inflammatory response via the alternative complement pathway. They can be seen using immunofluorescent stains as "lumpy-bumpy" glomeruli with subepithelial humps on electron microscopy. **Antistreptolysin O** titers may be high, and **serum C3** levels may be low. Both antistreptolysin O and serum C3 indicate a recent strep infection. Antibiotics are useful only if the patient has a persistent infection. Acute poststreptococcal glomerulonephritis is characterized by periorbital and peripheral edema in children and often resolves spontaneously.

Rapidly progressive (crescentic) glomerulonephritis (RPGN) can present with severe and progressive renal failure. Examples of RPGNs include Goodpasture's disease, microscopic polyangitis, and Wegener's granulomatosis. Light microscopy and electron microscopy often reveal a crescent-moon shape of the Bowman's capsule, wrapped around the glomerular capillaries.

Goodpasture's

- Type II hypersensitivity

- Anti-glomerular basement membrane that targets α3 chain of type IV collagen

- Key symptoms include hemoptysis and hematuria

- Linear IgG and C3 deposits seen on immunofluorescence

Microscopic polyangitis

- p-ANCA

Wegener's granulomatosis

- c-ANCA

- Involves oral/nasal mucosa as well as glomerulonephritis

IgA glomerulopathy (Berger's disease) is the most common cause of glomerulonephritis worldwide. It is due to increased IgA synthesis or decreased clearance of IgA, leading to mesangial IgA immune complex deposits. Berger's disease is often associated with mesangial hypercellularity and presents with upper respiratory infection symptoms or acute gastroenteritis.

Diffuse proliferative glomerulonephritis is predominantly associated with systemic lupus erythematosus (SLE). Light microscopy reveals 'wire looping' of capillaries and subendothelial immune complex deposits with granular appearance in immunofluorescence. Anti-DNA immune complexes activate the complement system and it is the most specific test for diffuse proliferative glomerulonephritis in setting of SLE.

Alport's syndrome is an X-linked disorder that affects the glomerular basement membrane due to defective type IV collagen. The syndrome is associated with sensorineural deafness. Treatment is dialysis and eventual kidney transplantation with renal failure.

Acute Interstitial Nephritis

Acute interstitial nephritis (AIN) is considered a hypersensitivity reaction that is often the result of drug-induced damage to the interstitial cells of the kidney. Numerous drugs including antibiotics, such as penicillin derivatives, aminoglycosides, amphotericin B, and nonsteroidal anti-inflammatory drugs, acetaminophen and diuretics, can cause AIN. Typically, AIN presents 7–10 days after drug administration with development of acute renal failure, rash, fever, and eosinophilia. Treatment requires removal of the offending drug and supportive care.

Transplant Rejection

Hyperacute rejection is immediate and presumably due to an ABO incompatibility.

Acute rejection occurs within the first 2 months after transplantation. The patient may develop fever, hypertension, graft tenderness, oliguria, and azotemia. The interstitium often shows an impressive **infiltration** by **lymphocytes**. Immunosuppressive agents can be attempted to prevent further damage to the graft.

Chronic rejection usually occurs after 2 months after transplantation. The symptoms are often the same as for acute rejection but much more insidious with abundant **plasma cells** in the interstitium. Intimal **fibrosis** of the cortical arteries can lead to renal ischemia, interstitial fibrosis, and tubular atrophy. At 5 years after transplantation, 5% of grafts are lost to chronic rejection.

TRAUMATIC AND MECHANICAL DISORDERS

Urolithiasis (Kidney Stones)

Most stones form when there is supersaturation of insoluble materials from either increased excretion or dehydration. **Calcium** is most commonly found in urinary stones and comprises 75–85% of all kidney stones. Urolithiasis is more common in men and often radiopaque upon imaging. Risk factors for urolithiasis include hypercalciuria, elevated BMI, recent weight gain and certain medications, such as triamterene, indinavir, and acetazolamide.

Struvite stones that are composed of ammonium magnesium phosphate are the second most common kidney stone at 10–15%. They are more common in women and are radiopaque. Urease-producing bacteria, such as Proteus, most often cause Struvite stones. Additionally, these stones are more likely to develop in alkaline urine, which contains more phosphate.

Uric acid stones make up just 5% of all kidney stones. They are radiolucent and more common in men. Uric acid stones are associated with gout and other conditions that can cause hyperuricosuria, such as myeloproliferative disorders or chemotherapy. Uric acid predominates in acidic urine with pH less than 5.5.

Lastly, **cystine** stones are very rare, radiopaque stones. They are primarily due to an autosomal recessive disorder of the cysteine transport system.

Signs and Symptoms

Renal colic can result when a stone blocks urine excretion. The pain is excruciating and usually starts in the flank, radiates around the side and into the groin. Renal colic is characterized by its waxing and waning nature, depending on the movement of stones and associated ureteral peristalsis. Symptoms for pyelonephritis, such as costovertebral tenderness, dysuria and hematuria may also be present.

Diagnosis

Presence of urolithiasis can be confirmed by radiologic tests. CT scan is the gold standard. However, abdominal X-ray, intravenous pyelogram (IVP), and ultrasonography are often utilized.

Treatment

Treatment of the renal colic often involves narcotics for pain control. Small stones may be shattered by ultrasound waves, or lithotripsy. If lithotripsy doesn't work, stones may be removed surgically. Drinking adequate water can prevent calcium stones. Patients with idiopathic hypercalciuria may benefit from thiazide diuretics. Struvite stones can be avoided by treatment of UTIs.

Ureteral Reflux

The most common cause of urinary reflux is misconnection between bladder and ureter during fetal development. As a result, hydronephrosis may develop from increased pressure in the ureter. Patient with ureteral reflux are at risk for pyelonephritis, renal scarring, hypertension, and chronic kidney disease. Children who present with persistent UTIs should be evaluated with a voiding cystourethrogram.

Treatment possibilities range from monitoring in mild cases to surgery. UTIs must be treated aggressively in this population.

Neurogenic Bladder

A neurogenic bladder is often due to abnormalities in cerebral control, sensation, or motor function. For example, diabetics have an associated neuropathy that prevents them from sensing when the bladder is full. It can also occur in the setting of acute spinal cord injury. Poliovirus can damage motor neurons, which inhibits proper detrusor muscle function.

Diagnosis

Urodynamic studies can evaluate the sensory loop, bladder capacity, and sphincter control. Urinary obstruction and reflux are picked up on a voiding cystourethrogram.

Treatment

Treatment may involve medications that enhance sphincter control, relax spastic detrusor, or stimulate the autonomic nervous system. The patient may opt for frequent catheterization or for surgical urinary diversion.

Trauma to the Urinary System

Fibrous capsules as well as a thick layer of fat protect the kidneys. However, trauma to the flank, near ribs 10–12 may result in kidney damage. The bladder and urethra are also at great risk for trauma during automobile accidents, as pelvic fractures often cause the bladder to shear off the urethra. These injuries should be suspected if blood is noted at the urethral meatus or if lower abdominal mass is present.

Grey Turner's sign refers to bruising of the flanks

RENAL FAILURE

Acute Renal Failure

Acute renal failure (ARF) is defined as the abrupt loss of kidney function, leading to retention of urea and other nitrogenous waste products.

The most common cause of acute renal failure is acute tubular necrosis secondary to ischemic damage, such as shock, rhabdomyolysis, surgery and toxins. Glomerulonephritis, renovascular disease, and interstitial nephritis can also lead to acute renal failure.

The causes of ARF can be categorized into three groups: Prerenal, intrinsic and postrenal. **Prerenal** azotemia is due to volume depletion or decreased effective arterial pressure leading to decreased GFR. **Intrinsic** renal disorders involve active renal pathology from necrosis, ischemia, or toxins. **Postrenal** ARF is due to urinary tract obstruction and often stems from stones, BPH, neoplasia, or congenital abnormalities.

Diagnosis

Patients will present with azotemia, or elevated BUN and creatinine, due to decreased GFR.

Treatment

Treatment requires close monitoring of fluid levels and electrolytes, decreased protein intake and lastly, dialysis.

Index	Prerenal	Postrenal	Tubular Injury	AGN
U/P osmolality	>1.5	1 to 1.5	1 to 1.5	1 to 1.5
Urine Na (mmol/L)	<20	>40	>40	>30
Fractional excretion of Na (FENa)	<0.01	>0.04	>0.02	<0.01
Renal failure index	<1	>2	>2	<1

Table 7 Diagnostic indices in acute kidney injury

Chronic Renal Failure

Due to an incredible functional reserve, symptoms of chronic renal failure often do not present until 90% of the nephrons are lost. The two major causes of renal failure in United States are diabetes and hypertension. Other causes include glomerulonephritis, adult polycystic kidney disease, obstructive uropathy, and tubulointerstitial disease.

Chronic renal failure (CRF) must last greater than 3 months to distinguish it from ARF. Complications of chronic renal failure are vast and include volume overload, hyperkalemia, metabolic acidosis, hyperphosphatemia, renal osteodystrophy, hypertension, anemia, dyslipidemia, and sexual dysfunction.

Diagnosis

Azotemia is usually the first sign of CRF. Because the failing kidneys cannot reabsorb Na^+, serum Na^+ is low. However, K^+ and H^+ remain high, leading to hyperkalemic metabolic acidosis. Moreover, decreased production of EPO leads to anemia and decreased activation of vitamin D leads to decreased Ca^{2+} absorption and phosphate retention. Renal osteodystrophy occurs when bones breakdown in an attempt to raise serum Ca^{2+}.

Treatment

Treatment includes restriction of dietary protein and correction of metabolic abnormalities. Dialysis and transplantation are reserved for refractory cases.

Uremic Syndrome

With chronic renal failure, the patient may present with neurologic symptoms including encephalopathy, drowsiness, seizures, peripheral neuropathy and **asterixis.** Cardiac abnormalities include hypertension and congestive heart failure from volume overload. Nausea, vomiting, and anorexia are common and patients often report a bad taste in the mouth. **Uremic frost,** or yellow-brown urea crystals from sweat may be seen and smelled on the skin.

> **Asterixis** is an involuntary hand flap that occurs when the patient has arms outstretched in front with palms facing away from the body

CORTICAL AND PAPILLARY NECROSIS

Diffuse Cortical Necrosis

Diffuse cortical necrosis results from infarction of the renal cortices without damage to the medulla. It's classically associated with **obstetric emergencies,** such as eclampsia and abruptio placentae, and may occur in the setting of septic or cardiogenic shock. End-organ vasospasm and disseminated intravascular coagulation ultimately lead to very poor prognosis in diffuse cortical necrosis.

Renal Papillary Necrosis (Necrotizing Papillitis)

Renal papillary necrosis occurs as the tips of the renal papillae develop ischemic necrosis, often secondary to diabetes mellitus. Less frequently, renal papillary necrosis can result from acute pyelonephritis or long-term use of phenacetin combined with aspirin.

Signs and Symptoms

Symptoms associated with phenacetin-induced papillitis include gastrointestinal disturbances, headache, hypertension, and anemia.

Diagnosis

Urinalysis shows pyuria and occasionally gross hematuria. The diagnosis can be made by IVP.

Treatment

Underlying infections should be treated and offending drugs removed.

Nephrotic Syndrome

Nephrotic syndrome results from increased basement membrane permeability and loss of plasma proteins. There must be **greater than 3.5 grams of protein** loss per day. **Hypoalbuminemia** occurs secondary to loss of proteins in the urine and generalized **edema** develops from decreased plasma oncotic pressure. **Hypercholesterolemia** can also occur from the overeager liver trying to compensate by making more proteins, but also ends up producing more cholesterol. Other symptoms may include ascites, pulmonary edema, and hypotension.

Nephrotic syndrome is caused by several glomerulopathies:

- **Minimal change disease (MCD)** is the most common cause of nephrotic syndrome in children and is often triggered by a recent infection. Although the glomeruli look normal on light microscopy, an electron microgram will reveal fusing of the epithelial podocytes. Corticosteroids are used for treatment with good prognosis.

- **Focal segmental glomerulosclerosis** occurs in older patients with clinical similarities to MCD. It is focal because only some of the glomeruli are affected, and segmental because only part of the glomerulus is affected. Immunofluorescence shows IgM and C3 deposition. Light microscopy shows hyalinosis.

Membranous glomerulonephritis (MGN) is a major cause of nephrotic syndrome in teens and young adults. MGN is associated with thickened capillary walls, intramembranous and subepithelial immune complex deposition, and the characteristic "**spike and dome**" appearance of immune complexes separated by thin spikes of basement membrane. Immunofluorescence reveals IgG and C3 in a granular distribution. MGN shows a poor response to steroid treatment. MGN is associated with the following:

- Infections, such as hepatitis B and syphilis

- Drugs, such as gold salts, penicillamine

- Malignancy

- Systemic lupus erythematosus

- **Membranoproliferative glomerulonephritis** involves subendothelial immune complexes with granular immunofluorescence. Type I is associated with HBV and HCV, and electron microscopy shows a characteristic "tram-track" appearance. Type II is associated with C3 nephritic factor, and electron microscopy reveals "dense deposits."

- **Diabetic glomerulonephropathy**

Diabetes, amyloidosis, and SLE may also cause nephrotic syndrome and are discussed separately.

TUBULAR DISORDERS

Acute Tubular Necrosis

Acute tubular necrosis (ATN) is the most frequent etiology of acute renal failure. ATN often occurs in setting of renal ischemia. It is also associated with rhabdomyolysis, myoglobinuria or direct toxic effects of numerous drugs and chemical substances. Quick removal of offending drug and appropriate supportive management can lead to complete recovery within 2 to 3 weeks. Granular **muddy brown casts** are seen in the urine.

Renal Tubular Acidosis

Renal tubular acidosis (RTA) is a result of dysfunctional tubules that are unable to either excrete H^+ or generate HCO_3^-. Urinary pH and serum K^+ can be used to differentiate between types of RTA, as shown in Table 8. All RTA result in hyperchloremic metabolic acidosis with variable levels of serum K+.

Type I RTA is a result of defective H^+ secretion in the DCT. As a result, more K^+ is excreted, leading to **hypokalemia**. In type I RTA, urine can't be acidified appropriately due to defective H^+ secretion, resulting in a urine pH exceeding 5.5.

Type II RTA is caused by a defective reabsorption of filtered. HCO_3^-. Increased HCO_3^- delivery to the DCT results in increased K^+ uptake into renal tubules and leads to **hypokalemia**. Thiazides may be used to induce volume contraction and stimulate HCO_3^- retention.Type III RTA occurs from decreased GFR and inability to produce enough NH_3. Serum K^+ is normal as type III RTA is not really a tubular process.

Type IV RTA is the only type of RTA that leads to **hyperkalemia**. Type IV RTA is associated with aldosterone deficiency, which can occur in the setting of hyporeninemia. Diabetes, hypertension, interstitial disease, and human immunodeficiency virus can contribute to hyporeninemia. In setting of type IV RTA, drugs that increase serum K^+, such as angiotensin-converting enzyme inhibitors and spironolactone should be avoided.

Type II RTA can occur iatrogenically with carbonic anhydrase inhibitors.

RTA types	Renal defect	GFR	Serum [K⁺]	Distal H⁺
I. Classic distal	Distal H^+ secretion	Normal	↓	> 5.5
II. Proximal	Proximal HCO_3^- re-absorption	Normal	↓	< 5.5
III. Glomerular insufficiency	NH_3 pro-duction]	↓	Normal	< 5.5
IV. Hyporenin-emic hypoal-dosteronism	↑ Atrial pressure	↓	↑	< 5.5

Table 8 Renal tubular acidosis

Nephrogenic Diabetes Insipidus

Nephrogenic diabetes insipidus (NDI) occurs when defective renal tubules allow large amount of urine to be passed. Key difference between central diabetes insipidus and nephrogenic diabetes insipidus is that in NDI, despite adequate ADH, the renal tubules fail to respond appropriately. NDI may be familial in origin or develop secondary to amyloidosis, sickle cell anemia, or drug use, such as lithium.

Signs and Symptoms

Patients develop polydipsia, polyuria with large amount of low osmolality urine and hypernatremia. Nephrotic diabetes indipidus patients do not respond to exogenous ADH.

Treatment

Thiazide diuretics can helpful as thiazides lower the circulating volume and induce more Na^+ and water reabsorption at the PCT, instead of reabsorption at the collecting tubules. Increased water resorption at PCT decreases urine volume and bypasses the ADH system.

Benign Prostatic Hyperplasia

Hyper**plasia**, not hypertrophy!

As men get older, many develop benign prostatic hyperplasia (BPH). As the prostate surrounds the urethra, BPH can impede flow of urine.

Signs and Symptoms

Symptoms include hesitancy, decreased force of urinary stream and dribbling of urine. Urinary retention may lead to urge incontinence and frequent nocturia. UTI can result from urinary retention.

Diagnosis

On digital rectal examination, the prostate may be large and fleshy. However, prostate may feel normal rectally, as BPH growth is often periurethral. Therefore, transrectal ultrasound may be a more sensitive test.

Treatment

Treatment with α-blockers, such as terazosin and prazosin reduces urinary bladder sphincter contractions, making it easier to void. Surgical treatment with a transurethral prostatectomy may be necessary to relieve the obstruction.

NEOPLASTIC DISORDERS

Bladder Carcinoma

The most common bladder cancer in the United States is transitional cell carcinoma. **Smoking, aniline dyes** and **schistosomiasis infection** are all risk factors. Men are diagnosed with transitional cell carcinoma three times more than women.

Signs and Symptoms

The most common presentation is painless hematuria. As the tumor gets larger, transitional cell carcinoma may cause obstruction and cystitis, as well as dysuria and pelvic pain.

Diagnosis

Malignant cells may be found in urine cytology and IVP may show a filling defect consistent with a tumor mass. A definitive diagnosis can be made by cystoscopy and biopsy.

Treatment

Treatment includes surgical resection, radiation and chemotherapy, depending on the stage of the tumor.

Renal Cell Carcinoma

Renal cell carcinoma (RCC) is an **adenocarcinoma** and the most common kidney tumor in adults. **Hematuria**, **flank pain**, and **abdominal mass** are the classic symptoms. Weight loss, fever, and hypertension can also occur. Hematuria is present in more than 70% of cases and may be the only sign. EPO production may be increased, leading to **polycythemia**. Ultrasound, IVP, CT and MRI scan can demonstrate tumor size and spread. Localized disease can be treated with surgery while advanced cases is often treated with chemotherapeutic agents, such as VEGF pathway inhibitors or mTOR inhibitors. RCC is ssociated with Von Hippel Lindau disease and has the characteristic metastasis to lung and bone via hematogenous route.

Wilms' Tumor

Wilms' tumor is the most common kidney tumor in children. Most cases are diagnosed before 10 years of age. Only 7% have bilateral kidney involvement. The key presentation of Wilm's tumor is abdominal mass that does not cross the midline and often present with abdominal pain, hematuria, and hypertension. Definitive diagnosis is biopsy. Treatment includes surgical resection and chemotherapy with good prognosis.

WAGR complex: **W**ilms' tumor, **A**niridia, **G**U malformations, mental **R**etardation

Prostate Carcinoma

Adenocarcinoma of the prostate usually develops in the peripheral regions of the prostate, compared to the periurethral location of BPH. Prostate cancer accounts for 18% of new cancers in men and is the second most common cancer in men after lung cancer.

Signs and Symptoms

Prostate cancer can present with obstructive BPH symptoms as well as hematuria and sometimes, erectile dysfunction. Some present with back pain from metastatic lesions to the spine.

Diagnosis

Serum prostate-specific antigen (PSA) and acid phosphatase levels are usually elevated. The prostate may be nodular, firm or irregular to palpation on digital rectal exam. Diagnosis can be made by ultrasound and biopsy. Metastatic lesions to the spine can be picked up with a bone scan.

In older males with back pain, think prostate cancer metastasis

Treatment

Treatment may include medical management with flutamide, radical prostatectomy, radiation, or 'watchful waiting'. If caught early, prognosis of prostate cancer is good. PSA levels can be used as a screening and monitoring test. However routine PSA measurements are discouraged, as PSA levels may also be high in patients with BPH.

VASCULAR DISORDERS

Renal Artery Stenosis

Although renal vascular disorders are uncommon causes of hypertension, they can result in poorly controlled hypertension that is refractory to medical therapy. Renal artery stenosis leads to decreased blood flow to the kidney. The affected kidney becomes confused and responds to the low blood pressure by stimulating the renin-angiotensin-aldosterone system, as an attempt to normalize the systemic blood flow. As a result, systemic blood pressure becomes elevated.

Fibromuscular dysplasia has the characteristic "string of beads" appearance on imaging.

While young patients can present with **fibromuscular dysplasia**, the most common presentation of renal artery stenosis in adult population is renal artery atherosclerosis. Renal artery atherosclerosis affects men twice as much as women and is often seen in the elderly population. Other unusual causes of renal vascular disease include aneurysm, Takayasu's arteritis, hypercoagulable states, external trauma, instrumentation, and compression of arteries from external sources, such as a tumor.

Signs and Symptoms

In addition to hypertension, patients present with abdominal bruit, hypokalemia, and metabolic alkalosis.

Diagnosis

IVP will demonstrate small kidney and a delayed appearance of contrast secondary to decreased delivery of blood to the affected kidney. Renal angiography can reveal the exact location of the lesion or obstruction. Another method is to measure the amount of renin in the renal veins, as the affected kidney will have higher levels of renin.

Treatment

Treatments include the use of antihypertensive medications, surgical correction, balloon angiography and stent placement.

Renal Arterial Embolism

Embolism in renal artery can occur from multiple sources. Blood clots from a cardiac source, such as mural thrombi from atrial fibrillation and atheromatous plaque, can travel to renal arteries. Infectious emboli can also lodge in renal arteries from an infective endocarditis or artificial heart valves. Trauma to abdomen, side or back can also precipitate renal artery embolism.

Signs and Symptoms

Acute renal artery occlusion may cause acute renal failure along with flank pain and hematuria.

Diagnosis

Lactate dehydrogenase may be elevated from tissue necrosis secondary to ischemic kidney damage. Diagnosis can be made by angiography.

Treatment

Treatment may require anticoagulation with heparin or stent placement.

Renal Vein Thrombosis

Etiologies of renal vein thrombosis include blood clots traveling from the IVC, tumor invasion of the renal vein, renal amyloidosis as well as diseases leading to nephrotic syndrome, such as membranous glomerulonephritis.

Signs and Symptoms

If the blood clot evolves slowly, the patient may be asymptomatic. However, an acute renal vein thrombosis can present with pain, costovertebral angle tenderness and hematuria.

Diagnosis

Diagnosis can be made with IVP, demonstrating a large affected kidney. In case of renal vein thrombosis, the blood has trouble leaving the kidney via renal vein, causing the affected kidney to become enlarged. Doppler ultrasonography may show an absence of blood flow in the affected renal vein.

Treatment

As in deep vein thrombosis, renal vein thrombosis can lead to pulmonary embolism. Treatment can consists of long-term anticoagulation with warfarin.

EFFECTS OF SYSTEMIC DISEASE ON THE KIDNEY

Diabetic Nephropathy

Five to 15% of all diabetic patients develop end-stage renal disease (ESRD). Over a third of patients with insulin-dependent diabetes develop ESRD in 20 years. Although the exact cause of diabetic renal disease is unknown, ESRD progression is fairly predictable. First, **microalbuminuria** occurs, followed by **gross proteinuria** after 15 years. Three to five years later, nephrotic syndrome and azotemia occurs, followed by ESRD in 1–5 years.

Pathology slides demonstrate thickening of the glomerular basement membrane and mesangium, or **diffuse glomerulosclerosis**. Nodular thickening within the glomeruli, or nodular glomerulosclerosis in diabetes patients are called, **Kimmelstiel-Wilson nodules**.

Disease progression may be slowed with tight control of serum glucose, a low-protein diet, **ACE inhibitors**, **ARBs**, and adequate management of hypertension. Ultimately, ESRD is treated by dialysis or transplantation.

Lupus Nephritis

Lupus nephritis refers to six different patterns or classes of glomerular disorders that are commonly seen in patients with SLE. Lupus nephritis present with a combination of proteinuria, hematuria, azotemia, nephrotic syndrome and renal insufficiency. Serologic studies reveal positive fluorescent antinuclear antibody, anti-DNA antibodies and decreased levels of C3 and C4. Remission occurs in one-third to one-half of patients, but relapses are common. Treatment involves the use of glucocorticoids with or without cytotoxic drugs. Lupus nephritis can present with six different classes of glomerular disorders listed:

- Minimal mesangial

- Mesangial proliferative

- Focal

- Diffuse

- Membranous

- Advanced sclerosing

Henoch-Schönlein Purpura

Henoch-Schönlein purpura is a systemic disease seen mainly in children. Vaccination, infection, or drugs precede clinical findings of Henoch-Schönlein purpura. The classic **palpable purpura** usually affects legs and buttocks. Nephritis occurs in 30% of cases with concomitant abdominal pain and GI bleeding. Immunofluorescent staining is positive for IgA in the mesangium.

Renal Amyloidosis

Renal amyloidosis can lead to nephrotic syndrome. The amyloid fibrils, Ig light chains or amyloid A, can be seen throughout the glomerulus, interstitium and in blood vessel walls. Amyloid may be seen with a Congo red stain examined by birefringence under polarized light. The glomeruli will eventually get obliterated, leading to renal failure and uremia. Treatment involves controlling the underlying amyloidosis and inflammation.

KIDNEY-RELATED ELECTROLYTE ABNORMALITIES

Hypernatremia

Serum Na^+ that is too high (> 155 mEq/liter) may be a result of dehydration from fluid losses, such as diarrhea, vomiting, sweating, burns, diabetes insipidus, or due to decreased fluid intake.

Signs and Symptoms

Lethargy, weakness, irritability and twitching can occur. If untreated, symptoms include central nervous system disturbances, such as coma, seizures and even death.

Treatment

Treatment is free water. ADH should be given to patients with central diabetes insipidus. The free water must be replaced slowly to prevent cerebral edema.

Hyponatremia

Serum Na⁺ that is too low (< 135 mEq/liter) often occurs when ADH levels are too high. SIADH is the primary cause of elevated ADH. Secondary causes include nephrotic syndrome, congestive heart failure, cirrhosis and use of diuretics. **Pseudohyponatremia**, or erroneous recording of hyponatremia, can occur with excessive hyperlipidemia.

Signs and Symptoms

Hyponatremic patients can present with nausea, malaise, headache, lethargy, obtundation, seizures, coma, and respiratory arrest.

Treatment

Serum Na⁺ needs to be replaced with hypertonic saline or fluid restriction. Hyponatremia should be corrected at a rate of no more than 8-10 mmol/L of sodium per day to prevent **central pontine myelinolysis**

Hyperkalemia

Serum K⁺ that is too high (> 5.5 mEq/liter) can occur due to decreased K⁺ excretion secondary to renal failure, defective renal secretory function, K⁺ sparing diuretics and hypoaldosteronism. Alternatively, excessive K⁺ release into the serum may result from massive cell damage from burn injuries or hemolysis. Pseudohyperkalemia occurs when K leaks out of the cells during a blood draw, causing an elevation in the measured serum K.

Signs and Symptoms

Hyperkalemia can lead to muscle weakness, paralysis, cardiac conduction abnormalities and lethal cardiac arrhythmias.

Treatment

Treatment involves removing serum K⁺ by diuretics, such as furosemide and thiazides or administering potassium-binding compounds to be excreted in the stool. K⁺ may also be shifted into cells with glucose by administering insulin. In setting of cardiac conduction abnormalities, calcium may be protective.

Hypokalemia

Serum K⁺ that is too low (< 3.5 mEq/liter) is a common problem in hospitalized patients. Hypokalemia may occur with diuretics, such as furosemide and thiazide, renal tubular diseases, hyperaldosteronism as well as vomiting and diarrhea. Alternatively, Anise-containing licorice can precipitate hypokalemia due to its ability to mimic aldosterone's effects. Patients receiving too much insulin may also drop their serum K⁺ as insulin drives potassium along with glucose into the cells.

Signs and Symptoms

Hypokalemic patients may present with muscle weakness, cardiac arrhythmias, renal abnormalities and glucose intolerance.

Treatment

Treatment is K⁺ replacement in oral or intravenous form. Intravenous K⁺ must be administered slowly as many patients experience burning.

PHARMACOLOGY

Table 9 lists the actions, indications, and toxicities of common diuretics.

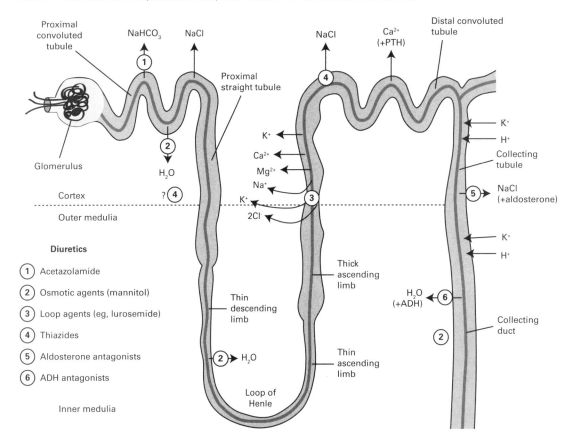

Figure 36 Diuretics and their sites of action
(Adapted from *Basic and Clinical Pharmacology*, 11th Edition)

Agents	Mechanism of action	Uses	Toxicities
Carbonic anhydrase (CA) inhibitors (acetazolamide)	Causes $NaHCO_3$ wasting at the PCT and blocks CA^{2+} in the eye	Glaucoma, metabolic alkalosis, urinary alkalinization, rarely used as a diuretic	Metabolic acidosis, paresthesias, hypokalemia
Loop diuretics (furosemide)	Inhibits Na+ re-absorption in the thick ascending limb, causes K^+ and Ca^{2+} wasting, may saturate the uric acid transporter	Volume overload (CHF, acute pulmonary edema, nephrotic syndrome, cirrhosis), hypertension, phyerkalemia, hypercalcemia	Hypokalemia (± metabolic alkalosis) hyponatremia, dehydration, hypotension, ototoxicity (especially if used in combo with aminoglycosides), hyperuricemia (± gout), interstitial nephritis/allergic reactions

Ethacrynic acid	Same	Same; tolerated by patients allergic to furosemide (a sulfa-containing drug)	Same, except no hyperuricemia or allergic reactions
Thiazide diuretics (hydro-chlorothiazide)	Blocks NaCl absorption in the DCT, causes K^+ wasting but stimulates Ca^{2+} reabsorption	Less effective than furosemide, but longer action; essentially the same indications as furosemide; also treats hypercalciuria and nephrolithiasis	Hypokalemia ($\pm$ meta-bolic alkalosis) hypo-natremia, dehydration, hypotension, hyperlipidemia, hyperglycemia, hyperuricemia, and allergic reactions
K^+-sparing diuretics (amiloride/ triamterene)	Directly acts on the DCT to increase Na^+ excretion, and decrease K^+ wasting	Weak diuretic used with other diuretics to prevent hypokalemia	Hyperkalemia, hyponatremia, dehydration
Aldosterone antagonists (e.g., spironolactone) (also happen to spare K^+)	Competitively blocks the actions of aldosterone on the DCT and collecting ducts	Hyperaldosterone states (e.g., cirrhosis, CHF)	Same as K^+ sparing plus endocrine disturbances (antiandrogen effects, gynecomastia, men-strual irregularities)
Antidiuretic hormone (ADH) antagonists (lithium)	Blocks ADH action on collecting ducts	SIADH, secondary causes of increased ADH (CHF, cir-rhosis, nephrotic syndrome)	CNS disturbances, interstitial nephritis, nephrogenic diabetes insipidus
Osmotic agents (mannitol)	Causes water and Na^+ diuresis by osmotic forces	Acute cerebral edema (from stroke or trauma), acute renal failure, acute glaucoma	Acute intravascular expansion may cause hypertension or pulmonary edema; dehydration later, nausea, vomiting, headache

PCT = proximal convoluted tubule;
DCT = distal convoluted tubule;
CHF = congestive heart failure;
CNS = central nervous system;
SIADH = syndrome of inappropriate ADH

Table 9 Diuretics

CHAPTER 18

REPRODUCTION

FETAL DEVELOPMENT

Overview of Embryogenesis

Fertilization defines the contact between a spermatozoa and an ovum, a process that can last an entire day! Generally, fertilization occurs while the ovum is still traversing the fallopian tube, which is why any scarring in the fallopian tube can predispose to an ectopic pregnancy. Initially, the sperm passes through the ovum's **corona radiata** by releasing **hyaluronidase**. Next the **zona pellucida** is penetrated, and the remaining enzymes are released from the spermatozoa's **acrosome** (Figure 1). Finally, the membranes of the sperm and ovum fuse, placing the sperm's contents in the ovum. This fusion produces metabolic signals which prevent any additional sperm from fertilizing the same ovum and that tell the ovum to complete its **meiotic** divisions.

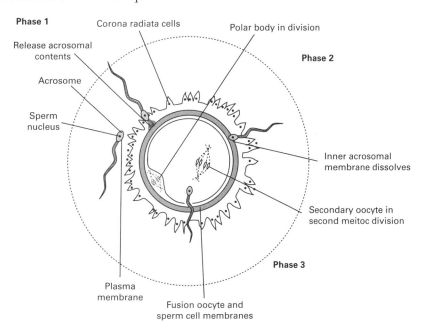

Figure 1 The phases of fertilization

Soon after fertilization is completed, **mitosis** begins. Initially, the overall mass remains the same, and each cell is **totipotent**, meaning that no differentiation has occurred and each individual cell can still develop into a mature organism. At approximately 16 cells, this quality is lost (i.e., differentiation begins), and the total cytoplasmic mass begins to increase. At this point the cell cluster is called a **morula** (Figure 2).

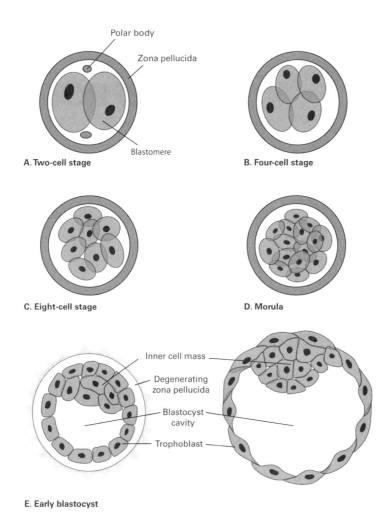

Figure 2 Embryonic development

Eventually, a cavity develops in the cell mass, creating a central area (**embryoblast**) that develops into the embryo, and a surrounding layer (**trophoblast**) that will comprise the fetal contribution to the placenta. The embryo is called a **blastula**, and it is at this stage that implantation into the uterine wall occurs (5–7 days post fertilization).

After implantation, both layers divide further. The trophoblast separates into the **syncytiotrophoblast** and the **cytotrophoblast**. The syncytiotrophoblast makes the lytic enzymes that allow for further burrowing into the endometrium. The cytotrophoblast layer is surrounded by blood from the maternal sinusoids, creating an early circulation.

Meanwhile, the embryo divides into an **ectoderm** and an **endoderm**. The endoderm surrounds the primitive yolk sac, whereas the endoderm forms part of the amnion cavity. The cells destined to become ectoderm also contribute to the **mesoderm**, which separates the original two layers. One cylindrical portion of mesoderm is known as the **notochord** (Figure 3). It induces formation of the neural tube from the ectoderm and later goes on to form the nucleus pulposus of the vertebral discs. Some other derivatives of these germ layers that are useful to know are listed in Table 1.

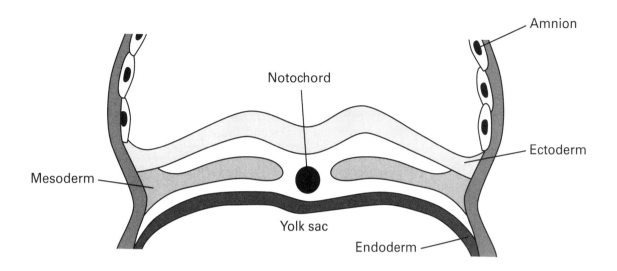

Figure 3 Trilaminar embryo

Ectoderm	Mesoderm	Endoderm
Epidermis (e.g., hair and nails)	Dermis	Gut epithelium
Nervous system	Cardiovascular structures	Glands
Brain	Lymphatics	Germ cells
Spinal cord	Connective tissue	Branchial pouches
Neural crest cells (e.g., autonomic nervous system, pia, melanocytes, chromaffin cells of adrenal medulla)	Muscle	Gut epithelium
Otic placode	Bone	
Otic cup	Genitourinary parenchyma	
Lens placode	Serous linings	
Branchial clefts	Dura	
	Spleen	
	Branchial arches	

Table 1 Adult derivatives of the trilaminar embryo

Branchial apparatus
levels:
1. think mastication
   and hearing
2. think facial
   expressions
3. think pharynx

Level	Cleft	Arch	Pouch
1	External auditory meatus	Muscles of mastication Anterior 2/3 of tongue CN V	Ear drum Eustachian tube
2	Cervical sinus (temporary only)	Muscles of facial expression, plus stapedius CN VII	Palatine tonsil
3	Cervical sinus (temporary only)	Posterior tongue Stylopharyngeus CN IX	Inferior parathyroids Thymus
4-6	Cervical sinus (temporary only) Persistence = branchial cyst	Extreme posterior tongue Throat cartilage Laryngeal muscles Fourth arch = CNX Sixth arch = recurrent laryngeal	Superior parathyroids Parafollicular cells of thyroid

Table 2 Derivatives of the Branchial Apparatus

REPRODUCTIVE TRACT DEVELOPMENT

Although the sex of a child is determined at conception, the development of the male and female reproductive systems does not begin until about 7 weeks gestation. The period before this is termed the "indifferent" stage of sexual development, when the **mesonephros** (precursor of the urogenital tract) develops sex cords, which can develop into either male or female organs.

Female Reproductive Development

If there is no Y chromosome present (e.g., the fetus is XX), the cortical sex cords begin developing into ovaries at about week 10. At 16 weeks, these break up to form primordial follicles, each of which carries a primordial **oocyte (oogonium)**. During this time, active division occurs to increase the number of oogonia. Note that once the child is born, no further oogonia production occurs. Unlike males, who produce new germ cells throughout life after puberty, **females are born with their full complement of germ cells**. This fact explains the concern about female exposure to radiation and mutagens even in a pediatric setting.

Two sets of ducts-the **wolffian (mesonephric)** duct and the **müllerian (para-mesonephric)** duct—are present in both sexes during development. If the embryo has ovaries, or no testes, the wolffian (mesonephric) duct regresses and the müllerian (para-mesonephric) duct develops into most of the female reproductive tract, including the uterus, the fallopian tubes, and upper third of the vagina. The lower two-thirds of the vagina develop from the **urogenital sinus**. The **gubernaculum**, a layer of tissue that follows during the descent of the ovaries, becomes the ovarian ligament and the round ligament of the uterus.

Male Reproductive Development

The presence of a Y chromosome causes the development of the sex cords into the testes and seminiferous tubules. The seminiferous tubules give rise to precursor **Leydig cells**, which secrete testosterone and determine development of the male external genitalia.

Müllerian inhibiting factor (MIF) or **Anti-Müllerian hormone (AMH)** is synthesized by precursor **Sertoli cells**. These two substances cause the mesonephric ducts to develop and the para-mesonephric ducts to regress (Figure 4). The lack of MIF causes the Müllerian ducts to automatically develop and the Wolfian ducts to automatically die, therefore leading to development of BOTH male and female internal genitalia and male external genitalia.

The mesonephric ducts eventually develop into the epididymis, vas deferens, ejaculatory duct, and seminal vesicles. Urogenital folds, under the influence of androgens, elongate and form the penis.

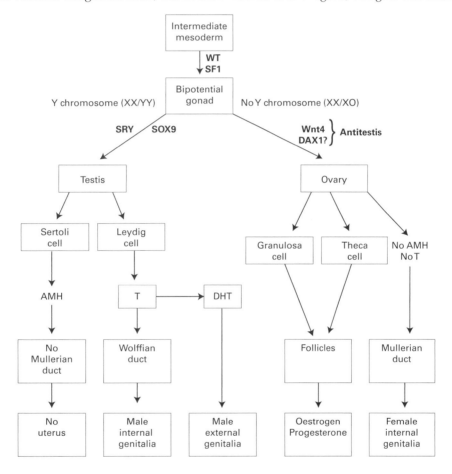

Figure 4 Normal Sexual Differentiation. SRY, sex determining region on Y chromosome; TDF, testis determining factor; AMH, anti-Müllerian hormone; T, testosterone; DHT, dihydrotestosterone; WT1, Wilms' tumour suppressor gene; SF1, steroidogenic factor 1; SOX9, SRY-like HMG-box; Wnt4, Wnt=a group of secreted signaling molecules that regulate cell to cell interactions during embryogenesis; DAX1, DSS-AHC critical region on the X chromosome.
(Adapted from *Early Assessment of Ambiguous Genitalia*)

ANATOMY

Female Reproductive Anatomy

The following are important structures of the female reproductive system (Figure 5).

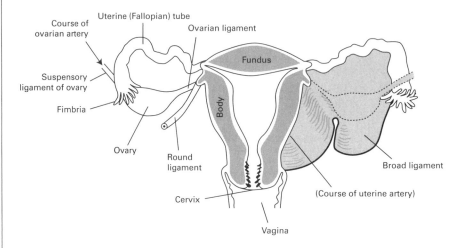

Figure 5 Female reproductive anatomy

- **Broad ligament**: Broad fold of peritoneum connects the uterus to the pelvic wall and floor. It contains the ovaries, uterine tubes (fallopian tubes), uterine artery, ovarian ligament, round ligaments of the uterus, and suspensory ligament of the ovary.

Note that although the fallopian tube and ovary both lie together in the broad ligament, the ovary does not connect directly to the fallopian tube. Instead, the **fimbriae** at the end of the fallopian tube "catch" the ovum released by the ovary. A miss could result in a peritoneal ectopic pregnancy.

- **Cardinal ligament**: Located at the base of the broad ligament of the uterus, it attaches the cervix to the lateral wall of the pelvis. It contains the uterine vessels (uterine artery and uterine vein).

- **Ovarian Ligament**: Connects the ovary to the lateral side of the uterus. It attaches just below where the uterine tube (fallopian tube) attaches to the uterus.

- **Round ligament of the uterus**: Connects the fundus of the uterus to the labia majora. It exits the pelvis via the deep inguinal ring, passing through the inguinal canal and on through to the labia majora. Contains no structures.

- **Suspensory ligament of the ovaries:** Connects the ovaries to the lateral wall of the pelvis. Contains the ovarian vessels (ovarian artery and vein), ovarian nerve plexus, and lymphatic vessels.

Cardinal ligament attaches to **C**ervix.

Round ligament: 0 structures

Male Reproductive Anatomy

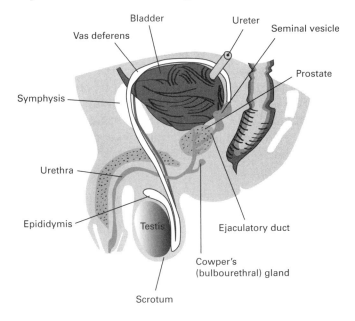

A.

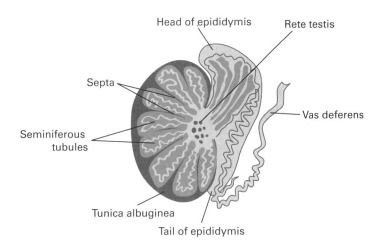

B.

Figure 6 A. Male Reproductive system **B.** Duct system of the testis (Adapted from *Ganong's Review of Medical Physiology*, 24th Edition)

Gonadal Drainage

Lymphatic Drainage

The ovaries and testes are supplied by branches of the descending aorta and drain to nodes in the posterior abdominal wall (the para-aortic lymph nodes). The distal ⅓ of the vagina, vulva and scrotum drain to the superficial inguinal nodes. The uterus, including the cervix, and proximal ⅔ of the vagina drain to the external iliac, obturator (part of the internal iliac), and hypogastric nodes.

Venous Drainage

The left ovary and testes first drain to the left gonadal vein, followed by the left renal vein, and then to the Inferior Vena Cava (IVC). This is similar to the left adrenal vein, which drains to the left renal vein before the IVC. Because there may be more venous congestion on the left side, varicoceles are more common on the left. In contrast, the right ovary and testes drain to the right gonadal vein, which then drains to the Inferior Vena Cava (IVC). The right side has a more direct route for blood flow to return to the heart. Note that this direct route makes it more common for the right testicle to be positioned anatomically higher than the left testicle.

REPRODUCTIVE ENDOCRINOLOGY

Hypothalamic and Pituitary Hormones

The hypothalamus is responsible for producing **gonadotropin-releasing hormone (GnRH)**, which is carried by the portal circulation to the anterior pituitary where it causes the release of **luteinizing hormone (LH)** and **follicle-stimulating hormone (FSH)**. GnRH only causes hormone release by the pituitary if secreted in pulsatile bursts. A steady infusion of GnRH actually causes pituitary suppression. GnRH gets feedback inhibition from **progesterone** and **testosterone** (Figure 7).

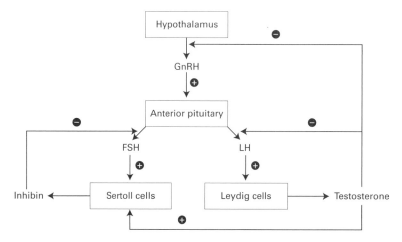

Figure 7 Male reproductive hormones. (GnRH = gonadotropin-releasing hormone; FSH = follicle-stimulating hormone; LH = luteinizing hormone)

In the male, FSH acts on the Sertoli cells to stimulate support of spermatogenesis. The Sertoli cells produce the hormone **inhibin**, which downregulates FSH in a feedback loop. LH acts on the Leydig cells to promote testosterone release. In feedback inhibition, testosterone not only suppresses GnRH, but it also directly lowers LH release from the pituitary.

In females, LH acts on the ovarian **theca cells** to promote progesterone production. Diffusion carries the progesterone to the neighboring granulosa cells, where it is converted first to testosterone and then to estrogen.

Androgens

There are three androgens worth mentioning. Perhaps the most well known is **testosterone**, but **dihydrotestosterone (DHT)** and **androstenedione** also play an important role in the human body.

In males, testosterone is mainly produced in the testis. Testosterone is converted to DHT, its most potent form, by **5-alpha-reductase** in various parts of the body including the testes, prostate, adrenal glands, and hair follicles (Figure 8). Besides the anabolic effects (increased muscle mass and bone density), these two androgen hormones have essential androgenic effects, playing a role in sexual differentiation, external virilization, and sexual maturation in puberty. Without testosterone/ DHT, the epididymis, vas deferens, and seminal vesicles would not differentiate, scrotal changes and phallic enlargement would not occur, and characteristic changes in male puberty (hair pattern, enlargement of sebaceous glands, deepening of voice) would be skipped. Testosterone is also essential in spermatogenesis, while DHT is involved in prostate hyperplasia and male-pattern balding.

Potency: androstenedione < testosterone < DHT

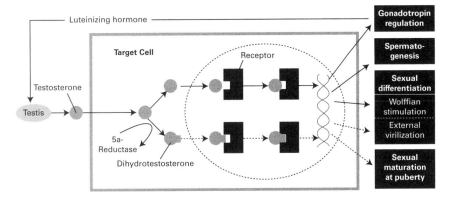

Figure 8 Actions of testosterone (solid lines) and dihydrotestosterone (dotted lines). The two hormones work on the same androgen receptor. (Adapted from *Steroid 5 alpha-reductase 2 deficiency*)

Androstenedione is produced mainly in the adrenal glands and is the least potent of the three androgens. Androstenedione and testosterone are converted to **estrogen** by **aromatase** in adipose tissue and Sertoli cells.

There are several pharmacological agents that are relevant here. Finasteride is a drug that inhibits 5α-reductase, causing lower levels of DHT. Flutamide is an antagonist at the androgen receptor, blocking the actions of testosterone and DHT. Ketoconazole is actually an antifungal drug (-azole) that blocks androgen synthesis by inhibiting **desmolase**. It is also worth noting that exogenous testosterone causes an increase serum testosterone level that through negative feedback leads to decreased local testosterone levels in the testes, leading to decreased testicular size and azoospermia.

Potency:
estriol
< estrone
< estradiol

Estrogen

Although estrogen and testosterone are in many ways analogous, estrogen has more varied effects. Estrogen is responsible for the development of both primary and secondary female sex characteristics. The estrogens include, **17-beta-estradiol**, **estriol**, and **estrone**. 17-beta-estradiol is produced by the ovary, while the placenta produces estriol, and aromatization of blood produces estrone. In addition to this, small amounts of estrogen are made in both the adrenal glands and testes. The order of potency from least to greatest is: estriol < estrone < estradiol.

Estrogen functions in the development of the genitalia and breast, as well as in female fat distribution. It is involved in the growth of the follicle, endometrial proliferation, and increases myometrial excitability. Estrogen functions not only its own receptor, but also those for LH and progesterone. Estrogen generally exerts a negative feedback on LH and FSH, but midway through the menstrual cycle, a positive feedback effect predominates, which causes a surge of LH and FSH that triggers ovulation. It demonstrates feedback inhibition of progesterone receptors. Estrogen, along with progesterone, is essential in maintaining pregnancy. Estrogen stimulates **prolactin** secretion, however it blocks prolactin action at the breast. This is why oral contraceptives are not given to women who are breastfeeding (You may give a progestin-only pill, however). Estrogen also increases the transport of proteins, sex hormone binding globulin (SHBG); as well as elevating HDL while lowering LDL levels. During pregnancy there is a 50-fold increase in the levels of both estradiol and estrone. There is also a 1000-fold increase in estriol, which comes from the placenta, and is an indicator of fetal well-being. Note that estrogen receptors are expressed in the nuclei of cells.

Progesterone

Progesterone plays a key role in maintaining the glandular activity of the endometrium during the latter half of the menstrual cycle. It also serves a developmental role in breast maturation. Progesterone always exerts negative feedback on GnRH, LH, and FSH.

Progesterone is produced by the corpus luteum, placenta, adrenal cortex, and testis. This hormone promotes changes related to gestation. It is involved in the stimulation of endometrial glandular secretions and spiral artery development. It is involved in the maintenance of pregnancy. It decreases myometrial excitability. Progesterone produces thick cervical mucus, which inhibits sperm entry into the uterus. It increases body temperature, making the environment inhospitable for sperm. This hormone inhibits the gonadotropins (LH and FSH). Progesterone relaxes the uterine smooth muscle, thereby preventing contractions. The hormone also causes a decrease in estrogen receptor expressivity. Elevation of progesterone is an indicator of ovulation. Some early miscarriages may be due to progesterone deficiency.

MALE REPRODUCTIVE PHYSIOLOGY

P comes before **S**; erection (parasympathetic) comes before ejaculation (sympathetic)

Male Sexual Response (Autonomic innervation)

- Erection is the result of the two tubular structures that run the length of the penis (the corpora cavernosa) becoming engorged with blood. Innervation is by means of the parasympathetic nervous system, via the pelvic nerve.

  NO → increased cGMP levels → smooth muscle relaxation → vasodilation → *stimulate erection.*

  Note: The drugs sildenafil and vardenafil inhibit the breakdown of cGMP thereby promoting erection.

  NE → increased intracellular Ca^{+2} concentration $[Ca^{+2}]$ in → smooth muscle contraction → vasoconstriction → *inhibit erection.*

- Emission occurs when the seminal fluid goes to the prostatic urethra. Innervation is by means of the sympathetic nervous system, via the hypogastric nerve.

- Ejaculation occurs when the sperm goes from the prostatic urethra to the outside world. Visceral and somatic nerve innervation, via the pudendal nerve.

Spermatogenesis and the Blood-Testis Barrier

Spermatogenesis occurs in the seminiferous tubules of the testes beginning when males start puberty (Figure 9). The key players are the Leydig cells and the Sertoli cells.

- **Leydig cells** are endocrine cells in the underlying interstitial tissue and influence spermatogenesis by secreting *testosterone.*

- **Sertoli cells** are non-germ cells that serve to support and nourish the developing spermatozoa and regulate spermatogenesis. They extend from the basement membrane to the lumen of the tubule, forming *tight junctions* with one another that comprise the blood-testis barrier, which isolates the gametes from autoimmune attack. Sertoli cells secrete inhibin, which inhibits FSH production. They also secrete *androgen-binding protein (ABP)* to maintain testosterone levels. In addition, the Sertoli cells produce anti-müllerian hormone (müllerian inhibiting factor), inhibiting the paramesonephric ducts (Müllerian ducts) in the male embryo.

An injury to the seminiferous tubules that exposes mature sperm to the blood can create an autoimmune reaction and lead to male infertility.

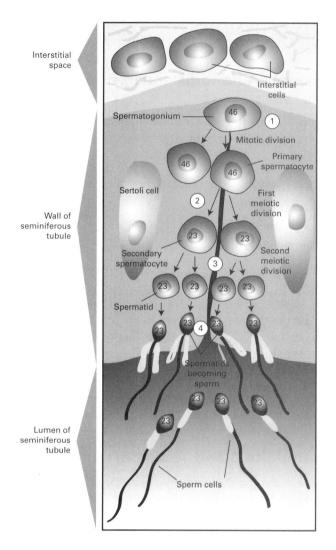

Interstitial space

Interstitial cells

Spermatogonium — 46 — ①

Mitotic division

46   46 — Primary spermatocyte

Sertoli cell

②   First meiotic division

Wall of seminiferous tubule

23   23 — Second meiotic division

Secondary spermatocyte

③

23 23 23 23

Spermatid

23 23 ④ 23 23

Spermatids becoming sperm

23 23 23

Lumen of seminiferous tubule

23

Sperm cells

Figure 9 Spermatogenesis and spermiogenesis
1) Spermatogonia undergo mitosis to become primary spermatocytes.
2) Spermatocytes undergo meiosis. 3) A second meiotic division results in spermatids.
4) Spermiogenesis = spermatids becoming sperm.
This entire process takes about 70 days to complete.
(Adapted from *Junqueira's Basic Histology: Text and Atlas*, 12th Edition)

The immature spermatogonia begin their journey from the basement membrane and make their way past the Sertoli cells (which provide structural and metabolic support) to the lumen of the seminiferous tubule. The spermatogonia serve to maintain the germ pool and go on to pass through the *blood-testis barrier* producing **primary spermatocytes**. After they undergo *meiosis I*, they become **secondary spermatocytes**. These secondary spermatocytes then undergo *meiosis II* before arriving at the tubule as **spermatids**. They are then transported from the rete testis to the efferent ductules, and finally to the epididymis, where they complete their maturation through *spermiogenesis*. The final product is the mature spermatozoan.

Hormonal regulation of spermatogenesis can be seen in Figure 10.

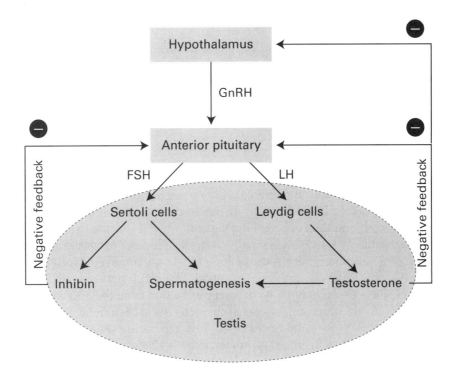

Figure 10 Hormonal regulation of spermatogenesis

Spermiogenesis

It is during the final phase of spermatogenesis, known as *spermiogenesis*, that the parts of the sperm are derived (Figure 11). (Note that the sperm feed on sugar in the form of fructose.)

- **Acrosome**—The cap-like structure derived from the Golgi apparatus. Covers the head of the sperm and contains enzymes important in ovum penetration.

- **Mid piece**—the neck of the sperm that contains a sheath of mitochondria

- **Flagellum/tail**—formed from the elongation of a centriole

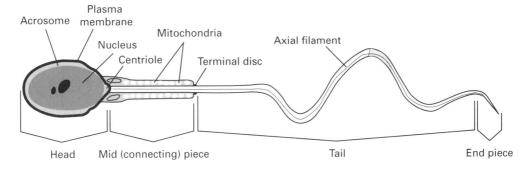

Figure 11 Parts of the sperm

Composition of Semen

The mature sperm are carried by the vas deferens and converge at the urethra at the site of the prostate, where the prostatic glandular tissue secretes up to 75% of the final ejaculate. The prostatic secretion is rich in citric acid and more important, *fibrinolysin*, which liquefies the semen.

FEMALE REPRODUCTIVE PHYSIOLOGY

Puberty

Although questions remain about the signals for the onset of puberty, it is clear that increased hypothalamic release of GnRH plays a key role. Two mechanisms appear to be responsible for suppressing GnRH release (and thus puberty) during childhood. First, the hypothalamus is acutely sensitive to negative feedback from even low levels of testosterone or progesterone. Second, central nervous system (CNS) inhibition plays a role. As these blocks are removed, GnRH is released at night. Initial release occurs only at night, but eventually the adult pattern—pulsatile releases approximately every 2 hours—takes hold. Androgen production from the adrenals also plays a role in initiating development of secondary sexual characteristics. **Menarche** defines the start of menstrual periods. The age at menarche varies by culture, geographic area, nutritional status and weight. In the Western world, the average age at menarche is 12.8 years.

Menstrual Cycle

Understanding the normal menstrual cycle hinges on interaction at four different levels: hypothalamus, pituitary, ovaries, and endometrium. An idealized cycle length is 28 days, although the range of normal includes somewhat shorter and longer cycles. Day 1 is defined as the first day of menstruation, with the first four days of the cycle comprising the menstrual phase. Days 5 through approximately day 14 are the **proliferative phase (follicular phase)**. The proliferative phase can vary in length from woman to woman and from month to month. This is followed by ovulation at about day 14, and then the **secretory phase (luteal phase)** from days 15-28. The luteal phase is usually a constant 14 days. Menstruation will occur 14 days after **ovulation** day (Figure 12).

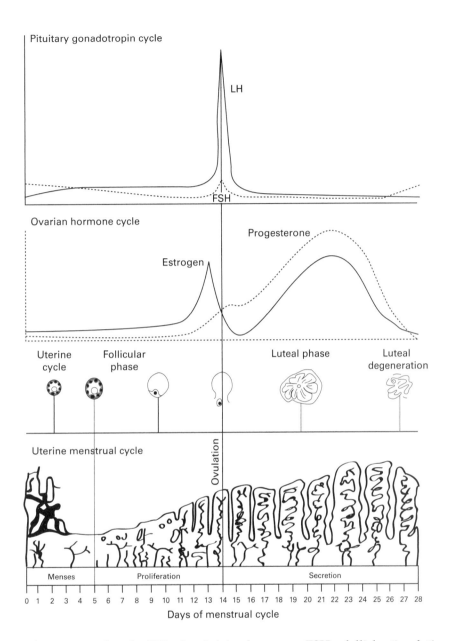

Figure 12 The menstrual cycle (LH = luteinizing hormone; FSH = follicle stimulating hormone)

The layers of the endometrium include the *stratum compactum*, *stratum spongiosum* (both of which are shed during menstruation), and the *stratum basale*. The proliferative (follicular) phase is primarily driven by estrogen, which stimulates endometrial proliferation. It is during the second week of the proliferative (follicular) phase that the follicle grows the fastest. Once the follicle has matured, it ruptures—ovulation has occurred. The secretory (luteal) phase is stimulated by estradiol and progesterone from the corpus luteum (see below). In the case that fertilization has occurred and *beta-hCG* is present, the corpus luteum maintains itself, and estrogen remains elevated, in order to maintain the endometrium to support implantation. This explains why a decrease in progesterone levels can lead to infertility. In contrast, if fertilization has not occurred, the corpus luteum regresses, and menstruation begins.

Phase	Hypothalmus or pituitary	Ovaries	Endomentrium
Proliferative	GnRH, LH, and FSH initially suppressed by estradiol, but then abruptly surge due to a positive feedback as estradiol increases	A primordial follicle matures to graafian stage; this mature follicle secretes increasing amounts of estradiol	Stimulated by estradiol, cellular proliferation and endometrical growth are maximized in preparation of a possible implantation
Ovulation	Surge of LH and FSH is the signal for ovulation	Oocyte released as mature follicle ruptures	
Secretory	LH causes luteinization of the ovarian follicle soon after ovulation, but then LH levels fall late in the cycle	Under the influence of LH, the ruptured follicle becomes a corpus luteum, which secretes high levels of progesterone, as well as estradiol	Progesterone stimulates glandular secretions
Menstrual	If pregnancy occurs, placental hCG takes over the role of maintaining the corpus luteum and suppressing menses	If no pregnancy occurs, corpus luteum recedes and estradiol and progesterone levels fall	Unsupported by estradiol and progesterone, endometrium undergoes involution and sloughing

LH = luteinizing horomone; FSH = follicle-stimulating horomone GnRH = gonadotropin-releasing horomone; hCG = human chorionic gonadotropin.

Table 3 Hormonal action throughout the menstrual cycle

Ovulation

As mentioned previously, estrogen generally exerts a negative feedback on LH and FSH, however, midway through the menstrual cycle, as estrogen levels rise, there is a *positive feedback effect* leading to an increase in GnRH receptors on the anterior pituitary. The estrogen surge causes the stimulation of LH release, causing ovulation—the rupture of the follicle. It should be noted that 24 hours prior to ovulation, progesterone levels begin to rise, leading to elevated body temperature in those 24 hours prior to ovulation. This rise in body temperature serves to accommodate the sperm during the time it needs to travel to the oocyte, making this the optimal time to conceive. *Mittelschmerz* is the term used when blood from the ruptured follicle causes irritation to the peritoneum, causing pain or discomfort.

Hypothalamic nucleus involved with ovulation = arcuate nucleus

Corpus Luteum

The corpus luteum is formed after ovulation. It produces progesterone and estrogen in the luteal phase. It has a lifespan of 13–14 days. If *beta-hCG* from the placenta is present, the lifespan will extend to 6–7 weeks, until the placenta is able to produce its own progesterone.

Oogenesis

As noted earlier, the ovary develops all its *oocytes* during embryogenesis and they lie dormant until puberty, *arrested in prophase of meiosis I.* Each oocyte is encapsulated by follicular cells and is known as a **primordial follicle (primary oocyte)**. Starting at puberty, approximately 10 follicles begin to grow under the influence of follicle stimulating hormone (FSH) during each menstrual cycle. Usually only one of these follicles develops to maturity, although we know there are exceptions (e.g., nonidentical twins). The follicle that becomes dominant **(the secondary oocyte)** suppresses the other follicles in a process known as *follicular atresia.* Meiosis I is completed (with the expulsion of polar bodies containing the unused DNA) and meiosis II begins. *Meiosis II is arrested in metaphase until fertilization.* The surrounding follicular cells also mature and become the **thecal layer** and **granulosa layer** (Figure 13). The granulosa cells produce progesterone and act in concert with the thecal cells to produce estrogen. If fertilization does not occur, the secondary oocyte degenerates (Figure 14).

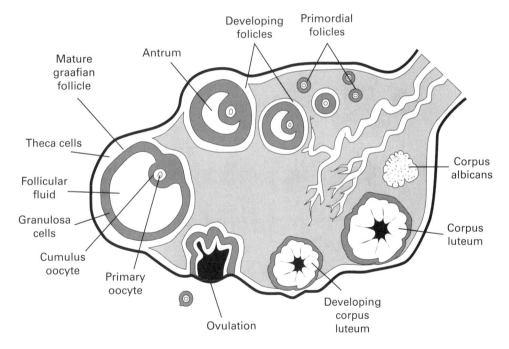

Figure 13 The stages of oogenesis

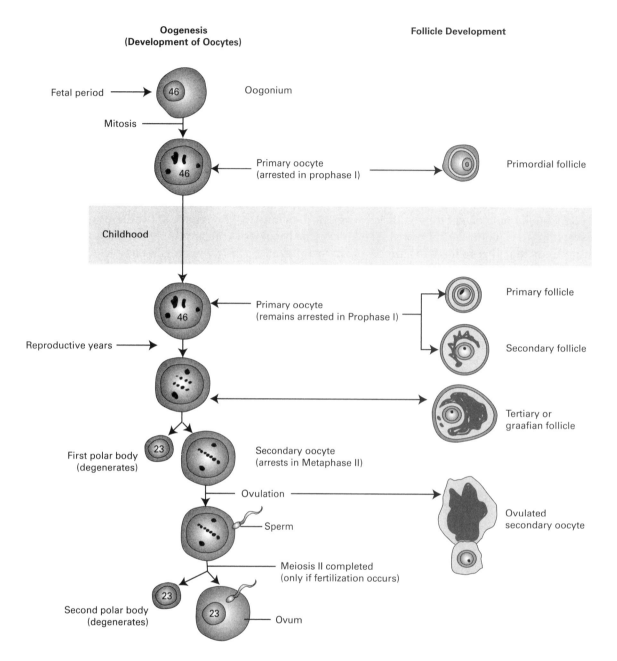

Figure 14 The stages of oocyte development
(Adapted from *Williams Gynecology*)

The Cervical Transition Zone

The cervix is divided anatomically into the **exocervix**, which projects into the vagina, and the **endocervix**. Histologically there is also a division that correlates roughly with the anatomic division but changes throughout life. The exocervix is lined by nonkeratinized, stratified squamous epithelium, whereas the endocervix is lined by mucin-secreting columnar epithelium. The **transition zone** refers to the border of these two epithelia, which makes a gradual transition rather than an abrupt one. The transition zone is the site of most cervical cancers, which are usually squamous cell carcinomas.

Conception

Conception and *fertilization* are used synonymously. Fertilization defines the contact between a spermatozoa and an ovum, a process which occurs within 12–36 hours of ovulation. This process most commonly occurs in the upper end (**ampulla**) of the fallopian tube. Generally, fertilization occurs while the ovum is still traversing the fallopian tube, which is why any scarring in the fallopian tube can predispose to an ectopic pregnancy. Initially, the sperm passes through the ovum's corona radiata by releasing *hyaluronidase*. Next the **zona pellucida** is penetrated, and the remaining enzymes are released from the spermatozoa's acrosome (Figure 1). Finally, the membranes of the sperm and ovum fuse, placing the sperm's contents in the ovum. This fusion produces metabolic signals that prevent any additional sperm from fertilizing the same ovum and that tell the ovum to complete its meiotic divisions.

With regard to the fertile period of each cycle, viability of the ovum is approximately 1 day, whereas the viability of sperm is about 3 days, so that maximal fertility is obtained when intercourse is timed within 1 day on either side of ovulation. In practice, this is often accomplished by charting female basal body temperature throughout the cycle because progesterone mildly raises core temperature after ovulation.

Pregnancy

Most of the changes that occur during pregnancy are related to hormonal signals, although the size and metabolic demands of the fetus also necessitate other physiologic changes. Approximately 5–7 days post-fertilization, implantation within the uterine wall takes place. The *placenta* must take over the role of the pituitary, producing LH to maintain the corpus luteum. This is a key function because the estrogen and progesterone produced by the corpus luteum are essential in maintaining the secretory response of the decidual cells of the endometrium (initially the chief source of nutrition for the developing embryo). The syncytiotrophoblast of the placenta produces a hormone that is analogous to LH called **human chorionic gonadotropin (hCG)**. This hormone can be detected in the blood 1 week post-conception and in the urine 2 weeks post-conception.

Eventually, the placenta (more specifically, the syncytial trophoblasts) overtakes the corpus luteum as a source of estrogen and progesterone. The placenta uses precursors produced by the maternal and fetal adrenal glands to produce these hormones. Estrogen is a signal for enlargement of the uterus and external genitalia. It also relaxes the pelvic ligaments for easier passage of the fetus through the birth canal. In addition, estrogen stimulates prolactin production. Together with progesterone, these hormones cause enlargement of the breast ductal system, although estrogen blocks the prolactin receptor so that lactation does not begin. Progesterone also decreases the contractility of the uterus to prevent spontaneous abortion. The incompletely understood hormone *human chorionic somatomammotropin* is also produced by the placenta in large amounts. One known action of this hormone is to decrease maternal insulin sensitivity so that more nutrients are available to the fetus.

The suggested weight gain associated with a pregnancy is approximately 25–35 lb. Some of this weight gain represents the need for stores of vitamins, calcium, and especially iron, which the fetus extracts from the mother. Maternal blood volume increases 30% by the end of the pregnancy. Cardiac output increases to supply the placenta adequately, and the extra blood compensates for normal blood losses during birth.

A normal pregnancy is considered to be 40 weeks, ±2 weeks on each side. Remember that by convention, these weeks are counted from the first day of the last normal menstrual period and not from the date of conception.

The Role of hCG

As mentioned previously, hCG is produced by the placenta, specifically by the syncytiotrophoblast. In addition to being used to detect pregnancy in the blood (1 week after conception) and in the urine (2 weeks after conception), hCG maintains the corpus luteum during the first trimester. It does so by simulating the actions of LH. Without its presence, there would be no luteal cell stimulation, resulting in abortion. In a normal pregnancy, beta-hCG levels double every two days during the first trimester. During the second and third trimesters, the placenta is able to synthesize its own progesterone and estriol, while the corpus luteum degenerates. In addition, there are some pathologic states in which hCG levels are elevated. These conditions include choriocarcinoma, hydatidiform moles, and gestational trophoblastic tumors.

Physiologic Changes of Pregnancy

During pregnancy, cardiac output increases 30–50% because plasma volume increases by 50% (causing a large increase in preload) and Red Blood Cell (RBC) volume increases by 30%. This increase in plasma volume to RBC volume leads to a *physiologic anemia*, and can cross over into *Iron-deficiency anemia*, which is common in pregnancy.

- In early pregnancy, blood pressure decreases, reaching its lowest at 16–20 weeks, which is when morning sickness worsens. Blood pressure returns to pre-pregnancy levels by term.

- There is an increase in minute ventilation, leading to a decrease in $P_A(CO_2)$ and $Pa(CO_2)$ and a mild respiratory alkalosis (so that CO_2 can be transferred more easily from fetus to mother).

- There is an increase in procoagulation factors, leading to a hypercoagulable state (preventing post-partum hemorrhage).

- Due to elevations in plasma volume, GFR increases, leading to decreases in BUN and creatinine.

- TSH and free T4 levels are normal, although total T4 might be elevated, due to more Thyroid Binding Globulin (TBG) causing more bound T4.

- There is an increase in peripheral resistance to insulin (due to *human placental lactogen*) that worsens throughout pregnancy, leading to hyperinsulinemia, hyperglycemia, and hyperlipidemia.

Labor

The exact mechanisms that signal the onset of labor (also called parturition) are not known, but the following factors are thought to contribute. Late in pregnancy, estrogen, which tends to increase uterine contractions, rises relative to progesterone, which suppresses contractility. The posterior pituitary hormone oxytocin increases uterine responsiveness, and its rate of production considerably increases during labor. Mechanical factors also play a role, as reflexive responses to the pain of contractions provide an urge to push. After delivery of the baby and the placenta, estrogen and progesterone levels decline rapidly. This *releases the prolactin receptor blockade*, and lactation can proceed. Suckling is required to maintain milk production, because the increase in nerve stimulation increases both **prolactin** and **oxytocin**. Prolactin will also decrease reproductive function, making it more difficult for breastfeeding mothers to get pregnant, by causing a temporary involuntary cessation of menses. Oxytocin plays a role in milk "let-down," with both oxytocin and prolactin being stimulated by suckling.

Menopause

Technically, **menopause** denotes the actual cessation of menstruation. In practical usage, it also refers to **perimenopause** (the 1- to 3-year phase of declining flow and decreasing frequency of menstruation) plus the cluster of responses that accompany a changing hormone balance. Physiologically, menopause can be understood to be due to the limited number of ovarian follicles that are able to respond to stimulation by FSH and LH. Follicles are lost either to ovulation or degeneration with each cycle so that, by the late 40s or early 50s, most women have a minimal number of follicles, and *estrogen and progesterone production by the ovaries decreases.*

The age of onset is earlier in smokers than in nonsmokers. With the removal of feedback inhibition from estrogen and progesterone, *levels of FSH, LH, and GnRH are elevated* (elevated FSH is useful for confirmation). Menopausal women may experience hot flashes (due to vasodilation), night sweats, insomnia, hirsutism, vaginal atrophy, and may develop osteoporosis and coronary artery disease. After menopause, the source of estrogen (estrone) is via the peripheral conversion of androgens, causing hirsutism. Elevated FSH and LH levels are used to diagnose premature menopause (*premature ovarian failure*), and low estrogen is implicated in *osteoporosis* and *atherosclerosis*.

Because hormone-replacement therapy (HRT) counteracts these changes, as well as lowers low-density lipoprotein (LDL) and increases high-density lipoprotein (HDL) cholesterol, it has received wide advocacy. It has been noted that administration of unopposed estrogen *increases the risk of endometrial cancer*, but the addition of *progestin* to the regimen alleviates this concern. There is also worry over an *increase in the incidence of breast cancer* associated with HRT. This has led to the recommendation that physicians should help the patient assess their relative individual risks regarding HRT. Side effects include breakthrough menstrual bleeding, weight gain, and fluid retention. Estrogen is metabolized in the liver, and HRT is contraindicated in patients with hepatic or gallbladder disease.

CONGENITAL REPRODUCTIVE DEFECTS

Klinefelter's Syndrome

Klinefelter's syndrome was the first sex chromosome abnormality to be recognized. It occurs in *phenotypic males* who are born with an extra X chromosome (47,XXY). This inactivated X chromosome is called a **Barr body** (Note that all XY females have one Barr body). It remains inapparent until puberty. The incidence is approximately 1 in 850 live births, but half of all 47,XXY conceptions result in spontaneous abortion. The female equivalent of this disorder, trisomy X, usually results in phenotypically normal females.

Signs and Symptoms

Klinefelter's syndrome is generally noted when secondary sexual characteristics fail to develop. These patients present with testicular atrophy (hypogonadism), eunuchoid body shape, are tall, have long extremities, and gynecomastia. These patients may also present with a developmental delay.

As might be expected, Klinefelter's syndrome results from *chromosomal nondisjunction*. This can occur in maternal or paternal meiosis I or meiosis II, or from a later mitotic error. The penetrance can vary due to *mosaicism*, usually through loss of one X chromosome. Dysgenesis of the seminiferous tubules causes a decrease in inhibin levels, which lead to *increased FSH* production. Additionally, abnormal functioning of the Leydig cells leads to decreased testosterone levels, which cause an *increased LH*, resulting in an elevation of estrogen levels (thereby causing female hair distribution and gynecomastia).

Physical examination and elevated levels of LH, FSH, and prolactin all increase suspicion of Klinefelter's, but karyotyping is the gold standard. Polymerase chain reaction (PCR) technique is also available.

As is the case with most congenital abnormalities, treatment is limited.

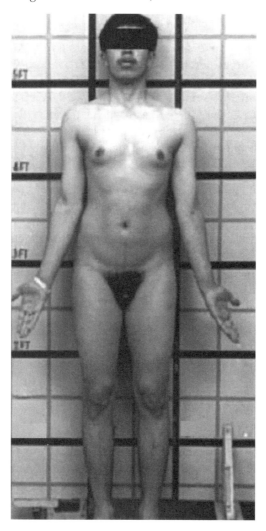

Figure 15 Klinefelter's syndrome
(Adapted from *Current Medical Diagnosis and Treatment*)

Turner's Syndrome

Turner's Syndrome is caused when the second sex chromosome is lost, and only an X chromosome remains, so that the karyotype is 45,X (45,XO) and contains no Barr body. It occurs in about 1 in 3000 live births. Although it is less common than some of the other sex chromosome aneuploidies, its classic features are often noticeable before the onset of puberty.

Signs and Symptoms

Typical findings include short stature (often under 5 feet tall if untreated), *ovarian dysgenesis* (usually streak ovaries), and typical facial and truncal abnormalities, including a low posterior hairline, webbing of the neck (*cystic hygroma*), and a broadened chest (shield chest) with widely spaced nipples, and cardiovascular abnormalities (preductal coarctation of the aorta; bicuspid aortic valve) (Figure 16). It is the most common cause of *primary amenorrhea*.

Turner's syndrome usually results from a nondisjunctional error that leaves either the ovum or sperm without a sex chromosome. In about 25% of cases, a mosaic pattern is noted, indicating that the chromosome was lost after fertilization.

Diagnosis

Diagnosis is usually by means of recognitions of physical findings, with subsequent karyotyping. Occasionally, this diagnosis is made prenatally by ultrasound or immediately after birth because many of the dysmorphologies are present. Decreased estrogen levels in this condition lead to elevations in LH and FSH levels. Some cases are not recognized until a workup for infertility take place.

Supplemental estrogen can restore the maturation of secondary sexual characteristics and initiate normal menses, but it does not confirm fertility. Growth hormone may help to increase stature if administered in youth.

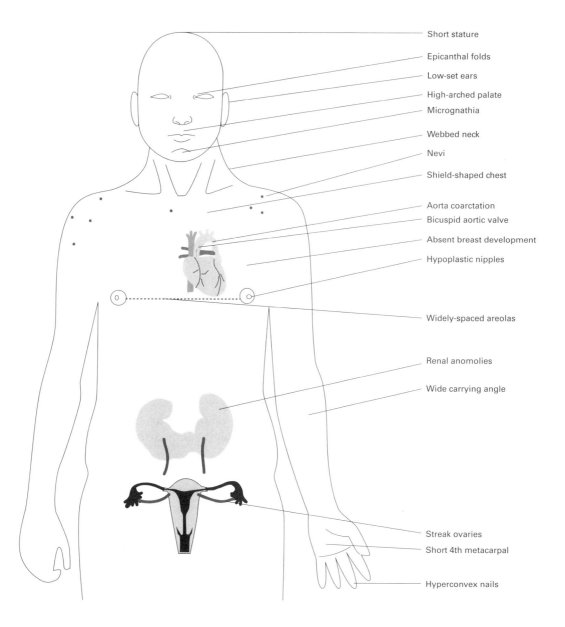

Figure 16 Classical phenotypic characteristics of Turner syndrome
(Adapted from *Williams Gynecology*)

Double Y Males

Double Y Males occur when a phenotypic male is born with an extra Y chromosome (47,XYY). The incidence is about 1 in every 1000 live births.

Signs and Symptoms

These are phenotypically normal males, who are very tall, and may have severe acne. Around 1–2% have a possible predisposition to displaying antisocial behavior. They have normal fertility.

This karyotype results form a nondisjunction during paternal meiosis II, leading to YY sperm.

Diagnosis

This karyotype is only noted during karyotype screening evaluations.

Behavioral problems, if present, are addressed individually.

True Hermaphrodite

This is a very rare condition in which both ovarian and testicular tissue types are present. This is very rare. The genotype in these cases are either 46,XX or 47,XXY. These individuals have ambiguous genitalia.

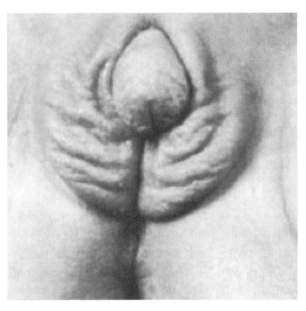

Figure 17 True hermaphroditism
(Adapted from *Current Medical Diagnosis and Treatment*)

Female Pseudohermaphroditism

Unlike the extremely rare cases of true hermaphroditism, where an individual is born with both testes and ovaries, **pseudohermaphroditism** occurs when the *phenotypic sex* (external genitalia) does not correlate with the *gonadal sex* (testes versus ovaries). In females, this is generally due to *virilization* resulting from abnormally elevated androgen levels, caused by enzymatic deficiency in biosynthetic pathways. These females are 46,XX genotype.

Signs and Symptoms

Female pseudohermaphroditism is generally discovered due to ambiguous genitalia, which are noted in the initial infant screening examination, but it may not become apparent until later in childhood. It also may be picked up from a salt-losing crisis, because often there is also a block in production of mineralcorticoids.

This condition is due to excessive exposure to androgenic steroids during early gestation. The most common cause of female pseudohermaphroditism is *congenital adrenal hyperplasia*, which is usually due to an autosomal recessive *defect in 21-hydroxylase* because this enzyme shunts precursors toward androgen production. The low levels of glucocorticoids exacerbate the problem by signaling for increased precursor synthesis. Another cause is in the case of exogenous exposure to androgens during pregnancy.

A diagnosis is made using anatomic investigation, including radiographic studies, with contributing evidence from measurements of various steroids, glucocorticoids, and precursors. Although ovaries are present, the external genitalia are virilized or ambiguous. In males with *21-hydroxylase deficiency* the more obvious anatomic evidence is absent, so that the first sign is a salt-losing crisis. This has led to increased use of heel-stick screening of both female and male infants for this deficiency.

Except for rare cases that are diagnosed late, gender assignment matches chromosomal sex, and surgery is performed to restore the normal female external genitalia. Emphasis is placed on early treatment because glucocorticoid administration can arrest virilization, maintain fertility, and prevent a salt-losing crisis.

Male Pseudohermaphroditism

Male pseudohermaphroditism results from undervirilization of a male embryo. During normal embryogenesis, the primary pathway produces female sexual characteristics; exposure to androgens alters differentiation towards a male phenotype. A breakdown in either androgen production or target tissue response can lead to male pseudohermaphroditism. Target tissue response is most often the cause and is called **androgen insensitivity syndrome** (formerly known as *testicular feminization).* The genotype here is 46, XY.

Signs and Symptoms

This disorder produces apparently normal female genitalia externally but with a blind-ended vagina (rudimentary vagina) and no uterus, ovaries, or fallopian tubes. No sexual hair is present. Functional testes develop (often located in the labia majora), which produce elevated levels of testosterone, and remain undescended in the abdomen or inguinal canal. There is minimal axillary or pubic hair.

Androgen insensitivity syndrome is an X-linked recessive disorder that results in failure to produce functional androgen-binding receptors. A similar phenotype occurs in the autosomal recessive inherited *defect of 5-alpha-reductase*, the enzyme that converts testosterone to its active form at the tissues.

Diagnosis

Prepubertal diagnosis is usually made when the testes are associated with hernias or mistaken for hernias. Otherwise, diagnosis is usually delayed until a postpubertal workup is done for primary amenorrhea. Testes are present, however the external genitalia are female or ambiguous. Testosterone, estrogen and LH levels are all elevated.

Removal of the testes is important because of the increased risk of cancer in undescended testes. This procedure generally is postponed until after puberty because the hormone production from the testes still leads to essentially normal female secondary sexual characteristics. Pain from the testes is an indication for prepubertal removal and hormone supplementation.

5-alpha-reductase Deficiency

The autosomal recessive deficiency of the enzyme 5-alpha-reductase results in the inability of males to convert testosterone to DHT. Ambiguous genitalia is often present until puberty, when elevated levels of testosterone causes masculinization and/or increased growth of external genitalia. The hormone levels of testosterone and estrogen are normal. LH level is normal or may be elevated. The penis may appear only at puberty (around age 12), however, the internal genitalia are normal.

Kallmann syndrome

Kallmann syndrome is an endocrine disorder in which GnRH release is totally blocked or significantly reduced. Development of the olfactory bulb is also incomplete. These individuals fail to develop secondary sexual characteristics and lack a sense of smell.

MALE REPRODUCTIVE PATHOLOGY

Priapism

Priapism is a condition in which there is persistent penile erection. This condition needs to be treated quickly, as failure to reduce the erection can lead to permanent penile damage. Sickle-cell anemia, spinal cord trauma, and the antidepressant *trazodone* are all associated with priapism.

Balanitis

Balanitis is the infection of the foreskin. It is most commonly caused by *Candida* infection. Treatment is with topical ointments or with a single dose of *fluconazole* (anti-fungal agent) given orally.

Penile Pathology

- **Carcinoma in situ.**

- **Bowen's disease**—The incidence of this disease is at its highest in those who are in their 40s and 50s. It presents with solitary, crusty plaques, that are grey in color and are usually found on the shaft of the penis or on the scrotum (in females, it can be found on the vulva). In fewer than 10% of cases, these lesions can progress to invasive squamous cell carcinoma (SCC). Diagnosis is made with biopsy.

- **Erythroplasia of Queyrat**—This is a form of Bowen's disease, in which the plaques are red and velvety, and usually involve the glans penis.

- **Bowenoid papulosis**—This condition usually affects younger age groups than the other subtypes. It presents with multiple papular lesions that usually do not predispose to SCC.

- **Squamous cell carcinoma (SCC)**—SCC is more common in Africa, Asia, and South America. It is commonly associated with Human Papilloma Virus (HPV) *types 16, 18, and 31,* particularly in males who have not been circumcised.

- **Peyronie's disease**—Acquired fibrosis within the corpus cavernosa causes the penis to be bent.

Orchitis

Viral orchitis is the leading cause of acquired testicular failure in adult men, and *mumps* should always be considered as a cause of testicular inflammation. The other classically important infection with a predilection for the testes is *syphilis*.

Signs and Symptoms

Unilateral or bilateral pain and swelling of the testes usually occurs about 1 week after the parotitis of mumps and is accompanied by systemic viral symptoms.

Viral orchitis is a rare finding in prepubertal males who develop mumps but occurs in about one-fourth of postpubertal cases. The inflammation usually remains interstitial and usually does not permanently disturb testicular function. However, direct viral involvement of the seminiferous tubules, or ischemia from excess pressure related to swelling, can lead to lasting damage. The syphilitic response is typical of that seen in other areas, with *gummas*, inflammation, and obliterative endarteritis.

Diagnosis

A diagnosis of mumps is generally made clinically, although saliva cultures and antibody titers can be confirmatory. Syphilis is diagnosed by the presence of an antibody reaction.

There is no antiviral medicine that is active against mumps, so treatment of orchitis focuses on pain control and the use of ice and corticosteroids to limit inflammation. Syphilis normally responds well to *penicillin*.

Cryptorchidism

Cryptorchidism refers to failure of the testes to descend into the scrotum, leading to undescended or partially descended testes, either unilaterally or bilaterally, although more often it is unilateral. Testicular descent is usually complete within the first year of life. Prematurity can increase the risk of cryptorchidism.

Signs and Symptoms

By definition, the chief finding is the lack of one or both testes in the scrotum. Cryptorchidism is frequently associated with inguinal hernias.

Cryptorchidism can involve the arrest of descent of one or both testes at any point in their developmental journey from the abdomen, through the inguinal canal, and down into the scrotum. Due to the temperature of the body being greater than that of the scrotum, it causes the lack of spermatogenesis. If a testis remains undescended for longer than about 2 years, germ cell development becomes compromised. There is an approximately 35-fold increase in the risk of testicular cancer (usually a germ cell tumor) in the undescended testicle, and this risk is not removed by surgical repositioning. Metastatic spread occurs via the *para-aortic lymph nodes*. The malpositioned testis is also more vulnerable to injury. Cryptorchidism in female pseudohermaphrodites has been previously discussed.

Diagnosis

The descent of the testes can be completed after birth, during the first year of life, particularly in premature infants. This can be observed on physical examination. Cryptorchidism must be distinguished from normal testis retraction reflexes on examination.

Surgical repositioning should be undertaken before spermatogenesis is compromised. Removal of a nonfunctional testis reduces risk for malignancy.

Testicular Torsion

Testicular torsion is the twisting of the spermatic cord, causing ischemia.

- Diagnosis is supported by lack of pain relief when the testis is supported.

- Treatment is by surgical detorsion within 6 hours to preserve the testicle.

Epididymitis

Epididymitis is inflammation of the epididymis. Chlamydia, gonorrhea, and tuberculosis are important infections that have a predilection for the epididymis. In addition, any urinary tract infection can extend to the epididymis and eventually may also cause orchitis.

Signs and Symptoms

Classically, patients present with unilateral testicular pain, swelling, tenderness, and fever. A concomitant urethritis may also be present.

Inflammation is due to a nonspecific neutrophil and lymphocyte response, in the case of sexually transmitted pathogens, and a typical granulomatous response in epididymal tuberculosis.

Diagnosis

Urethral swabs and urine culture may reveal the organism causing the epididymis. A purified protein derivative (PPD) should be placed to rule out tuberculosis. Especially in young men presenting with unilateral pain, torsion (twisting of the spermatic cord) must be ruled out because ischemic damage can rapidly result. Unlike in torsion, support of the testis in epididymitis provides some relief. Doppler ultrasound examination of nuclear scan with labeled erythrocytes can be used to demonstrate blood flow.

Treatment focuses on antibiotic coverage appropriate to the probable causative organisms. Lack of improvement raises suspicion for testicular cancer. *Gonorrhea* or *Chlamydia* should be suspected in patients less than 35 years of age, and should be treated with *ceftriaxone* (given intramuscularly) followed by *doxycycline* (for 10 days). In those older than 35, or with a history of anal sex, suspect *Enterobacter*, E. *coli*, *Klebsiella pneumonia*, *Proteus*, and *Serratia*, and treat with *fluroquinolones* (given for 10–14 days).

Tunica Vaginalis Lesions

These are lesions of the serous lining of the testis. They present as testicular masses filled with fluid, which can be transilluminated (unlike testicular tumors). In a hydrocele, there is an increase in fluid accumulation due to incomplete fusion of the processus vaginalis. Hydroceles are common in newborns. They often resolve themselves. A spermatocele is the dilation of the epididymal tract, and is not associated with any changes in infertility. Varicoceles dilated veins in the pampiniform plexus, giving the appearance of a "bag of worms". They are found in approximately 10–15% of normal men, and may lead to infertility.

Testicular Cancer

Although testicular cancer is uncommon, it is the most common neoplasm in men between 15 and 35 years of age. Testicular tumors are divided into *germ cell tumors* and *non-germ cell tumors*.

- **Testicular germ cell tumors** include about 95% of all testicular tumors. These can present as a mixed germ cell tumor (60%).

- **Seminoma**: 50% of testicular germ cell tumors are seminomas. They mostly affect males 15 to 35 years of age. These tumors are *malignant* and *painless*. They present with homogenous testicular enlargement. Histologically, they present with large cells in lobules with watery cytoplasm and a *"fried egg"* appearance. These tumors are radiosensitive. Metastasis presents late. The prognosis is very good. These are analogous to *ovarian dysgerminomas*.

- **Embryonal carcinoma**: These tumors are painful and often metastasize. Although pure embryonal carcinomas are rare, they make up some portion of 85% of mixed germ cell tumors found. Under the microscope, the cells show epithelial differentiation with clusters and sheets of atypical cells positive for cytokeratin. The architecture may be glandular, papillary, or solid. It may be associated with elevations of *alpha-fetoprotein (AFP)*, and *hCG*.

- **Yolk sac (endodermal sinus) tumor**: These are the most common testicular tumor in children up to 3 years old (infants). They are yellow and mucinous. Histological findings include *Schiller-Duval bodies* (which resemble primitive glomeruli). They are associated with elevations of AFP. These are analogous to *ovarian yolk sac tumors*.

- **Choriocarcinoma**: These tumors are *malignant*. Histologically, they present with disordered syncytiotrophoblastic and cytotrophoblastic elements. Metastasis is via hematogenous spread. They are associated with elevations of hCG.

- **Teratoma**: Teratomas consist of multiple tissues types. Mature teratoma in males is most often *malignant* (whereas in females it is more often benign). Although these tumors may commonly present in testicles, they may also be found in the sacro-coccygeal region as well.

- **Non-germ cell tumors (Sex cord/Gonadal stromal tumors)** account for 5% of all testicular tumors. These are mostly benign.

- **Leydig cell**: These tumors contain *Reinke crystals*. They usually produce androgen, resulting in *precocious puberty* in boys. This androgen can be peripherally converted to estrogen, which causes *gynecomastia* in these men. They are golden brown in color.

- **Sertoli cell**: 90% of these tumors are *benign*. Androblastoma develops from the sex cord stroma. On rare occasions, these tumors can elaborate androgens and estrogens.

- **Testicular lymphoma**: Often bilateral and aggressive. Large cell diffuse B-cell types make up most of these cases. Common in men over 60 years old.

Signs and Symptoms

Patients may note one or more of the following symptoms: a *unilateral* testicular mass that *may or may not be painful*; a sense of heaviness in the scrotum; sharp pain or a dull ache in the lower abdomen or scrotum, breast enlargement (gynecomastia) from hormonal effects of hCG, and low back pain resulting from tumor spread to the lymph nodes along the back. Metastasis to the lungs is most common, causing dyspnea, cough, or hemoptysis. About 10% of patients have pain at the time of presentation as a result of intratesticular hemorrhage.

Histologic classification of the tumor is important for treatment. Amongst the types of *germ cell tumors*, the division between *seminomas* and *non-seminomatous germ cell tumors (NSGCT)* is aided by serum tumor markers. *LDH* is elevated in both types of cancer, but alpha-fetoprotein and hCG are more elevated in NSGCT.

Diagnosis

Ultrasound may aid in diagnosis, but unilateral orchiectomy is ultimately done to make the tissue diagnosis.

Treatment has traditionally involved orchiectomy and chemotherapy. The standard chemotherapy protocol is three to four rounds of *Bleomycin-Etoposide-Cisplatin (BEP)*. However, more conservative approaches in low-grade tumors now involve using orchiectomy alone and following serial tumor marker levels to diagnose recurrence.

Prostatitis

The prostate can be infected by the same gram-negative GI bacteria (e.g., *E. coli*) that cause cystitis. Prostatitis may be caused by reflux of contaminated urine into the prostatic ducts. Acute cases are usually bacterial, whereas chronic cases are more commonly abacterial.

Signs and Symptoms

Symptoms include dysuria, urinary frequency and urgency, in addition to perineal or low back pain. In the acute setting, the patient may have a fever. Chronic cases present with recurrent UTIs. On examination, the prostate is tender and "boggy."

In acute cases: Gonorrhea or Chlamydia should be suspected in patients less than 35 years of age, while in those older than 35, suspect *Enterobacter*, *E. coli*, *Klebsiella pneumonia*, *Proteus*, or *Seratia*. A sample of the seminal fluid usually shows high bacterial counts and lots of WBCs.

Treatment is with *Floroquinolones* or *Trimethoprim-sulfamethoxazole* for 4 weeks.

Benign Prostatic Hyperplasia (BPH)

Hyperplasia of the prostate gland is common in men above 50 years of age. BPH is believed to be related to elevated estradiol levels and sensitization of the prostate to DHT, promoting growth. The result is nodular enlargement of the lateral and middle (*periurethral*) lobes of the prostate, causing compression of the urethra and urinary obstruction (Figure 18). BPH is NOT considered a premalignant lesion.

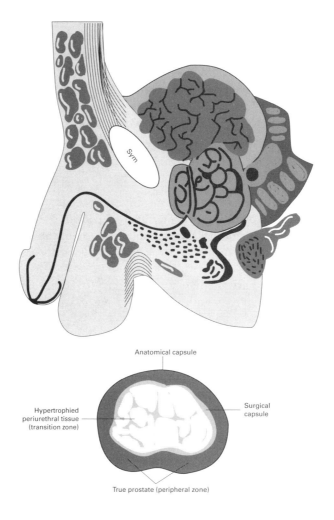

Figure 18 In benign prostatic hyperplasia, the enlarged periurethral glands are enclosed by the surgical capsule. (Adapted from *Current Medical Diagnosis and Treatment*)

Signs and Symptoms

Symptoms include increased urinary frequency (at day or night), hesitancy, decreased force of urine stream, difficulty starting and stopping the flow of urine, dribbling, and dysuria. Bladder distention and hypertrophy may result, leading to *hydronephrosis* and urinary tract infection (UTI) may occur with its associated symptoms.

Diagnosis

On rectal examination, the prostate may be large and fleshy, but it may be normal (because growth is often periurethral). Therefore, transrectal ultrasound may be a more sensitive test. ***Free prostate specific antigen (PSA) levels are elevated***.

Treatment with *alpha1-antagonists (terazosin, tamsulosin)* works within hours to days, causing relaxation of the smooth muscle, relaxing the urethra, therefore making it easier to urinate. *5-alpha-reductase inhibitors (finasteride, dutasteride)* work by inhibiting the conversion of testosterone to DHT, thereby reducing the size of the prostate. The *5-alpha-reductase inhibitors* take 3-6 months to decrease prostate volume, but are able to decrease PSA levels by about 50%. Surgical treatment with a transurethral prostatectomy (TURP) may be necessary to relieve the obstruction. In this procedure, the extra prostatic tissue in the periurethral zone is removed, improving flow through the prostate.

Prostatic Adenocarcinoma

Adenocarcinoma of the prostate is more common in men older than 50 years of age, and usually develops in the *posterior lobe (peripheral region)* of the prostate (compared to the periurethral location of BPH).

Signs and Symptoms

Patients may be asymptomatic but may have BPH symptoms (from urinary obstruction) as well as hematuria. Some patients may only present with bony pain from metastatic lesions. The presence of lower back pain may indicate osteoblastic metastasis in the bone.

Diagnosis

Diagnosis is most frequently made by digital rectal exam (DRE) indicating a prostate that is nodular, firm or irregular to palpation. Confirmation is by prostate biopsy. Serum *prostate-specific antigen (PSA)* and *prostatic acid phosphatase (PAP)* levels are good tumor markers. In prostatic adenocarcinoma, there is an *increase in total PSA* levels (bound and free), with a **decrease in the fraction of free PSA**. Metastatic lesions can be picked up with a bone scan. In cases of osteoblastic metastasis both the serum *alkaline phosphatase* and PSA levels are elevated.

Treatment may include *flutamide,* which inhibits testosterone at the receptor level. Radical prostatectomy, radiation, or "watchful waiting" (i.e., doing nothing, because tumor progression is fairly slow) are other possible treatment modalities. If caught early, prognosis is good.

FEMALE REPRODUCTIVE PATHOLOGY

Menstrual Disorders

- **Oligomenorrhea**: Infrequent menstruation that tends to involve sparse flow. Menstrual cycle lasts more than 35 days.

- **Polymenorrhea**: Menstrual bleeding more often than every 21 days (menstrual cycle is less than 21 days).

- **Hypomenorrhea**: Diminished menstrual flow during regular menses. Can include vaginal spotting.

- **Menorrhagia** (Hypermenorrhea): This refers to regular cyclic menses characterized by *abnormally heavy bleeding*, either due to increased flow or duration. This can be a sign of many abnormalities, including inadequate progesterone levels, clotting disorders, inflammation, and neoplasms.

- **Metrorrhagia**: Frequent but irregular menstruation. Also known commonly as *breakthrough bleeding*, it is bleeding or spotting that occurs at midcycle (between normal menses). Usually due to inadequate mid-cycle estrogen. This is a common problem with low-dose oral contraceptives.

- **Menometrorrhagia**: Heavy, frequent menstruation. Unusually heavy bleeding that occurs irregularly between menses.

• **Amenorrhea:** Amenorrhea is divided into two main categories: *primary amenorrhea*—a lack of menses onset by age 16, and *secondary amenorrhea*—the absence of menses for 3 consecutive months after menarche. There is a great deal of etiologic overlap between the two categories, and most of the causes can be understood in terms of the disturbances they cause in the endocrine system (Table 4). Pregnancy must always be considered as a cause of both primary and secondary amenorrhea. Administration of progestin is often used as a diagnostic test to see if the uterus is capable of responding normally on progestin withdrawal.

Partial moles are associated with a **partial** elevation of hCG, **partial** risk of malignancy and **parts** of a fetus upon ultrasound (Complete moles are characterized by extremely high hCG, greater risk of malignancy, and no fetal parts).

Hormonal state	Differential diagnosis
↓ estrogen	GnRH, LH, and FSH initially suppressed by estradiol, but then abruptly surge due to a positive feedback as estradiol increases
↓ FSH (central)	Reversible insults (e.g. illness, anorexia, stress, strenuous exercise) Turner's syndrome (primary)
↑ FSH (ovarian failure)	Hypothalamic or pituitary tumors Congenital GnRH deficiency (primary)
↑ androgen (adrenals vs. ovaries)	Female pseudohermaphrodism (primary) Premature menopause (secondary)
↑ prolactin	Adrenal tumor or hyperplasia Ovarian tumor Polycystic ovary syndrome Anabolic steroids

FSH = follicle-stimulating hormone;
GnRH = gonadotropin-releasing hormone

Table 4 Differential diagnosis of amenorrhea

• **Dysmenorrhea:** Dysmenorrhea is pain associated with menses. In younger women, the pain may or may not be associated with other pathologic findings. However, in older women, a secondary cause usually exists. Secondary causes of dysmenorrhea include PID, endometriosis, submucosal myoma, IUD use, and cervical stenosis.

The pain is usually in the lower midline of the abdomen and often occurs in conjunction with cramping, headache, nausea, diarrhea, and flushing. It may last for 1 or more days in the time leading up to or during menses.

Signs and Symptoms

The pain of primary dysmenorrhea is produced by constriction and anoxia in the uterus, due to cramping initiated by prostaglandins.

Diagnosis

Contrast imaging studies or laprascopy are sometimes necessary to rule out other causes and make this diagnosis. However, primary dysmenorrhea is a relatively common disorder, and in a younger woman with no other findings, a trial of nonsteroidal anti-inflammatory drugs (NSAIDs) can help to make the diagnosis.

NSAIDs are useful both for their analgesic and anti-inflammatory activity. The treatments for PID and endometriosis are discussed separately.

Infertility

Infertility is defined as failure to conceive after one year of unprotected intercourse. About one in five couples experience infertility. Approximately 40% of cases are due to "male factors," such as abnormal sperm function or the presence of a varicocele. Fifty percent of cases are due to "female factors," with about 30% due to tubal dysfunction, 15% due to ovarian dysfunction, and the remaining 5% due to cervical factors. About 10% of cases are unexplained.

Diagnosis

The first level of evaluation of infertile couples includes semen analysis, ovulation studies, and assessment of tubal function. Semen analysis involves testing for sperm count, motility, and morphology. Normal sperm count is greater than 20 million per ml. Ovulation studies include looking for signs of normal ovulation (e.g. regular menses and basal body temperature changes) as well as measurement of elevated progesterone during the luteal cycle. Tubal function is assessed by a contrast imaging study (hysterosalpingogram) and laparoscopy to assess patency of the tubes and look for pelvic adhesions.

The second phase of evaluation searches for cervical factors, luteal phase problems, and special sperm tests. Cervical factors are tested by the postcoital test, in which the woman's midcycle cervical mucus is tested 12 hours after intercourse for quality and quantity of surviving sperm.

Luteal phase insufficiency is treated with *clomiphene citrate* to trigger ovulation. Sperm are tested by the hamster egg penetration assay, in which the sperm are mixed with hamster eggs in which the zona pellucida has been removed, and the ability to fertilize is evaluated.

Treatment of infertility includes in vitro fertilization, surgical correction, and surrogacy, if the above factors cannot be easily corrected.

Gestational Trophoblastic Disease

Gestational trophoblastic disease (GTD) is a disorder associated with elevated beta-hCG and characterized by proliferation of placental trophoblastic epithelium of the mother, leading to tumors. GTDs are unique because they are maternal lesions but arise from gestational tissue! There are many types of GTDs including:

- **complete and partial hydatidiform moles (aka molar pregnancies)**

- **persistent/invasive gestational trophoblastic neoplasia**

- **choriocarcinoma**

- **placental site trophoblastic tumors**

Complete and partial hydatidiform moles are nonmalignant and make up 90% of GTDs. Complete moles consist only of paternal DNA, while partial moles result in triploidy (2 : 1 paternal to maternal DNA content). The other types are malignant and can arise from molar pregnancies, spontaneous or induced abortions, ectopic pregnancies, or normal pregnancies.

Treatment for all moles consists of *suction curettage*, and prophylactic chemotherapy for high-risk patients (extremes of age, previous history of GTD). Management also includes following beta-hCG levels afterwards.

Pregnancy-induced Hypertension (Preeclampsia and Eclampsia)

Pregnancy induced hypertension occurs in 7% of pregnant women from 20 weeks gestation to about 6 weeks postpartum. If it occurs prior to 20 weeks gestation, a molar pregnancy should be suspected. **Preeclampsia** is the condition consisting of the triad of *hypertension, proteinuria*, and *edema of the hands and face* during pregnancy. **Eclampsia** is when preeclampsia exists with the addition of *seizures*. Certain conditions increase the incidence of hypertension in pregnancy. These include: autoimmune disorders (ex: anti-phospholipid antibodies), chronic renal disease, diabetes, and preexisting hypertension. The condition can be associated with **HELLP syndrome** (Hemolysis, Elevated LFTs, Low Platelets). Cause of death is often due to cerebral hemorrhage and *Acute Respiratory Distress Syndrome (ARDS)*.

Signs and Symptoms

Characteristic symptoms include headache, blurred vision, facial edema, edema of the extremities, altered mental status, hyperreflexia, abdominal pain. Hemolysis (HELLP) may lead to anemia due to the breakdown of RBCs, causing hyperbilirubinemia and jaundice. Low platelet levels (HELLP) may cause hypercoagulability, resulting in easy bruising.

The condition is due to impaired vasodilation of the spiral arteries, causing **placental ischemia**.

Diagnosis

Lab findings may include hyperuricemia (increased uric acid levels due to renal disease), and thrombocytopenia.

Treatment involves delivery of the fetus as soon as it is viable. If this is not yet possible, then patients should be put on bed rest, salt restriction, and close monitoring and treatment of hypertension. *Nifedipine, hydralazine and Methyldopa* are a few of the possible drugs that can be used to treat pregnancy induced hypertension. Note that treatment of hypertension will not help with treatment of seizures in eclampsia. *IV Magnesium sulfate* and *Diazepam* (although controversial) can be given to prevent and treat seizures of eclampsia.

Recurrent Miscarriages

Miscarriages in the *first weeks of pregnancy* are usually attributed to low progesterone levels due to failure of the corpus luteum to respond to beta-hCG. In the *first trimester*, they are usually the result of chromosomal abnormalities, such as **Robertsonian translocation**. In the *second trimester* miscarriages are often secondary to the incomplete fusion of the paramesonephric ducts, causing a **bicornuate uterus**.

Complications of Pregnancy

- **Ectopic pregnancy**—Most often, ectopic pregnancies occur within the fallopian tubes. The presence of elevated hCG levels with sudden lower abdominal pain should raise suspicion of an ectopic pregnancy, with confirmation by ultrasound. Beta-hCG levels will often be lower than what should be expected for the current point in pregnancy. Patients may complain of pain with or without bleeding. The condition can mimic appendicitis. Risk factors may include pelvic inflammatory disease (*salpingitis*), history of infertility, ruptured appendix, prior surgery of the fallopian tube, and history of *Intrauterine Device (IUD)*, all of which can lead to scarring of the fallopian tube. Treatment includes *methotrexate* (which will terminate the pregnancy), and or surgical removal.

- **Abruptio placentae** is the premature detachment of the placenta from its point of implantation in the uterus. A hematoma develops between the uterus and the placenta causing pain. As a result, bleeding that is associated with pain often presents in the third trimester. Abruption may be present without bleeding if the cervical os is not disturbed. Complications include abrupt detachment and demise of the fetus. May be associated with *Disseminated Intravascular Coagulation (DIC)* in the mother. The risk of placental abruption is increased with hypertension, smoking, cocaine use, physical abuse and trauma, and anything causing severe vasoconstriction.

- **Placenta accreta**—Normally, the placenta attaches to the endometrium. In placenta accreta, a defective decidual layer allows for the placenta to attach to the *myometrium*. In other words, the placenta is essentially "encased in" the myometrium. There may be massive amounts of bleeding after delivery. However, there is no separation of the placenta after birth. Conditions that may predispose to placenta accreta include placenta previa, inflammation, and prior *cesarean section (C-section)*. Treatment is with hysterectomy because the placenta is not easily removed from the myometrium.

- **Placenta previa**—The placenta becomes attached to the lower segment of the uterus. There may be involvement of the internal os as well. Placenta previa may present as painless bleeding in any trimester, leading to poor oxygenation to the baby. Prior C-sections and multiparity are both factors that predispose to this condition. Should placenta previa be present in the third trimester, delivery by C-section is required.

- **Retained placental tissue**—If placental tissue remains within the uterus, it may cause postpartum hemorrhage.

Abnormalities of Amniotic Fluid

The levels of aminiotic fluid are usually assessed by ultrasound visualization or measuring amniotic fluid index. **Polyhydramnios** is characterized by too much amniotic fluid and usually caused by decreased fetal swallowing or increased fetal urination. This can be caused by fetal GI malformations (e.g. atresias) or maternal diabetes. **Oligohydramnios** is characterized by too little amniotic fluid and often has no identifiable cause.

Vulvovaginitis

Mild inflammation and infection of the vulva and vagina is typically caused by one of three organisms: *Candida, Trichomonas vaginalis*, and *Gardnerella*. More severe infections are caused by *Chlamydia* and other sexually transmitted diseases. Atrophic vaginitis has been previously discussed.

**CANdida:
CANt smell**

Signs and Symptoms

Patients may experience itching and burning with malodorous discharge, depending on the cause. *Candidal* infections are accompanied by a thick, curdly, non-odorous, white discharge, and *trichomonal* infections are accompanied by an odorous, greenish gray, frothy discharge. *Gardnerella* infections cause a grayish, malodorous discharge that is not as profuse as in trichomonal infections.

Diagnosis

Vaginal smears are treated with KOH and normal saline. Candidal infections show budding yeast with pseudohyphae. Trichomonal infections show motile flagellated organisms. *Gardnerella* infections show "**clue cells**," which are vaginal epithelial cells coated with coccobacilli.

Candida is treated with topical antifungals, such as *clotrimazole*. Both *Trichomonas* and *Gardnerella* are treated with *metronidazole*. Sexual partners should be treated as well to prevent reinfection.

Pelvic Inflammatory Disease

Pelvic inflammatory disease (PID), also known as *acute salpingitis*, is caused by ascending infection of the upper reproductive tract. Typically, microorganisms advance from the vagina and cervix to the uterus, fallopian tubes, and ovaries.

Signs and Symptoms

Symptoms include severe cervical motion tenderness, lower abdominal pain, and vaginal discharge.

The most common causative organisms are sexually transmitted, and include *Neisseria gonorrhoeae* and *Chlamydia trachomatis*. Risk factors for the development of PID include multiple sexual partners, sexually transmitted disease, and intrauterine device (IUD) use. Complications include chronic salpingitis, abscess formation, ectopic pregnancy, and infertility.

Diagnosis

Diagnosis is made by history and cultures, but should always include a pregnancy test to rule out ectopic pregnancy. Laparoscopy is sometimes needed to differentiate PID from appendicitis, a ruptured ovarian cyst, or an ovarian torsion.

Early and aggressive antibiotic administration is the mainstay of therapy. Depending on the degree of illness, it may necessitate hospitalization for intravenous antibiotics.

Ovarian Cysts

The blood is often brown, thus the term "chocolate"

- "**Chocolate cysts**" are cysts formed around the ovaries that are composed of endometrial tissue, and contain blood. These cysts vary with the menstrual cycle.

- **Corpus luteum cysts** occurs as a result of hemorrhage into a persistent corpus luteum. Often, these cysts regress spontaneously. Corpus luteum cysts are normal in pregnancy.

- **Follicular cysts** are the result of distention of the unruptured graafian follicle. Therefore, a woman can potentially have a follicular cyst every month, if ovulatory. It may be associated with hyperestrinism and endometrial hyperplasia.

- **Theca-lutein cysts** are due to gonadotropin stimulation. They are associated with choriocarcinoma and hydatidiform moles. More often they are bilateral and multiple.

Polycystic Ovary syndrome

Polycystic ovary syndrome is characterized by anovulation in the presence of steadily high levels of estrogen, LH, and androgen. Increased LH production leads to anovulation. Derangement of steroid synthesis by theca cells causes hyperandrogenism. This hormonal milieu can support the development of follicles, which become cysts because they are not ovulated. The cysts are therefore a consequence of the pathophysiology of the disease. This syndrome affects 2–5% of women of reproductive age.

Signs and Symptoms

Infertility, obesity, and hirsutism are present, and amenorrhea or abnormal menses are common.

Although the primary lesion leading to this syndrome is unknown, there are clues as to contributing factors. Elevated levels of androgen from adrenal hyperplasia or tumors are known to cause this syndrome. Presumably, obesity exacerbates this syndrome because androgens are converted to *estrone* in the fat. Estrone is believed to suppress FSH, with a relative increase in LH, leading to constant ovarian stimulation. Persistently elevated estrogen levels place these patients at higher risk for endometrial cancer.

Diagnosis

Diagnosis is made chiefly on the basis of history and hormone levels (elevated LH, estrogen and testosterone; low FSH), but transvaginal ultrasound is also diagnostic. Patients may have enlarged, bilateral cystic ovaries.

Current treatments include: weight loss, oral contraceptives (OCPs), gonadotropin analogs, *clomiphene*, *metformin*, *spironolactone*, and surgery. Oral contraceptives (OCPs) to restore normal cycling. OCPs will suppress LH, causing decreased synthesis of androgens, leading to lower than normal estrogen levels, thereby decreasing the risk of endometrial carcinoma. Gonadotropin analogs (such as *Luprolide* given in pulsatile form) are used in the treatment of infertility by stimulating ovulation and elevation of FSH. *Clomiphene* is also used to induce ovulation if fertility is desired.

Endometriosis

Endometriosis is the presence of non-neoplastic endometrial glands or stroma in places outside the uterus. The most common sites for implantation of endometrial tissue are the cul-de-sacs, ovaries, and fallopian tubes. However, sites as distant as the lung and kidney have been documented. It should be noted that during pregnancy, the endometrial tissue thickens and expands, which may lead to endometriosis in some cases. The term **adenomyosi**s specifically refers to endometrial tissue that has been implanted within the *myometrium*.

Signs and Symptoms

Notable mostly for an aching pain that begins up to a week before the onset of menses and becomes worse until menstrual flow occurs. It is characterized by cyclic, menstrual type bleeding from the ectopic tissue. The presence of endometrial tissue in the fallopian tubes, leads to the fallopian tubes being scarred, potentially preventing the egg from traveling to the womb or preventing the sperm from getting to the egg, both situations resulting in infertility. There may be signs specific to the site involved (e.g., bloody stools from gastrointestinal involvement). If endometrial tissues implants in the ovaries, it results in blood filled cysts, known as "**chocolate cysts**", being formed, which may rupture, causing their viscous fluid to spill to other parts such as the uterus, bowel and bladder.

Although the mechanism is unclear, possibilities include retrograde menstruation, ascending infection, spontaneous metaplasia, and vascular or lymphatic dissemination.

Diagnosis

Definitive diagnosis requires the documentation of endometrial glands and stroma in the tissue at the site under suspicion. Although the differential diagnosis for lower abdominal pain is broad, usually only PID and endometriosis consistently produce pain associated with menses.

A variety of 6- to 9-month hormonal regimens, often including GnRH analogues and oral contraceptives, are used with the goal of inhibiting ovulation and lowering overall hormone levels. During this time, it is hoped that the endometrial implants will recede. If unsuccessful, surgical removal can be performed. In women who still desire fertility, this involves systematic removal of the ectopic tissue, now often with laser surgery. Otherwise, hysterectomy with removal of the ovaries and fallopian tubes is usually performed.

Endometrial Hyperplasia

Endometrial hyperplasia is the abnormal proliferation of the endometrial gland. It is usually caused by excess stimulation of estrogen. Clinical presentation is usually as postmenopausal vaginal bleeding. Risk factors include anovulatory cycles, polycystic ovary syndrome, granulosa cell tumors (an estrogen secreting tumor), and hormone replacement therapy. It poses an increased risk for endometrial carcinoma. Any woman with increased menstrual bleeding after age 35 should have biopsy performed to confirm diagnosis.

Endometrial Carcinoma

Endometrial carcinoma is the *most common gynecologic malignancy*. It mainly occurs in women between the ages of 55 and 65. Endometrial carcinoma is usually preceded by endometrial hyperplasia. It presents clinically with vaginal bleeding. Risk factors include the prolonged use of unopposed estrogen (estrogen without progestins), diabetes, obesity, hypertension, nulliparity, polycystic ovary syndrome, and late menopause (causing prolonged endometrial estrogen exposure). The greater the invasion of the myometrium, the worse the prognosis.

Signs and Symptoms

Abnormal bleeding is usually the presenting symptom. Such bleeding in a post-menopausal female is a particularly ominous sign. In some cases, blockage of the cervix limits bleeding but predisposes to infection of the uterus and fallopian tubes.

Diagnosis

The majority of carcinomas are adenocarcinomas. Both stage and grade are important for prognosis.

Endometrial carcinomas are occasionally diagnosed by Pap smear, but the Pap smear is not designed to be specific for this cancer. Endometrial biopsy is the gold standard of diagnosis.

Treatment involves hysterectomy, with radiotherapy, unless the adenocarcinoma is low grade and confined to the uterine corpus. Prognosis for metastasis outside of the true pelvis is poor, with 5-year survival rates of about 5%.

Uterine Prolapse

Uterine prolapse refers to a weakening of support of the uterus, which leads to its descent into the vagina. Most commonly, this occurs as a delayed result of stretching during childbirth.

Signs and Symptoms

Patients typically note a vaginal mass. In severe cases, the prolapse can lead to pain or discomfort, usually most prominent when the patient is walking or sitting.

Weakness in the *transverse cervical and uterosacral ligaments* is the chief cause of uterine prolapse. The levator musculature and perineal body can help to compensate, so any damage to or weakness in these structures can contribute to prolapse.

Diagnosis

Diagnosis is with history and pelvic examination.

A surgical solution must be tailored to the reproductive desires of the woman and can range from hysterectomy with partial obliteration of the vagina, to plication (pleating/folding) of the suspensory ligaments. An inflatable vaginal counter-pressure device is available for women who do not desire surgery, or in whom surgery is contraindicated.

Urinary Incontinence

Urinary incontinence is the involuntary loss of urine. Traditionally, intermittent incontinence has been divided into three main categories: **urge** incontinence, **overflow** incontinence, and **stress** incontinence. Urge incontinence is caused by a hyper-reflexive bladder with or without diminished sphincter tone. Overflow incontinence results from prolonged urinary retention, often due to inability of the bladder nerves to detect stretching of the bladder. Stress incontinence is caused by laxity of the muscles making up the pelvic floor. Because it is seen mainly in multiparous women, stress incontinence is the focus of discussion.

Signs and Symptoms

Stress incontinence can usually be recognized by a history of urine loss with activities that increase intra-abdominal pressure, such as coughing, laughing, or lifting. These symptoms are more severe in upright than in supine positions.

Pregnancy and childbirth can cause damage to the normally strong suspensory ligaments that hold the urethra in close proximity to the pubis, increasing urethral resistance. Nevertheless, these changes are often not experienced until aging causes a weakening of the pelvic floor, and the urethra drops with relation to the pubis.

Diagnosis

Urinalysis should always be performed because subclinical urinary tract infection can be an easily treatable source of incontinence, especially in the elderly. The physician can perform a stress test, where the patient is observed while coughing with a full bladder, but the diagnosis can often be made on history.

Medical treatment focuses on improving sphincter tone with the use of alpha-adrenergic agonists. Estrogen replacement has also been shown to counteract atrophic changes. Anatomic resistance can be improved through the use of physical therapy, where the patient learns exercises to strengthen the pelvic diaphragm (*Kegel exercises*). Surgery also focuses on increasing anatomic resistance by stabilizing the urethra.

Myometrial Tumors

Also known as **fibroids**, **leiomyomas** are *benign* uterine neoplasms composed of smooth muscle. Malignant transformation is rare. They are the *most common of all tumors seen in women*. Leiomyomas may be estrogen-sensitive because they are most commonly seen during the reproductive years (and with pregnancy) and tend to shrink during menopause. However, contraceptive pills appear to have no effect of fibroid tissue. The peak incidence is between 20 to 40 years of age. There tends to be an increased incidence in African Americans.

Signs and Symptoms

Patients may be asymptomatic or experience pain. Leiomyomas may cause abnormal uterine bleeding, may lead to urinary disorders caused by pressure, or may result in miscarriage. Iron deficiency anemia may result from severe uterine bleeding.

Grossly, leiomyomas are firm, white, circumscribed nodules. They are found in three locations: *subserosal*, *intramural*, and *submucosal*. Submucosal fibroids compose only about 10% of leiomyomata but are the most symptomatic. Histologically, **a whorled pattern of smooth muscle bundle**s can be seen. Leiomyomas *do not* progress to leiomyosarcoma.

Diagnosis

Diagnosed via ultrasound.

Medical treatments include GnRH analogues and *mifepristone (RU-486)*, both of which have been found to shrink fibroids. *Leuprolide*, a GnRH analogue, induces a menopausal state by giving continuous GnRH, leading to suppression of FSH and LH. If bleeding or pain is severe, surgical removal of the tumor (myomectomy) or hysterectomy may be indicated.

Leiomyosarcoma

Leiomyosarcomas are tumors that are more commonly seen in middle aged women (40s to 60s). There is an increased incidence in African Americans. The tumor is a bulky and irregularly shaped tumor, having areas of hemorrhage, along with necrosis. These tumors *do not* arise from leiomyomas. The tumor may protrude out from the cervix, accompanied with bleeding. The tumor is highly aggressive, with a high recurrence rate. Diagnosis can be made by use of *desmin* to stain for this smooth muscle tumor. Treatment is with hysterectomy.

Cervical Intraepithelial Neoplasia (CIN) and Cervical Cancer

Cervical cancer is caused by **human papillomavirus (HPV)** *types 16 and 18*, which are sexually transmitted, but for which a vaccine is available. Risk factors for the development of cervical cancer include multiple partners, early age at first intercourse, smoking, HIV infection, and STDs. In essence, anything that increases exposure to HPV, increases the risk of cervical cancer. More than 75% are squamous cell carcinomas. The remaining cases are adenocarcinoma and are associated with mothers who used **diethylstilbestrol** during pregnancy.

Signs and Symptoms

Patients may be asymptomatic or may experience breakthrough or postcoital bleeding.

Grossly, the cervical lesion may be fungating or ulcerative. Microscopically, cells are evaluated both for precancerous dysplasia and evidence of invasive disease. Cervical dysplasia demonstrates disordered epithelial growth, which begins at the basal layer of the cervical squamo-columnar junction and spreads outward. The classification system of precancerous dysplasia is known as the **cervical intraepithelial neoplasia (CIN)** system. Atypia in the superficial cell layers is known as **koilocytosis** (in which there is perinuclear cytoplasmic clearing) and constitutes stage **CIN I**. Stage **CIN II** consists of atypia in both superficial and basal cell layers, and stage **CIN III** is atypia throughout with minimal maturation. CIN III is **carcinoma in situ** and is the same as stage 0 invasive carcinoma (Figure 19). Invasive carcinoma is often a squamous cell carcinoma, in which the peak incidence is 40 to 45 years of age.

16 and 18 types are high-risk HPV, which are most associated with cervical cancer. There are over 120 types.

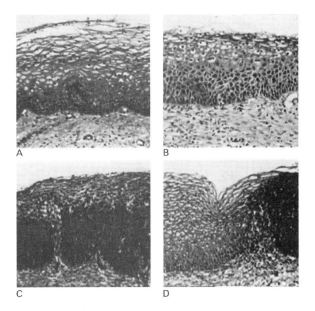

Figure 19 Cervical intraepithelial neoplasia (CIN). **A.** Normal ectocervix **B.** Moderate dysplasia—CIN II **C.** Severe dysplasia—CIN III **D.** Carcinoma in situ—CIN III
(Adapted from *Basic Histopathology. A Colour Atlas and Text*, 2nd Edition.)

Diagnosis

Asymptomatic patients are usually diagnosed by abnormal pap smear. The presence of *koilocytes* on a pap smear can identify *cervical dysplasia* before it progresses to *invasive carcinoma*. If invasive carcinoma spreads laterally, it can block the ureters, leading to renal failure. Abnormal Pap smears or symptomatic patients receive colonoscopy and biopsy, and excision if necessary.

Early detection through screening has led to excellent survival times. Stage 0 (carcinoma in situ) has a 100% cure rate, with stage I (confined to the cervix) rates at 85–90%. Stage IV (disseminated disease) has a 10-15% survival rate.

Vulvar Intraepithelial Neoplasia (VIN) and Vulvar Carcinoma

VIN I = hyperplasia
VIN II = dysplasia
VIN III = carcinoma in situ

Vaginal Intraepithelial Neoplasia is the precursor to vulvar and vaginal carcinoma. Carcinoma of the vulva is squamous in origin. It shares many similarities with cervical cancer, including an association with HPV infections and a classification system for vulvar intraepithelial neoplasia (VIN). Carcinoma is associated with prolonged irritation and genital warts caused by *HPV types 16, 18, and 31*.

Signs and Symptoms

Genital warts, pruritis, and bloody discharge are all early signs. Later lesions may appear as a mass or ulceration.

Koilocytosis can be seen in the superficial cell layers, as in CIN. If the basement membrane has been compromised, it is important to distinguish microinvasive carcinoma (stage Ia) from later stages because it can be treated less radically.

Diagnosis

Biopsy is essential for diagnosis. An abscess of the Bartholin's gland is a frequent cause of a tender vulvar mass not associated with cancer.

For carcinoma in situ and microinvasive carcinoma, local removal is usually sufficient. Later stages require radical vulvectomy with lymph node dissection.

Vaginal Pathology

- **Bartolin gland cyst**—This is a benign cyst that is infected (possibly due to a prior infection), and causes pain in the labia majora.

- **Squamous cell carcinoma (SCC)**—SCC is secondary to SCC of the cervix or VIN, both caused by HPV infection.

- **Clear cell adenocarcinoma**—Females born to mothers who have had exposure to *Diethylstilbestrol (DES)* while pregnant with them are often affected.

- **Sarcoma botryoides (rhabdomyosarcoma variant)**—This tumor affects girls under 4 years of age. Histologically, tumor cells are spindle-shaped and stain positive for *desmin* (which stains for muscle).

Premature Ovarian Failure

Premature ovarian failure occurs when women of reproductive age have premature atresia of the ovarian follicles. Estrogen levels are low, while FSH and LH levels are elevated. Affected patients show signs of menopause after puberty but prior to 40 years of age.

Anovulation

Anovulatory cycle—a menstrual cycle in which the ovaries do not release an oocyte, in which case, ovulation does not occur. Keep in mind that if a woman does not ovulate each menstrual cycle, she is not necessarily going through menopause. When anovulation becomes a chronic condition, it commonly leads to infertility. There are many possible causes of anovulation, including the following: hypothalamic-pituitary axis abnormalities, thyroid dysfunction (hyper- or hypo-), PCOS, hyperprolactinemia, excess weight loss or gain, Cushing's syndrome, and premature ovarian failure.

Ovarian Tumors

Tumors of the ovaries are divided into **ovarian germ cell tumors** and **ovarian non-germ cell tumors**. Table 5 shows a simple classification scheme for some ovarian tumors.

Type	Specific Neoplasms	Remarks
Surface epithelial	Serous Mucinous Endometrioid	Accounts for 75% of ovarian neoplasms but 95% of those leading to malignancy
Germ cell	Cystic teratomas are the only common neoplasms	15–20% of ovarian neoplasms but only 2–4% of malignancies; occurs mostly in young women
Sex cord gonadal stromal	Granulosa cell Thecal cell Sertoli or Leydig cell Lipid cell	5–10% of ovarian neoplasms but 1–3% of malignancies

Table 5 Classification of ovarian cancers

Ovarian Germ Cell Tumors

Because of the variety of tissues in the ovary, several types of neoplasms can arise. This is primarily attributable to the tendency of ovarian cancers to remain asymptomatic until significant growth has occurred.

- **Teratoma**: These make up 90% of ovarian germ cell tumors. Teratomas contain cells from 2 or 3 germ layers. There are three types of teratomas. *Mature cystic teratomas (dermoid cysts)* make up the most common type and are benign. *Mature solid teratomas* are unilateral and benign. *Immature teratomas* are malignant and make up 1% of ovarian teratomas.

- **Dysgerminoma**: These are *malignant* tumors. Histologically, they consist of sheets of uniform cells. Although they are analogous to the male seminoma, these are more rare. Tumor markers include hCG, and LDL.

- **Endodermal sinus (yolk sac) tumor**: Usually occur in young girls and women. Microscopy shows tubules lined by flattened cells and edematous stroma. **Schiller-Duval bodies** are found in some spaces. Serum AFP levels are elevated.

- **Mixed germ cell tumor**: contains some combination of the above three tumor types.

- **Choriocarcinoma**: These tumors are *rare but malignant*. Choriocarcinoma can arise from hydatidiform moles, the ovary, and from testicular tumors. During pregnancy, they can develop in both mother and/or baby. Histologically, they demonstrate hyperchromatic syncytiotrophoblastic cells (which make the placenta). Choriocarcinoma increases the frequency of *theca-lutein cysts*. The tumor marker is hCG. It is to be noted that **gestational trophoblastic neoplasia** consists of both *choriocarcinoma* and *hydatidiform moles*.

- **Other rare ovarian germ cell tumors**: pure embryonal carcinomas, pure polyembryomas.

Ovarian Non-Germ Cell Tumors (Surface Epithelial-Stromal):

This group of tumors makes up 90-95% of ovarian cancer.

- **Serous tumors**: Most common ovarian tumor—about 30%. 75% of serous tumors are benign and tend to be unilateral. The remaining 25% are malignant and usually bilateral. Serous tumors can be cystic and/or fibrous.

- **Mucinous tumors**: Make up 1/4 of ovarian neoplasms. Only 15% are malignant. Mucinous tumors are filled with mucin and thus, can get very big and multiloculated.

- **Endometrioid tumors**: Mostly malignant tumors that resemble endometrium. 40% are bilateral.

- **Clear cell tumors**: Cells have abundant clear cytoplasm. Associated with DES exposure.

- **Brenner Tumor**: Resemble bladder epithelia (transitional cell).

Stromal/Sex Cord Tumors:

- **Granulosa-stromal cell tumor**: These are large, unilateral, and sometimes malignant. Histologically they exhibit *Call-Exner bodies* (small clusters of cells around an eosinphilic-filled cavity). They secrete estrogen and thus, patients have signs of hyperestrogenism.

- **Sertoli-Leydig cell tumor:** These tumors produce androgens and 1/3 of women present with virilization. These may be benign or malignant.

- **Thecoma**: They are usually benign and may produce estrogen.

- **Gynandroblastoma**: Mixed tumors that are associated with androgen or estrogen production, causing virilization or signs of hyperestrogenism.

- **Sex cord tumor with annular tubules**: Can produce estradiol and progesterone. These are associated with *Peutz-Jeghers syndrome*.

Metastatic

- **Krukenberg tumor**: Derived from the GI tract as its primary site, this tumor often metastasizes to both ovaries. They are characterized by mucin-secreting **signet-ring cells**.

Signs and Symptoms

Specific cell type is determined by tissue examination and classified as benign, having low malignant potential, or malignant. Abdominal pain, bloating, ascites, and a palpable mass are symptoms of advanced disease.

Diagnosis

Most ovarian cancers are thought to arise from the surface of the ovary or germ cells, but some evidence suggests that the fallopian tube may also be a source. No reliable screening method for ovarian cancer exists. Ideally, diagnosis is made early by palpation of an ovarian mass on routine pelvic examination, and staging is done clinically based on extent of spread. An elevated level of **CA-125** is a tumor marker present in up to 80% of patients with epithelial ovarian cancer, but this value is traditionally used to evaluate effectiveness of treatment or recurrence.

Benign neoplasms involve removal of the tumor only or the entire affected ovary. Malignant neoplasms are usually treated with hysterectomy, bilateral oophorectomy, and chemotherapy.

BREAST PATHOLOGY

Common Breast Conditions

- **Acute mastitis**: A breast abscess that may develop during breastfeeding. There is an increased risk of infection through cracks and fissures that may develop in the nipple during nursing. The most common pathogen causing this condition is *Staphylococcus aureus*. Treatment involves the use of antibiotics, with continuation of breastfeeding.

- **Fat necrosis**: The benign, tender mass is usually a result of injury (trauma) to the breast tissue. Because it looks similar to cancer on physical exam and mammogram, biopsy is often required to establish diagnosis.

- **Gynecomastia (in males)**: This condition may be the result of *hyperestrogenic states* (such as cirrhosis, testicular tumors, and puberty), *Kleinfelter's syndrome*, or due to *drugs* (including *Spironolactone*, *Digitalis*, *Cimetidine*, Alcohol, *Ketoconazole*, estrogen, marijuana, heroin, and psychoactive drugs). Gynecomastia does not increase the risk of breast cancer.

Benign Epithelial Lesions of the Breast

- **Non-Proliferative Breast Changes**

- **Fibrocystic disease** of the breast is the most common cause of lumps in the breast from 25 years of age through menopause. It presents with premenstrual breast pain and multiple lesions, which are bilateral. The size of the mass may fluctuate throughout the menstrual cycle. Therefore, it is best to perform breast exams during or right after the menstrual cycle so as not to confuse a fibrocystic mass for a tumor. The presence of fibrocystic disease is usually not an indicator of an increased risk of carcinoma.

- **Fibrosis**: This is basically hyperplasia of the stroma of the breast.

- **Cystic**: The cysts appear as fluid-filled, blue domes. Ductal dilation is also present.

- **Adenosis:** In adenosis, there is an increase in the number of acini per lobule. Adenosis is physiologic in pregnancy. Fibroadenoma is a severe form of adenosis, and is the most common tumor in those under 25 years of age. **Fibroadenoma** presents as a small, firm mass with firm sharp edges, and is mobile. Elevations of estrogen, such as in pregnancy and menstruation, cause fibroadenomas to increase in size and tenderness. This tumor is not a precursor to breast cancer.

- **Phyllodes tumor (Cystosarcoma Phyllodes, Serocystic Disease of Brodie)**: Usually present as large quickly growing masses that form from the preductal stromal cells of the breast. Less than 1% of all breast neoplasms fall into this category. Tumor occurrence is most common between 40 to 50 years of age, and prior to menopause. Patients usually present with a firm, palpable mass that may be large and bulky. Histologically, it consists of connective tissue and cysts, and has *"leaf-like projections"*. These tumors grow quickly, potentially increasing in size within a matter of weeks. These tumors may become malignant.

Proliferative Breast Changes without Atypia

- **Sclerosing adenosis**: There is an increase in acini and the presence of intralobular fibrosis. It is associated with calcifications which compress the acini and distort the ducts.

- **Epithelial hyperplasia**: Epithelial hyperplasia occurs in women older than 30 years of age. This is an increase in the number of epithelial cell layers in the terminal duct lobule. The presence of atypical cells increases the risk of carcinoma.

- **Complex sclerosing lesion (radial scar)**: This is a scar with an irregular shape. It can look like invasive carcinoma, even with mammography.

- **Intraductal Papillomas**: It presents as a small tumor that grows in lactiferous ducts, and is usually located underneath the areola. Intraductal papilloma is the most common cause of fluid discharge from the breast, other than milk. The nipple discharge is straw-colored/yellowish and can be serous or bloody. The presence of this lesion leads to a very slightly increased risk of carcinoma.

Malignant Breast Tumors

Breast carcinoma is the most common malignant neoplasm in females. Risk factors include *increased exposure to estrogen*, increased total number of menstrual cycles (early menarche; late menopause), older age at first live birth, a history of breast cancer in the family, prior breast cancer in one breast, exposure to radiation, and obesity. In postmenopausal women, adipose tissue is a major source of estrogen. The conversion of *androstenodione* to *estrone* (a form of estrogen) occurs in the adipose tissue, accounting for the association between obesity and increased exposure to estrogen. Oral contraceptives and HRT are controversial as risk factors. Environmental factors are suspected because rates of breast cancer vary significantly across cultures.

Malignant breast tumors are common in women who are postmenopausal. They may arise from the mammary duct epithelium or the lobular glands. Overexpression of the *estrogen* and *progesterone* receptors or **erb-B2** gene (**human epidermal growth factor receptor 2—HER-2**, which is an **Epidermal Growth Factor Receptor—EGFR**) may have an effect on the prognosis and choice of treatment. The single most important prognostic factor is axillary lymph node involvement.

Signs and Symptoms

Masses may or may not be painful. Breast cancer can produce warmth and redness in the overlying skin (which is particularly true of cancers that arise during pregnancy). Some changes seen with breast cancer include:

- **Peau d'orange**—An eczematoid reaction giving the skin an orange-peel texture, and indicating the presence of edema from lymphatic blockage, as discussed previously.

- **Dimpling of the breast**—The presence of a new dimple may suggest that the cancer may involve the suspensory ligament of the breast.

- **New nipple retraction**—A newly formed nipple retraction is suggestive of lactiferous duct involvement.

Breast cancer spreads initially by local infiltration. Lymphatic spread is mainly to axillary lymph nodes but can involve the internal mammary chain. Hematogenous spread is mainly to the lungs and liver but can also involve bone, pleura, adrenals, ovaries, and brain.

Diagnosis

Mammographic screening is designed to diagnose clinically inapparent malignancies early. Ultrasound can be used to distinguish cysts from solid masses. Other diagnostic tools involve fine-needle aspiration, which has the advantage of allowing a diagnosis to be made before surgery. However, the test has a high false-negative rate. Open breast biopsy is the most sensitive diagnostic tool.

Initially breast cancer was treated with radical mastectomy, which consisted of removal of the entire breast, the pectoralis major and minor, and the axillary contents. It was later found that similar cure rates were achieved leaving the muscle intact, and this procedure, known as the *modified radical mastectomy*, became the standard. Studies are now demonstrating that local excision of small primary tumors ("lumpectomy"), followed by radiation therapy, can achieve similar results. Because it is now clear that breast cancer is often a systemic disease, adjuvant chemotherapy is now widely used at the time of presentation. In tumors that test positive for overexpression of estrogen receptors, therapy with *tamoxifen* (an antiestrogen) and *raloxifene* is proving to be beneficial. This is especially true in the elderly, who often cannot tolerate aggressive systemic chemotherapy. In tumors that are linked to overexpression of the **erb-B2 (HER-2 receptor)**, *trastuzumab* (a monoclonal antibody) is the current treatment being used.

In-Situ Breast Carcinomas

In-situ breast carcinomas are confined to the breast ducts and lobules. There are two types:

- **Ductal Carcinoma In Situ (DCIS)** results from ductal hyperplasia and fills the ductal lumen. Malignancy can present early, without basement membrane penetration. Comedocarcinomas are a subtype of DCIS that presents with ductal, caseous necrosis.

- **Lobular Carcinoma In Situ (LCIS)** involves atypical cells from the breast lobules. They are not associated with calcifications.

Invasive Carcinoma (70–85% of Breast Cancers)

Inflammatory Carcinoma: This is not a subtype, but rather a possible presentation of invasive carcinoma, in which there is dermal lymphatic invasion by breast carcinoma. The breast skin has a *Peau d'orange* (orange peel) appearance, which indicates edema and thickened skin from lymphatic blockage. Metastasis goes to the regional lymph nodes. Survival is 50% 5 years post diagnosis.

Invasive ductal (Infiltrating ductal): DCIS is the precursor. This is the *most common breast cancer,* accounting for about 3/4 of breast cancers. It is the worst and most invasive of the malignant breast tumors. It presents as a firm, fibrous, hard mass with sharp margins, and small, glandular, duct-like cells.

Invasive Lobular Carcinoma: LCIS is the precursor. This consists of an orderly row of cells (**Signet-Ring cells**). It is due to inactivation of the **E-cadherin** gene. The lesions are often multifocal and bilateral. Metastasis is to the peritoneum.

Paget's Disease: Often presents as eczematous patches on the nipple. *Paget cells* are large cells in the epidermis that have a clear halo. Paget's disease may suggest an underlying carcinoma. It may also present on the vulva.

Incidence of Gyneological Cancers within the United States:

Endometrial > Ovarian > Cervical (Most common worldwide)

Prognosis of Gyneological Cancers within the United States:

Ovarian cancer (worst prognosis), then cervical, followed by endometrial cancer

REPRODUCTIVE PHARMACOLOGY

	Mechanism	Clinical Use	Toxicity
Leuprolide	GnRH analog. Increases FSH/LH with pulsatile administration, decreases FSH/LH when continuous	Endometriosis, central precocious puberty, prostate cancer, fibroids	Hot flushes, gynecomastia, ↓ bone density
Estrogen (ethinyl estradiol, DES, mestranol)	Estrogen receptor agonist	HRT in postmenopausal women, menstrual abnormalities, hypogonadism, part of OCP	↑ risk of endometrial cancer
SERM	Mixed agonist/antagonist at estrogen receptor	Osteoporosis, breast cancer	Hot flushes, ↑ risk of thromboembolism
Anastrazole/ exemestane	Aromatase inhibitor	Breast cancer	Hot flushes, osteoporosis
Mifepristone	Progesterone receptor antagonist	Termination of pregnancy	Vaginal bleeding
OCP 1. combination 2. progestin only	Estrogen component— suppresses FSH Progesterone component—thickening of cervical mucus	contraception	Change in menstrual cycle, ↑ risk of blood clots, MI, stroke – CI in women > 35 who smoke
Dinoprostone	Synthetic prostaglandin	Induction of labor, termination of pregnancy	Vaginal bleeding/ discharge
Ritodrine/ Terbutaline	Beta 2-agonist, relaxes smooth muscles in uterus	Delay delivery of fetus	Hypotension, tachycardia, arrhythmia, fluid retention, hyperglycemia
Antiandrogens 1. finasteride 2. flutamide 3. ketoconazole 4. spironolactone	1. 5α-reductase inhibitor 2. nonsteroidal antiandrogen 3. inhibits androgen synthesis (by inhibiting desmolase) 4. aldosterone antagonist	1. male pattern hair loss, BPH 2. prostate carcinoma 3. prostate cancer 4. hyperaldosteronism	1. gynecomastia, sexual dysfunction 2. gynecomastia, decreased libido, blue-green urine 3. liver damage, ↓ sperm count 4. polyuria, gynecomastia, testicular atrophy, sexual dysfunction
Testosterone (methyltestosterone)	Testosterone receptor agonist	In males: hypogonadism, delayed puberty, impotence In females: breast cancer	Acne, accelerate prostate cancer
Sildenafil, Vardenafil	PDE-5 inhibitor	Erectile dysfunction	CI in patients on nitrates

DES = diethylstilbestrol; SERM = selective estrogen receptor modulator; HRT = hormone replacement therapy; OCP = oral contraceptive pills; PDE5 = phosphodiesterase type 5; BPH = benign prostatic hyperplasia; CI = contraindicated

Table 6 Reproductive Pharmacology

CHAPTER 19

SKIN AND CONNECTIVE TISSUE

BASIC STRUCTURE AND FUNCTION

The skin is the first line in the body's defense from harm. Acting as a physical barrier, the skin protects the internal organs from mechanical damage, environmental toxins, ultraviolet radiation, and infectious agents. It also importantly serves to protect the human body from electrolyte and water loss, which would otherwise compromise the resting state. Histologically, the skin is divided into two main layers: the epidermis and the dermis. The epidermis is the thick and avascular superficial layer of the skin. The epidermis is further subdivided into five layers that represent the process of maturing keratinocytes as they undergo active cell division at the dermo-epidermal junction differentiating and then moving superficially until they undergo apoptosis becoming the cornified outer layer of the skin. (See Table 1 & Figure 1.) The basement membrane zone separates and attaches the epidermis and the dermis. The dermis is a richly neurovascularized connective tissue layer composed of collagen fibers, elastic tissue, and ground substance. The dermis is further subdivided into the more superficial papillary dermis and the deeper reticular dermis. The dermis contains numerous sensory receptors as well as other skin appendages that provide thermoregulation and sensory perception. (See Table 2.) There are two major epithelial cell junctions maintaining the integrity of the epidermis, desmosomes and hemidesmosomes. Desmosomes function to connect keratinocyte cells within the layer of the stratum granulosum. Hemidesmosomes attach the deepest layer of the epidermis, known as stratum basale, to the basement membrane zone.

Burnt Skin Gets Less
Compliments.

Layers	Description	Associated Features
Stratum Basale (aka Stratum Germinatum)	Mitotically active single layer of stem cells	Melanocytes and melanin-containing melanosomes Tyrosinase Hemidesmosomes
Stratum Spinosum	Cells connective by intercellular bridges	Langerhans cells (antigen presenting cells) Desmosomes
Stratum Granulosum	Three to five layers of flat keratinocytes	Keratohyalin granules
Stratum Lucidum	Thin layer of dead keratinocytes only seen in acral skin	—
Stratum Corneum	Layers of flat anucleated dead keratinocytes	Keratin

Table 1 Epidermal Layers (deep to superficial)

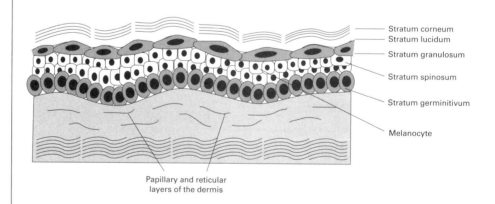

Papillary and reticular
layers of the dermis

Figure 1 Epidermal Layers

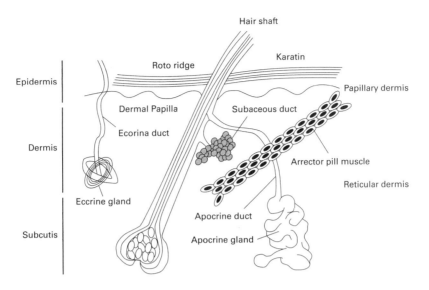

Figure 2 Dermal Appendages

TYPES OF COLLAGEN

Collagen is formed within fibroblasts and extruded into the extracellular environment as a triple helical structure of alpha chains known as procollagen. Procollagen is further modified in the extracellular space.

	Role	Location	Notes
Sensory			
Glomus Body	Thermoregulation	Nail beds Finger pads	Composed of arteriovenous shunts that shunt blood away from skin surface when exposed to colder temperatures Think glomus body tumor when patient presents with painful blue mass under fingernail
Free Nerve Endings	Temperature and Pain Sensation	Dermo-epidermal junction	—
Meissner's Corpuscles	Fine touch and Mechanoreception	Papillary Dermis	Ovalloid-shaped structure within papillae
Pacinian Corpuscles	Vibration and Mechanoreception	Reticular Dermis	"Onion skin" appearance
Adnexae			

Hair Follicles	Temperature insulation	Entire body except glaborous surfaces (palms & soles)	4 phases of cycle: Anagen (Growth), Catagen (Transition), Telogen (Rest), Exogen (Shed)
			Associated with arrector pili (smooth muscle involved in goosebumps phenomenon)
Sebaceous glands	Secrete sebum onto the hair follicles	Scalp, Face	Increased sebum production is associated with acne
Apocrine glands	Secrete sweat onto hair follicle	Axillae & Genitals	Malodorous sweat (odorless sweat is secreted, but bacterial involvement produces a malodor)
Eccrine Glands	Secrete sweat directly onto skin surface	Entire body	Odorless sweat
Nail	Protect distal fingers and toes	Distal fingers & distal toes	Keratinocytes regenerate in the basal cell layer of the nail matrix

Table 2 Dermal Appendage

Collagen Type	Tissues Found	Function
I	Bone, skin, tendon, teeth	Strength
II	Cartilage	Pressure-resistant
III	Blood vessels, skin, muscle	Volume expandable
IV	Basement membrane (all tissue)	Filtration

Table 3 Collagen Types

BIOCHEMISTRY OF SKIN PIGMENTATION

Melanin is the primary element involved in skin pigmentation. Melanin is produced by biochemical conversion of phenylalanine, an amino acid, in the epidermis.

Phenylalanine Hydroxylase   **Tyrosinase**   **Tyrosinase**

Phenylalanine -------------> Tyrosine ----------> Dopa -------------> Melanin

Phenotypic Tissue
Dyes Multicolored

Clinical Correlation

1. **Oculocutaneous Albinism** is an autosomal recessive deficiency of tyrosinase or defective tyrosinase transport. Patients typically have a normal number of melanocytes, but have deficient production of melanin.

2. **Ocular Albinism** is a X-linked recessive hypopigmentation limited to the eyes.

3. **Vitiligo** is an autoimmune destruction of melanocytes in skin causing patches of skin without pigment.

4. **Tinea versicolor** is a superficial *Malassezia* fungal infection that causes characteristic hypopigmented skin lesions due to the inhibition of tyrosinase.

EMBRYOLOGY

During the third week of embryogenesis, gastrulation occurs forming the three germ layers: ectoderm, mesoderm, and endoderm. The epidermis arises from a single cell layer of ectoderm. This epidermal layer originally forms a three-layered structure consisting of the mitotically active basal layer, the intermediate layer, and the overlying periderm. The dermis arises from the mesoderm. The dermis forms projections into the epidermis called dermal papillae. The dermis, which lies just deep to the epidermis, sends signals that induce the formation of the five epidermal layers: stratum basale, stratum spinosum, stratum lucidum, stratum granulosum, and stratum corneum.

Melanocytes arise from neural crest cells, where they migrate into the stratum basale and produce melanosomes, the pigmented granules containing melanin. Langerhans cells, the antigen presenting cells of the skin, migrate into the epidermis from the bone marrow. The mesoderm stimulates differentiation of epidermal appendages, like the hair follicle, which is derived from ectoderm. Nails also develop from the ectoderm. Mesodermal cells (also known as mesenchyme) secrete ground substance and differentiate into fibroblasts, which secrete collagen and elastic fibers. Mesodermal cells of the dermis encapsulate the hair follicles to form dermal root sheath as well as the arrector pili muscle.

IMMUNOLOGY

Hypersensitivity reactions occur when the immune system produces an exaggerated response to foreign antigens. These hypersensitivity reactions produce clinical effects that often manifest as various skin conditions. (See Table 4.) Atopy is the hereditary predisposition for certain patients to develop allergic reactions to environmental antigens, atopic dermatitis, allergic rhinitis, and asthma.

		Associations	Clinical Manifestation
Type I	Immediate	Certain foods (peanuts, shellfish, etc.) Cosmetics Medications	Urticaria Angioedema Anaphylaxis
Type II	Antibody-Mediated	Autoimmune	Bullous Pemphigoid Pemphigus Vulgaris
Type III	Immune Complex-Mediated	Small vessel vasculitis	Henoch-Schönlein Purpura
Type IV	Delayed	Poison Ivy Nickel	Contact Dermatitis

Table 4 Hypersensitivity Reactions

Skin Lesions

Below is a list of common terminology used when diagnosing various skin conditions. A small lesion is defined as being less than 0.5 cm in diameter and large lesion is defined as being greater than 0.5 cm in diameter.

Lesion	Definition	Example
Macule	A small, flat lesion of skin discoloration (hypo- or hyper- pigmented)	Ephelides
Patch	A large, flat lesion of skin discoloration (hypo- or hyper-pigmented)	Vitiligo
Papule	A small, solid skin lesion raised above the skin surface	Acne
Plaque	A large, solid skin lesion raised above skin surface	Psoriasis
Nodule	A palpable solid skin lesion that extends into the dermis	Acne
Pustule	A small, palpable pus-filled lesion	Impetigo
Crust	An area of dried purulent exudate (associated with the rupture of a pustule)	"Honey-colored" crust in impetigo
Wheal	A transient, raised skin lesion with irregular borders	Urticaria
Vesicle	A small, palpable fluid-filled lesion	Varicella Zoster
Bullae	A large, palpable fluid-filled lesion	Bullous pemphigoid
Keloid	A raised, irregular area of hypertrophic scar tissue in response to trauma	Pedunculated mass on ear after ear piercing

Table 5 Definitions of Skin Lesions

Ephiledes = Freckles

Urticaria = Hives

Varicella Zoster = Chickenpox

SKIN, CONNECTIVE TISSUE DISEASE

Hereditary

Osteogenesis Imperfecta

Osteogenesis imperfecta is a hereditary (most commonly Autosomal dominant) disorder of Type I collagen that presents with fragile bones, dental abnormalities, and progressive hearing loss.

SIGNS AND SYMPTOMS

Blue sclera, decreased bone mineral density on x-rays, repeat fractures after minimal trauma, translucent teeth, hearing loss

DIAGNOSIS

History and physical exam findings, genetic testing, skin biopsy

TREATMENT

Bisphosphonates (used off-label)

Ehlers-Danlos Syndromes

Ehlers-Danlos Syndromes are a group of heritable (most commonly autosomal dominant) connective tissue disorders characterized by skin hyperelasticity, tissue fragility, and joint hypermobility due to defective collagen. Classical Ehlers-Danlos Syndromes is associated with a defect in Type I collagen and presents with joint hypermobility and thin, hyperextensible skin. Vascular Ehlers-Danlos Syndromes is due to a defect in Type III collagen causing increased susceptibility to blood vessel rupture.

SIGNS AND SYMPTOMS

Thin, easily scarred skin, easy bruising, early-onset osteoarthritis, degenerative joint disease, mitral valve prolapse, scoliosis

INCREASED SUSCEPTIBILITY

Ascending aorta aneurysm, recurrent hernias, recurrent joint dislocations

DIAGNOSIS

History and physical exam

TREATMENT

Avoid contact sports and monitor for aortic aneurysms.

One Tiny Fractured Boy Sings Hymns (Type I, Teeth, Fractures, Blue Sclera, Hearing)

Osteogenesis imperfecta may be mistaken for child abuse.

Elder Dan lived in the circus as a contortionist.

Alport Syndrome

Alport syndrome is a hereditary (most commonly X-linked) disorder of Type IV collagen that presents with glomerular disease, sensorinerual deafness, and ocular abnormalities.

Signs and Symptoms

Glomerular disease (begins with childhood hematuria and progresses to end-stage renal disease in adulthood), progressive sensorineural hearing loss, cataracts, and other ocular abnormalities

Diagnosis

Skin or renal biopsy

Treatment

Kidney transplant if end-stage renal disease is present, otherwise none

> Multiples of 2: eyes, ears, kidneys, Type IV

Marfan Syndrome

Marfan Syndrome is an autosomal dominant connective tissue disorder characterized by ocular, cardiovascular, and skeletal abnormalities. This condition is associated with a mutation in the fibrillin gene resulting in defective elastin.

Signs and Symptoms

Characteristic body shape with long limbs and fingers, scoliosis, pectus excavatum, upward lens subluxation

Increased susceptibility

Ascending aortic aneurysms, mitral valve prolapse, berry aneurysms

Diagnosis

History and physical exam

Treatment

Beta blockers to slow aortic dilation, treat scoliosis, and lens subluxation

> **Marfan** is the **ELASTIC** man

Autoimmune

Systemic Lupus Erythematosus

Systemic Lupus Erythematosus (SLE) is a multi-system autoimmune disorder characterized by skin and mucosal involvement, renal disease, and hematologic abnormalities.

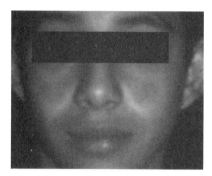

Figure 3 Malar rash of SLE
(Adapted from *The Color Atlas of Family Medicine*)

SIGNS AND SYMPTOMS

- Skin: Malar rash, photosensitivity, Raynaud's phenomenon, oral aphthous ulcers
- Other: Arthritis, serositis, glomerular disease, neurologic symptoms, hemolytic anemia, hypercoaguability (anti-phospholipid antibodies)

DIAGNOSIS

History and physical exam, elevated ESR, renal biopsy, immunoglobulins:

\+ anti-nuclear antibody (ANA) = sensitive

\+ anti-double stranded DNA (anti-dsDNA) & +anti-Smith antibodies (anti-Sm) = specific

TREATMENT

NSAIDs, corticosteroids (acute exacerbations), anti-malarial agents (hydroxychloroquine), cytotoxic agents (cyclophosphamide)

Scleroderma (Systemic Sclerosis)

Scleroderma is a multi-system autoimmune disorder characterized by diffuse skin fibrosis due to an overproduction of collagen from stimulated fibroblasts. There are two types of scleroderma: diffuse and limited. **Diffuse scleroderma** involves extensive skin fibrosis and early-onset visceral organ involvement.

Limited scleroderma involves fibrosis of the distal extremities only and late-onset visceral involvement. **CREST syndrome** is a variant of limited scleroderma that has skin involvement limited to the hands and fingers. CREST syndrome is characterized by calcinosis, Raynaud's phenomenon, esophageal dysmotility, sclerodactyly, telangiectasia, and positive anti-centromere antibodies.

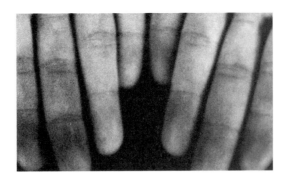

Figure 4 Raynaud's Phenomenon
(Adapted from *Fitzpatrick's Dermatology in General Medicine*, 8th Ed.)

Signs and Symptoms

Raynaud's phenomenon, skin tightening on face, fingers and toes, esophageal dysmotility and gastroesophageal reflux disease, pulmonary manifestations (pulmonary hypertension, interstitial fibrosis), renal symptoms, gastrointestinal symptoms

Diagnosis

Immunoglobulins

+ ANA = sensitive

+ anti-topoisomerase (anti-scl-70) antibodies = specific

+ anti-centromere antibodies = CREST syndrome only

Treatment

Supportive, calcium channel blockers (Raynaud's phenomenon)

Mixed Connective Tissue Disease

Mixed Connective Tissue Disease is an autoimmune connective tissue disease that combines the features of the well-known connective tissue disorders, such as scleroderma, systemic lupus erythematosus, etc.

Signs and Symptoms

Cutaneous rash (heliotrope or malar), photosensitivity, Raynaud's phenomenon, esophageal dysmotility, deforming arthritis

Diagnosis

Immunoglobulins

+ ANA = sensitive

+ anti-U1-RNP (ribonucleoprotein) antibodies = specific

Treatment

Corticosteroids

Bullous Disorders

Epidermolysis Bullosa

Epidermolysis Bullosa (EB) is a spectrum of heritable skin disorders characterized by bulla formation after minor skin trauma. Patients may also experience significant scar formation if bullae extend through the dermal layer (scars will not form if only the epidermis is involved). There are three main categories of Epidermolysis Bullosa depending on the level of the defect in the skin layer.

- Epidermolysis Bullosa Simplex (EBS) is the mildest form of EB and is associated with a defect in keratin at the level of the keratinocytes, causing intraepidermal cleavage. EBS patients are prone to develop blisters on sites exposed to trauma (hands, feet, elbows, knees) that typically heal without scar formation.

- Junctional Epidermolysis Bullosa (JEB) is associated with a defect in structural proteins of hemidesmosomes at the dermo-epidermal junction. JEB patients typically present in infancy with blisters at birth and other birth defects. These patients may not survive into childhood.

- Dystrophic Epidermolysis Bullosa (DEB) is the most severe form of EB and is associated with a defect in collagen fibrils in the dermis. Since the defect is below the basement membrane level, DEB patients typically present with widespread skin and mucosal blistering that heal with substantial scar formation and resultant anatomic deformities. Patients die early as the result of various complications.

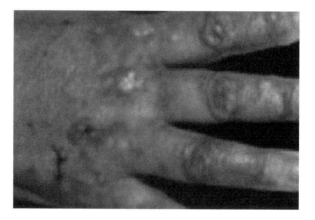

Figure 5 Epidermolysis Bullosa
(Adapted from *Fitzpatrick's Dermatology in General Medicine*, 8th Ed.)

Milia = small pearly-white papules.

SIGNS AND SYMPTOMS

Blistering of skin and mucosa, alopecia, milia, dental abnormalities, deformed fingernails

DIAGNOSIS

Skin biopsy for immunofluorescence to identify level of defect

TREATMENT

Supportive

Pemphigus Vulgaris

Pemphigus Vulgaris is a rare autoimmune skin disorder characterized by the production of autoantibodies against desmoglein proteins in desmosomes. By causing destruction of desmosomes, the antibodies damage the keratinocyte cell-to-cell junctions causing intraepidermal blister formation.

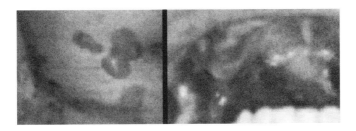

Figure 6 Pemphigus Vulgaris
(Adapted from *Fitzpatrick's Dermatology in General Medicine*, 8th Ed.)

SIGNS AND SYMPTOMS

Flaccid bullae (rupture easily) on skin and mucosal surfaces, erosions, + Nikolsky sign, vulnerable to secondary infections, may be fatal

DIAGNOSIS

Skin biopsy for immunofluorescence—antibodies are deposited between epidermal cells (fishnet-like pattern),

Immunoglobulins: + anti-desmoglein antibodies

TREATMENT

Supportive

Bullous Pemphigoid

Bullous Pemphigoid is a rare acquired skin disorder characterized by the production of autoantibodies against structural elements in hemidesmosomes, thereby destroying the dermo-epidermal junction and causing subepidermal blister formation. Less severe than pemphigus vulgaris.

Nikolsky Sign = skin separation occurs when lateral pressure is applied

Typical patient = middle age

Half (**hemi**) desmosomes = half the severity

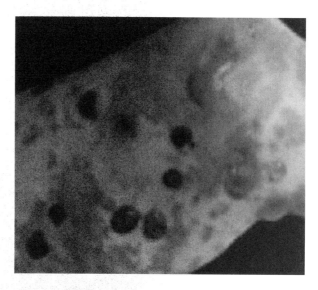

Figure 7 Bullous Pemphigoid
(Adapted from *Fitzpatrick's Dermatology in General Medicine*, 8th Ed.)

SIGNS AND SYMPTOMS

Tense bulla (stable) on skin only, pruritic inflammatory skin lesions, eosinophils within blisters, negative Nikolsky sign

DIAGNOSIS

Immunofluorescence—antibodies deposited at dermo-epidermal junction (linear pattern)

TREATMENT

Supportive

Nutritional

Vitamin A deficiency

Vitamin A deficiency may be the result of inadequate dietary intake or malabsorption syndromes.

SIGNS AND SYMPTOMS

Dry skin, xerostomia (squamous metaplasia of oropharyngeal mucosa), scaling, keratomalacia, and blindness

Hypervitaminosis A

Hypervitaminosis A may be the result of excessive dietary intake of vitamin A or by systemic accumulation of retinol-derived medications (e.g., isoretinoin). One notable dietary source of high levels of vitamin A is animal liver.

SIGNS AND SYMPTOMS

Dry skin that may be associated with scaling and desquamation, cheilosis, headache, fatigue, pseudotumor cerebri

Therapeutic levels of vitamin A are used to treat **measles** in developing countries.

Pellagra (Vitamin B3/Niacin deficiency)

Pellagra often occurs in cultures with a diet heavy in corn. Niacin deficiency may also occur when its precursor, tryptophan, becomes depleted such as in carcinoid syndrome, Hartnup disease, or malabsorption syndromes.

SIGNS AND SYMPTOMS

Dermatitis, Diarrhea, Dementia, Death

Scurvy (Vitamin C deficiency)

Scurvy is often the result of inadequate dietary intake of Vitamin C, especially in alcoholics and elderly patients. Since vitamin C acts as a cofactor in the hydroxylation of collagen, vitamin c deficiency causes the production of abnormal collagen.

SIGNS AND SYMPTOMS

Easy bruising, bleeding gums, impaired wound healing, "corkscrew" hairs

Dermatitis Herpetiformis

Dermatitis Herpetiformis is an autoimmune skin disorder characterized by pruritic vesicular lesions and gluten-sensitivity (celiac disease).

SIGNS AND SYMPTOMS

Papulovesicular rash located on elbows, knees, buttocks, and scalp

DIAGNOSIS

Skin biopsy for immunofluorescence—IgA deposited in dermal papillae

TREATMENT

Avoidance of dietary gluten

INFECTIOUS

Bacterial

Staphylococcus aureus and Streptococcal pyogenes

- **Folliculitis** is a purulent infection of the hair follicles limited to the epidermis. When multiple follicles are connected they form a **carbuncle**. When the infection extends deeper to involve the dermis, it is known as a **furuncle**. Folliculitis occurs in areas exposed to shaving (such as facial hair area). When folliculitis is associated with exposure to hot tubs or pools (**hot tub folliculitis**), pseudomonas aeruginosa is more commonly the causative agent. Folliculitis is typically self-limited, but may improve with application of warm compresses.

Pellagra = 4 Ds (Diarrhea, Dermatitis, Dementia, Death)

Typical patient = elderly woman with a "tea and toast" diet

- **Cellulitis** is a soft tissue infection involving the deep dermis and subcutaneous fat. **Erysipelas** is soft tissue infection of the superficial dermis and lymphatic vessels. These conditions occur when bacteria is introduced through a break in the skin barrier. Both conditions present with erythema, swelling and warmth of the infected region, which typically occurs in the lower extremities. Unlike cellulitis, erysipelas often affects children, may cause constitutional symptoms, and demonstrate a raised surface with a distinct line of demarcation. Treatment involves elevation of affected extremity and empiric parenteral antibiotic use.

- **Skin Abscess** is a soft tissue infection involving a well-circumscribed collection of purulent material.

- **Impetigo** is a superficial infection that causes vesicle formation with secondary formation of a honey-colored crust. Impetigo is highly contagious and is often observed in children and teens (especially wrestlers). **Nonbullous impetigo** may be caused by both *S. aures* and *S. pyogenes*. **Bullous impetigo** is caused exclusively by exfoliative toxin-producing S. aureus with a similar pathophysiology to that of pemphigus vulgaris. Bullous impetigo is typically localized to the trunk with few lesions. Treatment includes topical mupirocin if there are few non-bullous lesions. If lesions are extensive or are bullous, treatment should involve oral antibioitics (dicloxacillin, cephalexin, clindamycin). A sequela of streptococcal impetigo is poststreptococcal glomerulonephritis, regardless of antibiotic treatment.

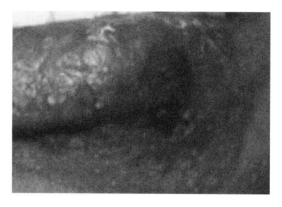

Figure 8 Impetigo with "honey-colored" crust
(Adapted from *The Color Atlas of Family Medicine*)

- **Staphylococcal Scalded Skin Syndrome** (SSSS), like bullous impetigo, is caused by exfoliative toxin-producing S. aureus. This syndrome typically affects infants and young children, beginning with constitutional symptoms (fever, malaise, irritability) and progressing to generalized blister formation and significant desquamation with a positive Nikolsky sign. SSSS is considered a dermatologic emergency and requires early intervention with intravenous fluids and penicillinase-resistant penicillin (e.g. nafcillin) or vancomycin.

- **Toxic Shock Syndrome** (TSS) is an invasive infection that is caused by the production of superantigens (TSST-1 exotoxin). This syndrome is characterized by a generalized nontender erythema of the skin that progresses to desquamation of the palms and soles and may result in multisystem organ failure and death. Factors that increase the risk of TSS occurrence include high absorbance tampons, nasal packing, recent surgery and skin trauma (burns or wounds). Severe TSS is a true emergency and requires close monitoring and supportive measures.

Streptococcus pyogenes (Group A Strep)

- **Scarlet fever** is caused by erythrogenic toxin- producing *S. pyogenes*. This infection consists of pharyngitis, "strawberry tongue" and an erythematous rash with a rough texture.

- **Necrotizing Fasciitis** is a rapidly progressing invasive soft tissue infection. This condition is characterized by significant tenderness, edema, and skin color changes (red to blue-gray) that spreads through the fascial planes. Tenderness may proceed to numbness prior to the development of tissue necrosis. Prompt intervention requires aggressive surgical debridement and use of empiric antibiotics.

OTHER

- **Cutaneous Anthrax** is caused by *Bacillus anthracis* after contact with livestock or animal hide. This skin lesion begins as a painless pruritic papule eventually progressing to a black eschar with surrounding edema and vesicles.

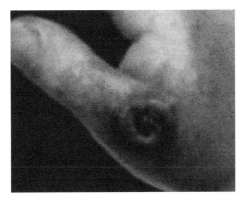

Figure 9 Cutaneous anthrax
(Adapted from *Fitzpatrick's Color Atlas & Synopsis of Clinical Dermatology*, 6th Ed.)

- **Cat Scratch Disease** is caused by *Bartonella henselae* after contact with flea-infested cats. This disease is characterized by regional lymphadenopathy, as well as a skin papule at the site of inoculation that may progress to a rash. More severe disease may also manifest with neurologic symptoms and visceral organ involvement.

- **Ecthyma gangrenosum** is an accompanying cutaneous feature that distinguishes *Pseudomonas aeruginosa* bacteremia from other infectious causes of bacteremia. The typical skin lesion consists of hemorrhagic bullae that progress to necrosis, due to perivascular invasion with subsequent tissue ischemia.

- **Leprosy**, caused by *Mycobacteria leprae*, is caused by acid-bacilli, Mycobacteria leprae. **Tuberculoid leprosy** is characterized by rapid onset of hypopigmented and hypoesthetic macular lesions with an asymmetric, limited distribution. **Lepromatous leprosy** demonstrates slowly progressive accumulation of nodular lesions and hair loss with a more diffuse distribution.

- **Lyme Disease** is a vector borne disease caused by *Borrelia burgdorferi* typically carried by a tick native to the northeast United States. The characteristic skin manifestion of early lyme disease is the bulls-eye lesions of **erythema chronica migrans**. As the disease disseminates, it may produces neurologic, cardiac, musculoskeletal symptoms.

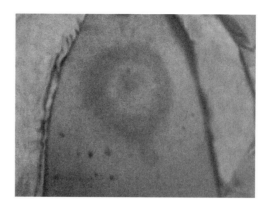

Figure 10 Erythema migrans of early lyme disease
(Adapted from *The Color Atlas of Family Medicine*)

Fungal

Tinea capitis or corporis patient:
Patient who participates in contact sports (especially wrestlers)

- **Dermatophytoses** are superficial fungal infections, typically caused by *Trichophyton* and *Microsporum*, with invasion limited to the stratum corneum and appendages. Lesions may manifest on the scalp (**tinea capitis**) and body (**tinea corporis** or **ringworm**) as single or multiple pruritic circular plaques with central clearing and raised edges. Dermatophytoses may also infect between the toe web space (**tinea pedis** or **athlete's foot**), the intertriginous folds of the groin (**tinea cruris**) or nails (**tinea unguium** or Onychomycosis).

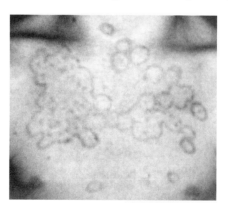

Figure 11 Tinea corporis

Tinea versicolor patient:
Patient who has just returned from vacation with a suntan (lesions become noticeable)

- **Tinea Versicolor** is a superficial fungal infection caused by *Malassezia* that causes either hypo or hyperpigmented skin lesions that may be associated with a scale. Lesions may be more noticeable after patient has gotten a suntan.

- **Seborrheic dermatitis** is a chronic skin condition that has been hypothesized to be associated with *Malassezia* infection. Patients typically present with thick yellowish scales on the scalp, nasolabial folds, ears or skin folds. In infants this condition is also known as **cradle cap** and in adults it can be considered **dandruff**.

- **Cutaneous candidiasis** (also known as **Candidal Intertrigo**) is a superficial fungal infection caused by *Candida albicans*. Since *Candida* thrives in moist warm areas, dermatitis typically occurs in intertriginous skin folds (inframammary, axillae, below pannus, intergluteal folds). Pruritic, erythematous plaques with satellite lesions characterize this infection. In infants this condition is known as **diaper rash**. This would be adequately treated with topical nystatin and drying agents.

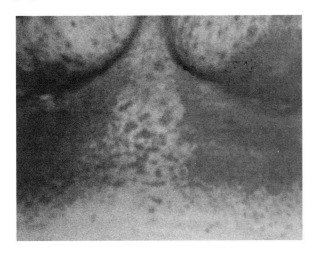

Figure 12 Inframammary candidal intertrigo
(Adapted from *Fitzpatrick's Dermatology in General Medicine*, 8th Ed.)

- **Sporotrichosis** is caused by *Sporothrix schenckii*, a dimorphic fungus found in soil or vegetation. This condition initially presents with a papule at site of inoculation, followed by the formation of nodular lesions dispersed along the lymphatic pathway from distal to proximal extremity (described as nodular lymphangitis).

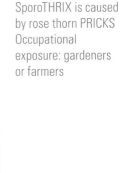

SporoTHRIX is caused by rose thorn PRICKS Occupational exposure: gardeners or farmers

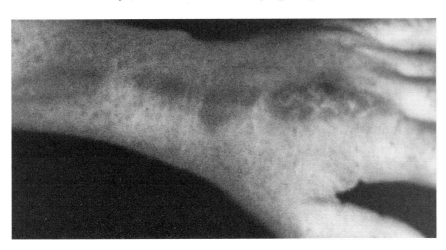

Figure 13 Nodular lymphangitis due to sporotrichosis
(Adapted from *Fitzpatrick's Color Atlas & Synopsis of Clinical Dermatology*, 6th Ed.)

Viral

- **Warts** are extremely common skin lesions in children and adults and are caused by Human Papilloma Virus. **Common warts** (also known as verruca vulgaris) are painless papules and nodules typically found on hands and fingers. **Plantar warts** have a thick scale that when scraped off reveal central black dots (signifying thrombosed blood vessels) and are located on soles of feet and toes. Anogenital warts begin as small papules that may progress to large outwardly growing lesions.

- **Herpes Simplex** is an infection characterized by vesicular skin lesions due to herpes simplex virus Type 1 (orofacial lesions) and Type 2 (genital lesions). Initial orofacial herpes infection is intensely painful and characterized by herpetic gingivostomatitis, while reactivation lesions are typically milder. Genital infections have mild reactivation lesions preceded by prodromal symptoms of burning, pruritis, and pain.

- **Molluscum contagiosum (poxvirus)** is an extremely contagious rash that is most commonly spread by auto-inoculation. The rash is characterized by flesh colored papules with central umbilication. While this condition is considered a sexually transmitted disease in adults, it is non-sexually transmitted in children.

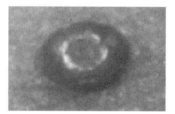

Figure 14 Molluscum contagiosum
(Adapted from *CURRENT Medical Diagnosis & Treatment*)

- **Varicella** (or **chickenpox**) is a common childhood illness caused by primary infection with varicella zoster virus. Beginning with a prodrome of fever and malaise, within 24 hours patients develop a pruritic maculopapular rash that proceeds to vesicle formation with a characteristic "dew drop on rose petal" appearance. At any time the rash will demonstrate lesions of different stages of healing.

- **Herpes zoster** (or **shingles**) is a common disease of adults that is caused by reactivation of the varicella zoster virus. Preceded by symptoms of localized pain and pruritis, patients soon develop an intensely painful unilateral vesicular rash in a dermatomal distribution. After resolution of the rash, patients commonly experience lingering localized pain (postherpatic neuralgia).

Herpetic whitlow
= fingertip vesicles and pustules due to direct skin inoculation from orofacial HSV-1 lesions

Typical patient = dentist/dental assistant

MOLLUSCum typically has a **PEARL**y papule
Umbilication = area of central depression

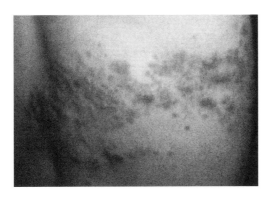

Figure 15 Herpes zoster lesion
(Adapted from *The Color Atlas of Family Medicine*)

- **Measles (Rubeola)**, caused by the measles virus, was once a common childhood illness that has become less common due to the invention of the MMR vaccine. This illness is characterized by an erythematous, maculopapular rash that begins on the head and moves caudally. Other presenting symptoms include cough, coryza, conjunctivitis and Koplik spots (small white spots on buccal mucosa).

- **Rubella (German Measles)**, caused by the Rubella virus, is another increasingly less common childhood illness due to the MMR vaccine. Similar to measles, rubella is characterized by a erythematous maculopapular rash with a cephalocaudal progression. Other distinguishing symptoms include upper respiratory symptoms and cervical/posterior auricular lymphadenopathy.

- **Roseola** is a common childhood illness caused by human herpesvirus 6. This illness is characterized by high fever that may be accompanied by febrile seizures that resolves in three to five days coinciding with the onset of a maculopapular rash.

- **Erythema infectiosum (or exanthem subitum)** is a common childhood illness caused by parvovirus B19. The classic presentation involves an erythematous facial rash with a characteristic "slapped cheek" appearance. This rash then spreads to the extremities with a reticular appearance.

Measles = 3 C's
(cough, coryza, conjunctivitis)

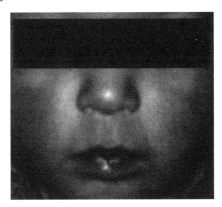

Figure 16 Fifth disease
(Adapted from *The Color Atlas of Family Medicine*)

- **Hand, foot, mouth disease** is a common childhood illness most often caused by coxsackie A virus. This illness manifests with a prodrome of fever, anorexia, and pain progressing to the development of oral ulcers as well as a vesicular rash localized to the palms, soles, and buttocks.

Parasitic

- **Scabies** is a skin infestation by the mite Sarcoptes scabei, often associated with crowded living conditions. The typical rash is characterized intensely pruritic papules and plaques that are most prominent in the web space between fingers, wrists, elbows, genitalia, and female areolae. Accompanying the rash may be significant excoriations as well as a burrow (a linear lesion which signifies the tunneling of the mite in the skin), which is pathognomic for scabies. Treatment includes topical permethrin cream or oral ivermectin.

- **Chigger** infestations are caused by the larvae of the mite Trombiculidae. These mites may be recognized as small red bugs on skin and cause intensely pruritic papulovesicular rash typically localized to an area of skin covered by tight fitting clothing, such as the elastic band of socks.

- **Lice** infestations are caused by pediculosis humanus capitis (scalp) or pediculosis humanus corporis (body) or Phthirus pubis (pubic hair). Lice infestation should be suspected when patients develop severe pruritis after sharing fomites (haircombs or clothing), living in crowded conditions or risky sexual behavior. This diagnosis is confirmed after visualizing lice or nits (lice eggs) within hair or clothing.

- **Hookworm** is caused by Ancylosotoma braziliense and typically occurs after contact with sand or soil that has been contaminated by dog feces. An initial papule forms at the site of larva penetration, with subsequent characteristic pruritic red/brown tortuous skin lesions on feet, legs, and buttocks. Treatment includes oral ivermectin or albendazole.

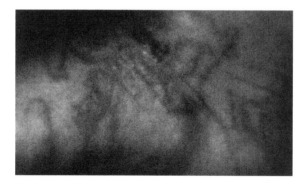

Figure 17 Hookworm
(Adapted from *The Color Atlas of Family Medicine*)

Hypersensitivity Reactions

Erythema Multiforme

Erythema multiforme is an acute, self-limited skin condition characterized by bulls-eye-shaped lesions that represents a spectrum of inflammatory skin eruptions. This skin eruption may be triggered by infectious agents (such as Herpes simplex virus, M. pneumoniae, Histoplasma, Borrelia, etc.) or medications (such as NSAIDs, penicillins, sulfa drugs or anti-epileptics).

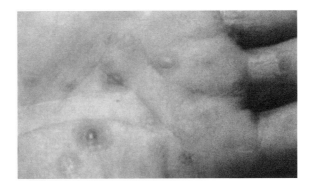

Figure 18 Erythema multiforme
(Adapted from *Lichtman's Atlas of Hematology*)

Signs and Symptoms

- **Erythema multiforme minor** represents localized skin lesions described by erythematous bulls-eye-shaped lesions with central pallor or bulla.

- **Erythema major** represents more diffuse skin lesions with systemic symptoms.

- **Stevens-Johnson syndrome** represents a more severe inflammatory reaction affecting the skin, as well as the mucous membranes. Stevens-Johnson Syndrome usually occurs as a reaction to medications. This syndrome begins with a prodrome of systemic symptoms followed by an erythematous rash with bulla formation involving less than 10% of body surface area.

- **Toxic epidermal necrolysis** is a more severe variant of Stevens-Johnson Syndrome with widespread rash and blister formation involving greater than 30% of body surface area. This condition has an increased mortality risk due to sepsis and shock.

Diagnosis

History and physical exam

Histology

Interface dermatitis (vacuoles at dermo-epidermal junction)

Treatment

Hospitalization and supportive treatment

Inflammatory

Acne Vulgaris

Acne vulgaris is a multi-factorial skin disorder with an increased prevalence amongst adolescence. The pathogenesis involves formation of comedones (cyst formation due to blocked follicles), proliferation of *Propionibacterium acnes*, androgen stimulation of sebaceous glands, and inflammation. While the condition is self-limited, significant lesions may leave behind permanent scars.

SIGNS AND SYMPTOMS

Closed (whitehead) or open (blackhead) comedones, erythematous papules, pustules or nodules located on face, back or chest

DIAGNOSIS

History and physical exam, rule out suspected hyperandrogenism (e.g., congenital adrenal hyperplasia or polycystic ovarian syndrome)

TREATMENT

Treatment aims to counteract each of the four main factors (individually or combined) involved in pathogenesis. First line treatment is with a topical benzoyl peroxide, which exerts its therapeutic effects as a powerful antimicrobial and anti-inflammatory agent.

1. Comedones—topical retinoic acid, systemic isotretinoin

2. *P. acnes*—topical benzoyl peroxide, systemic or topical antibiotics (clindamycin or erythromycin)

3. Androgen stimulation of sebaceous glands—systemic isoretinoin, oral contraceptives, spironolactone (anti-androgen)

4. Inflammation—corticosteroid (short term), topical benzoyl peroxide, topical retinoic acid

Rosacea

Rosacea is a chronic skin condition with a wide spectrum of presentations representing inflammation, dysfunctional sebaceous glands and telangiectasia formation over the face. While rosacea is of unknown etiology, it is considered to be a hereditary skin condition with known triggers including alcohol, certain foods, and sun exposure.

Facial erythema: SLE spares nasolabial folds, rosacea includes nasolabial folds

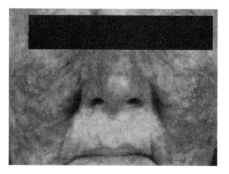

Figure 19 Papulopustular rosacea
(Adapted from *Fitzpatrick's Color Atlas & Synopsis of Clinical Dermatology*, 6th Ed.)

SIGNS AND SYMPTOMS

- **Erythemotelangiectic**—central facial erythema and telangiectasia formation

- **Papulopustular**—more severe facial flushing with formation of papules or pustules on face

- **Phymatous**—disfiguring plaques to nose, forehead or chin due to hypertrophy of sebaceous glands

- **Ocular**—periorbital skin lesions with ocular symptoms (foreign body sensation, vision changes, burning or pain)

Diagnosis

History and physical exam

Treatment

Topical metronidazole or azelaic acid (mild disease), oral antibiotics or oral isoretinoin (moderate disease), laser therapy (severe disease)

Hidradenitis suppurativa

Hidradenitis suppuritiva is a chronic inflammatory condition of apocrine glands in skin of axillae, scalp, and genital regions. This condition presents with tender erythematous nodules or abscesses that may form purulent draining sinus tracts and scar formation with possible secondary bacterial infection. Symptoms may range from mild to severe with complications (such as fistula formation). Therefore, patients may be treated with antibiotics (local or systemic), corticosteroids or may even require surgical management.

Psoriasis

Psoriasis is a chronic inflammatory skin disease represented by a complex interplay between immune system dysfunction with T-cell activation and epidermal hyperplasia. While various triggers have been identified to aggravate psoriasis, psoriasis is considered to predominantly be a genetic condition.

Auspitz sign = pinpoint bleeding seen when scale is removed

Koebner phenomenon = trauma induces the formation of linear lesions

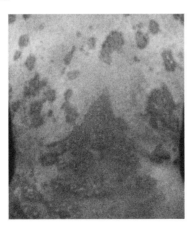

Figure 20 Psoriasis
(Adapted from *Fitzpatrick's Dermatology in General Medicine*, 8th Ed.)

SIGNS AND SYMPTOMS

Characteristic lesion is an asymptomatic erythematous plaque with a silvery scale, + Auspitz sign, + Koebner phenomenon

- **Plaque psoriasis:** intermediate to large size psoriatic plaques symmetrically distributed on elbows, knees, scalp, back, buttocks, and ear

- **Guttate psoriasis:** multiple small plaques (< 1 cm diameter)

- **Psoriatic arthritis:** seronegative spondyloarthritis with nail involvement (nail pitting, nail crumbling, beau lines)

DIAGNOSIS

History and physical exam

HISTOLOGY

Psoriasiform pattern (inflammatory infiltration and epidermal thickening)

TREATMENT

Topical corticosteroids, topical vitamin D analogs, topical coal tar, phototherapy (UVA + psoralen, UVB), systemic immunosuppressants (methotrexate, sulfasalazine), biologic modifying agents (TNF-alpha antagonists such as adalimumab)

Contact Dermatitis

Contact dermatitis is a skin condition that appears after exposure to a certain substance. Common substances that induce contact dermatitis include nickel in jewelry, laundry detergents, fragrances, latex products, poison ivy and poison oak. Timing of exposure as well as pattern of the rash gives a clue to the diagnosis of contact dermatitis.

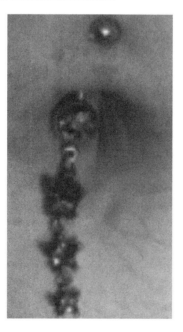

Figure 21 Contact dermatitis
(Adapted from *The Color Atlas of Family Medicine*)

SIGNS AND SYMPTOMS

- **Allergic contact dermatitis** occurs when the skin is exposed to a certain antigen (such as poison ivy) that produces a Type IV hypersensitivity reaction. Patients present with a pruritic erythematous rash.

- **Irritant contact dermatitis** occurs when the skin is exposed to an irritant (chemical or physical) that stimulates an inflammatory reaction. Patients present with skin redness, dryness and peeling.

DIAGNOSIS

History and physical exam, patch testing of allergens

TREATMENT

Avoid known triggers, topical corticosteroids or moisturizers (mild/moderate), systemic corticosteroids or antihistamines (moderate/severe)

Atopic Dermatitis (also known as Eczema)

Atopic dermatitis is a chronic inflammatory skin disease due to a complex interplay of environmental, immune, and genetic factors as well as dysfunction of the epidermal role as physical barrier. Atopic dermatitis is associated with other atopic disorders (such as allergic rhinitis and asthma). Patients typically complain of pruritis resulting in excoriations and exacerbations of the initial rash.

SIGNS AND SYMPTOMS

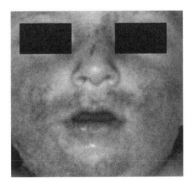

Figure 22 Atopic Dermatitis
(Adapted from *Fitzpatrick's Color Atlas & Synopsis of Clinical Dermatology*, 6th Ed.)

- Acute—erythematous papules or plaques typically located on face and extensor surface of limbs in children and flexor surface of limbs in adults, lesions are associated with edema and secondary infections

- Chronic—chronic scratching and rubbing of lesions leads to lichenification

DIAGNOSIS

History and physical exam

Lichenification = skin thickening with exaggeration of skin creases (leathery appearance)

Spongiotic pattern (inflammatory infiltrate and intercellular edema)

TREATMENT

Topical moisturizing lotions, topical corticosteroids, antihistamines, allergen avoidance, phototherapy

Lichen Planus

Lichen planus is an inflammatory skin condition that is characterized by the development of pruritic, violet papules most notable on the flexor surface of arms and wrists. Although considered to be of unknown etiology, lichen planus has been hypothesized to be associated with heptatitis C virus.

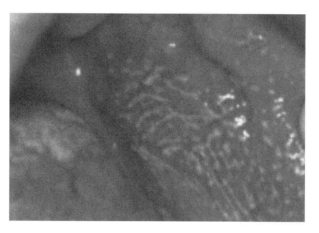

Figure 23 Wickham's striae in lichen planus
(Adapted from *Fitzpatrick's Dermatology in General Medicine*, 8th Ed.)

SIGNS AND SYMPTOMS

Intensely pruritic, violet-hued, papules on skin and oral mucosa, Wickhams striae (lace-like white lesion) overlaying skin and buccal mucosa lesions, + Koebner phenomenon, alopecia

DIAGNOSIS

History and physical exam

HISTOLOGY

Interface dermatitis (band-like inflammatory infiltrate and irregular epidermal hyperplasia)

TREATMENT

No consensus on appropriate treatments

Pityriasis Rosea

Pityriasis Rosea is an acute, self limited skin condition that is characterized by prodrome symptoms followed by the development of a characteristic truncal rash. While the exact etiology is unkown, pityriasis rosea has been hypothesized to be associated with HHV-7 infection.

Begins as a pink patch with thin scale on trunk followed by development of erythematous rash in a "Christmas tree" distribution on trunk

DIAGNOSIS

History and physical exam

TREATMENT

None (rash typically resolves within two months), topical corticosteroid to relieve pruritis

Pigmentation Disorders

Hypo

- **Albinism** is a deficiency of tyrosinase or defective tyrosinase transport leading to deficient or absent melanin production with resultant diffuse hypopigmentation.

- **Vitiligo** is an autoimmune destruction of melanocytes resulting localized patches of hypopigmentation.

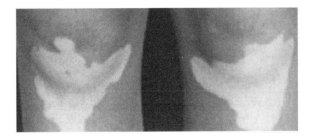

Figure 24 Vitiligo
(Adapted from *Fitzpatrick's Color Atlas & Synopsis of Clinical Dermatology*, 6th Ed.)

- **Piebaldism** is an autosomal dominant defect in embryologic differentiation or migration of melanocyte precursor cells from neural crest cells. Clinical features include white forelock (depigmented white patch of hair), areas with hypopigmented and normally pigmented macules.

- **Leukoderma** is typically a drug, chemical (e.g., liquid nitrogen) or disease (e.g., psoriasis, discoid lupus erythematous) induced destruction of melanocytes resulting in a localized severe hypopigmentation.

Hyper

- **Melasma** is localized hyperpigmentation of facial skin associated with increased levels of estrogen (pregnancy, hormone replacement therapy or oral contraceptives).

- **Ephelides** (freckles) are hyperpigmented brown macules that appear in childhood and increase with sun exposure.

- **Nevocellular Nevi** (moles) are hyperpigmented neoplastic proliferation of melanocytes that may be congenital or acquired.

- **Solar lentigo** is a hyperpigmented (light brown to black) macule located on sun-exposed skin that is acquired during adulthood due to ultraviolet radiation exposure.

- **Acanthosis nigricans** are thick brown lesions with a velvety appearance located on neck or intertriginous folds that are associated with hyperinsulinemia.

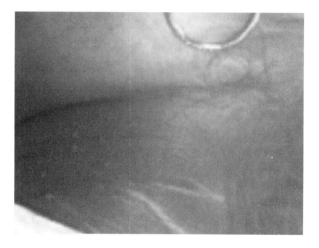

Figure 25 Acanthosis nigricans
(Adapted from *The Color Atlas of Family Medicine*)

Neurocutaneous Disease

Neurofibromatosis Type I

Neurofibromatosis is an autosomal dominant disorder of tumor suppression characterized by neurofibromas of the skin and the nervous system.

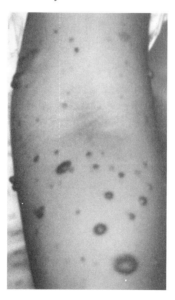

Figure 26 Neurofibromas in neurofibromatosis type I
(Adapted from *Fitzpatrick's Dermatology in General Medicine*, 8th Ed.)

Skin findings: Café-au-lait spots, neurofibromas

Sturge-Weber Syndrome

Sturge-Weber syndrome is a congenital disorder characterized by seizures, ocular abnormalities and facial capillary malformation with underlying leptomeningeal angiodysplasia.

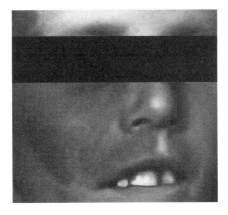

Figure 27 Port wine stain in Sturge-Weber syndrome
(Adapted from *Fitzpatrick's Color Atlas & Synopsis of Clinical Dermatology* , 6th Ed.)

Skin findings: unilateral port wine stain (nevus flammeus) in the distribution of the ophthalmic branch of the trigeminal nerve

Tuberous Sclerosis

Tuberous Sclerosis is an autosomal dominant disorder of tumor suppression characterized by seizures, progressive mental retardation, retinal hamartomas, renal angiomyolipomas, benign cardiac rhabdomyomas, and cutaneous manifestations.

Skin findings: Shagreen patches, hypopigmented "ash-leaf" lesions, adenoma sebaceum

Von Hippel Lindau Disease

Von Hippel Lindau Disease is an autosomal dominant disorder of tumor suppression characterized by cerebellar hemangioblastomas, retinal hemangioblastoma, renal cysts, and an increased propensity to develop renal carcinoma.

Skin findings: Cavernous hemangiomas of the skin

Immunocompromised Patients

- **Bacillary angiomatosis,** caused by Bartonella henselae, is a benign proliferative vascular disorder characterized by tan or dark proliferative masses on skin or organs.

- **Kaposi's sarcoma,** associated with HIV and Human Herpesvirus-8, is a common HIV-related malignancy that appears as reddish-purple nodules on skin or mucosa.

- **Oral candidiasis (thrush),** caused by the fungus *Candida albicans*, is a whitish plaque located on midline tongue, palate or gingivae that scrapes off.

- **Hairy leukoplakia,** caused by Epstein-Barr virus, is a whitish plaque located on the lateral tongue that does not scrape off.

Environmental

Since the skin acts as a physical barrier to the environment, skin is extremely vulnerable to trauma.

Wound Healing

When skin trauma occurs, various cells react immediately to perform the vital role of wound healing. The first step in wound healing involves vasoconstriction, platelet aggregation, and the coagulation cascade in order to diminish immediate blood loss. Following hemostasis, mast cells release chemotactic factors that recruit monocytes, macrophages and neutrophils to the wound site where they engage in wound debridement and signal epithelial cell migration. Tissue matrix metalloproteinases allow for the migration of epithelial cells to site of wound healing. The keratinocytes and other epithelial cells begin to replace the epidermal layers, fibroblasts produce the underlying connective tissue and vascular endothelial cells stimulate angiogenesis. Additionally myofibroblasts are recruited to contract the wound, allowing for wound closure. Over the following months, the scar tissue undergoes remodeling in order to regain tensile strength. Medical conditions, such as peripheral arterial disease and diabetes, and certain environmental exposures, such as tobacco use or malnutrition, may cause impaired wound healing.

Abuse

Physicians must always be aware of signs of abuse when evaluating skin trauma in children and the elderly. Bruising that occurs in certain patterns, such as in the shape of a belt buckle or hand print, should raise a red flag for possible abuse. Additionally, bruising that occurs on certain anatomical regions, such as areas typically covered by clothing, or are incompatible with age such as lower extremity bruises in a non mobile child may indicate abuse. Child abuse may also present as burns, especially if burns occur in cigarette burn pattern or a hot water burn with the absence of splash marks. If patients give a history of trauma that is inconsistent with the signs observed on physical exam, it should raise suspicion for abuse. Any form of child abuse is required by law to be reported to the authorities. Any elder suspected of abuse should be interviewed without the caregiver present.

Burns

Burn injuries are a common cause of skin trauma and may be due to chemical, radiation, electrical or thermal causes. Burns are classified by the degree of skin depth involved. Deeper burns, increased body surface area involved and sensitive anatomic locations (face, hands/feet, genitalia) indicate a worse prognosis.

- **First degree (superficial thickness)** burns involve injury to the epidermis only and demonstrate a tender, dry erythematous area.

- **Second degree (partial thickness)** burns involve injury to the epidermis as well as part of the dermis and demonstrate a tender, red area of skin with blister formation.

- **Third degree (full thickness)** burns involve injury to the entire depth of the dermis with or without injury to underlying deep tissues. Since the dermis contains blood vessels as well as free nerve endings, third degree burns are painless and appear pale or charred.

Complications of burn injuries include secondary infection (Pseudomonas aeruginosa), compartment syndrome with circumferential burns, hypotensive shock and multisystem organ failure. Mild burns may be treated on an outpatient basis with topical silver sulfadiazine or bacitracin, while severe second or third degree burns often require hospitalization with adequate fluid resuscitation and skin grafts.

Cold Injury

Similar to a burn injury, exposure to severe cold temperatures may cause cutaneous damage.

- **Chilblain (pernio)** is a nonfreezing injury caused by inflammation of blood vessels in the skin that may persist as a chronic condition. Like other cutaneous vasculitides, the injured areas are characterized by tender or red-purple lesions that may ulcerate or blister.

- **Cold panniculitis** is a cold injury to subcutaneous adipose tissue resulting in tender erythematous nodules that typically appear on face or lower extremities.

- **Trench foot (immersion injury)** occurs when patients are exposed to wet environments for extended periods of time (e.g., military officers walking in a river). Initially presenting as only a tender erythematous or swollen foot, the injured area progresses to liquifactive necrosis after days of prolonged exposure.

- **Frostnip** is a mild cold injury, demonstrating painful or numb pale skin on apical areas (such as nose or ears) that returns to normal with re-warming.

- **Frostbite** occurs when tissues become frozen resulting in ischemia and eventually tissue necrosis. Frostbite is classified by depth of tissue destruction with clinical symptoms ranging from erythema and blisters to dry gangrenous necrosis requiring amputation.

Any patients presenting with concern for localized cold injury require initial rapid rewarming in water.

frostNIP = small
frostBITE

Decubitus Ulcers

Decubitus ulcers are erosive lesions that develop over areas subject to increased pressure, typically in immobile patients who are unable to change positions frequently. When the skin is exposed to increased pressure for long periods of time, inadequate circulation and localized ischemic necrosis results. Inability to maintain a dry environment, such as with fecal or urinary incontinence, further contributes to maceration of the skin and ulcer development. Decubitus ulcers are classified based on clinical features and depth involved. They may be complicated by secondary local infection, bacteremia, osteomyelitis, fistula formation, sinus tract formation, malignant transformation (Marjolin's ulcer) or death.

Ultraviolet Light Radiation

Ultraviolet radiation in sunlight exists in three main forms classified by diminishing wavelengths: UVA, UVB, and UVC. UVA and UVB both penetrate the skin, while UVC is absorbed by the atmospheric ozone layer. When the skin is exposed to ultraviolet radiation, the energy (photons) may be reflected, transmitted to underlying structures or absorbed by chromophores. Chromophores, such as melanin, absorb photons and initiate biochemical changes. Acute UV exposure may result in the biologic response of sunburn, due to inflammation resulting from acute injury. Another biologic response to acute insult due to UV exposure is tanning, which is due to increased production and distribution of melanin in the epidermis. One beneficial effect of acute UV exposure is Vitamin D3 synthesis. Chronic exposure to ultraviolet radiation, causes photoaging and DNA damage which contribute to the development of benign and malignant neoplasms. Sunscreens are used to protect against the ultraviolet radiation by chemical (PABA derivatives) or physical barriers (zinc oxide). PABA sunscreen derivatives absorb UV and provide protection against UVB only, while zinc oxide reflects UV and protects against all UV and visible light.

Aging

As patients age, the skin undergoes histologic and clinical changes resulting from intrinsic factors and extrinsic stress. Intrinsic factors include thinning of the epidermal layers, a decrease in the number of Langerhans cells and melanocytes, decreased efficiency of sebum and sweat production, increased fragility of blood vessels, and degradation of elastic fibers. Extrinsic environmental stresses increase the susceptibility of the skin to the effects of aging, such as ultraviolet radiation, chronic friction forces, and smoking. Furthermore, aging of the immune system also contributes to skin aging by increasing susceptibility to the development of benign neoplasms (e.g., seborrheic keratoses) and skin cancer.

NEOPLASMS

Benign

Seborrheic Keratoses

Seborrheic keratoses are benign epidermal growths due to hyperproliferation of keratinocytes and melanocytes. These pigmented lesions increase with age and are common in the elderly. Although these growths are considered benign, sudden development of multiple lesions may be associated with an underlying malignancy (known as the sign of Leser-Trélat).

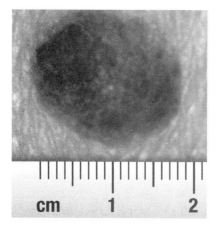

Figure 28 Seborrheic keratosis
(Adapted from *Fitzpatrick's Dermatology in General Medicine*, 8th Ed.)

SIGNS AND SYMPTOMS

Well-demarcated lesion with variable pigmentation (tan, brown, pink) that appears to be "stuck" onto the skin

DIAGNOSIS

History and physical exam, skin biopsy (if malignancy is suspected)

TREATMENT

Curettage, cryotherapy, laser therapy

Nevocellular Nevi (Moles)

Nevocellular nevi are benign neoplastic proliferation of melanocytes that may be congenital or acquired.

- **Congenital nevi** are large hyperpigmented lesions that present at birth that may become darker and hairier over time. Larger congenital nevi are associated with an increased lifetime risk of melanoma.

- **Acquired nevi** are smaller hyperpigmented nevi that develop in infancy or childhood. Development of extensive acquired nevi is associated with increased lifetime risk of melanoma.

- **Blue nevi** are blue-gray dome-shaped papules that may be mistaken for melanoma.

- **Spitz nevi** are pink-brown dome-shaped papules.

- **Halo nevi** are hyperpigmented macules circumscribed by a ring of depigmentation.

- **Dysplastic nevi** are acquired nevi that have ill-defined borders and irregularities in pigmentation. These nevi are associated with sun exposure and may precede the development of malignant melanoma.

Malignant

All cancers are staged by the size of the tumor, the number of nodes involved and the presence of distant metastases (TNM staging).

Basal Cell Carcinoma

Basal cell carcinoma (BCC) of the skin is an epithelial cell cancer due to the malignant proliferation of the deep basal cells of the epidermis. BCC is the most common cause of skin cancer, as well as the most common cancer overall. Risk factors associated with the development of basal cell carcinoma include fair complexion, cumulative sunlight exposure, ionizing radiation (X-rays), immunosuppression, and certain hereditary conditions (such as familial basal cell nevus syndrome). While the incidence of BCC is extremely high, the mortality rate is extremely low because it is locally invasive and rarely metastasizes.

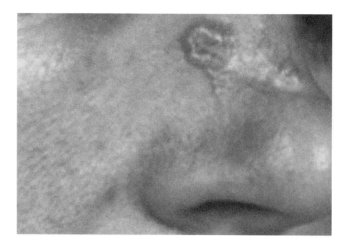

Figure 29 Basal cell carcinoma
(Adapted from *Fitzpatrick's Color Atlas & Synopsis of Clinical Dermatology*, 6th Ed.)

Signs and Symptoms

Shiny papule with raised edges located on sun-exposed skin of the head and neck (especially nose and periocular skin), may have telangiectasias or central ulceration

Diagnosis

Shave biopsy, excisional or punch biopsy if suspicious for malignant melanoma or a recurrent lesion

Histopathology

Cells with large blue nuclei (similar to basal layer of epidermis) form palisading pattern along tumor periphery, increased nuclus-to-cytoplasmic ratio

Treatment

Surgical excision (Mohs surgery), topical 5-fluorouracil or topical imiquimod for small and superficial lesions, radiation therapy for advanced and nonsurgical lesions

Squamous Cell Carcinoma

Squamous cell carcinoma of the skin is an epithelial cell cancer due to malignant proliferation of the superficial keratinocytes in the epidermis. Risk factors associated with the development of squamous cell carcinoma include fair complexion, cumulative sunlight exposure, chronic inflammation or irritation (e.g., Marjolin's ulcer), immunosuppression, xeroderma pigmentosum, tobacco and alcohol use, and exposure to certain chemicals (e.g., arsenic). Prior to developing squamous cell carcinoma, patients may present with **actinic keratoses** or a persistent non-healing wound. Unlike basal cell carcinoma, squamous cell carcinoma has a more significant risk of invasion and metastasis.

Actinic keratosis = pre-malignant lesion with a rough texture; associated with sun exposure

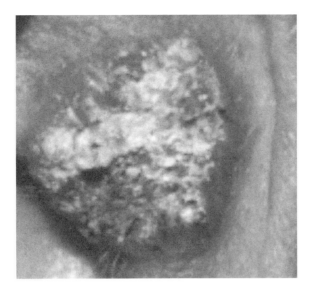

Figure 30 Squamous cell carcinoma
(Adapted from *Fitzpatrick's Color Atlas & Synopsis of Clinical Dermatology*, 6th Ed.)

Signs and Symptoms

Erythematous ulcerated lesion located on hands or face (especially vermillion border of lip, external ear, forehead and scalp), may be associated with a scale. **Keratoacanthoma** is a subtype of squamous cell cancer that is characterized by rapid growth of a dome shaped nodule with central ulceration or hyperkeratosis.

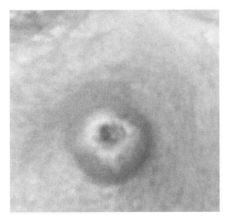

Figure 31 Keratoacanthoma
(Adapted from *Fitzpatrick's Color Atlas & Synopsis of Clinical Dermatology*, 6th Ed.)

Diagnosis

Excisional biopsy (full thickness), punch biopsy, or incisional biopsy (if smaller lesion or on cosmetically undesirable location)

Histopathology

Keratin "pearls", mitoses, increased nucleus-to-cytoplasmic ratio, abnormal keratinocytes in the dermis

TREATMENT

Topical 5-fluorouracil and imiquimod for noninvasive disease and actinic keratosis, surgical excision (Mohs surgery)

Malignant Melanoma

Malignant melanoma is neoplastic proliferation of melanocytes that predominantly affects sun exposed skin or mucosal membranes. Although melanoma is one of the less common causes of skin cancer, incidence has been increasing over the past century. Additionally melanoma has a significantly high mortality rate due to its predilection for distant metastases. Risk factors associated with the development of malignant melanoma include fair complexion, intense episodic sunlight exposure, phototherapy (such as psoralen + UVA for psoriasis), personal or family history of melanoma, immunosuppression, and dysplastic nevi. Melanoma demonstrates radial growth (increased diameter), followed by a vertical growth phase (increased depth). The most important prognostic factor is depth of invasion (the Breslow depth). There are various subtypes of malignant melanoma delineated by pattern of growth as well as clinical features.

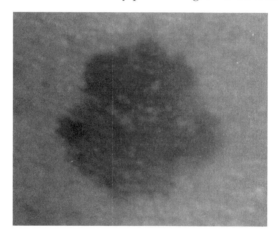

Figure 32 Malignant melanoma
(Adapted from *The Atlas of Emergency Medicine*, 3rd Ed.)

SIGNS AND SYMPTOMS

- **Superficial spreading melanoma**, the most common variant of malignant melanoma, typically presents as irregular pigmented lesions on unexposed skin (most commonly the upper back and lower extremities).

- **Nodular melanoma** is an aggressive variant of melanoma, characterized by pigmented nodules that may ulcerate. Since this variant lacks a radial growth phase, these lesions typically have a significant depth of invasion before identified.

- **Lentigo maligna melanoma** lesions have a long period of radial growth and are characterized by pigmented macules on the extremities.

- **Acral lentiginous melanoma** is the most common subtype of melanoma in African American patients. This form of melanoma typically presents with pigmented lesions on palms, soles or subungual (Hutchinson's sign).

DIAGNOSIS

ABCDE (Asymmetry, Border, Color, Diameter, Evolution) clinical features of lesion, dermoscopy (magnification of lesion to evaluate for suspected malignancy prior to biopsy), excisional skin biopsy with 1-2 mm margins

HISTOPATHOLOGY

Atypical melanocytes, increased nucleus-to-cytoplasmic ratio, mitotic figures

TREATMENT

Surgical excision with sentinel lymph node biopsy (if > 1mm thick and numerous mitotic figures)

Differential Diagnoses

PRURITIS

- Dermatologic Disorders—atopic dermatitis, contact dermatitis, urticaria, dermatophytoses, lichen planus, psoriasis, scabies, lice

- Non-dermatologic Disorders—renal disease (uremia), cholestasis, hematologic malignancy (Hodgkin lymphoma), Polycythemia vera, medications (opiates)

ALOPECIA

- Non-scarring: androgenic baldness, telogen effluvium, alopecia areata, trichotillomania, hyper/hypo-thyroidism, nutritional deficiency (e.g., iron), systemic lupus erythematosus, medications (e.g., chemotherapeutic agents)

- Scarring: trauma, infection (e.g., tinea capitis), discoid lupus erythematosus, scleroderma, lichen planus

PIGMENTATION DISORDER

- Hyperpigmentation: post-inflammatory change, melasma, acanthosis nigricans, nevocellular nevi (congenital, acquired, Spitz, halo, dysplastic), medications (e.g., minocycline), solar lentigo, tinea versicolor, neurofibromatosis

- Hypopigmentation: albinism, vitiligo, piebaldism, tinea versicolor, leukoderma (medication or disease induced), tuberous sclerosis

Photosensitivity

- porphyrias, systemic lupus erythematosus, discoid lupus erythematosus, medications (e.g., sulfonamides), albinism, xeroderma pigmentosum

REFERENCES

Alberts, Bruce et al. *Molecular Biology of the Cell*, 2nd Edition. New York: Garland Publishing, 1989. Print.

Barret Kim E., Barman, Susan M., Boltano, Scott. *Ganong's Review of Medical Physiology*, 24th Edition. New York: McGraw-Hill, 2012. Print.

Barret, Kim E. *Gastrointestinal Physiology*. New York: McGraw-Hill, 2005. Print.

Boron, Walter and Boulpaep, Emile L. *Medical Physiology*, 2nd Edition. Pennsylvania: Saunders, 2011. Print.

Brunton, Lawrence, Lazo, John, and Parker, Keith. *Goodman & Gilman's Pharmacologic Basis of Therapeutics*, 12th Edition. New York: McGraw-Hill Professional, 2010. Print.

CDC. *National Vital Statistics Report*. Volume 60:4. January 11, 2012. Print.

Cross, Patricia C. and Mercer, Lynne K. *Cell and Tissue Ultrastructure: A Functional Perspective*. New York: W.H. Freeman and Company, 1993. Print.

Cunningham F., Leveno Kenneth, Bloom, Steven. *Williams Obstetrics*, 23rd Edition. New York: McGraw-Hill, 2009. Print.

Darnell, James, Lodish, Harvey, and Baltimore David. *Molecular Cell Biology,* 2nd Edition. New York: Scientific American Books, 1990. Print.

Dudek, Ronald W. *High-Yield Gross Anatomy.* Baltimore: Williams & Wilkins, 1997. Print.

Feibusch, Kate C. et al. *Prescription for the Boards: USMLE Step 2*, 1st Edition. Boston: Little, Brown, 1996. Print.

Feldman, Mark, Friedman, Lawrence, and Brandt, Lawrence. Sleisinger and Fordtran's *Gastrointestinal and Liver Disease*, 9th Edition. Pennsylvania: Saunders, 2010. Print.

Goldman, Lee and Schaefer, Andrew. *Goldman's Cecil Medicine*, 24th Edition. Pennsylvania: Elsevier Saunders, 2012. Print.

Goldsmith Lowell, Katz Stephen, and Gilchrest Barbara. *Fitzpatrick's Dermatology in General Medicine*, 8th Edition. New York: McGraw-Hill, 2012. Print.

Hansen, John T. *Netter's Clinical Anatomy,* 2nd Edition. Pennsylvania: Saunders Elsevier, 2009. Print.

Kumar, Vinay et al. *Robbins and Cotran Pathologic Basis of Medicine*, 8th Edition. Pennsylvania: Saunders, 2009. Print.

Katzung, Bertram, G., Masters Susan B., Trevor Anthony J. *Basic & Clinical Pharmacology*, 11th Edition. New York: McGraw-Hill, 2009. Print.

Kauchansky, Kenneth, et al. *Williams Hematology*, 8th Edition. New York: McGraw-Hill Professional, 2010. Print.

Kliegman, Robert M. et al. *Nelson Textbook of Pediatrics*, 19th Edition. Pennsylvania: Saunders, 2011. Print.

Knoop Kevin, Stack Lawrence, and Storrow Alan. *The Atlas of Emergency Medicine*, 3rd Edition. New York: McGraw-Hill, 2010. Print.

LeBlond, Ricard, DeGowin, Ricard, and Brown, Donald. *DeGowin's Diagnostic Examination*, 9th Edition. New York: McGraw-Hill, 2008. Print.

Lichtman Marshall A. *Lichtman's Atlas of Hematology*. New York: McGraw-Hill, 2007. Print.

McPhee, Stephen J., and Hammer, Gary D. *Pathophysiology of Disease: An Introduction to Clinical Medicine*. New York: McGraw-Hill Medical, 2010. Print.

Mescher Anthony L. Junqueira's *Basic Histology: Text and Atlas*, 12th Edition. New York: McGraw-Hill Education, 2009. Print.

Morton, David, Forman, Bo K., and Albertine Kurt: *Gross Anatomy: The Big Picture*. Ohio: McGraw-Hill, 2010. Print.

Murray, Robert et al. *Harper's Illustrated Biochemistry*, 29th Edition. New York: McGraw-Hill Medical, 2012. Print.

Nelson, David and Cox, Michael. *Lehninger Principles of Biochemistry*, 5th Edition. New York: W. H. Freeman, 2008. Print.

Netter, Frank H. *Atlas of Human Anatomy*. Pennsylvania: Saunders Elsevier, 2006. Print.

Ogilvy-Stuart, A. L. and Brain, C. E. *Early Assessment of Ambiguous Genitalia*. Archives of Disease in Childhood, 2004. Print.

Papadakis Maxine, McPhee Stephen, J., and Rabow Michael W. *Current Medical Diagnosis & Treatment 2013*. New York: McGraw-Hill, 2013. Print.

Schorge John et al. Williams *Gynecology*, 2nd Edition. New York: McGraw-Hill, 2012. Print.

Shannon, Michael W., Borron, Stephen, W., and Burns, Michael. *Haddad and Winchester's Clinical Management of Poisoning and Drug Overdose*, 3rd Edition. Pennsylvania: Saunders, 2011. Print.

Stryer, L. *Biochemistry*, 2nd Edition. San Francisco: W.H. Freeman, 1981. Print.

Townsend, Courtney, M. et al. *Sabiston Textbook of Surgery*, 19th Edition. Pennsylvania: Saunders, 2012. Print.

Usatine, Richard, Smith, Mindy Ann, and Mayeaux, Jr. E. *The Color Atlas of Family Medicine*. New York: McGraw-Hill, 2009. Print.

West, John B. *Respiratory Physiology—The Essentials*, 4th Edition. Baltimore: Williams & Wilkins, 1990. Print.

Wheater, Paul R. and Burkitt, George. *Functional Histology: A Text and Colour Atlas,* Revised Edition. Edinburgh: Churchill Livingstone, 1987. Print.

Wheater, Paul R et al. *Basic Histopathology. A Colour Atlas and Text*, 2nd Edition. Edinburgh: Churchill Livingstone, 1991. Print.

Wilson JD, Griffin IE, Russell DW. *Steroid Sot-reductase 2 Deficiency*. Endocr Rev 1993; 14:77—93. Print.

Wolff, Klaus and Johnson, Richard. *Fitzpatrick's Color Atlas & Synopsis of Clinical Dermatology*. 6th Edition. New York: McGraw-Hill, 2009. Print.

Yanoff, Myron and Duker, Jay S. *Ophthalmology,* 3rd Edition. Missouri: Mosby Elsevier, 2008. Print.

Young, Barbara, Lowe James S., and Stevens, Alan. *Wheater's Functional Histology*, 5th Edition. Pennsylvania: Saunders Elsevier, 2006. Print.

BIOCHEMISTRY

Base Pairing of DNA and organization and condensation of DNA

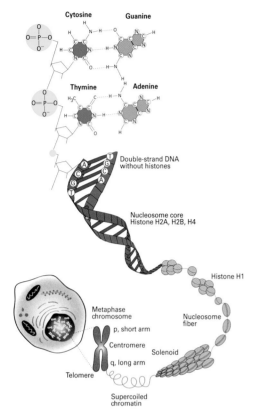

Cytosine Guanine

Thymine Adenine

Double-strand DNA without histones

Nucleosome core
Histone H2A, H2B, H4

Histone H1

Metaphase chromosome
p, short arm
Centromere
q, long arm
Telomere
Solenoid
Supercoiled chromatin
Nucleosome fiber

Osteogenesis Imperfecta	Type I collagen synthesis defect	Easy fractures, blue sclera, hearing loss, abnormal teeth
Alport Syndrome	Type IV collagen synthesis defect	Hematuria, sensorineural deafness, ocular abnormalities
Ehler-Danlos Syndrome	Various	Hyperextendibility, hypermobility, hyperfragility

Table of high yield facts for Glycogen Storage Diseases

Disease	Enzyme Deficient	Metabolic Effects	Results In	Notes
Type I: Von Gierke	Glucose-6-phosphatase	Increased amount of glycogen (normal structure) stored in liver, kidneys	Liver enlargement Severe Hypoglycemia Failure to thrive	Most important example of hepatic glycogenoses Autosomal recessive
Type II: Pompe	Lysosomal α-glucosidase (acid maltase)	Excessive deposition of glycogen (normal structure) in liver, heart, muscle	Massive cardiomegaly Pronounced hypotonia Cardiorespiratory failure often results in death by age 2	Autosomal recessive
Type III: Cori	Amylo- (1:6) glucosidase (debranching enzyme)	Increased glycogen (short outer branches) in muscle and liver	Like type I but milder	Autosomal recessive
Type V: McArdle	Skeletal muscle glycogen phosphorylase	increased amount of glycogen (normal structure) in muscle: cannot be broken down	Painful cramps on strenuous exercise Myoglobinuria	Autosomal recessive

High yield summary of Purine Salvage/Metabolism related diseases

Disease	Enzyme Deficient	Metabolic Effects	Results In	Notes
Gout	Many causes, affecting uric acid metabolism (uric acid is the product of purine degradation)	High uric acid levels in serum (hyperuricemia)	Uric acid crystals in joint, causing arthritis	Treatment: allopurinol, which inhibits xanthine oxidase to lower uric acid production
Lesch Nyhan syndrome	Hypoxanthine-guanine phosphoribosyltransferase (purine salvage)	Accumulation of hypoxanthine and guanine Excess uric acid production because salvage inhibition increases purine metabolism	Self-mutilation and aggression Mental and physical retardation Spastic cerebral palsy	Rare X-linked recessive disease, seen only in males Sometimes gouty arthritis develops
Adenosine deaminase (ADA) deficiency	ADA (purine degradation)	Accumulation of dATP, which inhibits ribonucleotide reductase (and DNA synthesis)	Severe combined immunodeficiency	Presents in neonatal period Children die from infection before age 2 Autosomal recessive

High yield summary of collagen synthesis defects

Disease	Defect	Symptoms
Scurvy	Vitamin C deficiency, cannot hydroxylate proline and lysine	Hemorrhage, bleeding from gums

Metabolism of Homocysteine

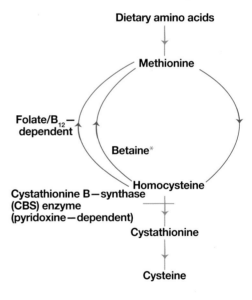

Dietary amino acids

Methionine

Folate/B$_{12}$—dependent

Betaine*

Homocysteine

Cystathionine B—synthase (CBS) enzyme (pyridoxine—dependent)

Cystathionine

Cysteine

High Yield Facts About Amino Acid Disorders

Disease	Enzyme Deficiency	Metabolic Effects	Results in	Notes
Phenylketonuria	Phenylalanine hydroxylase	Cannot convert phenylalanine to tyrosine	Mental retardation, "mousy odor," eczema,	Treatment: low phenylalanine and high tyrosine
Maple Syrup Urine Disease	Branched-chain α-ketoacid dehydrogenase	Cannot degrade branched chain amino acids	Maple syrup urine, mental retardation	Treatment: Avoid branched amino acids

Alkaptonuria	Homogentisate oxidase	Accumulation of homogentisate	Dark urine, dark connective tissue, arthritis	Urine that turns dark upon standing
Albinism	Tyrosinase	Cannot synthesize melanin from tyrosine	Pigmentation deficiency, visual problems, increased skin cancer risk	
Homocystin-uria	Various	Ammulate homo-cysteine	Mental retarda-tion, Marfans + Thrombosis	Treatment: Varies based on mutation
Cystinuria	Amino acid transporter	Excretion of COLA amino acids	Cystine kidney stones	Treatment: Alkanize urine
Canavan Disease	Aspartoacylase	Accumulation of -acetylaspartic acid	Hypotonia, seizures	Higher frequency in Ashkenazi Jews
Hartnup Disease	Neutral amino acid transporter	Tryptophan deficiency	Sun-induced pellagra	Mimics niacin deficiency

Vitamin Deficiencies/Excess

Vitamin	Function	Deficiency/ Excess	Signs/ Symptoms	Associated Conditions
Ai	Involved in synthesis of rhodopsin, bone growth, epithelial cell function	Deficiency	Night blindness, poor bone growth, poor tooth health, hyperkeratosis	Fat soluble vitamin deficiencies
		Excess	Hepatosplenomegaly, alopecia, yellow skin coloration, elevated intracranial pressure (bulging fontanelle, nausea and vomiting)	
B_1: thiamine	Cofactor in various reactions, synthesis of acetylcholine and GABA	Deficiency	Dry beriberi: periph-eral neuropathies, ptosis, muscle atrophy Wet beriberi: conges-tive heart failure, edema Wernicke's Encepha-lopathy: mental status changes, ophthal-moplegia, ataxia	Polished rice diet, alcoholics
B_2: riboflavin	Synthesis of FAD	Deficiency	Cheilosis (scaling and fissure on lips), glossitis (sore, red tongue)	
B_3: niacin	Part of NAD and NADP	Deficiency	Pellagra: 4Ds: dermatitis, diarrhea, dementia, death, "raw beef" swollen tongue	Anorexia, corn-based diet
B_6: Pyridoxine	Amino acid me-tabolism, glycogen metabolism	Deficiency	Peripheral neuritis, cheilosis, glossitis, seborrheic dermatitis	Isoniazid use
B_9: Folic Acid	Carbon transporter in various reactions including purine biosynthesis; needed in times of rapid growth	Deficiency	Megaloblastic anemia, neural tube defects (if low in mom)	Increased utilization (ie hemolytic anemias), decreased absorption (ie celiacs, alcoholics), decreased ability to use (ie convulsants, ethotrexate)

B_{12}: Cobalamin	Methylmalonyl-COA to succinyl-coa, homocysteine to methionine, purine synthesis	Deficiency	Megaloblastic anemia with elevated methylmalonyl-COA, peripheral neuropathy	Vegan diet, Pernicious anemia, Crohn's disease, ileal resection
Biotin	Carboxylase reactions	Deficiency	Alopecia, dermatitis	Raw egg white consumption
C	Hydroxylation of proline and lysine in collagen synthesis	Deficiency	Scurvy: poor wound healing, bleeding gums, petechiae, iron, folate, and B_{12} deficiency	Lack of fruit in diet
D	When converted to 1,25–hydroxyvita-min D: Intestinal ab-sorption of calcium, bone resorption (increases serum calcium)	Deficiency	Rickets (children): bowing of legs Osteomalacia (adults): gait instability, bone pain, muscle weakness Paresthesia, muscle cramping, hypocal-cemia (can lead to seizures), tetany (Chvostek, Troussea sign)	Lack of sunlight, Fat soluble vitamin deficiencies
		Excess	Hypercalcemia: "Stones (kidney stones), bones (bone pain), groans (constipation, nausea, vomiting), psychiatric overtones (confusion, coma)"	
E	Antioxidant	Deficiency	Hemolysis from increased oxidative stress on red blood cells, truncal ataxia, myopathy	Fat soluble vitamin deficiencies
K	Cofactor in synthesis of clotting factors II, VII, IX, X and anticoagulants protein C and S	Deficiency	Hemorrhage, all newborns are given Vitamin K shot to pre-vent hemorrhage	Long term broad spectrum antibiotic use

EPIDEMIOLOGY & BIOSTATISTICS

The Bell Curve

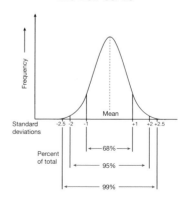

Prevalence is a measure of how many individuals have the diagnosis of a specific disease within a given population.

Incidence measures the rate of diagnosis of a disease within a given population. It is expressed in terms of the number of new cases diagnosed during a specific period of time in a given population. It is important to remember that the period of time needs to be specified in order to calculate incidence. Distinction between prevalence and incidence is a commonly tested question on USMLE, as many confuse the two.

The **sensitivity** of a test refers to how likely the test is to be able to detect if the disease is present:

$$\text{SeNsitivity} = A/(A + C)$$

The **specificity** refers to the test's ability to detect when the disease is absent.

$$\text{Specificity} = D/(B + D)$$

Positive predictive Value (PPV) refers to the likelihood of the patient actually having the disease if the test has a positive result.

$$\text{PPV} = A/(A + B)$$

Negative Predictive Value (NPV) refers to the likelihood of the patient not having the disease if the test has a negative result.

$$\text{NPV} = D/(C + D)$$

	Disease Present	**Disease Absent**
Exposed group	A	B
Unexposed group	C	D

CARDIOLOGY

Fetal Circulation

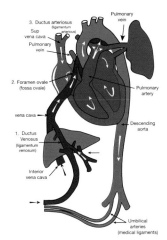

Cardiac Cycle

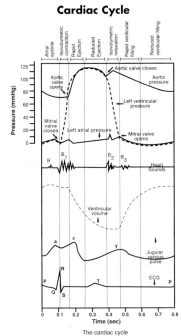

The cardiac cycle

Cardiac Output Graph

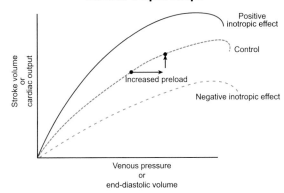

Venous Return Graph

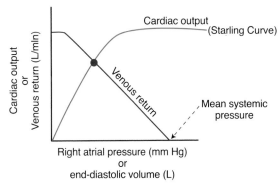

Regulation of Mean Arterial Pressure

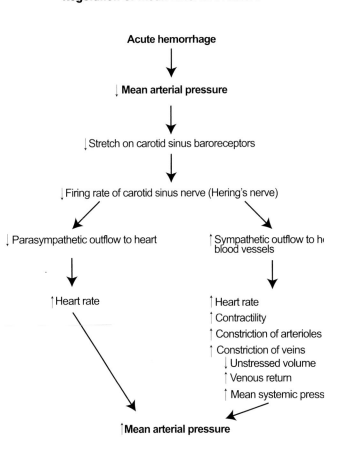

EKG

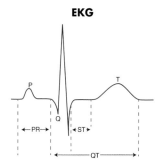

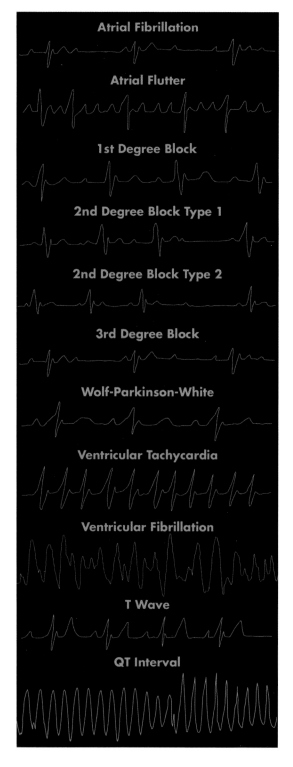

Valvular Abnormalities

Lesion	Symptoms	Signs
Mitral stenosis	Dyspnea, orthopnea, PND	Diastolic rumble Concomitant MR
Mitral regurgitaiton (MR)	Pulmonary edema, fatigue right heart failure (secondary to left heart failure)	Holosystolic blowing murmur at the apex
Mitral prolapse	Chest pain, similar to MR	Midsystolic click, late systolic murmur
Aortic stenosis	Chest pain, syncope, presyncope, LV failure	Harsh systolic crescendo murmur at the right upper sternal border
Aortic regurgitation	LV failure, arrhythmias	High pitched diastolic murmur at the right upper sternal border
Austin-Flint mumur Quincke's	Widened	Pulse pressure; pulses; water-hammer pulse; Duroziez's sign
Tricuspid stenosis	RV failure, lower extremity edema, hepatic congestion	Tricuspid opening snap at the left lower sternal border
Tricuspid regurgitaiton	RV failure, lower extremity edema, hepatic congestion	Large v wave on JVP; blowing systolic murmur at the left lower sternal border

PND- paroxysmal nocturnal dyspnea; LV- left ventricle; RV- right ventricle; JVP- jugular

Calcium Channel Blockers

Drug	Mechanism	Uses	Toxicities
Nifedipine	Class IV	Coronary and peripheral vasodilation, hypertension, Prinzmetal's angina	Hypotension; nausea and vomiting, bradycardia, left ventricular failure
Diltiazem	Class IV	Supraventricular tachyarrhythmias	Same as nifedipine
Verapamil	Class IV	Supraventricular tachyarrhythmias	Same as nifedipine
Long-acting agents: Amlodipine Felodipine	Class IV	Long-term treatment of hypertension	Same as nifedipine

Vasodilators

Drug	Mechanism	Toxicities
Nitroprusside	Similar to nitric oxide; direct smooth muscle relaxant	Hypotension; prolonged use leads to cynanide toxicity
Nitrates Nitroglycerin Isosorbide dinitrate	Similar to nitric oxide; direct smooth muscle relaxant (used for hypotension and angina)	Hypotension
Hydralazine, minoxidil	Direct smooth muscle relaxant	Hypotension
Terazosin	α-antagonist	Orthostatic hypotension, loss of sympathetic tone, synoope
Clonidine	CNS α_1 agonist	Hypotension

Angiotensin-Converting-Enzyme (ACE) Inhibitors

Drug	Mechanism	Toxicities
Nitroprusside	Blocks ACE, disrupting the renin-angiotensin system	Hypotension; prolonged use leads to cynanide toxicity
Losartan	Angiotensin II receptor inhibitor	Vasodilation, decreased venous return; less cough than ACE inhibitors

Classes of Antiarrhythmics

Class	Mechanism	Effects
Class IA	Na⁺ channel blocker	Prolongs the action potential duration
Class IB	Na⁺ channel blocker	Reduces maximum velocity of AP upstrokes
Class IC	Na⁺ channel blocker	Prolongs retractory period
Class II	β-Blockers	Slows conduction through the AV junction
Class III	K⁺ channel blockers	Prolongs action potential
Class IV	Ca⁺² channel blocker	Blocks slow inward current

CELL BIOLOGY

Action Potential

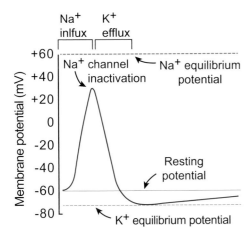

P-450 enzyme interactions

Inducers of P-450 enzymes	Inhibitors of P-450 enzymes
Barbituates	Acute alcohol use
Carbamazepine	Cimetidine
Chronic alcohol use	Erythromycin
Griseofulvin	Grapefruit juice
Phenytoin	HIV protease inhibitors: e.g. Indinavir
Quinidine*	Isoniazid
Rifampin	Ketoconazole
St. John's wort	Sulfonamides

Mnemonic: Inducers		Mnemonic: Inhibitors
Cars and **C**hronic Alcohol use at **B**ars **GR**eatly **ST**ains **P**eople's **Q**uiet **R**eputations	**C**hronic Alcohol **B**arbituates **G**riseofulvin **St.** John's wort **P**henytoin **Q**uinidine **R**ifampin	I'm **SICK** of **AGE**-ing. I wish I could **in**hibit the **Pro**cess. **S**ulfonamides **I**soniazid **C**imetidine **K**etoconazole **A**cute alcohol **G**rapefruit juice **E**rythromycin **P**rotease **in**hibitors (HIV medication)

*Quinidine may also act to inhibit P-450 enzymes, but to a lesser effect.

Lysosomal storage diseases

Lysosomal storage disease	Defective lysosomal enzyme	Accumulated substrate	Characteristics
Sphingolipidoses: accumulation of sphingolipids			
Gaucher's disease* most common -AR	β-glucocere brosidase	Glucocerebroside	Hepatospleno-megaly, bone pain and fractures, Gaucher's cells (macrophages resembling crumpled tissue paper), neuro-dysfunction
Niemann-Pick disease* -AR	Sphingomyelinase phingomyelinase	Sphingomyelin	Cherry-red spot on macula, foam cells (macrophages in liver and spleen), progressive neuro-dysfunction, death usually before age 3
Tay-Sachs disease* -AR	Hexosamindase A	GM2 ganglioside	NO hepatospleno-megaly, cherry-red spot on macula, lysosomes with "onion skin," progressive neuro-dysfunction, developmental delay delaydelayhepatosplenomegaly, cherry-red spot on macula, lysosomes with "onion skin," progressive neuro-dysfunction, developmental delay
Farber disease -AR	Ceramidase	Ceramide	Granulomas and nodules in skin and around joints, neurological deficits
Krabbe's disease -AR	Galactocerebrosidase	Galactocerebroside	Peripheral neuropathy, developmental delay, globoid cells (multinucleated macrophages)
Metochromatic leukodystrophy -AR	Arylsulfatase A	Cerebroside sulfate	Central and peripheral neuropathy (demyelination), dementia, hereditary ataxia
Fabry's disease -XR	α-galactosidase A	Ceramide trihexoside	Peripheral neuropathy, cardiovascular, renal disease, angiokeratomas
Mucopolysacharidoses: accumulation of glycosominoglycans (GAGs)			
Hurler's syndrome -AR	α-L-iduronidase	Heparan sulfate, dermatan sulfate	Clouding of corneas, coarse facies (gargoylism), developmental delay
Hunter's syndrome -XR	Iduronate sulfatase	Heparan sulfate, dermatan sulfate	NO clouding of corneas, developmental delay, coarse facies, aggressive behavior

* = more common in Ashkenazi Jews; AR = autosomal recessive; XR = x-linked recessive

Types of Collagen

Type of Collagen	Associated with	
Type I (Strongest and most common form of collagen—90%)	Bone, Skin, Tendon, Dentin, Fascia, Cornea, Late wound repair	Affected in Osteogenesis Imperfecta

Type II	Cartilage, vitreous body, nucleus pulposus	
Type III (reticulin)	Skin, blood vessels, uterus, fetal tissue, granulation tissue	Affected in Ehlers Danlos
Type IV	Basement membrane: especially of kidneys, ears and eyes	Affected in Alport's syndrome
Elastin	Skin, large arteries, vocal cords and lungs	Affected in Marfan's syndrome Affected in Emphysema

ENDOCRINE SYSTEM

Steroid Synthesis

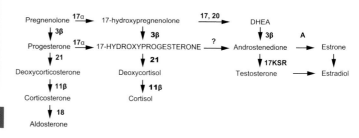

Pituitary Hormones

Anterior Pituitary	Posterior Pituitary
FSH	Oxytocin
LH	Vasopressin (ADH)
GH	
TSH	
Prolactin	
ACTH	
MSH	

MEN Syndrome

Syndrome	Characteristics
MEN 1 (Wermer's syndrome)	Parathyroid adenomas Pancreatic adenomas Pituitary adenomas
MEN 2A (Sipple's syndrome)	Parathyroid adenomas Pheochromocytomas Medullary thyroid carcinoma
MEN 2B	Medullary Thyroid carcinoma Pheochromocytoma Neuromas

Calcium regulation

Effects	Serum Calcium	Serum Phosphate	Bone	Kidney	Intestine	Stimulus for Activity
PTH	Increase	Decrease	Increased resorption	Increased calcium reuptake, decreased phosphate reuptake	Increased calcium update (indirect through Vitamin D)	Decreased serum calcium
Vitamin D	Increase	Increase	Stimulates osteoclasts and osteoblasts; increased resorption in Vitamin D intoxication	Increased calcium reuptake, increased phosphate reuptake	Increased calcium update	Decreased serum calcium, increased PTH, decreased serum phosphate
Calcitonin	Decrease		Decreased resorption			Increased serum calcium

Mineral & Vitamin Deficiencies & Toxicities

Mineral	Deficiency	Toxicity
Calcium (Ca)	Nerve and muscle excitability (cramps, tetany, laryngospasm, convulsions and paresthesias) Chvostek's sign (contraction of facial muscle when facial nerve is tapped) Trousseau's sign (carpal spasm with occlusion of brachial artery with blood pressure cuff)	Polyuria, renal failure, constipation, neurological symptoms
Sodium (Na)	Nausea, headache, seizures, respiratory arrest, encephalopathy	See hyponatremia
Potassium (K)	Muscle weakness, fatigue, cramps, constipation, ileus, flaccid paralysis, tetany, cardiac arrest	Muscle weakness, fatigue, cramps, diarrhea
Iron (Fe)	Microcytic anemia	GI upset, vomiting, acidosis
Phosphorus (P)	Hypocontractility, impaired tissue oxygenation (due to decreased RBC 2,3-DPG), platelet dysfunction, muscle pain, bone fractures	Symptoms related to underlying disorders (hypoparathyroidism, chronic renal failure)
Magnesium (Mg)	Neuromuscular and CNS hyperirritability (cramps, weakness, tremors)	Muscle weakness, neurologic syndromes-cardiac arrest
Zinc (Zn)	Dysgeusia (altered taste), anosmia (altered smell), impaired wound healing, growth retardation	
Fluoride (F)	Tooth decay	Tooth mottling
Iodine (I)	Goiter, cretinism	

Adrenal Gland

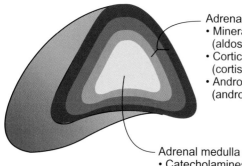

Adrenal cortex
- Mineralocorticoids (aldosterone)
- Corticosteroids (cortisol)
- Androgens (androstenedione)

Adrenal medulla
- Catecholamines (epinephrine)

GASTROINTESTINAL SYSTEM

Histological Features of the Gastrointestinal Tract

Location	Histologic Features
Esophagus	Mucosa is comprised of nonkeratinized stratified squamous epithelium Upper 1/3 is composed of skeletal muscle only Middle 1/3 is composed of both skeletal and smooth muscle Last 1/3 is composed of smooth muscle only
Stomach	Mucosa is comprised of columnar epithelium, which secretes mucus to form a protective layer against gastric acid Parietal cells secrete HCl and intrinsic factor Chief cells secrete pepsinogen D cells secrete somatostatin G cells secrete gastrin
Small intestine	Entire small intestinal mucosa is comprised of columnar epithelium
Duodenum	Only segment with Brunner's submucosal glands, which secrete bicarbonate to neutralize stomach acid Goblet cells secrete mucus Villi and crypts
Jejunum	Goblet cells secrete mucus Villi and crypts
Ileum	Goblet cells secrete mucus Peyer's patches (lymphoid nodules) Villi and crypts
Colon	Entire large intestinal mucosa is comprised of columnar epithelium Many goblet cells Only crypts, lack villi

Hormones of the Gastrointestinal Tract

GI Hormone	Origin	Action	Regulation
Cholecystokinin (CCK)	I cells of small bowel	↓ gastric emptying to help digestion ↑ pancreatic secretions to help digestion ↑ gallbladder contraction for bile production	↑ fat- or protein-rich chyme ↓ by somatostatin
Gastrin	G cells of stomach	↑ acid production and gastric motility ↑ Zollinger-Ellision Syndrome	↑ by amino acids (esp. tryptophan and phenylalanine) ↑ vagal stimulation by VIP ↓ stomach distention and acid in the stomach
Gastric inhibitory peptide (GIP)	K cells of small bowel	↑ insulin release ↓ acid secretion by parietal cells	↑ by protein, fat, carbohydrate
Motilin	Enterochromaffin cells of small bowel	Promotes migrating motor complexes (MMC) in the stomach and intestine	↑ during fasting states

Secretin	S cells of small bowel	Role is to decrease acidity in the lumen of small bowel ↑ pancreatic bicarbonate secretion ↓ bile secretion ↓ acid production by parietal cells	↑ by fatty acids and acid in lumen
Somatostatin	D cells of stomach, small bowel, and pancreas	↓ release of other GI hormones: CCK, gastrin, GIP, motilin, VIP ↓ gallbladder contraction ↓ pancreatic hormones: insulin, glucagon, secretin	↑ by acid secretion in GI lumen ↓ by vagal stimulation
Vasoactive intestinal polypeptide (VIP)	Parasympathetic ganglion of the GI tract	Stimulates relaxation of GI smooth muscle and lower esophageal sphincter ↑ bicarbonate secretion from pancreas ↓ acid release from stomach	↑ by gastric distention and parasympathetic stimulation ↓ by sympathetic stimulation

Stomach Hormones

Cell Type	Location	Secretory Product
Chief cells	Body	Pepsinogen
Parietal cells	Body	HCl Intrinsic factor
G cells	Antrum	Gastrin
Mucous cells	Antrum	Mucus

Manifestations of Cirrhosis

Lab findings	↑ AST, ALT, GGT (gamma-glutamyl transferase) ↑ Bilirubin ↓ Albumin ↑ PT
Clinical manifestations	Spider nevus Hepatic encephalopathy Jaundice Esophageal varices and hematemesis Gynecomastia Splenomegaly Ascites Melena Palmar Erythema Tremor and asterixis Edema Hepatorenal syndrome

GENETICS

Autosomal Dominant Diseases

Disease	Mutation	Characteristics
Achondroplasia	Fibroblast Growth Factor Receptor 3	Dwarfism. Associated with advanced paternal age. Normal-sized head, short limbs.
Autosomal dominant polycystic kidney disease (ADPKD)	PKD1	Bilateral, massive, cystic enlargement of kidneys. Features include flank pain, hematuria, renal failure, berry aneurysms, mitral valve prolapse, and polysistic liver disease. Presents during adulthood. There is a recessive form that presents during infancy.

Familial adenomatous polyposis	APC gene (chromosome 5)	Multiple adenomatous colonic polyps. Colon resection is needed to stop advancement to colon cancer.
Familial hypercholesterolemia	LDL receptor	Marked elevation in LDL. Heterozygotes have cholesterol of 300+, homozygotes with cholesterol 700+. Associated with tendon xanthomas (often Achilles), and early MI.
Hereditary hemorrhagic telangiectasia (Osler-Weber-Rendu syndrome)	Endoglin (ENG)	Most common genetic vascular disease associated with telangiectasias, recurrent epistaxis, arteriovenous malformations (AVMs).
Huntington's disease	CAG trinucleotide repeat	Decreased levels of GABA and ACh in the brain and atrophy of the caudate nucleus lead to findings of dementia and depression in 30–50 year old individuals.
Hereditary spherocytosis	Spectrin or ankyrin defect	Spectrin or ankyrin defect causes spheroid erythrocytes, hemolytic anemia, increased MCHC. Cured by splenectomy.
Marfan syndrome	Fibrillin	Fibrillin mutation causes a connective tissue disorder. Characteristic long extremities, tall stature, hyperextensive joints, pectus excavatum, arachnodactyly, cystic medial necrosis of the aorta causing dissecting aortic aneurysms, lens subluxation and mitral valve prolapse.
Multiple endocrine neoplasias (MEN)	Ret gene (MEN 2A and 2B)	Tumors of the pancreas, parathyroid, thyroid, adrenal medulla, and pituitary glands.
Neurofibromatosis type I	NF1	Café au lait spots, neural tumors, Lisch nodules, scoliosis, optic gliomas, pheochromocytomas. Chromosome 17.
Neurofibromatosis type II	NF2 (merlin)	Bilateral acoustic neuroma. Chromosome 22.
Osteogenesis imperfecta	Type I collagen	Easily fractured bones with minimal trauma, blue sclerae, deafness and tooth defects, can be confused with child abuse.
Tuberous sclerosis	TSC	Seizures, mental retardation, renal failure. Hamartomas ("tubers") in multiple organ systems, including the brain, retina, kidneys, and heart.
Von Hippel Lindau disease	VHL	Hemangioblastomas of the central nervous system, bilateral renal cell carcinomas, pheochromocytomas. Caused by a gene deletion in a tumor suppressor gene (VHL) on chromosome 3.

Autosomal Recessive Diseases

Disease	Mutation	Characteristics
Albinism	Tyrosinase	Lack of melanin, increased skin cancer risk.
Alkaptonuria	Homogentisic oxidase	Dark urine, ochronosis, brittle articular cartilage.
Childhood polycystic kidney disease		Collecting duct dilation, progressive renal insufficiency early in life
Cystic fibrosis	Cystic fibrosis transmembrane conductance regulation gene on chromosome 7 (defective chloride pump)	Thick secretions, pneumonia, pancreatic insufficiency. Diagnosis by sweat electrolyte test.
Gaucher disease	Glucocerebrosidase deficiency	Accumulation of glucocerebroside in macrophages (leading to Gaucher's cells), hepatosplenomegaly.
Hurler syndrome	Lysosomal alpha-L-iduronidase (leading to accumulation of glycosoaminoglycans)	Developmental delay, abnormal facies (gargoylism, coarse facial features), cloudy corneas, deafness, claw hand, hepatosplenomegaly, heart valve abnormalities.

Krabbe disease	Arylsulfatase A	Accumulation of cerebroside sulfate, leading to peripheral neuropathy and developmental delay, along with severe seizures, vision loss, and hearing loss.
Metachromatic leukodystrophy	arylsulfatase A	Central and peripheral demyelination, seizures, developmental delay and behavioral problems, dementia.
Niemann-Pick disease	Shingomyelinase	Hepatosplenomegaly, "cherry-red" spot on macula, foam cells, progressive intellectual decline, seizures, tremors
Phenylketonuria	Phenylalanine hydroxylase	Mousy odor, mental retardation, eczema, convulsions.
Tay-Sachs disease	Hexosaminidase A deficiency	Mental deficiencies, blindness, "cherry-red" spot on macula.

HEMATOLOGY & ONCOLOGY

Causes of Prolonged PTT

PTT	PT	Both
Factor VIII, IX, XI, or XII deficiency/inhibitor	Factor VII deficiency/inhibitor	Combined Deficiency
Heparin	Vitamin K deficiency	DIC
vWF inhibitor	Liver Disease	Direct Thrombin Inhibitor
Antiphospholipid Ab	Warfarin	Combined Heparin and Warfarin use
Liver Disease		Overdose of heparin or warfarin alone
		Liver Disease

IMMUNOLOGY

Cytokines

Name	Produced by	Function
Interleukin 1 (IL-1; lymphocyte-activating factor)	Activated mononuclear phagocytes	Similar properties to tumor necrosis factor (TNF)
		Immunoregulatory effects at low concentrations, activation of CD4 cells, and B-cell growth and differentiation
		At high systemic concentrations, causes fever, induces synthesis of acute phase plasma proteins by the liver, and initiates metabolic wasting (cachexia)
IL-2 (T-cell growth factor)	CD4+ T-cells	Major autocrine growth factor for T-cells
		Amount of IL-2 produced by CD4+ T-cells is a principal factor in determining the strength of an immune response
		Stimulates the growth of NK cells and stimulates their cytolytic function
		Acts on B-cells as a growth factor and a stimulus for antibody production
IL-3 (multilineage colony-stimulating factor)	CD4+ T-cells	Stimulates growth and differentiation of bone marrow stem cells
IL-4 (B-cell growth factor)	CD4+ T-cells	Regulates allergic reactions by switching B-cells to IgE synthesis and enhancing IgE production
		Inhibits macrophage activation and stimulates CD4+ cells
IL-5 (B-cell differentiation factor/B-cell-stimulating factor II)	CD4+ T-cells and mast cells	Facilitates B-cell growth and differentiation
		Stimulates growth and activation of eosinophils

IL-6 (B-cell differentiation factor/B-cell-stimulating factor II)	Mononuclear phagocytes, vascular endothelial cells, fibroblasts, activated T-cells, and other cells	Synthesized in response to IL-1 or TNF Serves as a growth factor for activated B-cells late in the sequence of B-cell differentiation Induces hepatocytes to synthesize acute-phrase proteins, such as fibrinogen
IL-7	Bone marrow stromal cells	Feciliates lymphoid stem cell differentiation into progenitor B-cells
IL-8 (neutrophil-activating protein 1)	Macrophages and endothelial cells	Powerful chemo-attractant for T-cells and neutrophils
IL-10 (cytokine)	T-cells, activated B	Inhibits T-cell-mediated immune inflammation Also inhibits cytokine production and development of Tn-1 cells and drives the system toward a humoral immune response
IL-12	Activated monocytes and B-cells	Potent stimulator of NK cells, stimulates the differentiation of CD8+ T-cells into functionally active CTLs Regulates the balance between Tn-1 and Tn-2 cells by stimulating the differentiation of naïve CD4+ T-cells to the Tn-1 subset
IL-13	Produced by activated T-cells	Has a pleiotropic action on mononuclear phagocytes, neutrophils, and B-cells, which produces an anti-inflammatory response and suppresses cell-mediated immunity
Interferon g (IFN-g)	CD4+ T-cells, CD8+ T-cells, and NK cells	A potent activator of mononuclear phagocytes Facilitates differentiation of T and B-cells, activates cascular endothelial cells and neutrophils, stimulates the cytolytic activity of NK cells, up-regulates HLA class I expression, and induces many cell types to express HLA class II molecules
TNF-a	Mainly, macrophases stimulated with bacterial endotoxin but also activated T-cells, NK cells, and other cell types	Principal mediator of the host response to gram-negative bacteria At low concentrations, it stimulates leukocytes, mononuclear phagocytes, and vascular endothelial cells At high concentrations, it induces fever, cachexia, and septic shock
TNF-b (lymphotoxin)	Activated T-cells	Has similar actions to TNF-a and binds to the same cell surface receptors, although it is usually a locally acting paracrine factor and not a mediator of systemic injury Like TNF-a, a potent activator of neutrophils and an important regulator of acute inflammatory reactions
Transforming growth factor b (TGF-b)	Activated T-cells and endotoxin-activated mononuclear phagocytes	Acts as an "anticytokine," which antagonizes many responses of lymphocytes Inhibits T-cell proliferation and maturation of macrophage activation Acts on other cells, such as polymorphonuclear leukocytes and endothelial cells, to counteract the effects of proinflammatory cytokines Promotes wound healing, synthesis of collagens, bone formation, and angiogenesis

Granulocyte-macrophage colony stimulating factor (GM-CSF)	Produced by activated T-cells, activated mononuclear phagocytes, vascular endothelial cells, and fibroblasts	Promotes growth of undifferentiated hematopoietic cells and activates mature leukocytes Recombinant GM-CSF is administered clinically to promote hermatopoesis

Deficiencies of Phagocytic Cells

Inheritance	Deficiency	Mechanism	Signs/ Symptoms
Chronic Granulomatous Disease			
X-linked/ autosomal recessive	NADPH oxidase	Decreased intracellular microbial killing.	Increase susceptibility to catalase positive organisms, including normally nonpathogenic types (s. epidermis, etc).
Chédiak-Higashi Syndrome			
Autosomal recessive	Microtubule polymerization	Failure of lysosomal emptying.	Recurrent pyogenic bacterial infection, association with albinism
Leukocyte Adhesion Deficiency			
Autosomal recessive	LFA-1 integrin	Neutrophils are unable to adhere to vessel walls and extravasate to participate in acute inflammation	Recurrent bacterial and fungal infections. Associated with delayed separation of the umbilicus.

Summary of Hypersensitivity Reactions

Mechanism	Chronology	Signs/ Symptoms	Examples	Treatment
Type I				
Cross-linking of IgE antibodies on masT-cells/ basophils releases histamine and other anaphylactic factors	Immediate	Erythema, hives, respiratory distress	Bee stings, Food allergies, Penicillin allergy	Epinephrine, antihistamines, corticosteroids
Type II				
IgG or IgM directed toward cellular antigens. May be cytotoxic (through activation of complement/ NK cells) or noncytotoxic.	Variable	Cytotoxic: loss of tissue function.	Goodpasture's syndrome, Pernicious anemia, Pemphigus vulgaris.	Corticosteroids
		Noncytotoxic: may mimic the effects of that given tissue	Grave's disease	
Type III				
IgM forms complexes with soluble antigen and fall out of solution and deposit on tissues. Deposition initiates local inflammatory response.	5–12 hours	Presentation is dependent largely on the primary site of immune complex deposition Vasculitis Glomerulonephritis Arthritis.	Arthus reaction (from tetanus vaccine), Serum sickness	Corticosteroids

Type IV				
T-cells become sensitized on primary exposure to antigen. On secondary exposure, cell-mediated damage takes place.	24–48 hours	Localized rash (Contact dermatitis). Loss of tissue function.	Diabetes mellitus type 1, Multiple sclerosis, PPD test, Contact dermatitis (ex. Poison ivy)	Corticosteroids

MICROBIOLOGY

Gram Positive & Gram Negative

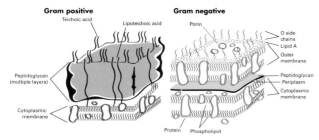

Four Phases Of Bacterial Growth

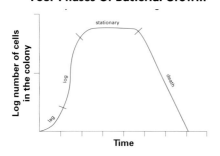

CMV Cytopathic Effect (CPE)

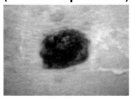

Kaposi's sarcoma skin lesion (Human Herpesvirus 8)

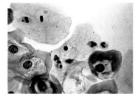

Koilocytes (HPV)

Roseola skin lesions (Human Herpesvirus 6)

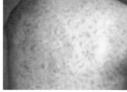

Hepatitis B Serologies

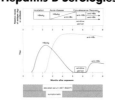

Koplic lesions of buccal mucosa (Measles/Rubeola)

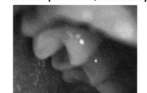

Multinucleated giant cells in Respiratory Syncytial Virus (RSV)

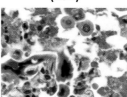

Negri body (Rabies virus)

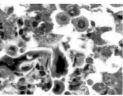

Hantavirus

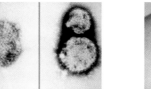

Skin scrapping associated with Tinea

MR image reveals multiple "ring-enhancing" lesions

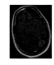
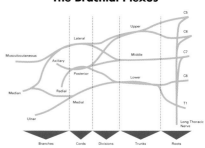

MUSCULOSKELETAL SYSTEM

The Brachial Plexus

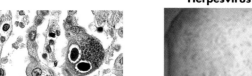

Common Nerve Injuries

Nerve	Common Injury	Motor Deficit	Sensory Deficit
Radial nerve	Midshaft humerus fracture	Wrist drop—flaccid hand flexion, difficulty with hand extension	Decrease sensation on posterior and lateral arm, posterior forearm, and dorsum of hand
Musculocutaneous nerve		Difficulty flexing elbow	Decrease sensation on lateral forearm via lateral cutaneous nerve of forearm
Axilliary nerve	Shoulder dislocation	Difficulty abducting the arm greater than 90°	Numbness over the dome of the shoulder
Median nerve	Carpal tunnel syndrome, wrist fracture, or Supracondylar humerus fracture	Decrease thumb function, can't abduct or oppose thumb, Pope's blessing sign/hand of benediction: unopposed radial nerve, lack of flexion for index and middle finger.	Numbness or decrease sensation over palmar aspect of the thumb, index, middle, and medial half of the ring finger.
Ulnar nerve	Fractures of medial epicondyle of the humerus, wrist fracture	Clawhand sign—inability to adduct thumb + inability to abduct or adduct fingers.	Numbness and decrease sensation over both palmar and dorsal aspect of lateral half of the ring finger and pinky

Long thoracic nerve	Mastectomies with axillary node dissection, thoracic nerve impingement	Winged scapula—medial border of scapulae protrude like wings due to reduced contraction of the serratus anterior muscles on the anterior-medial aspect of the scapula.	None
C5 C6 root	Traction or tear of the upper trunk, blow to shoulder, trauma from delivery	Erb-Duchenne palsy/ Waiter's tip: paralysis of the abductors, lateral rotators, and loss of biceps. Arm will be medially rotated, with forearm pronated and hanging by the side.	None
Inferior trunk, C8 T1	Thoracic outlet syndrome—subclavian artery and inferior trunk are compressed	Atrophy of the interosseous muscle, thenar eminence, and hypothenar eminence	Decrease sensation over the medial aspect of the hand and forearm

Sarcomere Structure

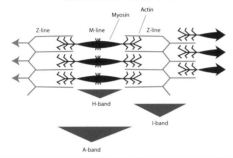

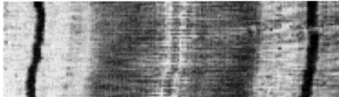

Dark lines wherever there is *any* myosin. Light lines where there is *only* actin. **A**-band = d**A**rk band **I**-band = L**I**ght band. **M**yosin is anchored to the **M**-line. **A**ctin is anchored to the **Z**-line (think "A to Z").

Contraction of a Sarcomere

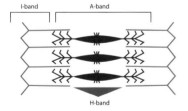
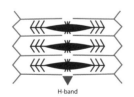

(Note: H-band and I-band shorten, while the A-band does not change.)

A. Action of Myosin B. Release and Recocking of Myosin

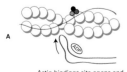
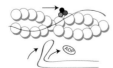

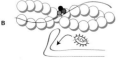

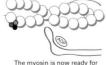

Actin bindings site opens and myosin head attaches.

When ADP is kicked off, myosin head moves and actin shifts (contraction).

ATP binds to myosin, knocking it off the actin and recocking the head.

The myosin is now ready for another round of contraction.

NEUROLOGY & NEUROANATOMY

Neurotransmitters

Neurotrans-mitter	Role In Pathology	Location	Drugs
NE (norepinephrine)	Lower in depression Higher in anxiety	Higher in anxiety Locus ceruleus	TCA's, maprotiline and mirtazapine are NE reuptake inhibitors
Dopamine	Increased in schizophrenia, decreased in Parkinson's and depression	Ventral tegmentum and substantia nigra pars compacta (SNc)	Levodopa and carbidopa increase level of dopamine while selegiline prevent dopamine breakdown
Serotonin (5-HT)	Decreased in anxiety and depression	Raphe Nucleus	SSRI's
Ach	Reduced in Alzheimer's, Huntington's, REM sleep	Neuromuscular junction, Basal nucleus of Meynert	Organophosphates and nerve agents inhibit breakdown of Ach
GABA	Reduced in anxiety, Huntington's	Nucleus accumbens	Benzodiazepines are GABA agonists and reduce anxiety

Cerebellar Signs

PINARD'S: **P**ast pointing, **I**ntention tremor, **N**ystagmus, **A**taxia, **R**ebound, **D**ysdiadokinesia, **S**lurred speech

Homunculus

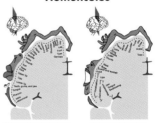

Somatosensory cortex in right cerebral hemisphere

Motor cortex in right cerebral hemisphere

Dermatomes

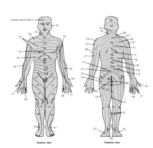

C2: top of head
C3: Turtleneck
T4: Nipples
T7: Xyphoid process
T10: Belly butTEN
L1: Inguinal L1gament
L4: Down on alL 4 knees
S2,S3,S4: Erection & penile/anal sensations

Upper Motor Neurons vs. Lower Motor Neuron

STORM BABY!	UMN	LMN
S: Strength	Lowers	Lowers
T: Tone	Increases (spastic)	Decreases (flaccid)
O: Others	Superficial reflexes absent	Fasciculation
	Clonus	Fibrillation
		Reaction of degeneration
R: Reflexes	Increases	Decreases
M: Muscle mass	Only slight loss	Atrophy
B: Babinski sign	Positive	Negative

Circle of Willis

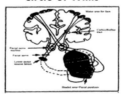

Epidural Hematoma

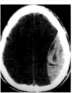

Subdural Hematoma

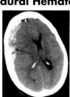

Subarachnoid Hematoma

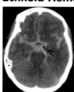

PHARMACOLOGY

Volume of distribution: V_d (liters) = $D/(C_p)$

Where D = total amount of drug in the body and C_p = concentration of drug in plasma.

Michaelis-Mentin and Linweaver-Burke Plot

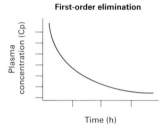

First-order elimination

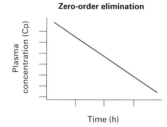

Zero-order elimination

Clearance: CL = rate of elimination/concentration of drug in plasma

$$CL = V_d \bullet K_e$$

Where K_e is the elimination constant

Half life: $t_{1/2} = (0.693 \bullet V_d)/CL$

Where $t_{1/2}$ = half life, V_d = volume of distribution, and CL = clearance

Therapeutic index: TI = LD50/ED50

Where LD_{50} is the median lethal dose and ED_{50} is the median effective dose.

Loading dose: $C_p \bullet V_d$

Maintenance dose: $C_p \bullet$ Clearance

Dose Response Curves for Partial Agonist, Full Agonist, Agonist Plus Competitive Antagonist, and Agonist Plus Noncompetitive Antagonist

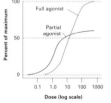
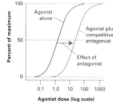
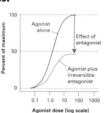

Autonomic Nervous System Effects by Organ System

Area	Sympathetic		Parasympathetic	
	Receptor	Effect	Receptor	Effect
Heart				
Sinoatrial node	β_1	Increases firing	M_2	Decreases firing
Ectopic pacemakers	β_1	Increases firing	None	
Contractility	β_1	Increases firing	M_2	Decreases
Blood vessels				
Splanchnic vessels	α	Contraction	M	Relaxation
To skeletal muscle	β_2	Relaxation	M_3	Relaxation
	α	Contraction		
	M	Relaxation		
Gastrointestinal tract				
Smooth muscle	α	Relaxation	M_3	Contraction
	β_2	Relaxation		
Sphincters	α_2	Contraction	M	Relaxation
Myenteric plexus	α	Inhibition	M_3	Activation
Secretion	None	None	M_1	Increases
Lungs: bronchi	β_2	Relaxation	M_3	Contraction

Genitourinary tract				
Bladder	β_2	Relaxation	M_3	Contraction
Sphincter	α_1	Contraction	M_3	Relaxation
Uterus	β_2	Relaxation	M_3	Contraction
	α	Contraction		
Penis	α	Ejaculation	M	Erection
Eye				
Radial muscle	α_1	Contraction	None	None
Circular muscle	None	None	M	Contraction
Ciliary muscle	β	Relaxation	M_3	Contraction
Skin				
Pilomotor muscles	α	Contraction		
Sweat glands	α (apocrine)	Activation	M (thermoregulatory)	Activation

G_s protein activates the cAMP-dependent pathway

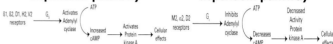

G_i protein inhibits the cAMP-dependent pathway

G_q protein activates phospholipase C, releasing DAG/IP3

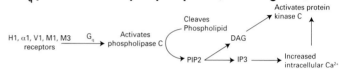

Lipoprotein Metabolism

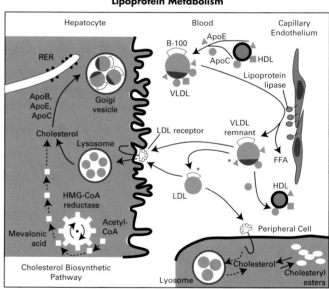

Coagulation Cascade and Clot

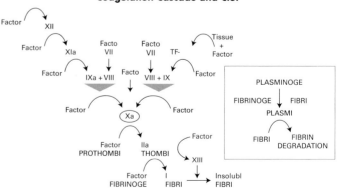

Biosynthesis of the Four Families of Eicosanoids

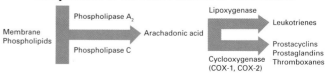

PSYCHIATRY

Sleep Cycles

Sleep Stage	% total sleep	Characteristics of EEG pattern	Comments
Awake		Low amplitude, high frequency Beta waves (NO sawtooth waves)	
Relaxed wakefulness		Rhythmic alpha waves	
Stage 1 (light sleep)	5%	Low amplitude, mixed frequency Theta waves	Usually short duration (1–7 min)
Stage 2	45%	Slower waves with bursts of rapid sleep spindles and K complexes	
Stage 3–4 (deep sleep)	25%	High amplitude, low frequency (slow) delta waves	Sleepwalking and night terrors; bedwetting; aging, depression and benzodiazepines decrease this stage
REM sleep	25%	Low amplitude, high frequency Beta waves AND sawtooth waves (similar to awake state)	Dreams and nightmares, rapid extraocular muscle movements, loss of motor tone, penile and clitoral tumescence; ACh is the main neurotransmitter, but NE decreases REM

Developmental Milestones

2 months	moves extremities, coos, looks at faces, tracking moving objects, turns to sound
4 months	holds head up, rolls over tummy to back, hands to mouth, social smile
6 months	sits assisted, grasps objects, rolls over both directions, responds to name/sounds
9 months	sits alone, crawls, pulls to stand, transfers objects, mama/dada, stranger anxiety
12 months	cruises, picks up objects with thumb and forefinger, shakes/bangs objects
18 months	walks, drinks from cup, scribbles, points, uses single words, separation anxiety
2 years	runs, climbs, kicks ball, 4-block tower, lines/circles, object permanence
3 years	tricycle, conversation, core gender identity, parallel play
4 years	hop 1 foot, simple drawing, cooperative play, names colors
5 years	uses fork and spoon, toilet trained, counts to 10, wants to be like friends
6-11 years	same sex friends, identifies with same sex parent, develops conscience
puberty	abstract reasoning, formal operations, formation of personality

Signs of Depression

SIG E CAPS = **S**uicidal ideation, **I**nterest decreased, **G**uilt, **E**nergy decrease, **C**oncentration decreased, **A**ppetite change, **P**sychomotor change, **S**leep disturbances

Suicide Risk Factors

SAD PERSONS = **S**: sex (male), **A**: age (elderly or adolescent), **D**: depression, **P**: previous attempt, **E**: ethanol abuse, **R**: rational thinking loss, **S**: social support lacking, **O**: organized plan, **N**: no plan, **S**: sickness

PULMONOLGY & RESPIRATORY SYSTEM

Representation of Lung Volumes

Functional residual capacity (FRC): FRC = ERV + RV. The volume left in the lungs after normal expiration. Inspiratory capacity (IC): IC = VT + IRV. The amount of air that can be sucked in after a normal expiration.
Vital capacity (VC): VC = ERV + VT + IRV. Total lung capacity (TLC): The whole shebang. TLC = RV + ERV + IRV + VT.

Lung Volumes in Obstructive & Restrictive Lung States

Disease Pattern	FEV1	FVC	FEV$_1$/FVC	FEF$_{25–75\%}$	TLC
Normal	—	—	-0.8	—	—
Restrictive	↓	↓	– or ↑↑	↓	↓↓
Obstructive	↓↓	↓	↓↓	↓↓	– or ↑

Oxygen-Hemoglobin Dissociation Curve

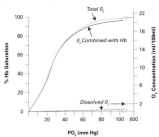

Factors Influencing Oxygen-Hemoglobin Dissociation Curve

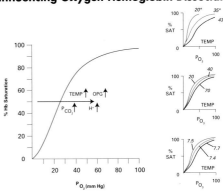

Arterial Blood Gas Analysis In Acid-Base Disorders

Condition	pH	PCO$_2$	Bicarbonate
Normal	7.40 (7.38-7.42)	40 (35-45)	24 (22-26)
Respiratory acidosis	< 7.40	> 40	Compensated ↑
Metabolic alkalosis	< 7.40	Compensated ↓	< 24
Respiratory alkalosis	> 7.40	< 40	Compensated ↓
Metabolic alkalosis	> 7.40	Compensated ↑	> 24

Causes of Metabolic Acidosis with an Anion Gap

MUDPILES:
M – **M**ethanol (formic acid)
U – **U**remia
D – **D**iabetic ketoacidosis (DKA)
P – **P**araaldehyde
I – **I**ntoxication (ethyl alcohol)
L – **L**actic acidosis
E – **E**thylene glycol (antifreeze),
S – **S**alicylates (aspirin)

Clearance Formula

Clearance (C) = (U $\cdot$ V)/P
  Where C = clearance (ml/min), U = concentration in urine (mg/ml), V= volume of urine made per minute (ml/min), and P = concentration in plasma (mg/ml).
C = GFR = (U$_{inulin}$ $\cdot$ V)/P$_{inulin}$

Starling Equation

GFR = K$_f$({P$_{glom}$ – P$_{BS}$) – ($\neq_{glom}$ – $\neq_{BS}$)]
  Where K$_f$ = filtration coefficient, P$_{glom}$ = hydrostatic pressure in the glomerular capillary, P$_{BS}$ = hydrostatic pressure in Bowman's space, $\neq_{glom}$ = oncotic pressure in the glomerular capillary, and $\neq_{BS}$= oncotic pressure in Bowman's space.

Effects of Changes in Renal Vascular Resistance with a Constant Renal Perfusion

Renal arteriolar vascular resistance					
↑	Efferent	RPF (ml/min)	GFR (ml/min)	FF	Examples
↑		↓	↓	-	NSAIDS
↓		↑	↑	-	Prostaglandins
	↑	↓	↑	↑	Angiotensin
	↓	↑	↓	↓	Ace inibitors

Filtered load = GFR (ml/min)   P (mg/dl)

Excretion rate = U (mg/dl)   V (ml/min)

FWC = $V - C_{osm}$

Remember, $C_{osm} = (U_{osm} - V)/P$

Alterations in Extracellular Fluid (ECF) and Intracellular Fluid (ICF) Under Different Physiological Stressors

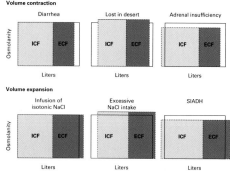

Flowchart of Acid/Base Physiology

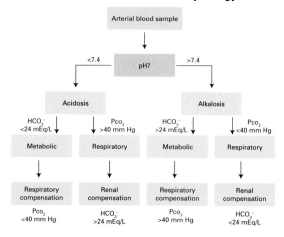

Summary of Hormones that Act on the Kidney

Hormone	Stimulus for secretion	Actions on kidneys	Location
PTH	↓ Plasma[Ca²⁺]	↓ Phosphate reabsorption ↑ Ca²⁺ reabsorption Stimulates 1α-hydroxylase	Proximal and distal tubules
ADH	↑ Plasma osmolarity ↓ Blood volume	↑ H₂O permeability	Distal tubule and collecting duct
Aldosterone	↓ Blood volume (via renin-angitensin II) ↑ Plasma [K+]	↑ Na+ reabsorption ↑ K+ secretion ↑ H+ secretion	Distal tubule
Atrial natriuretic factor	↑ Atrial pressure	↑ GFR ↓ Na+ reabsorption	
Angiotensin II	↓ Blood volume (via renin)	↑ Na+-H+ exchange and HCO₃⁻ reabsorption	Proximal tubule

Diuretics and Their Sites of Action

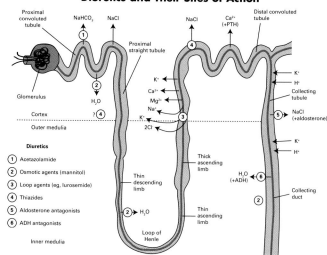

REPRODUCTIVE SYSTEM

Normal Sexual Differentiation

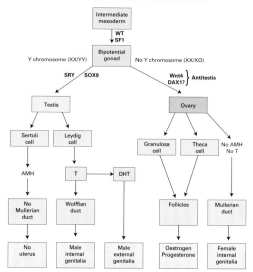

Spermatogenesis and Spermiogenesis

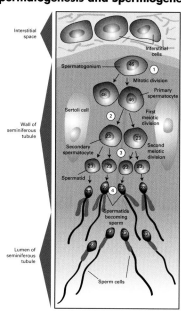

The Menstrual Cycle

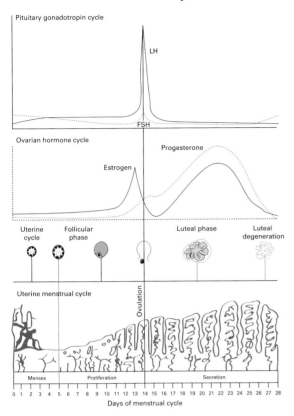

Day 1: First day of Menstruation

Days 1–4: Menstrual Phase

Days 5–approximately 14: Proliferative Phase (Follicular Phase). Length varies.

Day 14: Ovulation

Days 15–28: Secretory Phase (Luteal Phase). Length is constant at 14 days.

The stages of Oocyte Development

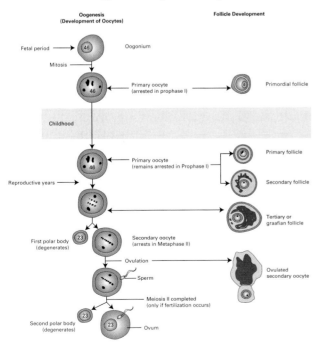

Oogenesis

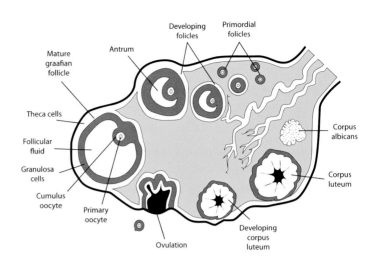

Spermiogenesis

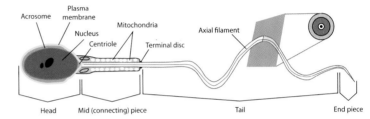

Benign Prostatic Hyperplasia (BPH)

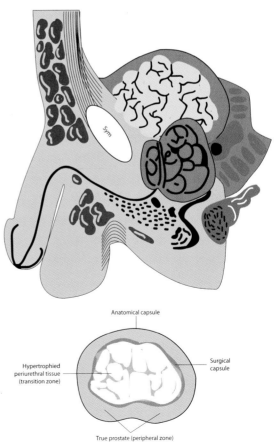

Cervical intraepithelial neoplasia (CIN)

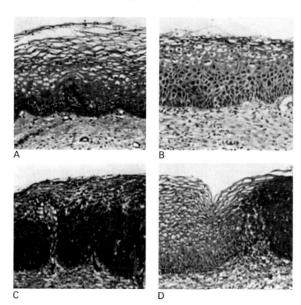

A. Normal ectocervix B. Moderate dysplasia—CIN II
C. Severe dyplasia—CIN III D. Carcinoma in situ—CIN III

Differential Diagnosis of Amenorrhea

Hormonal State	Differential Diagnosis
↓ estrogen	GnRH, LH, and FSH initially suppressed by estradiol, but then abruptly surge due to a positive feedback as estradiol increases
↓ FSH (central)	Reversible insults (e.g. illness, anorexia, stress, strenuous exercise) Turner's syndrome (primary)
↑ FSH (ovarian failure)	Hypothalamic or pituitary tumors Congenital GnRH deficiency (primary)
↑ androgen (adrenals vs. ovaries)	Female pseudohermaphrodism (primary) Premature menopause (secondary)
↑ prolactin	Adrenal tumor or hyperplasia Ovarian tumor Polycystic ovary syndrome Anabolic steroids

SKIN & CONNECTIVE TISSUE

Collagen Types

Collagen Type	Tissues Found	Function
I	Bone, skin, tendon, dentin	Strength
II	Cartilage	Pressure-resistant
III	Blood vessels, skin, muscle	Volume expandable
IV	Basement membrane (all tissue)	Reticular Dermis
X	Epiphyseal plates	

Biochemistry of Skin Pigmentation

Phenylalanine Hydroxylase   Tyrosinase   Tyrosinase

Phenylalanine ⟶ Tyrosine ⟶ Dopa ⟶ Melanin

Hypersensitivity Reactions

		Associations	Clinical Manifestation
Type I	Anaphylactic (Immediate)	Certain foods (peanuts, shellfish, etc.) Cosmetics Medications	Urticaria Angioedema Anaphylaxis
Type II	Cytotoxic	Autoimmune	Bullous Pemphigoid Pemphigus Vulgaris
Type III	Immune-Complex Mediated	Small vessel vasculitis	Henoch-Schonlein Purpura
Type IV	Cell Mediated (Delayed)	Poison Ivy Nickel	Contact Dermatitis

SLE Criteria = ONE MAD RASH In Person

Oral ulcers
Neurologic symptoms
ESR
Malar rash
Antinuclear antibodies
Discoid rash
Renal symptoms
Arthritis, Serositis
Hematologic symptoms
Immunoglobulins (anti-ds-DNA, anti-Sm)
Photosensitivity.

Typical Patient: 20–40 year old female with facial rash after sun exposure.

Malar rash = nontender erythematous rash with butterfly distribution over cheeks and nose.

Discoid rash = erythematous oval shaped lesions that may be complicated by scar formation or hair loss.

anti-SCL 70 = Skin/Swallow, Collagen, Lungs.

Raynaud's phenomenon = cold weather or strong emotions cause vasospasm in fingers characteristic color changes (white blue red).
Typical patient: 30–50 year old female with shiny wrinkle-free skin.

Malar rash of SLE

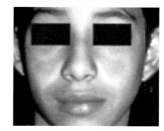

Raynaud's Phenomenon

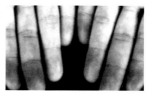

Epidermolysis Bullosa

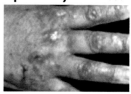

CREST Syndrome

C: Calcinosis; anti-Centromere-antibody
R: Reynaud's phenomenon
E: Esophygeal dysmotility
S: Sclerodactyly
T: Telangiectasia